The half century between 1885 and 1935 witnessed a significant improvement in the health of the British people and an unprecedented expansion of preventive and therapeutic services offered by the state through its local authorities. Behind the expansion in public services were profound changes in attitudes toward poverty and dependency and toward the political and cultural significance of health; changes in social policy and administration; and changes in the understanding of the causes of disease. This book examines the era through the ideas and experiences of one prominent participant, Sir Arthur Newsholme, who rose to become a leading public health authority in Britain.

Professor Eyler draws particular attention to Newsholme's tenure as the Medical Officer of the Local Government Board in Whitehall, where he helped to launch some of its boldest measures, including national health insurance and programs for tuberculosis, venereal disease, and infant welfare. Eyler also details Newsholme's postretirement studies of international health systems; his statistical and epidemiological studies and their connection to his policy recommendations; and his conflicts with biometricians over these studies.

Sir Arthur Newsholme and State Medicine, 1885–1935

Cambridge History of Medicine

Edited by

CHARLES ROSENBERG, Professor of History and Sociology of Science, University of Pennsylvania

Other titles in the series:

Continued on page following the Index

Sir Arthur Newsholme and State Medicine, 1885–1935

JOHN M. EYLER

University of Minnesota

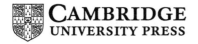

CAMBRIDGE
UNIVERSITY PRESS

PUBLISHED BY THE PRESS SYNDICATE OF THE UNIVERSITY OF CAMBRIDGE
The Pitt Building, Trumpington Street, Cambridge, CB2 1RP, United Kingdom

CAMBRIDGE UNIVERSITY PRESS
The Edinburgh Building, Cambridge CB2 2RU, United Kingdom
40 West 20th Street, New York, NY 10011-4211, USA
10 Stamford Road, Oakleigh, Melbourne 3166, Australia

First published 1997

Printed in the United States of America

Typeset in Bembo

Library of Congress Cataloging-in-Publication Data
Eyler, John M.
Sir Arthur Newsholme and state medicine, 1885–1935 / John M.
Eyler.
p.   cm. – (Cambridge history of medicine)
Includes bibliographical references and index.
ISBN 0-521-48186-4
1. Newsholme, Arthur, Sir, 1857–1943.   2. Health officers – Great
Britain – Biography.   3. Medicine, State – Great Britain – History.
I. Title.   II. Series.
[DNLM: 1. Newsholme, Arthur, Sir, 1857–1943.   2. Public Health –
biography.   3. Public Health Administration – history – Great
Britain.   4. Health Services – history – Great Britain.   WZ 100 N558e
1997]
RA424.5.N4E95   1997
362.1'092 – dc20
[B]
DNLM/DLC
for Library of Congress   96-18932
                                                                          CIP

*A catalog record for this book is available from
the British Library.*

ISBN 0 521 48186 4 hardback

For Audrey

CONTENTS

ILLUSTRATIONS

PREFACE

The half century between 1885 and 1935 witnessed a significant improvement in the health of the British people. Crude death rates offer the easiest, if least sensitive, measure. When this fifty-year period opened (1881–5) the crude annual mortality rate for England and Wales was 19.4 deaths per thousand population. By the turn of the century that rate had fallen to 17.7 per thousand (1896–1900), and by 1930 to 12.1 (1926–30).[1] Even more revealing is the downward trend in the death toll from the chief epidemic diseases which had been the focus of the nineteenth-century public health movement – cholera, typhus, typhoid or enteric fever, smallpox, measles, scarlet fever, diphtheria, whooping cough, diarrhea, and dysentery. During the last two decades of the nineteenth century the collective rate at which these diseases killed fell by more than a third (3,408 deaths per million annually in 1871–80 to 2,142 per million annually in 1891–1900).[2]

These same decades also saw an unprecedented expansion of preventive and therapeutic services offered by the state through its local authorities. In 1885 the public health activities of most British local authorities were rudimentary. Even the most active confined themselves, for the most part, to environmental sanitation. Among civil authorities only the Poor Law Guardians offered medical treatment paid for by taxes or by rates, local property taxes. By 1935, on the other hand, almost the entire population of England and Wales had access to a wide range of both sanitary and clinical services offered by local authorities and supported by the rates and by grants from the national Treasury. These new services included not only those that the nineteenth century had struggled to provide – sewage and garbage disposal, a protected water supply, supervision of milk and food, smallpox vaccination, and isolation or quarantine facilities – but also medical consultation and clinical services through a network of outpatient clinics and residential institutions and home health services offered by visiting nurses, social workers, and medical officers. In addition a substantial portion of the population was covered by national health insurance. Scholarly interest in these municipal medical services has quickened recently as historians have begun to reconsider the

---

1 *Annual Report of the Registrar-General of England and Wales,* 63 (1900): lxi, hereafter cited as *Ann. Rep. Reg.-Gen.;* & *Statistical Abstract for the United Kingdom,* B.P.P. 1932–3, XXV, Cmd. 4233, 7.
2 *Ann. Rep. Reg.-Gen.,* 63 (1900): civ.

role of such services as preventive agents and to reassess Thomas McKeown's interpretation of fall of mortality in the nineteenth century.[3] In making such judgments, a knowledge of the extent and use of these services is essential. That information can be obtained only from local studies.

Behind this expansion in public services stand profound changes in attitudes toward poverty and dependency and toward the political and cultural significance of health; changes in social policy and administration; and changes in the understanding of the causes of disease. Illustrative of the speed and magnitude of these changes is the identification of health problems between the Boer War and the First World War that were considered so critical to the national interest that new public services were encouraged – sometimes mandated – by Parliament and supported by the national purse. Historians have studied a number of these themes topically. Still others remain to be explored. This book takes a somewhat different tack. It examines the career of one prominent participant in these innovations.

Arthur Newsholme rose to become a leading public health authority in Britain. He was for four years (1884–8) a part-time Medical Officer of Health (M.O.H.) in the London vestry of Clapham, dividing his time between public health activity and private general practice. For twenty years (1888–1908) he was full-time M.O.H. in Brighton, where he helped build what his contemporaries regarded as a model local authority health program. If Newsholme had never left Brighton, his career as a public health administrator and epidemiologist still would have great historical interest, illustrating as it does a variety of social and intellectual forces then operating in local public health work. But in 1908 Newsholme left Brighton to become the nominal head of the English public health service. As Medical Officer of the Local Government Board (L.G.B.) in these years he was in Whitehall when most of the social welfare initiatives of the prewar Liberal governments were enacted during the Great War. During his tenure at the L.G.B., Britain launched some of its boldest initiatives in public medical services: national health insurance and special programs for tuberculosis, venereal disease, and infant welfare. Newsholme's career was involved with each of these. Following his retirement from the civil service in 1919, Newsholme remained active for another fifteen years, serving on the faculty of the newly created Johns Hopkins School of Hygiene and Public Health and as a consultant and elder statesman on both sides of the Atlantic. His most important work in these years was the prolonged study of national health schemes he undertook for the Milbank Memorial Fund of New York.

This book is a study of the professional activities and the ideas of one individual. It is not intended to be a biography. There is no reason to think that Newsholme's personal life would be particularly interesting to others or that, if available sources

---

3 For an answer to McKeown which places particular stress on the work of municipal medical services, see Anne Hardy, *The Epidemic Streets: Infectious Disease and the Rise of Preventive Medicine, 1856–1900* (Oxford: Clarendon Press, 1993). As representative of McKeown's arguments, see his *The Role of Medicine: Dream, Mirage, or Nemesis?* (Princeton, N.J.: Princeton Univ. Press, 1979).

allowed a better look at the man or a reconstruction of his personality we would view the health problems and policies of his generation any differently. Nor do I claim that Newsholme typifies the public health world of the late nineteenth or early twentieth centuries. That is a doubtful historical proposition for any individual, but, as Newsholme's strong disagreements with some of his contemporaries show, it is especially doubtful for him. A career study does offer the historian certain advantages. It grants the luxury of a highly focused and comprehensive investigation of the products of one mind and the activities of one individual over an entire professional lifetime. When that individual was an articulate and prolific administrator involved in important policy changes, a historical study of that career offers a promising opportunity to observe the integration of intellectual and institutional forces in policy making and administration. In addition careful attention to Newsholme's attitudes and recommendations allows us to amplify and to correct some generalizations found in certain topical histories of public health or health policy, which, of necessity, are based on more selective, if broader, reading. His example demonstrates that public health experts were not necessarily as close to unanimous in their opinions as some historians have claimed and that their ideas were capable of substantial change. The perspective adopted in this book emphasizes the evolution of ideas over time and the role that experience with one health problem may have had in conditioning the responses to others. It is important to bear in mind how diverse were the responsibilities of Medical Officers of Health (M.O.H.). None could be concerned exclusively with waterborne diseases, with infant mortality, with tuberculosis, or with any other disease or health problem.

A study of Newsholme's career offers an excellent opportunity to observe the workings of an active and efficient local authority health program in the late nineteenth and early twentieth centuries. Through the unpublished Proceedings of the Brighton Sanitary Committee, through Newsholme's annual reports and scientific papers, and through newspapers, it is possible to investigate how the permissive health legislation of the late Victorian era could be translated into local services and to observe how a successful Medical Officer of Health administered a department, conducted research, and labored to expand local health services. Historical attention has only recently been directed at the activities of local health authorities, yet it was at the local level that most services were provided, if they were provided at all. The activities of the central health authority have received more historical attention, but the Local Government Board in the period of the Liberal social welfare initiatives, 1906–14, has not received the historical attention that it deserves. The Board has often been portrayed as a hidebound, conservative bureau that subjected its medical staff to the stultifying supervision of laymen schooled in the traditions of the Poor Law. While there is certainly a historical basis for that stereotype, it is also true that in these years the Board's Medical Department played an innovative role in the formation of new health policy, sometimes initiating change, sometimes reacting to initiatives begun elsewhere.

Administrative records in the Public Record Office, L.G.B.'s annual reports, and Newsholme's annual reports, special investigations, and circulars throw considerable light on the health initiatives of the Liberal and Coalition governments during the Local Government Board's last dozen years of life. Since Newsholme moved directly from an active local authority to the central health authority at a time of critically important change, his career provides an instructive example of how local experience and experiments in health administration affected national policy. Relations between central and local authorities or agencies in public health at the turn of the century were more complex and bidirectional than sometimes has been assumed.

Newsholme's writings also offer the opportunity to study some important conceptual changes. His amazing production of statistical and epidemiological studies is a fruitful source for historical investigations of this sort. Newsholme's career demonstrates that the close connection between vital statistics and public health reform that began in the early Victorian period continued unabated in the Edwardian age. Many of the same techniques that William Farr and John Simon used were also employed by Arthur Newsholme in Brighton and in Whitehall. Newsholme's epidemiological research illustrates not only this continuity of statistical techniques and the productive uses to which mathematically simple procedures could be put, but it demonstrates a very close connection between epidemiological research and administration. Administrative need suggested topics for statistical research. The results of that research were used in turn to defend existing health policies and sometimes to help initiate new ones.

Newsholme's studies also demonstrate how the understanding of the cause of disease and the focus of public health initiatives changed during his career. From the beginning of his career Newsholme resisted a reductionist approach to disease prevention. Epidemics, even those of diseases known to have microbial agents, could not be adequately explained by knowledge of the agent and host alone. It was essential, Newsholme insisted, to have adequate knowledge of the environment. His epidemiological investigations did much to clarify the circumstances which produced high infant mortality. They helped to document the means by which known agents, such as the typhoid bacillus, were transmitted. They also helped to clarify the nature and the transmission of diseases such as scarlet fever, whose cause was still not established. But Newsholme's goals as well as his understanding of disease changed. If we include his retirement years in our perspective, we can document a transformation in Newsholme's vision on a very broad front: from acute infectious diseases to chronic diseases, from sanitation to personal health services, from prevention to health promotion, from public health narrowly conceived to state medicine.

While I adopt a somewhat different approach from my colleagues and predecessors who have written topical histories, I would be the first to acknowledge my indebtedness to their research and interpretations. I have attempted to draw on their work to place Newsholme's ideas and activities in historical context, and in the first twelve chapters of this book I provide the reader with many references to the secondary historical literature. In the final chapter of this book, I discuss how I believe my study of Newsholme's career is related to current historical understanding of British public health, state medicine, and social policy. The remainder of this book is focused unapologetically on Newsholme's writings and the records of his work. We follow the paper trail relentlessly wherever it leads, trying to understand as fully as possible the nature and significance of one career.

During the course of my study I have grown to respect Newsholme, although I understand why some of his contemporaries disagreed with him and I recognize traits that some found annoying. One must admire his mental energy and vigor. His bibliography is testimony to his creative powers, ceaseless labor, and prolific habits. One can also admire his humanity and his commitment to the improvement of human health and welfare. He insisted that humans be treated as free moral agents, and while he placed upon individuals some responsibility for their physical condition and that of their families and those around them, he resisted attempts to blame most victims for their plight and showed remarkable understanding of the problems working-class families had in procuring the necessities of a healthy, decent life. In Newsholme's view the primary responsibility for health and welfare lay with the state acting through its local authorities. He opposed those who resisted public intervention on either political or biological grounds, and he was particularly troubled by those who did so wielding bogus scientific authority. He is an example of the technical experts who had a hand in creating the system of state services that so transformed the relationship between the British people and their state. But while he admired the way a technocratic state could set priorities and marshal resources, his was not a technocratic agenda. Newsholme regarded social reform and health improvement not primarily as tools to serve economic, political, or strategic ends but as moral imperatives. A civilized, liberal society could not tolerate the preventable human suffering and the premature loss of life his investigations demonstrated were occurring. Similarly there were limits to what the state could do. In spite of his admiration for the goals and the comprehensive nature of the Soviet health care system, his respect for human rights kept him from sharing John Kingsbury's or Sidney Webb's enthusiasm for the Soviet system. Similarly his insistence on individual moral accountability made him rather unsympathetic toward certain classes of people – alcoholics, drug addicts, adult males infected with venereal disease – and left him open, especially after the Great War, to charges of prudery and rigidity. It is a feature observed in many who are driven by a strong sense of moral purpose. Newsholme could persevere. He had a harder time compromising.

I owe a large debt of gratitude to those institutions and individuals who have helped me in the preparation of this work. Thanks belong first to the libraries and archives I used. I am particularly indebted to Roger Davey and his staff at the East Sussex Record Office, who in the close quarters of their former facility tolerated for many weeks my presence in their basement map room and the stacks of manuscript reports I needed in their hallway. I am grateful especially to Margaret Whittick, who went out of her way to help me find local records I would otherwise surely have missed. I am also grateful for permission to use the library of the Post-Graduate Medical Center at Brighton, which, to my knowledge, holds the only complete series of Newsholme's annual reports from Brighton, and the archives of the British Medical Association in London. I am also eager to acknowledge the help I received in being allowed to consult the Webb/ Passfield Papers at the British Library of Political and Economic Science and the collection of Newsholme papers preserved by the library of the London School of Hygiene and Tropical Medicine. Mary E. Gibson of the latter institution located five uncatalogued boxes of Newsholme letters, notes, and reprints and reconstructed the history of how they came into the library's possession in 1965. Like any student of British administration, I have been heavily dependent on the Public Record Office. Alice Prochaska, then at the P.R.O., brought critical classes of records to my attention when I was beginning this project, saving me countless hours, and she has offered many helpful suggestions along the way.

The U.S. National Institutes of Health through the National Library of Medicine provided a grant (LM03765) which permitted me to visit libraries and archives in Britain, and the University of Minnesota has given me a single quarter leave and a sabbatical furlough to finish the research and to prepare the manuscript. I am pleased to acknowledge this support. Anthony Wohl, David Smith, and John Hutchinson have read parts of the manuscript and made valuable suggestions. I was also assisted by two anonymous readers for Cambridge University Press who gave the manuscript a thorough review and recommended helpful changes.

ABBREVIATIONS

Ann. Rep. Chief Med. Off. Board of Education	*Annual Report of the Chief Medical Officer of the Board of Education*
Ann. Rep. L.G.B.	*Annual Report of the Local Government Board*
Ann. Rep. Reg.-Gen.	*Annual Report of the Registrar-General of England and Wales*
B.L.	British Library
B.M.A., C.M.W.A.	British Medical Association Central Medical War Committee
B.M.A., Med. Pol. Comm.	British Medical Association, Medico-Political Committee
B.P.P.	British Parliamentary Papers. House of Commons Sessional Papers unless otherwise noted
Brighton, Proc. San. Comm.	Brighton Corporation, Proceedings of the Sanitary Committee
Brighton, *Proc. Town Council*	Brighton Corporation. *Proceedings of the Town Council*
Brighton, *Proc. Town Council, Proc. Comm.*	Brighton Corporation. *Proceedings of the Town Council, Proceedings of Committees*
D.N.B.	*Dictionary of National Biography*
D.S.B.	*Dictionary of Scientific Biography*
H.L.R.O.	House of Lords Record Office
L.G.B.	Local Government Board
L.S.E.	London School of Economics

M.O.H.   Medical Officer of Health, or
                                        Medical Officers of Health

Med.-Chir. Trans.   *Medico-chirurgical Transactions*

Newsholme, *Ann. Rep.* (Brighton)   Brighton Corporation. Medi-
                                        cal Officer of Health, *Annual
                                        Report on the Health, Sanitary
                                        Condition, &c. of the Borough of
                                        Brighton*

Newsholme, *Ann. Rep. Med. Off. L.G.B.* *Annual Report of the Medical Of-
                                        ficer of the Local Government
                                        Board*

Newsholme, *Q. Rep.* (Brighton)   Brighton Corporation, *Quar-
                                        terly Report of the Medical Officer
                                        of Health*

Newsholme, *Rep.* (Clapham)   Board of Works for the Wands-
                                        worth District, *Report on the
                                        Sanitary Condition of the Several
                                        Parishes . . . by the Medical Offi-
                                        cers of Health,* "Report on
                                        Clapham."

P.R.O.   Public Record Office

PART I

The Medical Officer of Health and the Local Sanitary Authority

1

The Medical Officer of Health and his town

THE APPOINTMENT OF A NEW M.O.H.

On May 17, 1888, the Town Council of Brighton met to select the town's first full-time Medical Officer of Health (abbreviated M.O.H.). The position had been advertised the previous month, and there was a large field, seventy-four medically qualified men in all.[1] A committee of councillors and aldermen cut that number first to fifteen and then to six, all of whom were then serving elsewhere as Medical Officers of Health (also abbreviated M.O.H.). After interviewing these six, the committee placed two names before the Town Council: Henry Tomkins, M.D., M.O.H., for Leicester, and Arthur Newsholme, M.D., M.O.H., for the London vestry of Clapham. At age thirty-two Newsholme was slightly younger, and unlike Tomkins, he had served only part-time for a vestry not full-time for a borough. But Newsholme made a stronger initial impression, and his supporters on the Council contended that his was the more impressive set of academic credentials. The Council was not used to judging professional qualifications, and there was much joking in the meeting about brainpower and cleverness:

We ought to take their age a little into consideration. My candidate, Arthur Newsholme, is running Henry Tomkins very close. Well, but he is five years younger (several Voices: 'No'). Yes, he is 31, and Henry Tomkins – (after whispering with several Councillors near him) – well, he is 32, and Henry Tomkins 36, four years difference. Well, if he is 32, where will he be when he be 36? (roars of laughter). I wish him to be in Brighton (applause). A man with all those degrees at 32 is a clever man and we want the cleverest.[2]

Tomkins's backers acknowledged that Newsholme looked and talked like a gentleman. "He had seldom seen a better looking man (laughter). He was gentle-manly and kindly in his manner, and in that way he carried all before him."[3]

---

1 For the selection process, see Brighton, Proc. San. Comm. 6 (3 May 1888): 52–5; ibid. 6 (8 May 1888): 57–8; ibid. 6 (11 May 1888): 70–1; and "Report of the Sanitary Committee," 11 May 1888, Brighton, Proc. Comm., Report Book, 6 (11 May 1888): 224–5. See also *Sussex Daily News* (12 May 1888): 6.
2 Councillor Dell in the report of the Council meeting *Sussex Daily News* (18 May 1888): 3.
3 Alderman Reeves, ibid.

Tomkins did not make as good an impression on first meeting, but his champions were convinced that he was the more experienced and the more practical candidate. But Newsholme's degrees, his academic prizes, and his publications in public health won him the appointment. He was elected by the margin of twenty-nine to seventeen votes.[4] He came to Brighton at once to take up his new duties at an annual salary of £500, a typical salary for a full-time M.O.H. in that year.[5] In the late 1880s public health was struggling to establish itself as a medical speciality, and he would soon rise to be one of its leaders.[6]

Newsholme was a Yorkshireman. He had been born in 1857 in Haworth, the fourth son of Robert Newsholme, a wool stapler or merchant, who had served as churchwarden to the Reverend Patrick Brontë.[7] While Patrick Brontë, the last of the family, died when Arthur Newsholme was only four years old, young Arthur grew up among people who thought they knew the Brontës well. The Newsholmes lived near the Haworth parsonage, and their family lore included many stories about their eccentric and gifted neighbors. Newsholme's mother delighted in identifying the local inspiration for characters and incidents in Charlotte Brontë's novels. As a young boy Newsholme overheard his elders reminiscing disapprovingly about Branwell Brontë's dissipation, and as an old man Newsholme claimed to still have in his possession the tumbler from which Branwell drank his beer when visiting the Newsholme home.[8]

Although while he was young his family attended the Haworth Church, Newsholme believed that the most formative influences in his early life came not from Church, but from chapel, from the strong local Wesleyan tradition.[9] His mother came from a Wesleyan family, and to satisfy her, the Newsholme family attended chapel Sunday evenings after attending the Church in the morning. After his father's early death, before Arthur was five years old, his mother reared the children in a strict Evangelical environment and sent young Arthur to the local Wesleyan Sunday school. As we will see in examining his adult moral and social attitudes, Arthur Newsholme bore the marks of this upbringing throughout his

---

4 Brighton, *Proc. Town Council,* 17 May 1889: iii.
5 A study by the Local Government Board in 1885 showed that these salaries ranged from £350 to £900 with most falling between £400 and £600. Dorothy Porter, "Stratification and Its Discontents: Professionalization and Conflict in the British Public Health Service, 1848–1914," in *A History of Education in Public Health: Health That Mocks the Doctors' Rules,* ed. Elizabeth Fee and Roy M. Acheson (Oxford and New York: Oxford Univ. Press, 1991), 96.
6 For the professionalization of public health in Britain, see Dorothy [Watkins] Porter, "The English Revolution in Social Medicine, 1889–1911" (University of London: unpublished Ph.D. dissertation, 1984), esp. 58–315.
7 There is no biography of Newsholme, and sources of information about his personal life are sparse. The primary source about his early life are the early sections of his autobiographical reflections of public health work: Arthur Newsholme, *Fifty Years in Public Health: A Personal Narrative with Comments* (London: George Allen and Unwin, 1935), pp. 17–48. See also his more important obituaries: "Sir Arthur Newsholme, K.C.B., M.D., F.R.C.P.," *Br. Med. J.,* (1943), no. 1: 680–1; "Arthur Newsholme, KCB, M.D. Lond, F.R.C.P.," *Lancet* (1843), no. 1: 696; and "Sir Arthur Newsholme, K.C.B.," *Nature* 151 (1943): 635–6
8 Newsholme, *Fifty Years,* 18.   9 Ibid., 23–7.

life. The public wit he cultivated in adulthood went only part way in tempering the moral earnestness and rigidity his upbringing had fostered. As an adult he emphatically defended Evangelicalism as a potent historical force for individual and social improvement and for political and social stability.[10]

Robert Newsholme's death left his family in economic difficulty. His son Arthur was among the small group of Victorian professionals who rose from obscurity by brilliant academic performance, winning by prizes and scholarships opportunities family wealth and connections could never have provided. His formal education began at a free grammar school near his home. After six years there he transferred for a year to Keighley Grammar School. The following year, 1872, he went to London to live with an uncle, a schoolmaster and the executor of his father's estate, and attended matriculation classes for University College. At this time he aspired to join the Indian Civil Service. His intelligence and intellectual curiosity were already evident. Rather than sticking to the subjects he would have to master to enter University College, the young Newsholme also attended advanced classes in Anglo-Saxon, English literature, and chemistry. In the autumn of 1873, at the age of sixteen, he entered University College, but family troubles, probably financial, soon forced him to return to Bradford, where his mother was then living.

It was only at this time that he began to consider medicine as a career. His mother's physician agreed to take him on as a dispenser and surgery assistant, and for more than a year he helped out in a successful provincial general practice, learning some anatomy and physiology from the doctor's assistant. By the fall of 1875, arrangements had been made to allow Newsholme to take his small inheritance before his majority so that he could pursue his education, and he returned to London. This time he entered St. Thomas's Hospital Medical School, where he had an exceptional career, earning prize money in competition each year. These prizes combined with earnings from tutoring allowed him to pay his way. He qualified early at Apothecaries Hall, becoming a Licentiate of the Society of Apothecaries (L.S.A.) in 1876 and thereby becoming a registered practitioner. He was examined for his M.B. in 1880, earning both a gold medal in medicine and a two-year University Scholarship. The following year he became M.D., earning first class honors and another gold medal. He would eventually become a Member of the Royal College of Physicians (M.R.C.P.) in 1893 and a Fellow (F.R.C.P.) in 1898. Immediately following his M.D. highly prized house officerships came his way at St. Thomas's: House Physician, House Surgeon to Outpatients, and Resident Accoucheur.[11] He also served as House Surgeon at Tottenham Hospital and Registrar at the Evelina Hospital for Children.

In other circumstances such a promising beginning might have led to a career as a medical consultant, with an appointment at a London hospital and a special-

10 Ibid., 25–7.
11 "Sir Arthur Newsholme, K.C.B., M.D., F.R.C.P.," *St. Thomas's Hospital Gazette*, 41 (1943): 92.

ized private practice. But such professional advancement was difficult, uncertain, and achieved by only a few.[12] Despite his success in examinations he lacked the personal connections with the leaders of the London medical establishment which still counted for much in the making of a consultant's career, and he did not have the resources to survive the period of waiting on the fringes of London's hospital world. He also had by this time greater financial needs. In 1881 he had married Sara Mansford from Marlborough, Lincolnshire. Their marriage was happy, childless, and lasted until her death in 1933.[13] In the early eighties his marriage provided an added incentive to end his training and enter practice.

Rather than buy a practice, he risked trying to establish a new one in the London suburbs. He found a place on High Street, Clapham, and hung up his shingle in 1883.[14] Like most other beginning practitioners, he supplemented his fees from patients. He tutored medical students, wrote articles, and edited a series of science textbooks for schoolchildren, writing two of the volumes himself.[15] For a while he had a club practice, providing prepaid medical services for members of a local chapter of the Manchester Unity of Oddfellows. This was an experience he would draw on again and again much later in his career when discussing national health care schemes. He also accepted part-time institutional posts: physician to the City Dispensary and medical officer to the Westminister and Southlands Training Colleges for Teachers.[16] According to his own account he quickly built a successful practice with an income from practice of just under £900 by the end of his fifth year. He came to Brighton for a smaller, if more secure, income.

We do not know how Newsholme's interest was first drawn to hygiene and public health. St. Thomas's had, it is true, the first lectureship in hygiene among British medical schools,[17] but hygiene did not play a very significant part in its curriculum.[18] In Newsholme's student days the lecturer on hygiene was Alfred Carpenter, M.O.H. of Croydon and a busy general practitioner, who gave twelve lectures on hygiene in the summer. Newsholme attended these but later could recall only Carpenter's pleasant manner as a lecturer, the social event he held for the students at his home, and a field trip to see the sewage treatment farm at

---

12 For an account of the problems of establishing a practice in Victorian Britain and of the process of becoming a consultant, see M. Jeanne Peterson, *The Medical Profession in Mid-Victorian London* (Berkeley, Los Angeles, London: Univ. of California Press, 1978), 90–138.

13 "Newsholme," *Br. Med. J.* (1943), no. 1: 680.

14 For his experience as a private practitioner, see Newsholme, *Fifty Years*, 129–32. The *London Suburban Directory, Southern Suburbs*, 1884 reports Newsholme's address as 39 High Street.

15 Richard Balchin, *Hughes's Science Readers*, No. 1 for Standard III, ed. A[rthur] Newsholme (London: Joseph Hughes, 1883); Richard Balchin, *Hughes's Science Readers*, No. 2 for Standard IV, ed. A[rthur] Newsholme (London: Joseph Hughes, 1883); A[rthur] Newsholme, *Hughes Science Readers*, No. 3 for Standard V (London: Joseph Hughes, 1884); and A[rthur] Newsholme, *Hughes's Science Readers*, No. 4 for Standards VI and VII (London: Joseph Hughes, 1884).

16 Newsholme's testimony, *Report of the Royal Commission on the Poor Laws and Relief of Distress*, Appendix vol. 9, B.P.P. 1910, XLIX [Cd. 5068], p. 155.

17 Royston Lambert, *Sir John Simon 1816–1904 and English Social Administration* (London: MacGibbon and Fee, 1963), 261–2.

18 The following information is drawn from Newsholme, *Fifty Years*, 43–4.

Beddington. The M.B. examination dispensed with hygiene in a brief and perfunctory way. Newsholme was able to pass with distinction, although he had done no preparation on hygiene other than reading through a short textbook during a train ride to the Isle of Wight. As a student Newsholme did have contact with a leading Victorian public health authority. In 1880 he was house physician to John Syer Bristowe.[19] Bristowe was then M.O.H. of Camberwell and the President of the Society of Medical Officers of Health. He had undertaken a number of important investigations for John Simon, Medical Officer first of the Privy Council and then of the Local Government Board.[20] While the young Newsholme was impressed with Bristowe's clinical teaching and especially with his general textbook on medicine,[21] as a student he did not take any interest in Bristowe's work in preventive medicine.

It seems that Newsholme's initial interest in hygiene was partly the result of financial need, for he found in hygiene a lucrative supplemental income. Beginning in 1882 and for several years thereafter, he lectured one evening a week on elementary physiology and hygiene for a six-month term at the central Y.M.C.A. on the Strand to a large class of elementary school teachers preparing to shepherd their pupils through the Science and Art Department's examinations, which included questions on hygiene.[22] Newsholme soon became an examiner on this subject for the Science and Art Department. In 1884 he exploited this education market even further by publishing a textbook intended for those preparing for the advanced South Kensington examination in hygiene.[23] This book, like most British hygiene manuals of the period, was modeled on Edmund Parke's *Manual of Practical Hygiene,* which had first appeared in 1864.[24] Newsholme's *Hygiene* was followed within three years by another on school hygiene,[25] and later by elementary hygiene texts for young schoolchildren and for domestic economy classes in teacher training schools.[26] These publications were very successful. His *Hygiene* sold over 12,000 and his *Domestic Hygiene* over 40,000 copies, and his *School Hygiene* went through fifteen editions before 1918.[27]

19 For a sketch of Bristowe, see C. Fraser Brockington, *Public Health in the Nineteenth Century* (Edinburgh and London: E. & S. Livingstone, 1965), 257–9.

20 For Newsholme's reminiscences of Bristowe, see Newsholme, *Fifty Years,* 35–7.

21 John Syer Bristowe, *A Treatise on the Theory and Practice of Medicine* (London: Smith, Elder, & Co., 1876).

22 Newsholme, *Fifty Years,* 147. See also the title he claimed for himself, Lecturer on Physiology and Hygiene at the Exeter Hall Science Classes, on the title page of his *Hygiene: A Manual of Personal and Public Health* (London, 1884).

23 Arthur Newsholme, *Hygiene: A Manual of Personal and Public Health* (London: George Gill & Sons, 1884).

24 For a discussion of British hygienic textbooks, see Porter [Watkins], "English Revolution," 340–73.

25 Arthur Newsholme, *School Hygiene: The Laws of Health in Relation to School Life* (London, 1887).

26 The former began as *Lessons on Health: Containing the Elements of Physiology and Their Application to Hygiene* (London, 1890). It was republished as *Elementary Hygiene,* new ed. (London, 1893). The latter is Arthur Newsholme and Margarot Eleanor Scott, *Domestic Economy: Comprising the Laws of Health in Their Application to Home Life and Work* (London: Swan Sonnenschein & Co., 1902).

27 Newsholme, *Fifty Years,* 147, 150.

Newsholme moved from popularizer to participant in 1884, when he became part-time M.O.H. for Clapham at an annual salary of £80.[28] Clapham was then one of six subdistricts of the Metropolitan District of Wandsworth.[29] Health and sanitation were then the responsibility of the Board of Works for the Wandsworth District. Its Sanitary Committee had a subcommittee for each subdistrict, and each subcommittee employed a part-time M.O.H.[30] Newsholme was the only one of these M.O.H. who was not also employed by the Poor Law Guardians as District Medical Officer to provide medical services to paupers.[31] The year following his appointment Newsholme returned to London University to acquire his Diploma in Public Health. But his education in public health depended much less on the modest syllabus for this diploma than on his private study.[32] In Clapham he discovered William Farr's and John Simon's annual reports. Reading these reports by the former Statistical Superintendent of the General Register Office and by the Medical Officer of the Privy Council proved to be Newsholme's primary education in public health and epidemiology. As we will see in the next chapter, Newsholme was particularly indebted to Farr.

THE TOWN AND ITS REPUTATION

When Newsholme arrived, Brighton was a prosperous seaside resort with a population of 115,000. Over the last century and a third, an enthusiasm first for the medicinal use of sea water and then the fashion of taking the sea air had transformed the former fishing village into the largest British resort and the eighteenth largest town in England and Wales, excluding greater London.[33] The patronage of the Royal Family, beginning in the 1760s but particularly the regular visits beginning in 1783 of the Prince of Wales, the future Regent and King,

---

28 For his autobiographical comments on his work as M.O.H. of Clapham, see ibid., 133–43.
29 The other subdistricts were East Battersea, West Battersea, Putney, Streatham, and Wandsworth.
30 See Board of Works for the Wandsworth District, *Minutes of Proceedings.*
31 In this book the Poor Law refers to the New Poor Law of 1834, the welfare system that served England for the remainder of the century. Funds for relief were raised through local property taxes – the poor rate, or the rates – and were administered by the locally elected Board of Guardians. Relief might consist of food and shelter, of money, and of medical care. If given in a poor law institution, it was known as indoor relief; if outside of such an institution, outdoor relief. Relief was given on terms intended to deter applications. Those in receipt of relief were pauperized and suffered conditions that were frequently harsh and stigmatizing as well as the loss of certain civil rights.
32 For a very useful discussion of the curriculum for the DPH, see Roy Acheson, "The British Diploma in Public Health: Birth and Adolescence," in *A History of Education in Public Health: Health that Mocks the Doctors' Rules,* ed. Elizabeth Fee and Roy M. Acheson (Oxford: Oxford Univ. Press, 1991): 55–78.
33 For the social history of Brighton, see Edmund W. Gilbert, *Brighton: Old Ocean's Bauble* (London: Methuen & Co., 1954); Anthony Dale, *Fashionable Brighton 1820–1860,* 2nd ed. (Newcastle-upon-Tyne: Oriel Press, 1967); and Clifford Musgrave, *Life in Brighton from Earliest Times to the Present* (London: Faber and Faber, 1970).

George IV, had made Brighton the foremost sea resort, eclipsing even Bath as the provincial center of fashion and recreation.[34] By the second third of the nineteenth century, however, royal patronage had dwindled. Victoria visited for the last time in 1845. Thereafter the Royal Pavilion, the fantastic Oriental pleasure palace the Regent had built for himself, stood empty.[35] But by that time Brighton had found other sources of prosperity. Its pleasant climate and setting, its elegant buildings, and the reputation for fashion and rakishness that it had acquired in the Regency all continued to lure many wealthy visitors. By some accounts the decades 1830–60 marked the peak of Brighton's fashion, but in the 1870s the town was probably its most prosperous, and it continued to attract large numbers from the upper classes.

Equally important for Brighton's future was the completion of the railroad from London in 1841. The rail link to the Metropolis changed Brighton's character as a resort. First it rapidly increased the number of visitors and stimulated the growth of the town itself. In 1837, four years before the coming of the railroad, at a time when Brighton could boast of good coach service, stage coaches brought to Brighton 50,000 visitors during the entire year, but in 1850 the railroad brought 73,000 visitors in a single week.[36] Brighton's population also grew rapidly, from 46,000 to 65,000, in the first decade after the completion of the main line to London, and within three decades its population had nearly doubled.[37] It was soon one of the nation's largest provincial towns, and it acquired during the century powers of self-government. It gained parliamentary representation in 1832 and was incorporated as a borough in 1854.[38] In the last quarter of the century this urban growth slowed, in part because the town was running out of vacant land and was unable to annex the adjacent community of Hove. Between the censuses of 1851 and 1881 Brighton had experienced the largest incremental growth of any English or Welsh seaside resort, but between 1881 and 1911 it ranked fifth in incremental growth and ninety-fifth in percentage growth.[39]

The railroad also helped change the social composition of Brighton's resort trade. Cheaper and faster rail travel attracted visitors from lower down the social scale. During the second half of the century Brighton developed two seasons, the official season in the autumn months, which continued to attract the fashionable classes, and a summer season, which drew ever larger crowds of middle- and

34 E. W. Gilbert, "The Growth of Brighton," *Geographical J.*, 114 (1949): 37–42.
35 Dale, 15, 17.
36 John K. Walton, *The English Seaside Resort: A Social History 1750–1914* (Leicester: Leicester Univ. Press, 1983), 22.
37 Gilbert, "Growth," 43–4. For a discussion of the development of Brighton's districts after the coming of the railroad, see Sue Farrant, "The Growth of Brighton and Hove 1840–1939," in *The Growth of Brighton and Hove 1840–1939*, ed. Sue Farrant, K. Fossey, and A. Peasgood (Falmer, East Sussex: The Centre for Continuing Education, University of Sussex, 1981), 25–30.
38 B[enjamin] W[ard] Richardson, "The Medical History of England: The Medical History of Brighton," *Medical Times and Gazette* (1864), no. 1: 651; Gilbert, *Brighton*, 153.
39 Walton, 61, 65, 66, 68.

lower-middle-class families for summer holidays, and eventually working-class visitors and day-trippers.[40] By the later decades of Victoria's reign Brighton was feeling the competition for the most fashionable trade from other resorts, especially those on the South Coast such as Eastbourne, Hastings, and Bournemouth. These smaller and newer resorts could promise quieter surroundings and a more uniformly privileged resident social set.[41]

But Brighton was not only a resort. Its reputation as a healthy and fashionable place and its proximity to London – it was closer to the Metropolis than any other seaside resort – made Brighton a natural choice of location for boarding schools. By the 1880s there were some 125 of them, more than in any other South Coast resort town.[42] Its economy also had an industrial component, relying most heavily in the later decades of the century on its railway manufacturing works. In 1891 the railroad employed directly more than 2,600 of Brighton's residents.[43] A host of small manufacturers and the building trades were also important sources of employment, but the dominance of its resort trade and schools meant that Brighton had primarily a service economy. As the resort trade was seasonal, there were regular periods of unemployment for many of the town's laboring residents. Despite its great wealth, Brighton experienced many of the same problems with poverty as other nineteenth-century British towns.[44] As we shall see in considering the slum clearance projects in the last two decades of the century, the proximity of opulence and squalor could be very striking in Victorian Brighton.

Newsholme came to Brighton at a time when local government was becoming more active. One can trace the municipal activism of the last quarter of the century to a variety of forces, among them economic growth, interurban competition, and the formation of a municipal gospel, an ideology of social reform which successfully transferred the labor of rescue and moral uplift from Church, chapel, and missionary society to the local authority.[45] Resort towns had particularly strong incentives to undertake municipal improvements and to engage in municipal trading. By the 1870s many English resorts were willing to spend public money to provide amenities and entertainments for visitors in order to promote the local tourist trade.[46] In the last quarter of the century they, like some northern

40 This social change occurred at most resorts. See ibid., 59–60.
41 See the comparative measures of social status of the resorts' residents in ibid., 78, 79, 80, 81.
42 Gilbert, *Brighton*, 197–200; and Walton, 97.   43 Musgrave, 312; and Gilbert, *Brighton*, 156–7.
44 For a short description of poverty and working-class life in Brighton, see Musgrave, 312–14, 319–24. For a useful autobiographical account of an early twentieth-century working-class childhood, see John Langley, *Always a Layman* (Brighton: Sussex Society for Labour History, 1976). In the early twentieth century Brighton's Sanitary Committee provided public works jobs for the unemployed. See Brighton, Proc. San. Comm. 22 (16 Nov. 1905): 305–6; and ibid. 23 (11 Oct. 1906): 183–4. Newsholme described the provisions for medical relief in Brighton in his testimony of the *Report of the Royal Commission on the Poor Laws and Relief of Distress*, Appendix Vol. 9, B.P.P. 1909, XLIX, [Cd. 5068], 155–8.
45 This role that a municipal gospel played has been effectively argued for the case of Birmingham in E. P. Hennock, *Fit and Proper Persons: Ideal and Reality in Nineteenth-Century Urban Government* (Montreal: McGill-Queens Univ. Press, 1973), see esp. 61–169.
46 Walton, 140–55.

industrial towns, provided water, gas, electricity, and tramways either by buying private companies or by initiating publicly owned utilities.[47] Street lighting and paving, pleasure piers, promenades, town bands and orchestras, parks, pleasure gardens, and winter gardens all made their appearance as municipal projects in the last three decades of the century.

Brighton acted earliest and on a grand scale by buying the Royal Pavilion in 1850 and remodeling it as a public attraction. Half a century later the Corporation purchased the Aquarium and continued to run it, even though the facility incurred major financial losses. But more characteristic of this late Victorian municipal activism were the Corporation's efforts beginning in 1872 to buy up the private water companies serving the town and to build new pumping stations.[48] As a result of these efforts the number of homes receiving pumped water increased rapidly. The Corporation soon found other uses for its public water supply, adding public drinking fountains, public baths, a swimming pool, and public toilets. By the middle 1890s the Corporation also was spending public money to maintain public parks and gardens, a race track, a cricket ground, the beach, the Dome – the former stables of the Royal Pavilion which had been converted and enlarged to provide an assembly hall, a library, a museum, and a gallery – and to provide street cleaning and lighting.[49] By 1900 only Blackpool among the English seaside resorts provided all four basic public utilities: water, gas, electricity, and tramways, but Brighton was one of three resorts which provided three of the four.[50] A year later it added the fourth, when its tramway system began to operate.[51]

Although Brighton's economy depended upon its reputation as a healthy place, and although it had early proven its willingness to spend on ornaments and attractions, the town was not in the vanguard in investing in the invisible infrastructure of modern urban life, which included a proper sewage system. The Corporation was content to trust the health of the town to the natural advantages of Brighton's site. By 1860 only about a quarter of the houses of Brighton were drained into the town's 8½ miles of sewers.[52] The remaining three-quarters relied on cesspools, estimated by unfriendly critics to number around 10,000. Moreover,

47 Malcolm Falkus, "The Development of Municipal Trading in the Nineteenth Century," *Business History,* 19 (1977): 134–61; and Anthony Sutcliffe, "The Growth of Public Intervention in the British Urban Environment during the Nineteenth Century: A Structural Approach," in *The Structure of Nineteenth Century Cities,* ed. James H. Johnson and Colin G. Pooley (London: Croom Helm, 1982): 107–24.
48 Gilbert, *Brighton,* 166–7.
49 "Estimate of Money Required on the District Fund Account for the Service of the Half-Year Commencing 1st January and Ending 30th June 1893." Brighton, *Proc. Town Council,* 31 Oct. 1892; and "London-by-the Sea," *London,* 6 June 1895: 430–2.
50 Walton, 145.
51 Adrian Peasgood, "Public Transport and the Growth of Brighton 1840 to 1940," in *The Growth of Brighton and Hove 1840–1939,* ed. Sue Farrant, K. Fossey, and A. Peasgood (Falmer, East Sussex: University of Sussex Centre for Continuing Education, 1981), 49.
52 "Report on the Drainage of Brighton, with a Chemical and Microscopical Analysis Illustrative of the Pollution of the Sea and Well Waters," *Lancet* (1862), no. 2: 397; and "Report of The Lancet Sanitary Commission on the Drainage of Brighton," *Lancet* (1868), no. 2: 383.

the sewers then simply discharged their contents from three large iron pipes into the sea opposite the sea front. By the late 1850s visitors were beginning to notice and to complain about disgusting odors and discoloration of the sea water.

Building a sewer system was an expensive proposition with a technologically unproven outcome. Like many Victorian towns, Brighton found it difficult to muster political will and the capital to do so.[53] As early as the 1850s one of the town's mayors, himself a medical practitioner, unsuccessfully urged the Council to appoint a Medical Officer of Health and to build proper sewers for the town.[54] The Town Council hired two engineers to draw up plans and to make estimates for building a comprehensive sewer system, but a majority could not be found in the Council to support the expensive plan, and the project had to wait almost two decades.

The reform party would eventually triumph by exploiting the town's fear of losing its resort trade. In this campaign the reformers found a powerful ally in *The Lancet,* which intermittently over a period of twenty years dramatically publicized the sanitary inadequacies of this famous health resort. Its campaign began in November 1860 when it published under the provocative title "The Death Drains of Brighton" a letter, soon to be republished in *The Times,* from a London surgeon who blamed illness in his household on the faulty drains of the house he rented while on a Brighton holiday.[55] The medical journal was soon providing lurid descriptions of the town's sewers and cesspools and editorial warnings to visitors and their medical practitioners.

How often has it happened that the jaded denizen of London and his drooping children have met with sickness, and perhaps death, where they had sought for health from the invigorating breezes of the sea! The autumnal flight to the sea-shore is, in too many instances, an exchange of well-drained, commodious, and cleanly dwellings, for the hidden abominations of cesspools, and elaborate disguises of household dirt in many forms. The free air inhaled by day upon the beach, or in the neighbouring fields, but poorly compensates for the deadly nightsoil malaria that steals throughout the bedrooms and empoisons the unconscious sleepers.[56]

In editorials and leading articles during the decade the medical journal urged the construction of an intercepting sewer to divert the town's sewage from the sea front and its disposal, preferably on land as sewage manure or, failing that, into the sea at a distance from the town.[57] It pointed out what Brighton's rivals, Eastbourne

53 For an illuminating account of the problems of providing sewers for Victorian cities, see Wohl, *Endangered Lives,* 80–116.
54 This practitioner was undoubtedly J. Cody Burrows, who was Mayor of Brighton in 1857, 1858, and 1871. B[enjamin] W[ard] Richardson, "The Medical History of England: The Medical History of Brighton," *Medical Times & Gazette* (1864), no. 1: 651; and *Friend's Brighton Almanack* (1894): 20. His complaint to a London surgeon about this episode is recorded in William Acton, "The Death Drains at Brighton," *Lancet* (1860), no. 2: 522.
55 Acton, "Death Drains;" and "The Drains at Brighton," *The Times,* 23 Nov. 1860: 10.
56 Leading editorial, 8 Dec. 1860, *Lancet* (1860), no. 2: 566.
57 In addition to the editorials already cited, see leading editorial 9 Nov. 1861, *Lancet* (1861), no. 2: 415 [actually 451]–2; untitled editorial, ibid., (1862), no. 2: 334–5; and "Brighton Drainage," ibid. (1869), no. 1: 621.

and Hastings, had already done to construct proper sewers,[58] and it castigated the Town Council for its delay, myopia, and incompetence. "There is probably no town in the United Kingdom which is blessed with a greater set of dunderheads than Brighton."[59] Town officials and local newspapers at first responded with denials and accusations of slander and foul play.[60] They next sought lesser solutions in extending the discharge pipes at the sea front farther out into the sea and in the testimony of hired consultants about the purifying power of sea water.[61] Finally, driven by the fear that visitors would go elsewhere if drastic measures were not taken, the Council was forced to act. It hired the engineer John Hawkshaw and between 1871 and 1874 constructed intercepting sewers and a sewer outfall four miles to the east of town.[62]

But the new sewer did not put the issue of the town's drainage to rest. Hawkshaw's design was defective.[63] The intercepting sewer and its outlet were built at low elevation, below the level of high tide. Hawkshaw had installed gates at the outlet to prevent the influx of sea water, but the result was that for as long as thirteen hours in every twenty-four the discharge of sewage was prevented, and the lower third of the intercepting sewer became a reservoir of putrefying sewage. Despite the existence of one-way valves in the lower third of the intercepting sewer and a ventilating furnace kept constantly burning, sewer gas issued from the town's street drains and gullies causing concern to the health conscious.

The Lancet took up the issue again in November 1881 as the town was preparing to host a Health Congress. In April 1882, when a coroner's jury determined that sewer gas had caused a death from blood poisoning, the journal jumped to the offensive, warning the town it faced an epidemic induced by sewer gas.[64] This time the town was even more defensive than it had been in the 1860s. The Town Council hired experts. Sir Joseph Bazalgette, the engineer who had built London's interception sewers, inspected and reported on Brighton's drainage, and the prominent medical sanitarian Benjamin Ward Richardson reported on the health and sanitary condition of the town.[65] Finally in June 1882 the Mayor and Corporation

58 "Report of The Lancet Sanitary Commission on the Drainage of Brighton," ibid. (1868), no. 2: 382; and "Brighton Drainage," ibid. (1869), no. 1: 476–7.
59 "Brighton Drainage," ibid. (1869), no. 2: 526.
60 See, for example, the letter by William Kebbell, Physician to the Sussex County Hospital, "The Drainage of Brighton," ibid. (1862), no. 2: 404; and letters by Philip Lockwood, the Borough Surveyor, and P. R. Wilkinson, the estate agent, which appeared under the title "The Drains at Brighton," *Times,* 27 Nov. 1860: 4. See also *Brighton Gazette,* 29 Nov. 1860: 5, and "Brighton and Its Slanderers," ibid., 4.
61 Farrant, "Growth of Brighton," 29; "The Drainage of Brighton," *Lancet* (1864), no. 2: 186–7; and Untitled editorial, 29 May 1869, ibid. (1869), no. 1: 751–2.
62 "Brighton Sewerage: Report of Sir Joseph Bazalgette, C.B., C.E., June 27, 1882," ibid. (1882), no. 2: 34.
63 For descriptions of the sewer system and its problems, see "Brighton Sewerage: Report of Sir Joseph Bazalgette, C.B., C.E.," ibid. (1882), no. 2: 33–4; and Benjamin Ward Richardson, "Report on the Sanitary Condition of the Borough of Brighton," ibid., (1882), no. 2: 757–8, 763.
64 "Blood-poisoning at Brighton," ibid. (1882), no. 1: 536.
65 Bazalgette's report is reprinted in "Brighton Sewerage: Report of Sir Joseph Bazalgette, C.B., C.E.," ibid. (1882), no. 2: 33–5. Richardson's report is reprinted as "Dr. Richardson's Report on the Sanitary Condition of the Borough of Brighton," ibid. (1882), no. 2: 747–63.

sued *The Lancet* for damages its reports and editorials had done to the town's reputation and resort trade.[66] But such defensive acts were to no avail. Now the advantages were all on the side of those who wanted sanitary improvement. In announcing its suit, the town felt obliged to promise to follow any recommendations that its experts would suggest. *The Lancet* turned the suit into additional bad publicity for the town, and it hired its own engineer to evaluate Brighton's sewer system and to suggest changes.[67] The town eventually dropped the suit in a face-saving maneuver, after *The Lancet* published the full text of Richardson's report, a masterpiece of diplomacy.[68] But in the end it was forced to make the type of changes in the sewers its sanitary critics had been demanding.[69]

The fight over the town sewers goes some way toward explaining the environment, physical and political, Newsholme found, when he came to Brighton. He found a modern and adequate system of main drainage and a recently quickened sensitivity in the Town Council about public sanitation. The public criticism *The Lancet* had helped mobilize reflects an important change in public opinion. At the national level important legislation of the early 1870s, which we will consider in the next section, encouraged a more active and uniform public health policy. In Brighton the pressure of criticism from beyond the town's boundaries not only insured that better drainage would be provided but helped subdue and discredit those forces in the Town Council which favored above all else low rates and minimal public intervention. Appeal to public opinion in London remained one of the strongest weapons in the hands of those who favored a strong sanitary policy in Brighton. We will see it employed in particularly difficult political circumstances during Newsholme's tenure in Brighton.

Each of the two major battles over public sanitation in the 1870s and 1880s resulted not only in major drainage construction but also in an expansion of regular public health activity. It is no coincidence that regular meetings of the Sanitary Committee and the appointment of the town's first Medical Officer of Health follow the public controversy of the early seventies and regular reports of the Sanitary Committee first appear in the wake of the next storm of the town's sewers.[70] Fear of continued bad publicity and a recognition that the prosperity of the town depended on the public's faith that everything that could be done to make Brighton healthy was being done drove the Town Council to ensure a continual surveillance of the town's health. A substantial increase in the size of the

66 "The Corporation of Brighton v. 'The Lancet,' " ibid. (1882), no. 1: 1093.
67 J. Bailey-Denton, C. E., "Report on the Brighton Sewerage," ibid. (1882), no. 2: 196–8.
68 Part of the letter from the solicitors is reprinted in the untitled leading editorial, ibid. (1882), no. 2: 811.
69 Richardson, for example, had suggested the use of steam pumping to ensure the constant discharge of sewerage from the outfall and the improved ventilation of sewers. "Dr. Richardson's Report," 762–3.
70 Prior to the early 1870s the Sanitary Committee was inactive, meeting only when summoned. It thereafter met fortnightly, just prior to each meeting of the Town Council. The regular reports of the committee begin only in 1882.

Sanitary Department in 1885 and Newsholme's appointment as the town's first full-time M.O.H. in 1888 can be seen as additional reflections of the new political consensus in Brighton.[71] The day was now past when it was necessary to argue that the local authority might and properly should act to prevent disease and to ensure the existence of a healthy environment. The question had become one of means. Newsholme was fortunate in this respect. Discussions of public health were now conducted in terms which gave the technical expert an advantage. The question was how best to promote the public health, not whether it was proper to act for that purpose.

THE LOCAL HEALTH AUTHORITY

Recent historians have dated the beginning of a meaningful national public health program in Britain from the passing of the Public Health Act, 1872.[72] This legislation saw to it that every place in England and Wales had one and only one sanitary, or health, authority and that each of these authorities appointed a Medical Officer of Health. Prior to this time the appointment of an M.O.H. was optional, and few local authorities had made such appointments. Hereafter preventive measures that had been adopted in only a few places were more actively encouraged by the central authority and were applied on a much wider scale at the local level. In a county borough like Brighton, the Sanitary Authority was the Town Council. Brighton Town Council, like most other local authorities, delegated much of its responsibility for health and sanitation to its Sanitary Committee, one of about a dozen permanent committees comprising Councillors and Aldermen that framed proposals for the whole Council and supervised the work of the town's officials. The Sanitary Committee, in turn, acted through the Sanitary Department, headed by the Medical Officer of Health.

Under normal conditions Brighton's Sanitary Committee met every two weeks.[73] Since the Committee acted for the Council, the Committee's actions were subject to approval at the next Council meeting. Ordinarily Council approval was obtained with little or no discussion. However, at times, objections were raised and occasionally heated debate ensued. At such times the Council might except part of the Committee's proceedings from its approval, thus overturning a Committee decision. In most instances, however, decisions made by the Sanitary Committee on matters of public health were final. The Committee initiated all

---

71 The Sanitary Committee appointed four additional Assistant Sanitary Inspectors in August 1885. Brighton, Proc. San. Comm. 4 (10 Aug. 1885): 115–16.

72 35 & 36 Vict. C. 79, sect. 3–5 and 10. For insight on the early implementation of the Act, see *Ann. Rep. L.G.B.* 2 (1872–3): xxxix–1. This interpretation is convincingly argued in Anthony S. Wohl, *Endangered Lives: Public Health in Victorian Britain* (Cambridge, Mass.: Harvard Univ. Press, 1983), 181–2.

73 For the unpublished records of the Committee see Brighton, Proc. San. Comm. A published, edited portion of these records is found in the Proceedings of the Committees section of the Proceedings of the Town Council: Brighton, *Proc. Town Council, Proc. Comm.*

changes in public health policy. If Council approval was withheld, the matter was returned to the Committee for further consideration.

The Medical Officer of Health was an employee of the local authority. The Local Government Board orders which specified the duties of the M.O.H. made it clear that the M.O.H. was to be the technical adviser of the local sanitary authority and the administrator of the local sanitary department.[74] He was to be prepared to advise the sanitary authority on all matters relating to the public health. In order to do this he was expected to keep himself informed on the health and sanitary condition of his district by inspection and investigation. He was to supervise the work of the Inspectors of Nuisances and other employees of the Sanitary Department and to enforce the local sanitary bylaws in a manner directed by the sanitary authority. He was also required to investigate immediately any outbreak of contagious or dangerous disease, to report that outbreak to the local sanitary authority and to the Local Government Board, and to advise "the persons competent to act" what might be done to prevent the spread of the disease. He was to keep records of his activities and to prepare an annual report to be submitted to the local sanitary authority and to the L.G.B. Thus while the M.O.H. had some latitude in carrying out the Committee's directives, and while he could suggest new departures in services or procedures, he could not initiate policy changes or make even minor staff appointments on his own authority. Furthermore until 1921, when M.O.H. serving outside the Metropolis received security of tenure, most served at the pleasure of their Sanitary Authority and might be easily dismissed.[75] But an M.O.H., particularly one serving a local authority where municipal pride was high, had advantages denied even to the head of the nation's public health service, the Medical Officer of the Local Government Board. The local M.O.H. had administrative responsibility – he was the head of the Sanitary Department – and direct access to the public authority – he attended meetings of the Sanitary Committee and the Town Council, where decisions were made.

A successful M.O.H. learned how to manage his Committee. Both his technical expertise and his intimate knowledge of the day-to-day workings of the Sanitary Department gave him an advantage in dealing with the Committee members, who had other interests and pursuits. In Newsholme's day, the Brighton Town

---

74 "Urban Sanitary Authorities. – Appointments and Duties of Medical Officers of Health, and Inspectors of Nuisances. Circular Letter" and "Urban Sanitary Authorities. – General Order," *Ann. Rep. L. G. B.* 2 (1872–3): 29–36; and "General Order (Urban Sanitary Authorities). – Regulations as to Medical Officers of Health, No Portion of Whose Salaries Is Repaid out of Moneys Voted by Parliament," ibid., 10 (1880–1): 25–8. The Sanitary Committee of Brighton had these regulations before them when they considered Newsholme's appointment, "Report of the Sanitary Committee," Brighton, Proc. Comm., Report Book, 6 (22 March 1888): 180–8.

75 Wohl, *Endangered Lives,* 190. In London the M.O.H. received tenure in 1891; Anne Hardy, "Public Health and the Expert: The London Medical Officers of Health, 1856–1900," in *Government and Expertise: Specialists, Administrators and Professionals, 1860–1919,* ed. Roy MacLeod (Cambridge: Cambridge Univ. Press, 1988), 130.

Council contained some members who were identified simply as gentlemen.[76] A small number of professionals, mainly doctors and solicitors, were also elected to the Council. Labor representatives entered the Council in greater numbers from the mid-1890s.[77] But the dominant force on the Council came from the town's commercial and business interests. In 1895, for example, the Council contained two gentlemen, one physician, one solicitor, a signalman, an engine driver, a bricklayer, an engineer, and a painter.[78] The remaining members that year were in trade or commerce. Most conspicuous were the nine builders, including the Mayor, and several hotel keepers and caterers. Newsholme would have some clashes with the trade interests on the Council, most seriously, as we will see in Chapter 3, with the Butchers' Association in 1893 and 1894. But in general he was wisely solicitous of local business interests and was careful to avoid raising unnecessary trade opposition.

Newsholme's greatest asset in dealing with the Sanitary Committee was his ability to persuade. His credentials, his growing output of scientific and professional papers, and the professional honors, which he saw came to his committee's attention, all helped bolster his credibility.[79] But it was critical that he be able to frame explanations that Committee Members would find comprehensible and convincing. This was a difficult task in the late nineteenth century, when the understanding of the infectious diseases was changing rapidly and when the results of public policies were not always what had been expected. Newsholme was well prepared for the task of educating and reassuring the Committee. The popular health manuals he had written over the last few years gave him experience presenting current hygienic knowledge in terms that any literate person could understand.[80] He also learned how to use vital statistics for argumentative purposes in dealing with his committee.

A successful M.O.H. like Newsholme, particularly one from a resort town, had to balance his need to expose health risks and to occasionally remind his Committee and the Council what bad publicity and public doubts about the town's salubrity could cost the borough while at the same time leaving no room for doubt that he had the best interest of the town at heart. In his annual reports he routinely compared to the borough's advantage Brighton's vital statistics to those of other towns.[81] This was an annual exercise in reassuring the Committee and

---

76 For a list of candidates and their occupations, see *Brighton Gazette* (29 Oct. 1903): 3.
77 For press coverage of the changes brought about by the increase in Labour members and evidence of friction in the Council caused by this change, see *Brighton Gazette* (7 July 1894): 5; untitled editorial, *Brighton Herald* (28 July 1894): 2; and *Sussex Daily News* (4 Aug. 1894): 6–7.
78 "London-by-the-Sea," *London,* 6 June 1895: 429.
79 See, for example, the Committee's pride in Newsholme's selection as an examiner in state medicine at London University and in preventive medicine at Oxford. Brighton, Proc. San. Comm., 14 (13 May 1897): 377; ibid., 15 (12 May 1898): 349–50; and *Brighton Herald* (21 May 1898): 2. See also the Committee's congratulations upon his election as Milroy Lecturer at the Royal College of Physicians, Brighton, Proc. San. Comm. 11 (26 April 1894): 271.
80 See in particular Newsholme, *Hygiene,* and Newsholme, *School Hygiene.*
81 Newsholme first did this in Newsholme, *Ann. Rep.* (Brighton), 1889, 7.

the Council that their investment of health was paying good dividends. In his first year on the job and on at least one other occasion he also wrote illustrated pieces extolling the virtues of Brighton as a health resort.[82] Such boosterism must have pleased his Committee. Newsholme also learned early the value of exploiting the sense of competition between resorts to obtain the Committee's consent to innovations he proposed. One of the first changes he made in the Sanitary Department was to establish a weather station and to subscribe to the Meteorological Office's weather chart service.[83] Newsholme would put the station to research uses, but the Committee funded it to permit him to publicize the town's favorable climate, and it encouraged him to send a daily report by telegraph to the *Daily Mail*.[84]

While Newsholme knew the importance of appealing to local pride and interests, it would be wrong to paint him as a mere propagandist or to suggest that his use of evidence with his committee was duplicitous. He was prepared to educate even when the lesson was not always welcome. Soon after arriving in Brighton he took on the vexed question of Brighton's health relative to other towns. Sanitary reformers, Edwin Chadwick, Benjamin Ward Richardson, and recently editors of *The Lancet,* had compared the crude mortality rates of towns to gain public attention and to demonstrate how badly reform was needed. The practice brought protests from some industrial and resort towns who considered that they were being unfairly treated.[85] In a sort of primer on vital statistics, Newsholme defended the use of mortality data as a measure of health, and he demonstrated how deceptive the use of crude mortality rates could be and the importance of correcting for differences of age composition in comparative studies.[86] But he went on to show that Brighton's recorded mortality rates were actually understated. Rates corrected for the demographic peculiarities of Brighton, for the unusual age and sex distribution of its population, would actually be higher than the figures usually used to rank the nation's towns.

A successful M.O.H. also found powerful political allies. Newsholme's most important in Brighton was Joseph (after 1895, Sir Joseph) Ewart, M.D., a retired Deputy-Surgeon-General of the Indian Army, and a former President of the medical faculty of Calcutta University.[87] Even in retirement Ewart was a promi-

82 Arthur Newsholme, "Brighton as a Health Resort," *Illustrated Medical News,* 5 (5 Oct. 1889): 2–4; and Arthur Newsholme, *The Climate and Other Advantages of Brighton* (Brighton: Brighton Publicity Association, [c. 1906]).
83 Brighton, Proc. San. Comm. 6 (30 Aug. 1888): 141–4.
84 Ibid., 13 (11 June 1896): 434–8; and ibid. 14 (9 July 1896): 11. The same proceedings are printed in Brighton, *Proc. Town Council, Proc. Comm.* (18 June 1896): 24–5, and ibid. (16 July 1896): 22.
85 For background on this debate, see John M. Eyler, "Mortality Statistics and Victorian Health Policy: Program and Criticism," *Bull. Hist. Med.,* 50 (1976): 335–55.
86 Arthur Newsholme, "On Some Fallacies of Vital Statistics, especially as applicable to Brighton," Brighton, Proc. Town Council, 6 (15 Nov. 1888): 205–17, or Brighton, *Proc. Town Council, Proc. Comm.* (22 Nov. 1888): 15–19.
87 For biographical sketches of Ewart, see *Sussex Daily News* (10 Nov. 1891): 5; and *Brighton Gazette* (7 July 1893): 8. See also D. D. Friend's and Company's *Brighton Almanack* (1894), 20, 84, 95.

nent member of the profession, both as a consultant and in medical societies.[88] He had strong interest in epidemiology and public health. He was a founder of the Sussex and Brighton Sanitary Association, a President of the Epidemiology Society of London and, on at least one occasion, the co-chairman of a section at the annual meeting of the Sanitary Institute.[89] While in India he had published on vital statistics and public health.[90] His two inaugural addresses to the Epidemiological Society show that in the early 1890s he had an amateur's enthusiasm for recent discoveries in bacteriology, a detailed knowledge of current health legislation, and a sympathy for Medical Officers of Health who worked under what he regarded as unreasonable legal and financial constraints.[91] Ewart was chairman of the Sanitary Committee when Newsholme was selected M.O.H. It was he who had nominated Newsholme for the post. So strong was Ewart's advocacy of his candidate that it provoked objections from his peers in the Council.[92] Ewart would soon rise from Councillor to Alderman and would serve as Mayor from 1891 to 1894. He remained on the Brighton Sanitary Committee until 1900. While the full discussions of the Committee were not recorded, ample evidence remains in the manuscript proceedings of the Sanitary Committee and in the published proceedings of the Town Council to prove that Ewart was an invaluable ally to Newsholme, especially in the first four or five years of Newsholme's tenure.

When Newsholme arrived in Brighton, authority for local public health initiative rested on several statutes, the most important by far the Public Health Act of 1875, a comprehensive codification of previous legislation.[93] It should be seen as one of Parliament's attempts to carry out the recommendations of the Royal Sanitary Commission (1868–71) for the consolidation of legislation and authority in sanitary work. Among the other results of the Commission's recommendations were the Public Health Act, 1872, which we have considered already, and the establishment of the Local Government Board itself.[94] Together these enactments set the stage for a more rapid development of public health services in the last quarter of the century.

The Public Health Act, 1875, placed a statutory obligation on local authorities to perform certain functions: to enforce emergency orders issued by the L.G.B. to deal with major epidemics (sect. 134–9), to maintain minimum standards of

88 He was a consultant to the Royal Alexandria Hospital for Sick Children, a founder of the Throat and Ear Hospital, a member of the Council of the South Eastern Branch of the British Medical Association, and in 1894 President of the Brighton and Sussex Medico-Chirurgical Society.

89 *Public Health* 12 (1899–1900): 23–4.

90 Joseph Ewart, *A Digest of the Vital Statistics of the European and Native Armies in India; Interspersed with Suggestions for the Eradication and Mitigation of the Preventable and Avoidable Causes of Sickness and Mortality amongst Imported and Indigenous Troops* (London, 1859); and Joseph Ewart, *The Sanitary Condition and Discipline of Indian Jails* (London, 1860).

91 Joseph Ewart, "A Brief Review of Recent Sanitary Legislation," *Trans. Epidem. Soc. Lond.* 10 (1890–1): 1–21; and Joseph Ewart, "Inaugural Address of Session 1891–2," ibid. n.s. 11 (1891–2): 1–26.

92 *Sussex Daily News* (18 May 1888): 3.   93 38 & 39 Vict. C. 55.

94 Jeanne L. Brand, *Doctors and the State: The British Medical Profession and Government Action in Public Health, 1870–1912* (Baltimore: Johns Hopkins Univ. Press, 1965), 8–21.

sanitation (sect. 13–15, 23–5, 35–7, 46–7, 64, 91–102), to take rudimentary precautions to protect the public from exposure to infected persons and objects (sect. 120, 126–9), and to assume very limited responsibility for the condition of working-class housing (sect. 71–8, 80, 82). Stated this way, these statutory obligations sound more sweeping than they were, for effects of the Act were weakened by the considerable latitude local officials had in interpreting the act and in the generous protection the Act gave to private property (sect. 91, 94–6, 99). For public health activists much more significant were the Act's permissive powers, those powers a local Sanitary Authority might, but was not required to, employ. A Sanitary Authority might, subject to certain conditions, undertake major capital investment in infrastructure: build sewers, establish a public water supply, or construct an isolation hospital (sect. 27–32, 51–60, 131–3). In the name of better health it could provide public services: street cleaning, rubbish collection, ambulance service, disinfection services, and on a temporary basis free medical care and drugs to the poor (sect. 42, 121–4, 133). And it could intervene in the marketplace by inspecting, seizing, and condemning meat unfit for human consumption, by requiring factories and workshops in sewered towns to provide toilets for their workers, and by regulating divided and sublet houses (sect. 116–19, 38–9, 90).

Local authorities might obtain additional powers through private legislation, although this was a difficult, costly, and unpredictable process.[95] Brighton obtained such additional powers on several occasions and during Newsholme's tenure considered doing so again. The Brighton Improvement Act, 1884[96] was the most significant piece of private legislation in this regard. In addition to authorizing capital improvements to markets, streets, and sea front this Act restated more explicitly and specifically a number of powers contained in the Public Health Act, 1875. It also authorized the borough to ban houses of prostitution and advertisements for cures of venereal diseases. Most significant for Newsholme's career is the wider latitude this private legislation gave Brighton's M.O.H. in the supervision of the trade in milk, meat, and other food stuffs (sect. 55, 119–23). We will consider the use Newsholme made of these important provisions and his attempts to gain their extension in Chapters 3 and 5.

In the last quarter of the nineteenth century the local Sanitary Authority thus had enormous latitude in its activities. It might, provided it obtain L.G.B. approval for some actions, act on a wide front and offer both environmental and personal services and supervision. However, an authority that was not committed to active intervention might get by through doing little more than appointing a part-time M.O.H. and a part-time Inspector of Nuisances, performing perfunctory sanitary inspection, and receiving and forwarding to the L.G.B. an annual report from its M.O.H. Important general legislation was passed early in Newsholme's tenure in

95 Local authorities nevertheless made much use of private legislation in public health work. For a discussion see Christine Bellamy, *Administering Central–Local Relations, 1871–1919: The Local Government Board and Its Fiscal and Cultural Context* (Manchester: Manchester Univ. Press, 1988), 196–8.
96 47 & 48 Vict. C. 262.

Brighton that broadened the powers of local sanitary authorities. But that legislation was usually either permissive – that is, it came into effect in an area only when the local authority formally adopted the act, as in the case of Infectious Disease (Notification) Act, 1889,[97] and the Infectious Disease (Prevention) Act, 1890,[98] or its provisions depended on initiation by the sanitary authority and its M.O.H., as in the case of the Housing of the Working Classes Act, 1890.[99] We will consider the terms of these acts in later chapters.

The actions of the local sanitary authority were subject to the scrutiny of the L.G.B. In addition to the power to issue emergency orders in serious epidemics, the L.G.B. was empowered to send inspectors to meetings of any sanitary authority, to collect information on the local authority's activities, and to hold a local inquiry and to issue provisional orders in cases where there were complaints that the local sanitary authority had neglected its duty or where the sanitary authority's actions were contested or challenged.[100] But the greatest leverage the L.G.B. had with local authorities came from its oversight of the local authority's use of tax money, funds from the national treasury. To encourage the appointment of M.O.H., Parliament made funds available to pay part of the salaries of these officers. But in accepting such money the local authority subjected itself to greater scrutiny by the L.G.B. in the appointment, salary, and dismissal of the M.O.H.[101] Like many local authorities, Brighton Corporation sought to retain full control of its M.O.H., refusing this offer of Imperial funds and paying his full salary out of the local rates.[102] But local authorities could not so easily escape one other source of L.G.B. influence. This was the power of the L.G.B. to approve or sanction applications for loans local authorities made for public works.[103] The L.G.B. became the gatekeeper for the low-cost, long-term, government loans made by the Public Works Loans Commissioners, loans that were essential for building the modern public municipal infrastructure and which financed the great expansion of public health work in the late nineteenth century. Between 1871 and 1891 the Public Works Loan Commissioners, with L.G.B. sanction, loaned £50 million to local authorities, £2.5 million for housing projects and the rest for sanitary improvements.[104] By 1908 that cumulative sum exceeded £184 million.[105] Brighton's experience with the construction of an isolation hospital and its experience with slum clearance projects show how great an influence the L.G.B. could exercise in local public health work through the imposition of conditions for its

97 52 & 53 Vict. C. 72.   98 53 & 54 Vict. C. 34.
99 53 & 54 Vict. C. 70.
100 35 & 36 Vict. C. 79, sect. 15; and 38 & 39 Vict. C. 55, sect. 33–4, 293–7, 299.
101 "General Order (Urban Sanitary Authorities). – Regulations as to Medical Officers of Health, Whose Salaries Are Partly Repaid out of Moneys voted by Parliament," *Ann. Rep. L.G.B.*, 10 (1880–81): 13–19.
102 "Report of the Sanitary Committee," Brighton, Proc. Comm., Report Book, 6 (22 March 1888): 179.
103 38 & 39 Vict. C. 55. sect. 233–44.   104 Wohl, *Endangered Lives*, 114.
105 *Ann. Rep. L.G.B.* 38 (1908–9), II: xxxv.

sanction to borrow money. But in spite of all we have said about the power of the L.G.B., the initiative for public health work remained at the local level. Law and custom gave the L.G.B. some influence over the way the local sanitary authority undertook its public health work once it had decided to act. But beyond a power to enforce a bare minimum of activity, the L.G.B. could do little to force a reluctant local authority into action.

Brighton Corporation was not among the local authorities which appointed a M.O.H. before 1872, in those years when such appointments were permitted but not required. Its first M.O.H., R.P.B. Taaffe, was not appointed until 1874.[106] Taaffe seems to have been an able officer. He saw that routine sanitary inspections were undertaken; he enforced local sanitary regulations, and he foresaw the need for many of the major expansions in Sanitary Department activity that would only occur under Newsholme's administration: the compulsory notification of infectious diseases; the building of a public abattoir; the construction of a modern isolation hospital; the demolition of slums and the rebuilding under local authority supervision of working-class housing.[107] But Taaffe worked at a disadvantage. His time was divided; he continued to practice medicine, working for the local authority only part-time. Furthermore, his sanitary authority had not yet been convinced that major expansions of public health activity were necessary. Newsholme's undivided attention, his energy and ability, and growing support in the Town Council for sanitary intervention would substantially alter the tempo and scope of local authority health activity in Brighton.

For assistance Newsholme inherited a staff of ten Inspectors of Nuisances.[108] This was a large staff for a town of 115,000 people. A number of Metropolitan sanitary authorities at about this time had only one Inspector of Nuisances for between 50,000 and 100,000 people, and even at the end of the century, after a considerable growth in the staff of the Metropolitan sanitary authorities, there was still only one Inspector of Nuisances for every 20,000 people for the whole of London.[109] Brighton's size and prosperity made closer sanitary supervision possible. Within the Sanitary Department the M.O.H. was the only medically qualified employee. The Inspectors were, as a rule, former artisans, and Newsholme believed they stood in the same relation to the M.O.H. as a trained nurse stood to a physician.[110] Under his prodding the Sanitary Committee encouraged the Inspectors to obtain special training, offering to pay tuition for evening classes in building

106 Taaffe was chosen from a field of four local doctors and appointed at a salary of £200. "Report of the Sanitary Committee," Brighton, Proc. Comm., Report Book, 3 (11 Dec. 1873): 262–3, 266; ibid. (1 Jan. 1874): 270; and ibid., 6 (22 March 1888): 180.
107 For Taaffe's frustrated reform efforts, see R.P.B. Taaffe, *Quarterly Report*, 1874, no. 3: 3; R.P.B. Taaffe, *Annual Report*, 2 (1875): 4; ibid. 6 (1879): 4; and Beatrice Webb's notes on the Brighton Town Council meetings of 5 Jan. 1876 and 19 April 1888 in Webb, Local Government Collection, London School of Economics, vol. 241.
108 *Page's Brighton Directory, 1888*, 846.   109 Wohl, *Endangered Lives*, 195.
110 Arthur Newsholme, "The Duties and Difficulties of Sanitary Inspectors," *The Sanitary Record*, n.s. 10 (1888–9): 411.

construction and hygiene at the local polytechnical school, and offering financial rewards to those who earned certificates in these classes or the more prestigious Certificate of the Sanitary Institute.[111] The Sanitary Department also modified its pay scale to favor longevity of service, hoping to retain those with special training and experience.[112] Judging from the employment record of the male Inspectors of Nuisances, the strategy was effective. During Newsholme's tenure in Brighton, twenty men were at one time or another employed as Inspectors. Four of these resigned during Newsholme's first two years. Four others Newsholme hired worked for the Department fewer than two years. But after the first couple of years, Newsholme's staff was remarkably stable. In fact, for the last twelve years he was M.O.H. there was only one resignation among these employees. When Newsholme left Brighton for Whitehall in 1908 the ten Inspectors then working for the Sanitary Department averaged over fifteen years of service each, and the four senior Inspectors had been employed by the Sanitary Department on average more than nineteen years each.[113] Such longevity speaks well for Newsholme's qualities as an administrator.

Thus for most of his career in Brighton, Newsholme had a staff that was well trained and experienced. He promoted from within the Department, rewarding dedicated service and special training. As opportunities permitted and the work of the Sanitary Department became more varied, he sought to make specialized appointments to senior employees. By 1895 one Inspector was assigned to meat inspection and was Superintendent of the town's new abattoir; another was designated Inspector under the Factory and Workshops Act and Shop Hours Act, and another had special responsibility for cases of infectious disease. They thus had interesting work, a sense of specialized authority, and a reasonably good salary – after 1897, £156 per year.

However, the few women who worked for the Department in these years as Inspectors of Nuisances did not have the same satisfying experience. Newsholme first recommended hiring a woman to fill a vacant Inspector's post in September 1892.[114] He argued that such an appointee would be a special aid in helping to reduce infant mortality. She would visit homes of the poor where births had been registered to teach hygiene and infant feeding, carrying on work already begun in Britain by voluntary agencies. She might also do home visiting to oversee the care of children suffering from measles. A woman, Newsholme argued, would also be better than a man at obtaining food samples in the market for testing under the

111 Brighton, Proc. San. Comm. 6 (25 Sept. 1889): 52–3; and ibid. 14 (23 June 1897): 439–44, or Brighton, *Proc. Town Council, Proc. Comm.*, 1 July 1897: 19–22.

112 See, for example, Brighton, Proc. San. Comm. 7 (9 Oct. 1890): 466–7; and ibid. 14 (23 June 1897): 439–44. The same information was published in Brighton, *Proc. Town Council, Proc. Comm.*, 16 Oct. 1890: 15–16; and ibid. 1 July 1897: 19–21. See also *Sussex Daily News*, 2 July 1897, 2.

113 This information has been compiled from the list of Sanitary Department employees in Newsholme, *Ann. Rep.* (Brighton) in each year beginning in 1889.

114 Brighton, Proc. San. Comm., 9 (1 Sept. 1892): 322–3 or Brighton, *Proc. Town Council, Proc. Comm.*, 15 Sept. 1892: 14–15; Newsholme, *Fifty Years*, 335–7.

Food and Drug Acts. As he frequently did in such situations, he pointed to what other towns were doing. Both Glasgow and Manchester had recently hired female Inspectors. While the Sanitary Committee endorsed the idea, there was opposition in the Town Council and delay while support for the idea was raised in the community.[115] An appointment was not made until February 1893, when Alice Ramsden, an experienced, thirty-five-year-old nurse was hired.[116] Prior to joining the Sanitary Department staff she had been at St. Bartholomew's Hospital in London, at the Sussex County Hospital, and the Brighton Workhouse, and had worked as a district nurse for a voluntary society. She thus seems to have been an ideal candidate. But Ramsden worked for the Department only two years, quitting in May of 1895.[117] She was succeeded by Caroline Gammage, who remained only a year and was replaced in turn by Elizabeth Beesley, who lasted only nine months.[118] Beesley's resignation is recorded as due to ill health. But the rapid attrition among these women suggests that they did not find their lot in the Sanitary Department a very happy one. The precise reasons are not recorded, but salary was undoubtedly one of them. Although male Inspectors in these years began at twenty-five shillings per week, the Sanitary Committee and Town Council sanctioned a weekly salary for Alice Ramsden of only twenty shillings (20s) plus cloak and bonnet. The *Brighton Herald* called this a "meagre and inadequate" wage and predicted that although the Department would undoubt-edly find someone to accept it, since the labor market for women was so full, a woman with the "tact, discretion, and intelligence" called for was worth more than this "pittance."[119] Gammage and Beesley worked for the same wage, £52 per year. At the time of Beesley's resignation the lowest paid male Assistant Inspector, who had worked for the Department only two years, received £72 16s, and the most highly paid Assistant Inspector with eight years' seniority received £142.

The Sanitary Committee now reconsidered its position. Due to the "difficulty of obtaining the right class of person for this wage," Newsholme recommended that no one be hired and that the position be downgraded.[120] It was combined

115 For example, the Sanitary Committee received a resolution favoring the appointment of a woman as Inspector from the Brighton Women's Liberal Association. Brighton, Proc. San. Comm. 10 (17 Dec. 1892): 62.

116 Brighton, *Proc. Town Council*, 15 Sept. 1892: iv; *Brighton Herald*, 17 Sept. 1892, 3; and *Brighton Gazette*, 18 Feb. 1893, 5. For Newsholme's continued support of the idea, see Brighton, Proc. San. Comm., 10 (29 Dec. 1892); 72–87 or Brighton, *Proc. Town Council, Proc. Comm.*, 5 Jan. 1893, 26–31. For Ramsden's qualifications, see Brighton, Proc. San. Comm., 10 (9 Feb. 1893): 144–5 or Brighton, *Proc. Town Council, Proc. Comm.*, 16 Feb 1893: 21.

117 Brighton, Proc. San. Comm. 12 (30 May 1895): 370, or Brighton, *Proc. Town Council, Proc. Comm.*, 6 June 1895, 27.

118 Brighton, Proc. San. Comm. 12 (13 June 1895): 400; ibid., 14 (9 July 1896): 20; ibid., 14 (30 July 1896): 35; and ibid. 14 (19 April 1897) 359. The same information is also available in Brighton, *Proc. Town Council, Proc. Comm.*, 20 June 1895, 21; ibid., 16 July 1896, 20; ibid., 7 Aug. 1896, 36; and ibid., 6 May 1897, 29.

119 *Brighton Herald*, 17 Sept. 1892, 2.

120 Brighton, Proc. San. Comm. 14 (23 June 1897): 439–44; or Brighton, *Proc. Town Council, Proc. Comm.*, 1 July 1897: 19–22.

with the post of Ambulance Nurse, and the incumbent was expected to give most of her time to the Sanatorium, providing occasional service to the other Inspectors. The incumbent would receive board and room in the institution, and her annual salary was reduced from £52 to £20. The money saved by reducing her salary and that of the junior clerk paid for most of the salary increase the senior male inspectors received that year. Although the committee again considered appointing a woman as Inspector in 1907, it did not make another such appointment during the years Newsholme was in Brighton.[121] It would be helpful to know more about this episode in Brighton. Unfortunately the historical record is meager.[122]

In addition to the Inspectors of Nuisances, the work of the Department was conducted by the matron, nurses, and servants of the Sanatorium, by the Department's disinfector, who was hired in 1895,[123] and by a series of Deputies to the M.O.H. and House Physicians of the Sanatorium. The last were unpaid positions, staffed for short terms by physicians working to fulfill the requirements of the Diploma in Public Health. Their appointments in Brighton begin in 1898. Thus there was considerable growth in the Sanitary Department under Newsholme, but that expansion came about through the addition of employees other than Sanitary Inspectors, mainly through the addition of lower-paid workers and from the free labor of physicians training to become M.O.H. As we consider in greater detail the work of the Sanitary Department under Newsholme's administration, it is important to retain some sense of proportion. Despite this expansion in the work of the Sanitary Department, operating expenses, leaving aside the capital expenses of the new isolation hospital, of the Sanitary Department remained relatively small. Its staff, for example, was tiny in comparison with that of the municipal police department with its five Police Stations, its 149 Constables, 12 Sergeants, and 16 other officers and inspectors of higher grades.[124]

This steady expansion and diversification in Newsholme's staff is merely one indication of the transformation of public health work in Brighton during Newsholme's tenure as M.O.H. Another is the change he made in the *Annual Reports* of the town's M.O.H. Taaffe's last reports were very simple productions. Four pages in length, they merely summarized the vital statistics of the town, compared the town's annual death rates to those of the other large British towns, and listed

121 Brighton, Proc. San. Comm. 23 (14 Feb. 1907): 327; ibid., 25 April 1907: 385; ibid., 8 May 1907: 402; and ibid. 24 (10 Oct. 1907): 91.
122 The position of women sanitary inspectors is still an unexplored historical field, but for a good beginning, see Celia Davies, "The Health Visitor as Mother's Friend: A Woman's Place in Public Health, 1900–14," *Social History of Medicine* 1 (1988): 39–59. Also useful is F. J. Greenwood, "Women as Sanitary Inspectors and Health Visitors," in *Women Workers in Seven Professions: A Survey of Their Economic Conditions and Prospects,* ed. Edith J. Morley (London: George Routledge & Sons, 1914), 221–34.
123 Brighton, Proc. San. Comm. 13 (26 Sept. 1895): 93–5; and Brighton, *Proc. Town Council,* 3 Oct. 1895: iii.
124 *D. B. Friend & Co,'s Brighton Almanack for 1893* (Brighton, 1883), 25.

the number of sanitary inspections conducted during the year. Starting from this modest scale Newsholme's reports rapidly grew in size, averaging 76 pages for each of his full years in Brighton and exceeding 120 pages in 1902 and 1904. But his reports were not only vastly longer, they differed in kind, presenting not only administrative and statistical summaries, but the results of original epidemiological investigations, careful analyses, and intelligent discussions of the leading causes of death and illness and recommendations for public intervention, and careful documentation of the adoption and effects of new public health initiatives. These reports are a valuable source for studying the history of British public health at the local level. We will consider them closely in the next six chapters, in which we trace the development of Newsholme's ideas and analyze his role in the evolution of the public health enterprise in a unusually prosperous and active local authority.

2

Fact, theory, and the epidemic milieu

THE METHODS OF EPIDEMIOLOGY AND THE WORK
OF THE M.O.H.

While still a comparatively young Medical Officer of Health, Arthur Newsholme became an authority on vital statistics and an important epidemiologist. His *The Elements of Vital Statistics,* which first appeared in 1889 shortly after he arrived in Brighton, seems to have been the first practical textbook of statistics for Medical Officers of Health.[1] It was widely used during his career and remained a standard source for many years, appearing in a new edition as late as 1923.[2] As a perusal of Newsholme's bibliography shows, his publications in vital statistics and epidemiology are both numerous and varied. He did intensive local investigations as well as sweeping international comparisons. He studied old scourges like smallpox and typhoid fever as well as diseases that had received little attention from statisticians, such as cancer. He traced epidemics, identified long-term trends in mortality, morbidity, and fertility, and he tried to identify the causes for these changes. We will consider examples of his statistical and epidemiological investigations in several of the following chapters.

I will argue that Newsholme's epidemiology and his administrative work were intimately related. The latter frequently suggested the subjects for the former and often supplied the data. The former provided the direction and credibility for the latter. It was Newsholme's view that "epidemiology is the centre and main spring

---

1 Arthur Newsholme, *The Elements of Vital Statistics* (London, 1889). Noel Humphreys, William Farr's former associate at the General Register Office was apparently preparing a text of his own which he set aside when he learned that Newsholme was about to go to press. Newsholme, *Fifty Years,* 274. Newsholme also wrote summary articles on vital statistics in medical and financial encyclopedias. See "Vital Statistics," *Encyclopaedia Medica,* 14 vols. (New York: Longmans Green & Co., 1899–1904), vol. 13: 398–413. Newsholme's papers also contain the page proofs of an article "Vital Statistics," for the *Encyclopedia of Accounting, Insurance and Finance* (1904), a publication which I have not been able to locate, Newsholme Papers, London School of Hygiene and Tropical Medicine, uncatalogued materials. Hereafter this collection will be cited simply as Newsholme Papers.
2 Arthur Newsholme, *The Elements of Vital Statistics in Their Bearing on Social and Public Health Problems,* new ed. (London: George Allen & Unwin, 1923).

of all public health work."[3] That assessment was made in 1918 in the midst of planning the postwar reorganization of the central British health authority, the planning that led to the creation of the Ministry of Health. Newsholme's plan, a road not taken, would have restructured the central authority to emphasize statistical surveillance of health and epidemiological research over routine administrative supervision. Such a scheme was in keeping with Newsholme's long-held view that public health work was a scientific as well as an administrative task. Medical Officers of Health, he wrote in 1896,

> do not desire to degenerate into mere empiricists concerned with the performance of certain ceremonies of sprinkling and washing and with the enforcement of isolation of Mosaic rigidity. That is the view that some, alas! take. If we are to maintain our standing and reputation this view must not be allowed to spread. The scientific and purely medical aspects of our work must be kept in the forefront. We are concerned not solely with individual cases of disease, but also with the conditions producing and controlling entire epidemics. It is part of our duty to study the influence of every personal and environmental condition on the evolution of each disease, in order that by so doing we may arrive at a less empirical and more rational conception of its causation.[4]

In this view the M.O.H.'s primary task was applied epidemiology: the surveillance of a population's health, the investigation of the causes of illness and premature death, and the assessment of the effectiveness of intervention. This activity not only assured the status of the M.O.H., elevating him above the Inspector of Nuisances or the Sanitary Inspector, for example, but it made public health an intellectual pursuit. The M.O.H. was not only to enforce the law and to administer the sanitary department, he was to contribute to the advancement of knowledge, especially of the natural history of disease. As we shall see, Newsholme did all of these things.

But it is also clear that Newsholme was first and foremost a practical health officer for whom statistical methods were tools. When statistical results and administrative experience or his commitment to certain reforms conflicted, he was prepared to ignore the statistics. We find this response most often when statistical trends fail to confirm the value of work he was convinced was effective. As the invited guest at the American Red Cross conference on child welfare work held in Paris in 1922 he observed that

> As regards child welfare work and how to obtain major results, it is quite axiomatic that child welfare work has been a chief means of bringing about a reduction in infant mortality. Even in the absence of corroborative statistics, it is certain that such work decreases infant mortality. To think otherwise would be to assert that ignorance is as good as knowledge;

3 Arthur Newsholme, "On the Post-bellum requirements for 'Carrying on' in the Medical Department," memorandum to the President of the Local Government Board, 17 Dec. 1918, P.R.O. MH 78/90.
4 Arthur Newsholme, "A National System of Notification of Sickness," *Br. Med. J.* (1895), no. 2: 529.

that care of infants is no better than carelessness; and that educated skill, added to maternal instinct, is no better than maternal instinct alone.[5]

It was on issues of this sort that Newsholme's differences from the new statistical authorities, the biostatisticians such as Karl Pearson and Raymond Pearl, were most marked and their disputes most heated. Those differences, which came to the fore after 1900, were both methodological and political. They will occupy our attention in later chapters. In this chapter we consider Newsholme's use of statistics during the 1890s, when his enthusiasm was uncompromised by criticism of rival authorities who employed newer mathematical methods and who challenged his faith in the power of public intervention to improve human health and welfare.

Newsholme was self-taught in statistics. As a fledgling M.O.H. in the middle 1880s he had the help of two acquaintances in launching his statistical studies: a fellow M.O.H. in the Metropolitan District of Wandsworth and an actuary who was a neighbor and a member of the Clapham vestry.[6] But his education came principally from the *Annual Reports* of the Registrar-General. His careful study of these reports became a lifelong habit. In midcareer he described himself as "a zealous and persistent student" of the Registrar-General's reports.[7] Many late Victorian Medical Officers of Health could have said the same. The General Register Office (G.R.O.), the Registrar-General's bureau, collected, arranged, and published the vital data on which public health administration depended, and its scheme for classifying the causes of death, its statistical nosology, became, de facto, the national and international standard for reporting and classifying disease and death.[8] The G.R.O.'s data and many of its statistical conventions were adopted in turn by the Medical Officer of the Local Government Board. In this way they entered public health administration directly.

Newsholme's textbook on vital statistics demonstrated how the methods developed in the G.R.O. by its Statistical Superintendent, William Farr, could be applied in local health administration. Newsholme's indebtedness to Farr is obvious in that book and in much of his statistical work. His writings are full of praise for Farr, whom he considered "the father of sanitary science."[9] His interest in

5 American Red Cross, *American Red Cross European Child Health Program 1921–1922: Medical Conference at Paris Headquarters, February 2–3, 1922* (Paris: Medical Department of the American Red Cross, 1922). Bibliotheque Nationale, Paris, VII J 1. Thanks to John Hutchinson for this quotation.

6 Newsholme, *Fifty Years*, 136–7, 149, 273–4.

7 Arthur Newsholme, "A Contribution to the Study of Epidemic Diarrhoea," *Public Health*, 12 (1899–1900): 139.

8 For the development of this nosology, see John M. Eyler, *Victorian Social Medicine: The Ideas and Methods of William Farr* (Baltimore: Johns Hopkins Univ. Press, 1979): 53–60.

9 Arthur Newsholme, *The Elements of Vital Statistics*, 3rd ed. (London, 1899), 9. Unless otherwise stated, citations to this work will be to the third edition. See also Arthur Newsholme, "A National System of Notification and Registration of Sickness," *J. Roy. Statist. Soc.* 59 (1896): 1; and Arthur Newsholme, "The Measurement of Progress in Public Health with Special Reference to the Life and Work of William Farr," *Economica* 3 (1923): 186–202.

Farr's work and the importance he attached to it may perhaps best be seen in the fact that Newsholme was an unsuccessful candidate for Farr's former post at the G.R.O. in 1893, long after he had achieved prominence in the Medical-Officer-of-Health world, and in the fact that he retained an interest in that position for another decade, until, in other words, he had succeeded to John Simon's former position at the L.G.B.[10]

The vital data which the General Register Office collected and made available came from two primary sources during Newsholme's career: the census returns of population and the civil registration of births, deaths, and marriages.[11] From its beginning in 1801 the census was taken every ten years, not nearly often enough for late-nineteenth-century epidemiologists like Newsholme who wanted a quinquennial census.[12] The early enumerations were plagued with glaring problems of inaccuracy and inconsistency, but beginning with its transference to the G.R.O. in 1841, the census was designed for greater scientific utility. Hereafter its reports offered more and better information on the size, geographical distribution, and age structure of the population and also returns for occupation, housing, and occasionally for other topics such as physical handicap.

The system of civil registration had been created in 1836.[13] The first registration acts permitted the registration of marriages and births and required the registration of all deaths in England and Wales. These vital events were registered with the local Registrar, from whom records made their way periodically via a Superintendent Registrar to the General Register Office in London. At the G.R.O. the data were analyzed by Registration Districts and Registration Counties, and the returns were published quarterly and annually. The registration system, like the early census enumerations themselves, was based upon the geographical units of the Poor Law. The local Registrar's subdistrict was usually a division of the Poor Law union. For that reason the Registration Districts and Counties, which were composites of these subdistricts, often failed to correspond with local authority boundaries, and local officials, other than the Guardians, the elected body that administered the Poor Law locally, seldom found published vital statistics for precisely their jurisdiction. This fact was a constant source of frustration to

10 Newsholme remembered the year incorrectly as 1898. Newsholme, *Last 30 Years*, 28–29.
11 History of the census and of civil registration has received much attention, and it is a subject which cannot be dealt with adequately here. For useful discussions, see D. V. Glass, *Numbering the People: The Eighteenth-Century Population Controversy and the Development of Census and Vital Statistics in Britain* (Farnborough, Hants.: D. C. Heath, 1973); M. J. Cullen, "The Making of the Civil Registration Act of 1836," *J. Ecclesiastical Hist.* 25 (1974): 39–59; Simon R. S. Szreter, "The Genesis of the Registrar-General's Social Classification of Occupations," *Br. J. Sociology*, 35 (1934), 522–46; Edward Higgs, "The Struggle for the Occupational Census, 1841–1911," in *Government and Expertise: Specialists, Administrators and Professionals, 1860–1919*, ed. Roy MacLeod (Cambridge: Cambridge Univ. Press, 1988), 73–86; Eyler, *Victorian Social Medicine*, 39–46, 52–3, 60–2; A. J. Taylor, "The Taking of the Census, 1801–1951," *Br. Med. J.* (1951), no. 1: 715–20.
12 Newsholme, *The Elements*, 8–9; Newsholme, *Ann. Rep.* (Brighton) 1889: 5; and ibid. 1891: 13.
13 "An Act for Marriages in England," 6 & 7 Wm.IV C. 85; and An Act for Registering Births, Deaths, and Marriages in England," 6 & 7 Wm.IV C. 86.

Medical Officers of Health like Newsholme, who wanted to see the data collection services consolidated with the public health service. He suggested that the census enumerators and the local registrars should be appointed by the local sanitary authority and work under the supervision of the M.O.H. and that the census and registration data should be collected and published for individual sanitary districts, boroughs, or counties.[14]

Medical interest in registration centered on the returns of the cause of death. From the very beginning this information had been required at the time of registration, but initially anyone – medical practitioner, coroner, or layman – could decide what had caused the death and report the same to the registrar, and the returns were often medically useless. Farr and the Registrar-General worked to encourage certification of cause of death by medical practitioners, and the G.R.O. began to provide practitioners with printed forms for that purpose in 1845. By 1870, 92 percent of English and Welsh deaths were medically certified, although the quality of that certification was sometimes still poor.[15]

The same years, the early 1870s, that saw a consolidation of public health legislation, and greater pressure on local authorities for action in public health also witnessed a stiffening of registration requirements and efforts to make the registration system more responsive to local administrative needs. The Births and Deaths Registration Act, 1874, required medical certification of the causes of death and made the registration of births compulsory.[16] It also made concessions to the demands of Medical Officers of Health. The act empowered local authorities to require Registrars to supply regular, usually weekly, returns from the birth and death registers and immediate notification of the death from a dangerous infectious disease.[17] Thus while the nation's vital record-keeping system had not been designed to support the type of local health administration that had evolved in England, by the time Newsholme entered the public health service some of the incompatibilities between the two systems had been ironed out.

The census and civil registration provided the raw data from which Victorians attempted to measure relative health. Edwin Chadwick and a few early sanitary activists had compared mean age at death in town and country districts of England

14 Arthur Newsholme, "On the Death Rates and Causes of Death in Enumeration Districts, with Special Reference to the Conditions of Housing," *Public Health* 4 (1891–2): 226; and Brighton, Proc. San. Comm. 8 (29 Jan. 1891) 88; ibid., 16 (26 Jan 1899): 158–9; and Newsholme, *Ann. Rep. Med. Off. L.G.B.* 38 (1908–9): v–vi.
15 William Farr, "Letter to the Registrar General on the Causes of Death in England," *Annual Report of the Registrar-General of Births, Deaths, and Marriages in England,* 33 (1870): 408. The most comprehensive Victorian discussions of the problems with the registration system and the inaccuracies in English vital statistics is Henry W. Rumsey, *Essays and Papers on Some Fallacies of Statistics Concerning Death, Health and Disease with Suggestions Towards an Improved System of Registration* (London, 1875).
16 "An Act to Amend the Law Relating to the Registration of Births and Deaths in England, and to Consolidate the Law Respecting the Registration of Births and Deaths at Sea," 37 & 38 Vict. C. 88.
17 See also Newsholme, *The Elements,* 22–3.

and among different social classes to provide shocking illustration of the waste of human life due to removable causes.[18] This was effective propaganda but poor statistics. The statistically more astute quickly discredited this approach by pointing out that such comparisons ignored the different age distributions in the populations chosen. The heavy immigration of young adults to industrial cities and high birth rates there gave those towns high concentrations of young lives. For that reason alone the towns could be expected to record much lower figures for mean age at death than did the rural areas Chadwick used for comparison. Chadwick was not justified in implying that the low average age of death in towns was due entirely to sanitary defects. But while his critics might reject his methods, they shared both Chadwick's assumption that length of life was a reflection of the healthiness of the environment in which that life was spent and his desire to show numerically how much an unhealthy environment shortened human life. The statisticians insisted, however, that life expectancy, not mean age at death, was the proper vital index, and they argued that the expectancy of life could only be computed accurately from a life table.

Life tables had made their appearance in the eighteenth century in efforts to rationalize the highly speculative insurance and annuity business. They were applied to public health problems in the 1830s and 1840s, and in the hands of statisticians like William Farr, they became the most powerful demographic and epidemiological tools available. From the national registration and census data Farr constructed three national life tables, a table for the Healthy Districts of England, those districts having crude mortality rates below 17 per 1,000, and a number of other life tables for more select geographical areas or for occupational groups.[19] He called the life table a "biometer," explaining that it measured the vitality of a population just as a barometer measured atmospheric pressure or a thermometer measured temperature.[20] Farr used these life tables to trace the improving health of the nation over the decades and to compare the longevity and health of different places and social groups. His example helped make the life table the most trusted measure of health and vitality. Newsholme was merely expressing the consensus of his generation when he wrote that a life table is "the only absolutely trustworthy means" of comparing the health of two communities or monitoring the health of one population over time.[21]

But the construction of a life table in the nineteenth century was a laborious

---

18 For a discussion of this topic, see Eyler, "Mortality Statistics," 339–46.
19 Eyler, *Victorian Social Medicine,* 72–83, 141. For the context of these early hygienic applications of life tables, see also John M. Eyler, "The Conceptual Origins of William Farr's Epidemiology: Numerical Methods and Social Thought in the 1830s," in *Times, Places, and Persons: Aspects of the History of Epidemiology,* ed. Abraham M. Lilienfeld (Baltimore: Johns Hopkins Univ. Press, 1980), 1–21.
20 *Annual Report of the Registrar-General of Births, Deaths, and Marriages in England,* 5 (1841), xxiii–xxiv. This section appears over the Registrar-General's signature, but it was certainly written by Farr.
21 Arthur Newsholme and T.H.C. Stevenson, *The Second Brighton Life Table* (Brighton: Brighton Corporation, 1903), 3.

exercise in logarithmic computation. It was a task beyond the patience and the competency of most administrators and public officials. Faced with the job of computing one, even those who could do the construction sought substitutes most of the time. Mortality or death rates (the ratio of deaths to years of life at risk) computed directly from the census and registration figures were taken as second-best indices of physical well-being. The most commonly used rate was the general or crude death rate. This was the rate for deaths from all causes among the entire population, recorded conventionally as an annual rate per 1,000 people. Crude mortality rates dominated the reports of the Registrar-General and of the central and local health authorities. The Registrar-General published quarterly a table ranking the largest towns in the kingdom by prevailing annual crude mortality rates, and soon newspapers were republishing this list just as they published weather and stock market reports. Although local officials from industrial cities and resort towns, places that usually did poorly in this ranking, sometimes protested, crude death rates entered popular usage as the measure of public health.[22]

As mid-Victorian statisticians and epidemiologists realized, the protesting local officials had grounds for complaint. Comparisons of these crude rates could be misleading. Such rates might be fairly used to monitor the risk of death in one population over a short time period, but they were not a valid way of comparing the health of two different populations or even of monitoring the experience of one population over a long period of time. Victorians recognized two fundamental problems. First, not all deaths that occurred in some districts should be credited to those districts. When they raised this objection, they most frequently followed it with the example of deaths that occurred in large institutions such as hospitals and work houses to which sick or invalids were brought from outside district boundaries. But an even more important objection sprang from the realizations that different populations might have very different age structures and that the risk of dying varied greatly with age and to a lesser extent with gender. To overcome these objections, mid-Victorian epidemiologists, William Farr most notably, devised schemes to transfer deaths occurring in institutions to the deceased's place of residence before comparing local mortality rates. To deal with differences in the age and sex profiles of the populations being studied, Farr taught public health workers the importance of using standardized mortality rates.[23] As standard populations, he preferred the nation as a whole or the Healthy Districts.

But like life tables, standardized mortality rates were troublesome to compute and not well understood. They were not in common use in the public health literature of Victorian Britain. Farr used them frequently only after 1860 and then only in his more careful studies. The alternative for those who wanted to avoid

22 Eyler, "Mortality Statistics," 348–50; Simon Szreter, "The GRO and the Public Health Movement in Britain, 1837–1914," *Social Hist. Med*, 4 (1991): 436–40.
23 Eyler, *Victorian Social Medicine*, 83.

some of the pitfalls of the crude mortality rates but were unable to construct life tables or to standardize their rates was to use more specialized mortality rates. These rates were either for deaths at particular ages – as we shall see, infant mortality became an important such index – or they were for deaths from specific causes. William Farr popularized the zymotic disease mortality rate. The zymotic diseases were the first division of his statistical nosology and comprised the epidemic, endemic, and contagious diseases. As Farr understood them, these diseases thrived in conditions of filth, crowding, and human misery. For that reason they provided a convenient way of identifying places where sanitary conditions were defective. The zymotic mortality rate remained in common use for the rest of the century. Even more specialized disease mortality rates were used as well. In his influential study of the health in select registration districts published in 1857 for the Privy Council, Edward Headlam Greenhow stressed the value of mortality from pulmonary disease and from "alvine flux" (diarrhea, dysentery, and cholera) as sanitary indices.[24] Mortality from diarrheal diseases became in fact another important sanitary index in the second half of the century. Finally the study of epidemics and investigations of disease transmission encouraged the use of mortality rates for individual diseases. Victorian authors using these more selective rates sometimes recognized that such rates might need correction for peculiarities in the composition of the population. Most often, however, such refinements were lacking, and cause-specific mortality rates were taken at face value.

The use of all these mortality rates and of life tables as indices of health and well-being assumed that length of life reflected quality of life. Mid-Victorian statisticians and epidemiologists recognized, however, that a long life might not be a healthy one, and that without knowledge of the sickness prevailing in a community one could not speak with certainty about its health. It was often assumed that there was a fairly constant ratio between cases of illness and deaths from those illnesses, between morbidity and mortality. But this convenient assumption did not bear rigorous scrutiny, and as early as the 1840s there were demands from medical spokesmen and public health advocates for the registration of sickness.[25] The Metropolitan Association of Health Officers, the Epidemiological Society of London, the Manchester and Salford Sanitary Association, the Social Science Association, and, after 1867, the British Medical Association favored the registration of sickness. But even its most enthusiastic advocates recognized that such registration would incite popular and professional resistance. To ease the way, registration advocates suggested beginning with the registration of illness in people who were powerless to object, those treated in poor law practice and in hospitals.

24 Edward Headlam Greenhow, "The Results of an Inquiry into the Different Proportions of Death Produced by Certain Diseases in Different Districts in England," *Papers Relating to the Sanitary State of the People of England*, B.P.P. 1857–8, XXIII, 1–164.
25 For a short history of the movement for sickness registration see Newsholme, "A National System," *J. Roy. Statist. Soc.*, 3–9. See also Eyler, *Victorian Social Medicine*, 63.

Local experiments on such lines were tried and usually failed. But beginning in 1877 a number of private acts were passed requiring the notification of a select number of infectious diseases among the entire population of a particular town. The successful working of these local acts encouraged the passage of important permissive legislation. The Infectious Disease (Notification) Act, 1889, required the Metropolitan local authorities and permitted provincial local authorities adopting the Act to demand the prompt notification to the M.O.H. of all cases of smallpox, Asiatic cholera, diphtheria, "membranous croup," erysipelas, or any of a list of fevers: typhoid, typhus, enteric, relapsing, continued, puerperal, and scarlet.[26] The local authority was to pay the notifying physician 2 shillings 6 pence (2s 6d) for each notified case from his private practice and 1 shilling (1s) for cases notified in a poor law or other public practice. Subject to L.G.B. approval, a local authority could also add other diseases to the list. Unlike the registration of deaths and their causes, registration of sickness was confidential. Beginning in 1889 the L.G.B. began a voluntary system of pooling this information.[27] Local authorities which agreed to send a table of their registered cases would receive a printed confidential return of the cases of all participating towns. In the 1890s most towns adopted the Act, and in 1899 its terms were extended to the entire nation.[28] It was thus not until the 1890s that local authorities obtained accurate information about some of the nonfatal illness appearing in their jurisdictions. This information made possible epidemiological studies of a sort that had previously been very difficult to undertake.

As a local administrator Newsholme made use of all the conventional statistical indices and comparisons. His annual reports from Brighton normally give crude mortality rates for the borough and for each of its wards. They compare the rate from one ward to another, and compare the town's current rate to its rates for past years and to the rates for the other large towns of the kingdom. He also used for such comparative purposes Farr's zymotic disease mortality rate, and, as he grew suspicious that that rate was too inclusive and indiscriminate, he began to use with increasing frequency infant mortality rates and mortality from typhoid or enteric fever.[29] When mortality from all causes changed suddenly, he drew attention to the fact and looked to more specialized mortality rates for part of the explanation.[30] In

26 "An Act to provide for the Notification of Infectious Disease to Local Authorities," 52 & 53 Vict. C. 72.
27 The Local Government Board took over a scheme of pooling morbidity data begun in Salford the year before. Newsholme, "Registration and Notification," *J. Roy. Statist. Soc.,* 13.
28 "An Act to extend the Infectious Disease (Notification) Act, 1889, to Districts in which it has not been adopted," 62 & 63 Vict. C. 8.
29 He would eventually hold that typhoid mortality was the best measure of sanitary progress and that infant mortality was the best index of combined sanitary and social condition; Newsholme, *Ann. Rep. Med. Off. L.G.B.* 47 (1917–18): vii. He expressed suspicion of the use of the zymotic rate much earlier, since the zymotic diseases had nothing in common except contagion, Newsholme, *Ann. Rep.* (Brighton), 1889, 13. In listing this rate in his annual reports, he substituted the term "infectious" in 1898, and by 1901 this rate had disappeared from his annual reports.
30 See for example his discussion of the high quarterly rate in Newsholme, *Q. Rep.* (Brighton), 1890, no. 4: 1–3.

this he was doing what was expected of an M.O.H. What distinguished News-holme's statistical writings in the years he was in Brighton were his resourceful employment of the data from sickness notification, his use of life table techniques in local health assessment, and his preference for standardized rather than crude rates. We consider each in turn.

The Infectious Disease (Notification) Act, 1889, received Royal signature soon after Newsholme came to Brighton. Almost at once he recommended its adoption by the Corporation, but it took some months to overcome opposition from keepers of lodging houses and from members of the local medical profession, so the Act was not adopted until January 1891, with notification beginning the following March.[31] Newsholme had already initiated a system of household sur-veillance. The year before notification of disease began he had started a log of Brighton streets and houses, noting for each house the name, age, sex, and cause of death for each deceased resident.[32] After the registration of infectious diseases became compulsory, the Sanitary Department began to visit the home of every notified case, to conduct a sanitary inspection, and to gather information on the case and on other family members.[33] It initially ascertained the number, age, and gender of those living in the house and inquired whether other family members had previously suffered from the reported disease. As his understanding of the causes and transmission of disease evolved, Newsholme added other questions such as the source of the family's milk supply. The scale of this work grew very rapidly. The Department conducted 1,560 household visits following an illness the year notification came into force. The next year, 1892, that number had grown to 5,757.[34] Such visitation was an aid to administration. It turned up unreported cases. It identified disease contacts. As we will see in subsequent chapters, it also permitted Newsholme to undertake some of his most interesting epidemiological studies. As he would explain much later, the notification of a case was a pointer for future research, the starting point for epidemiological investigation.[35]

Newsholme soon began campaigning for an extension of sickness notification. In a series of papers to medical and statistical colleagues in the middle 1890s and

31 Brighton, *Proc. Town Council* (15 Jan. 1891), ii; and *Sussex Daily News* (16 Jan. 1891): 3. For the Town Council's previous rejection of the proposal and the campaign to secure its adoption see Brighton, Proc. San. Comm. 7 (26 Sept. 1889): 42–50; ibid. (21 Nov. 1889): 111–12; ibid. (13 Feb. 1890): 210–11; ibid. 8 (11 Dec. 1890): 42–6; Brighton, *Proc. Town Council* (5 Dec. 1889): ii; and *Sussex Daily News* (6 Dec. 1889), 3. Newsholme, *Ann. Rep.* (Brighton), 1889, 18.

32 Arthur Newsholme, "Special Report on the Mortality and Causes of Mortality in Eight Districts in Brighton," Brighton, Proc. San. Comm. 9 (28 April 1892): 158, or ibid. Brighton, *Proc. Town Council, Proc. Comm.* (5 May 1892): 19. This report was republished as "On the Death Rates and Causes of Death in Enumeration Districts, with Special Reference to the Conditions of Housing," *Public Health* 4 (1891–2): 226

33 Arthur Newsholme, "The Epidemiology of Scarlet Fever in Relation to the Utility of Isolation Hospitals," *Trans. Epidemiology Soc. Lond.* n.s. 20 (1900–1): 64.

34 Newsholme, *Ann. Rep.* (Brighton), 1892, 14.

35 Arthur Newsholme, "Disease Records as an Indispensable Means of Disease Prevention," *Proc. International Conference on Health Problems in Tropical America* (Boston: United Fruit Co., 1924): 943.

in occasional remarks in the next two decades, he argued for the immediate extension of registration to all illness attended in Poor Law and charity practice, for a further extension of the reporting of accidents and illnesses in industry, and for a significant increase in the number of infectious illnesses in the general population notifiable to the M.O.H.[36] Even some of his most sympathetic listeners regarded these proposals as hasty and politically impossible, so sensitive were the issues of personal privacy and added burdens on the rates.[37] In view of his interest in notification and his persistent advocacy of its extension, it is somewhat surprising to find Newsholme opposing the L.G.B.'s scheme to circulate privately weekly notification data among participating sanitary authorities. At his suggestion Brighton did not participate in the voluntary scheme until 1899. Newsholme's stated reason for recommending nonparticipation was a fear that the information shared in this fashion would not remain confidential.[38]

Newsholme was among a handful of Medical Officers of Health to construct life tables for their jurisdictions in the 1890s. His first Brighton Life Table was based upon the censuses of 1881 and 1891 and the deaths registered in the intervening decade.[39] He constructed a second table a decade later on the same principles employing another census and decade of death registration.[40] Such local life tables were not simply records of observed events. They were abstract constructs tracing through life a hypothetical group of 100,000 infants born simultaneously, assuming that these infants would spend their entire lives in their place of

---

36 Arthur Newsholme, "A National System of Notification of Sickness," *Br. Med. J.* (1895), no. 2: 529–31; Arthur Newsholme, "A National System of Notification of Sickness," *Public Health* 8 (1895–6): 106–8; and Arthur Newsholme, "A National System of Notification and Registration of Sickness," *J. Roy. Statist. Soc.* 59 (1896): 1–28. Abstracts of the latter were published under the same title in *Lancet* (1895), no. 2: 1560–4; and *Medical Press,* n.s. 60 (1895), 658–61. In 1902 he repeated the substance of these demands adding to them, as a result of his experience with scarlet fever and diphtheria, the call for the registration of suspect cases, Arthur Newsholme "Vital Statistics and Their Relation to Sanitary Reform," *Proceedings of a Conference on Sanitary Progress and Reform* (Manchester: Manchester and Salford Sanitary Association, 1902), 61–74. The text of this paper was reprinted under the same title in *Lancet* (1902), no, 1: 1755–8; and in *Medical Magazine,* n.s. 11 (1902): 360–72. For a late reiteration of these views, see Arthur Newsholme, "Memorandum by Dr. Newsholme, Medical Officer to the Local Government Board," Royal Commission on Venereal Diseases, *Final Report,* B.P.P. 1916, [Cd. 8189], XVI, 101–2; Arthur Newsholme, testimony, Royal Commission on Venereal Diseases, *Appendix to Final Report,* B.P.P. 1916, [Cd. 8190], XVI, 219.
37 See, for example, the comments of Lord Thring at the meeting of the Royal Statistical Society when Newsholme's paper was discussed, *J. Roy. Statist. Soc.* 59 (1896): 32. The year before the editor of the *British Medical Journal* thought Newsholme's proposals were laudable but premature. Registration would have to be extended piecemeal, "A National System of Registration of Sickness," *Br. Med. J.* (1895), no. 2: 1631.
38 Brighton, Proc. San. Comm. 8 (26 Feb. 1891): 129–30. For later accommodation to the scheme see ibid. 13 (27 Feb. 1896): 298–9; and ibid. 16 (10 Aug. 1899): 387–8. In 1901 the Committee agreed readily to send quarterly returns to the G.R.O. for inclusion in the Registrar-General's *Quarterly Reports,* ibid. 18 (28 March 1901): 184–5.
39 Arthur Newsholme, *The Brighton Life Table* (Brighton, 1893).
40 Arthur Newsholme and T.H.C. Stevenson, *The Second Brighton Life Table* (Brighton: Brighton Corporation, 1903).

birth and during that time be subject to the risks of death at each age of life which the real population of the place had experienced during one decade. Newsholme explained to fellow Medical Officers of Health how a local life table could be constructed from the census and registration returns.[41] The task involved dealing with the peculiarities of the nation's vital statistics we have already noticed – the incompatibility of municipal and registration boundaries and local disturbances caused by immigration and the presence of large institutions – as well as a further difficulty posed by the fact that census returns were made only for age groups not for individual years of life. To make the process accessible to Medical Officers of Health few of whom knew calculus, Newsholme championed the use of a graphical method of interpolating the numbers living or dying at each year of life. See Illustration 2.1. Such a graphical approach was sometimes used by actuaries and had been used by Joshua Milne in his construction of the famous Carlisle Table (1815). Newsholme argued that his graphical method put the construction of a life table for his jurisdiction within the reach of every M.O.H., and he attempted to demonstrate that the results obtained by this method were as accurate as those obtained from the same data by more analytical means.[42] The Brighton Life Tables permitted Newsholme to measure accurately the mortality and life expectancy of the people of his town and to draw valid comparisons with the experience of other populations for which a recent life table existed.[43]

We conclude this section by considering Newsholme's use of standarized rates. Newsholme championed the use of these rates when he recognized that differences in the age structure of populations to be compared would make the use of crude rates fallacious. One such occasion was the paper he wrote with the actuary George King on the much discussed question whether the increase in cancer mortality recorded in the Registrar-General's Reports was due to a real increase in the incidence of cancer or merely to improving diagnosis and registration.[44] Newsholme and King insisted that since cancer was much more common in older people, it could be very deceiving merely to compare the crude rates of mortality from cancer. These authors calculated instead standardized cancer death rates for time periods since 1860 for England and Wales, Scotland, Ireland, and for the policyholders of the Scottish Widow's Fund Life Office, a commercial life insurance company, which had for a long time kept particularly good records of the causes of death of its members. To standardize these rates they applied the age-

41 In addition to the two tables themselves see Arthur Newsholme and T.H.C. Stevenson, "The Graphic Method of Constructing a Life Table Illustrated by the Brighton Life Table, 1891–1900," *J. Hygiene* 3 (1903): 297–324; and Newsholme, *The Elements*, 255–89.

42 Newsholme and Stevenson, "Graphic Method," 314–24.

43 See, for example, his comparison of rates from the Brighton, Glasgow, and Manchester tables, the only life tables then existing for the experience of British towns in the period 1881–90. Newsholme, *Q. Rep.* (Brighton), 1894, no. 3: 15.

44 George King and Arthur Newsholme, "On the Alleged Increase of Cancer," *Proc. Roy. Soc. Lond.* 54 (1893–4): 209–42. See also Arthur Newsholme, "The Statistics of Cancer," *Practitioner,* 62 (1899): 371–84.

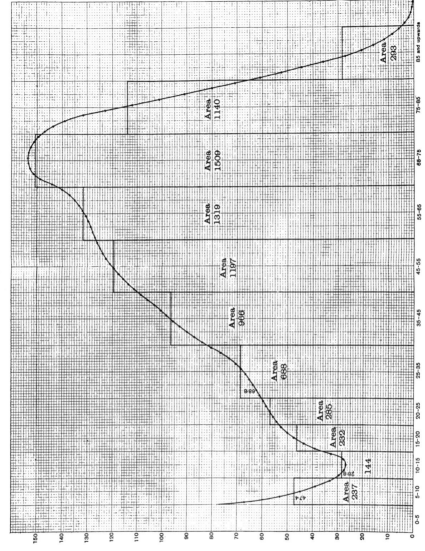

Illustration 2.1. Life Table Calculations without Calculus. From Newsholme, "The Graphic Method of Constructing a Life Table...," *Journal of Hygiene*, 3 (1903): between pp. 302 and 303.

specific cancer mortality rates for these populations to a population of a million distributed by age according to Farr's last national life table. The comparison of these standardized rates sometimes gave a very different impression from the comparison of crude rates. Newsholme and King showed that when crude cancer death rates were used, Ireland recorded a rate consistently higher than England and Wales for the period 1860–90, but when standardized rates were compared, Ireland's rates were consistently lower. The reason why the comparison of crude rates was so deceptive, of course, was that Ireland had a much older population than England. Standardized rates corrected for the effects of differing age structures. There is a strong similarity of approach in this study to the methods Newsholme used in his life table calculations. In fact the authors employed the same method of interpolating graphically that Newsholme had just used to construct his first Brighton life table.[45]

We find the same care to correct for population differences in the study of Britain's declining crude birth rates which Newsholme prepared with T.H.C. Stevenson, his former Deputy Medical Officer of Health, who was then employed at the General Register Office.[46] These authors reminded their readers of the difference between a birth rate – the ratio of births to population – and a fertility rate – the ratio of births to women aged 15 to 45. To illustrate how values for these ratios vary from place to place they reprinted a table Newsholme had first prepared for his *Elements of Vital Statistics* showing for the London boroughs of Kensington and Whitechapel the legitimate birth and legitimate fertility rates in 1891.[47] The excess of Whitechapel's rate was 83 percent when inhabitants were the denominator, 177 percent when women aged 15 to 45 were the denominator, and only 53 percent when married women aged 15 to 45 were used. They warned that the differences in fertility during a woman's reproductive life and the differences in the age distribution of women and the proportion who marry in different communities all mean that crude birth rates are untrustworthy measures of fertility and that both fertility and birth rates have to be corrected for the age distribution and marriage rates in the communities compared. In this example the authors used the age-specific fertility rates in Sweden to calculate a standard birth and fertility rate for the counties of England and Wales and then computed factors of correction (the ratio of the standard rate for England and Wales to the standard rate for the county), for each rate which, when used to multiply the rates for each county, permitted the resulting corrected rates to be fairly compared county by county. In this way Newsholme and Stevenson could demonstrate that in every county there had been a significant real drop in fertility since the 1881 census.[48]

45 King and Newsholme, "Alleged Increase," 216–20. Newsholme may have learned this technique from King. He gives King credit for showing that it was the method Milne had used in constructing the Carlisle table in Newsholme, *Brighton Life Table*, "Preface," n.p.

46 Arthur Newsholme and T.H.C. Stevenson, "An Improved Method of Calculating Birth-Rates," *J. Hygiene* 5 (1905): 175–84, 304–10.

47 Newsholme and Stevenson, "Improved Method," 176; and Newsholme, *The Elements,* 72.

48 Newsholme would return to this subject in a few years. See Arthur Newsholme, *The Declining*

While Newsholme recognized many of the pitfalls of using raw vital data and crude rates, as a practical local official with diverse administrative responsibilities, he did not always bother making the sorts of corrections we have been discussing. Consider, for example, a very interesting study of housing density and mortality he published in his *Annual Report* for 1892.[49] In this report he grouped the ninety-two enumeration districts from the 1891 census into eight groups according to their ranking by crude mortality rate. He recognized the need to correct these rates for differences in the composition of their populations, but, when he wrote, he did not have the age distribution for the enumeration districts at the 1891 census, the midpoint in his period of observation. As a proxy he used the age distribution of the four registration subdistricts for the previous census, 1881. Assuming that the age structure of each subdistrict had remained unchanged and using the experience of the entire nation for the period 1871–80 as his standard, he computed in turn a standard death rate, a factor of correction, and a corrected death rate for each of the four registration subdistricts in the years 1890–1. All this was done simply to allow him to argue that he could ignore disturbances caused by differences in age structure of the population inhabiting the groups of enumeration districts he was comparing. He estimated that the error caused by ignoring these differences would not be more than 3 per 1,000 for any one of his eight groups of enumeration districts. That was small in comparison to the range of crude mortality rates in these eight groups, 8.7 to 27.9 per 1,000. Hereafter in this study he relied on crude rates for mortality from all causes and from separate groups of diseases. Numerical precision was much less important than the policy implications of the relative differences in risks of death.

THE CAUSES OF EPIDEMICS

One might read Newsholme's writings during the 1880s and the 1890s as exemplifying the way in which the findings of bacteriology were received by the public health community in the generation after Koch announced the discovery of the tuberculosis bacillus. If one chooses to read them this way, one must conclude that the process of intellectual change was much more gradual than is sometimes glibly asserted and that older hygienic notions had remarkable longevity.[50] It comes as no surprise to find in Newsholme's textbooks on hygiene from the middle 1880s

Birth-Rate: Its National and International Significance (London, New York: Cassell & Co., 1911). We will discuss this work later.

49 Arthur Newsholme, "Special Report on the Mortality and Causes of Mortality in Eight Districts in Brighton," Brighton, Proc. San. Comm. 9 (28 April 1892): 158–76. This was republished as "On the Death Rates and Causes of Death in Enumeration Districts, with Special Reference to the Conditions of Housing," *Public Health* 4 (1891–2): 226–31.

50 Anne Hardy documents not only the longevity of the notion that sewer gas caused typhoid fever but also the role of that idea in stimulating sanitary reform. Anne Hardy, *The Epidemic Streets: Infectious Disease and the Rise of Preventive Medicine 1856–1900* (Oxford: Clarendon Press, 1993), 165–9.

long discussions of air and ventilation and warnings of the debilitating effects of an atmosphere contaminated with the products of respiration or combustion or polluted with sewer gas or with the air from mines or marshes.[51] In these works he even repeated a favorite example of the anticontagionists in the 1830s and 1840s, the Black Hole of Calcutta, admittedly an extreme case, but one which demonstrated, he believed, the power of airborne poison to depress vitality and render the human body susceptible to disease. Although he predicted in his textbook on hygiene of 1884 that the contagia of specific diseases would be found to consist of specific microbes, he also considered that the contagia of some diseases, including typhoid fever, might be generated de novo under proper physical conditions and held that other diseases such as erysipelas, puerperal fever, summer diarrhea, and diphtheria, were caused by inhaling sewer gas or by ingesting it dissolved in water or milk.[52]

It will probably come as more of a surprise to those who would like find a bacteriological revolution in preventive medicine to read in Newsholme's handbill from the middle nineties advising the citizens of Brighton to dispose properly of household rubbish as a way of preventing summer diarrhea, his warning that diarrhea in children was caused by "poisonous smells" absorbed by milk and food and that such smells were generated by decomposing household refuse.[53] At the time he composed that handbill he accepted several microbes as causes of specific disease. However, he still retained the old division of epidemic diseases into those that were strictly infectious, such as measles and whooping cough, those that were purely miasmatic, like ague, and those that were miasmatic-contagious like typhoid fever or cholera.[54] His statements about typhoid fever typify the change in his attitudes during the 1890s. In the late 1880s he concluded that only a few cases in Brighton were caused by infected ingesta, water or milk. Most were caused by exposure to sewer gas or to the products of organic decomposition. "If there is one fact more certain than another in Sanitary Science," Newsholme insisted, "it is that Enteric Fever occurs chiefly and almost solely when there is an excrement-sodden condition of the soil."[55] He then went on to discuss the evils of cesspools. By the midnineties his views had undergone substantial changes. The essential cause of typhoid fever was now the typhoid bacillus, while secondary causes

51 Arthur Newsholme, *Hygiene: A Manual of Personal and Public Health* (London, 1884), 148, 158–60, 162–4; and Arthur Newsholme, *School Hygiene: The Laws of Health in Relation to School Life* (London, 1887), 21–3, 24–5.

52 Newsholme, *Hygiene* (1884), 154–5, 163–4. See also his attribution of isolated cases of typhoid fever in Clapham to sewer gas from defective plumbing. Newsholme, *Report* (Clapham), 23 June 1886: 3 and 14 Sept. 1887: 3; and Arthur Newsholme, "Typhoid Fever from Defective Workmanship," *Sanitary Record*, n.s., 6 (1884–5): 351–2.

53 Arthur Newsholme, "As to the Emptying of Dustbins and Ashpits," reprinted in Newsholme, *Q. Rep.* (Brighton) (1895), no. 1: 12.

54 Arthur Newsholme, "The Natural History and Affinities of Rheumatic Fever: A Study in Epidemiology," *Lancet* (1895), no. 1: 664.

55 Newsholme, *Ann. Rep.* (Brighton) (1889), 21.

included individual susceptibility or resistance and vehicles for contagion such as milk, water, or shellfish.[56] While he still believed that typhoid fever might be acquired by inhalation, he now insisted that it was much more often conveyed by food or drink. At the turn of the century he sometimes sounded quite dismissive of faulty drainage as a cause of typhoid, but on occasion he fell back on this old explanation, as when he reported three cases he could account for in no other way.[57]

Intellectual inertia and the difficulties of changing long-held notions go only part way to explain the reason for this lasting concern with drains and smells, privies and cesspools, soil and air. We can also read Newsholme's writings of the 1880s and 1890s as reflecting the problems he faced as an administrator and an epidemiologist. As a local official he had to investigate and explain the appearance of individual cases of infectious disease. As an epidemiologist he described and accounted for the incidence of these diseases in the aggregate. He could not accomplish those tasks in the 1890s without recourse to nonspecific, environmental causes, the sorts of causes which lay and medical sanitarians had been relying on for a half century.

Newsholme believed this problem was most acute when one tried to account for epidemic phenomena. Knowledge of the microbe seemed incapable of explaining the timing, magnitude, or other essential features of epidemics. To illustrate, he presented a homily. Consider an episode in which a drunken man dies of a broken neck after being thrown from a restive horse.[58] Viewing the incident narrowly one might attribute his death to his broken neck. While it is true that he might have died if he had not been drunk or if his horse had been docile, his death can only be adequately explained by resort to all three causes: his drunkenness, his horse's restiveness, and his broken neck. This example is brought forward in his epidemiology of diphtheria in 1898. In that study the Klebs–Loeffler bacillus is accepted as the *causa causans* of diphtheria. But he quickly points out that the presence of the bacteria is not an adequate explanation for epidemics of the disease. Not only do sporadic cases, harboring the microbe in their throats and noses, appear without an epidemic's ensuing, but healthy individuals may be found in whose throats the bacillus is present. To explain the prevalence of disease in human communities the *causa efficiens* and the *causa movens*

---

56 Arthur Newsholme, "An Address on the Spread of Enteric Fever by Means of Sewage-Contaminated Shellfish," *Br. Med. J.* (1896), no. 2: 639–40. See also Newsholme, *Ann. Rep.* (Brighton) (1897), 20–1.

57 See, for example, Newsholme, *Ann. Rep.* (Brighton) (1900), 51; and Arthur Newsholme, "The Spread of Enteric Fever and Other Forms of Illness by Sewage-Polluted Shellfish," *Br. Med. J.* (1903), no. 2: 296.

58 Arthur Newsholme, *Epidemic Diphtheria: A Research on the Origin and Spread of the Disease from an International Standpoint* (London, 1898), 162–4. Newsholme's medical readers would have been familiar with distinctions among types of causes he was trying to draw. For a useful account which uses both historic and contemporary examples to explain the issues, see Lester S. King, *Medical Thinking: A Historical Preface* (Princeton, N.J.: Princeton Univ. Press, 1982), 187–223.

must also be sought, and these will be found in environmental circumstances, in the epidemic milieu.[59]

In the closing years of the nineteenth century, he undertook a series of epidemiological investigations of individual infectious diseases of which we will consider three: rheumatic fever, diphtheria, and diarrhea. These studies were similar in approach. They all presupposed a specific microbial cause. They all used data from different locations to chart the rise and fall of incidence over a long time period. And they all demonstrated that only in certain environmental circumstances were the infectious diseases in question liable to occur in epidemics.

The earliest of these was his study of rheumatic fever which he presented as his Milroy Lectures to the Royal College of Physicians in March 1895.[60] In these lectures he had two purposes. First, by relying on analogies to other diseases and on acute rheumatic fever's clinical characteristics, he argued that this disease was a specific infectious disease, even though its agent was as yet unknown and although some authorities had recently argued that it was a constitutional disease, either the result of reflex nervous irritation or of lactic acid excess. Second, and of greater interest to us here, he attempted to determine its epidemic milieu. Since in Britain rheumatic fever was not a reportable disease, there were no civil morbidity statistics he could use. Even if it had been a reportable disease, compulsory disease reporting was too recent in Britain to provide the long-term data he needed. Mortality statistics were not very useful, because rheumatic fever had a low case fatality. So he turned instead to the records of the hospitals of Great Britain and of a few American and Continental cities. He was certainly aware of many pitfalls in this procedure. Fashions in diagnosis and classification might change. The appearance of the salicylates might mean that recently more cases were nursed at home rather than admitted to a hospital. The number of hospital beds might not keep pace with population growth. Still, he was convinced that hospital records, particularly the ratio of rheumatic fever cases to all medical admissions, provided sufficiently reliable data to trace the rise and fall of the disease from year to year. To supplement these hospital records, he obtained the records of certain Scandinavian towns where rheumatic fever had been compulsorily notifiable since the 1860s.

He had to work slowly, tentatively, comparing himself to a paleontologist reconstructing an ichthyosaurus from a few bone fragments. The curves he drew for individual places showed that rheumatic fever occurred either in explosive epidemics lasting from one to three years or, especially in larger towns, in more protracted epidemics which, he thought, might represent the combination of two or more outbreaks.[61] In the intervening years the disease continued at a lower

59 Newsholme cites at this point Leon Colin, "Epidémies," *Dictionnaire Encyclopedique des Sciences Medicales* 35 (1887): 35–7 in ibid., 163. The same distinctions among causes appear earlier in Newsholme, "Natural History . . . Rheumatic Fever," 589.
60 Newsholme, "Natural History . . . Rheumatic Fever," 589–96 and 657–65. He later presented his results in abbreviated form in Arthur Newsholme, "The Epidemiology of Rheumatic Fever," *Practitioner* 66 (1901): 11–21.
61 Newsholme, "Natural History . . . Rheumatic Fever," 594.

endemic level. There was no fixed period between epidemics, but periods of maximum incidence commonly occurred in three-, four-, or six-year cycles. Finally there were certain great epidemic periods in which the disease was pandemic.

What determined whether a year was epidemic? Because rheumatic fever was endemic, it could not be chance importation of the contagium. Nor, did Newsholme believe, were changes in human behavior or physiology probable causes. He suspected environmental changes and considered local records of temperature of air and soil, humidity, barometric pressure, and rainfall. High temperature and low rainfall seemed to favor rheumatic fever, but these associations were not very convincing. So Newsholme turned to groundwater.[62] The choice was not accidental and certainly no surprise to his contemporaries. Medical Officers of Health in Newsholme's generation had encountered in their training and in reading the reports of the central health authority the groundwater theory for cholera and typhoid fever of the famous Professor of Hygiene from Munich, Max von Pettenkofer. John Simon, Medical Officer of the Privy Council, had given Pettenkofer's theory prominent consideration in his own discussion of the 1866 cholera epidemic and had offered the remarkable prediction that "henceforth no local health-officer will be properly up to the standard of his scientific duties, unless he thoroughly knows the distribution and stratification of soils in the district for which he acts, nor unless he also maintains such systematic and exact observation of the height of wells as will enable him always to speak with precision as to the movements of water-level in the soil."[63] There was no rush to install floats in English wells, because when Newsholme inquired in the mid-nineties, he could find few records of groundwater levels. But Pettenkofer's ideas were known, and a few British observers had kept careful records of groundwater and had attempted to use them in explaining epidemic trends.[64]

Thus when Newsholme turned to groundwater, he was operating in a viable if minor tradition in British epidemiology. At a much later time he recalled that his approach in the mid- and late nineties had been "determined" by Pettenkofer's theory.[65] Both men believed that although the diseases they were considering might have specific contagious principles, the presence or absence of the specific contagion alone could not explain observed fluctuations in incidence in time or place. Both contagion and a suitable environment were requisites for a disease outbreak. It was Pettenkofer's notion, a notion he defended for four decades, that cholera and typhoid fever were not directly transmissible from person to person

62 Ibid., 658–61.

63 John Simon, *Report of the Medical Officer of the Privy Council* 9 (1866): 458. Newsholme was certainly familiar with this section, because he quoted from it in his autobiography in discussing his research on rheumatic fever, Newsholme, *Fifty Years,* 110.

64 The most dedicated British proponent of a groundwater explanation at the time Newsholme studied the problem was probably Baldwin Latham. See his "The Relation of Ground Water to Disease," *Q. J. Roy. Meteorological Soc.* 17 (1891): 1–18.

65 Newsholme, *Fifty Years,* 107.

even though a disease germ was expelled from the sick in both diseases.[66] The germ was not the cause of new cases. One did not contract cholera or typhoid fever by swallowing their germs any more than one became drunk by swallowing yeast cells. Just as yeast needed to undergo a period of preparation in appropriate conditions to produce the cause of drunkenness, cholera and typhoid germs needed to ripen in an appropriate soil to produce the cause of new cases, a cause which Pettenkofer usually conceived as an airborne product, a miasma. Pettenkofer's extensive researches convinced him that the proper environment for this ripening was porous soil containing organic material at the right temperature and moisture. Groundwater was a convenient indicator of soil moisture. Pettenkofer found that when cholera was epidemic, groundwater levels were falling. He suggested that the falling water table left an enlarged layer of moist but not saturated soil which seemed to be an ideal breeding ground for the cause of cholera.

Pettenkofer represented, then, one of many compromise positions between a strict contagionist and a strict miasmatic or localist stance. Newsholme never committed himself to Pettenkofer's explanations for cholera or typhoid, but he found in Pettenkofer's model two attractive features: the idea that epidemics may be related to the exogenous life of microbes in the soil, and the notion that groundwater might serve as an indicator of epidemic periods. Although he could find records of water levels in only a few wells in and around London and in the south of England, Newsholme was sufficiently impressed with what he discovered to conclude that the incidence of rheumatic fever and the level of groundwater were inversely related.[67] He could not quantify this relationship, and he found a few years in which epidemics did not occur when groundwater was low. But he was convinced that low groundwater was an important determinant of epidemics of rheumatic fever and that such epidemics never took place when groundwater was high.

Like Pettenkofer, Newsholme saw groundwater levels as indicators of environmental conditions suitable for the generation of epidemic rheumatic fever. Those environmental conditions were only one cause of epidemic rheumatic fever. The others were the as yet undiscovered microbe, and personal factors determining susceptibility or resistance.[68] The personal factors included strictly biological ones: age, sex, heredity, and also environmentally influenced ones: occupation, fatigue, diet, chill. Newsholme emphasized the influence of the environment on the microbe of rheumatic fever. This microbe must, he reasoned, be omnipresent, since rheumatic fever is endemic. Certain environmental conditions, of which

66 For a summary of Pettenkofer's ideas on the causation of typhoid and cholera, see Edgar Erskine Hume, *Max von Pettenkofer: His Theory of the Etiology of Cholera, Typhoid Fever, and Other Intestinal Diseases, A Review of His Arguments and Evidence* (New York: Paul B. Hoeber, 1927), 45–106; and Claude E. Dolman, "Max Josef von Pettenkofer," *D.S.B.*, X, 558–60. See also Charles-Edward Amory Winslow, *The Conquest of Epidemic Disease: A Chapter in the History of Ideas* (Princeton, N.J.: Princeton Univ. Press, 1944), 311–36.

67 Newsholme, "Natural History . . . Rheumatic Fever," 658–61.   68 Ibid., 589, 660–1.

groundwater is the best indicator, enable the microbe to "assume sufficient malignancy to fit it for aggressive parasitic life."[69] Recent discoveries about the tetanus organism made it plausible to argue that the rheumatic fever agent might exist saprophytically in the soil, infecting humans in large numbers when it left the soil in conditions of heat and dryness.

By 1901, in drawing on recent discoveries about malaria's transmission, Newsholme was suggesting that the rheumatic fever organism might be carried from the soil to humans by an insect, probably a domestic insect like the housefly.[70] His original notion was, however, much more in keeping with the miasmatic or atmospheric models of the nineteenth century. What he first had in mind can be seen clearly in his epidemiology of diphtheria, where the methods and notions he employed in his study of rheumatic fever received fullest development.[71] Working this time from uncorrected mortality figures extending back to the mid–nineteenth century for British, Colonial, American, and European cities, he identified epidemic years and then sought climatic determinants of diphtheria's incidence. He found that in general high diphtheria mortality occurred in dry years and dry places, and was higher in continental than in island climates and in the drier parts of nations.[72] Because diphtheria sometimes became epidemic only after two or more years of dry weather and the great epidemics almost always occurred in this way, Newsholme suspected drought was important mainly in causing the level of groundwater to fall. The limited records of groundwater levels confirmed his hunch. Newsholme conceded that his personal experiences as a Medical Officer of Health were consistent with the common medical belief that diphtheria was associated with damp soil and damp houses. Damp houses, he suggested, favored colds and sore throats which left the occupants more susceptible to the Klebs–Loeffler bacillus. It also seemed that the first rains after a drought became a dangerous time for diphtheria. These apparently conflicting observations could, Newsholme believed, be explained by assuming that the diphtheria organism, like that for rheumatic fever, and he postulated, like those for enteric fever, scarlet fever, and erysipelas, had two phases of existence. One was passed saprophytically in the soil, the other parasitically in the human body. Long periods of damp soil favored the former. Dry soil favored the latter.[73] He imagined that in warm, dry soil the organism would reproduce rapidly. Certain environmental changes, including a sudden rise in groundwater, would force from the soil ground air and with it these microbes. Newsholme had long imagined that groundwater and the air in the soil played a role in disease causation. In 1884 he had warned that soil air containing the emanations of cesspools and drains might be aspirated into those

---

69 Ibid., 663.   70 Newsholme, "Epidemiology of Rheumatic Fever," 21.
71 Newsholme, *Epidemic Diphtheria*. He repeated his argument in "The Epidemiology of Diphtheria," in *The Bacteriology of Diphtheria*, ed. G.H.F. Nuttall and G. S. Graham-Smith (Cambridge: Cambridge Univ. Press, 1908), 53–81.
72 Newsholme, *Epidemic Diphtheria*, 157–60.   73 Ibid., 175–6, 184–7.

homes that did not have impervious basements or floors, as changes in barometric pressure or rising groundwater forced air from the soil.[74] By the mid-nineties his theory included microbes, but he succeeded in grafting new bacterial ideas onto the old stock of environmental and sanitary notions. It was a clever if short-lived synthesis. By suggesting that pathogenic microbes might live and reproduce freely in the environment, he retained a wide sphere in which climatic and other environmental forces might operate.

In his administration Newsholme took the association of air, climate, and infectious disease seriously. In 1896, the year following his Milroy Lectures on rheumatic fever, he had a float installed in a well in North Street so that he could monitor groundwater levels.[75] The same year he began plotting the date every notified case of disease began against data from the borough weather station, and soon he felt confident that he could predict when notifications, especially those for diphtheria and scarlet fever, would become more numerous.[76] Barometric pressure and rainfall were his best indicators.

As a final example of Newsholme's attempts to identify the epidemic milieu let us consider his extensive study of epidemic or summer diarrhea, presented in 1899 as his Presidential Address to the Incorporated Society of Medical Officers of Health.[77] Diarrhea was an important cause of death, especially of infants. It was prevalent in late summer and early autumn and was a subject of growing concern for Medical Officers of Health. We will consider diarrhea again in discussing infant mortality; our interest for the moment, however, is the role Newsholme assigned the environment in its causation. Epidemic diarrhea was a difficult subject for statistical study. While he believed there was a disease properly called epidemic or infantile diarrhea having a specific bacterial cause, Newsholme recognized that the Registrar-General's mortality statistics for diarrhea probably included deaths from a variety of conditions.[78] As fashions of diagnosis changed, it was hazardous to compare for long periods rates of death attributed to diarrhea. It was, however, reasonable to compare rates for shorter periods from different places. This comparison would illuminate the conditions in which diarrhea thrived. Newsholme recognized however, that the ordinary diarrhea mortality rates published for the large towns in the Registrar-General's Quarterly Reports could not be used for these comparative purposes.[79] Because three-quarters of diarrheal deaths occurred

---

74 Newsholme, *Hygiene* (1884), 292.

75 Brighton, Proc. San. Comm. 13 (11 June 1896), 434–8; or Brighton, *Proc. Town Council, Proc. Comm.* (18 June 1896): 24–5.

76 Newsholme, *Epidemic Diphtheria,* 169. Newsholme retained his belief in the relevance of rainfall to the prevalence of scarlet fever for some time. See his "The Utility of Isolation Hospitals in Diminishing the Spread of Scarlet Fever. Considered from an Epidemiological Standpoint," *J. Hygiene* 1 (1901): 148–9.

77 Arthur Newsholme, "A Contribution to the Study of Epidemic Diarrhoea," *Public Health* 12 (1899–1900): 139–211. As was often the case he also prepared a shortened version; see his "The Public Health Aspects of Summer Diarrhoea," *Practitioner* 69 (1902): 161–80.

78 Newsholme, "Study of Epidemic Diarrhoea," 140–3, 154, 159.   79 Ibid., 144.

in the first year of life, comparisons of diarrhea mortality rates calculated as the Registrar-General did (all diarrhea deaths per 1,000 population) penalized towns with high birth rates. The correct mortality figure for his purposes was diarrhea deaths in the first year of life to 1,000 births. But the information needed for that ratio was not available from published returns. So Newsholme again turned to a proxy and used the rate of all diarrhea deaths to 1,000 births. It was not an ideal index, but it did go some way toward correcting for differences in the age distribution of the populations compared. In this study he employed the annual and quarterly diarrheal mortality rates, usually from 1882 to 1898 for thirty-one large British towns.

At the time Newsholme wrote, the most extensive and influential study of epidemic diarrhea was a provisional report published in 1889 by Edward Ballard at the Medical Department of the Local Government Board.[80] Ballard in 1880 had begun investigating the high mortality from diarrhea in Leicester but soon expanded his scope to include other towns as well. Although he died before he could prepare a final report, his provisional report identified an extensive list of conditions he thought favored epidemic diarrhea: poor sanitation and ventilation; high population density; warm, dry weather; loose soil easily permeated by air or water; sewer or cesspool emanations; and poor infant care.[81] The list was so inclusive it read like a catalogue of the preoccupations of sanitarians and was little help in focusing thought or action. The novelty of Ballard's report, however, was the suggestion that the timing of diarrhea epidemics was related to the temperature of the subsoil. He had plotted local climatic observations and local records of diarrhea and observed that diarrheal mortality did not begin to rise in summer until the temperature of the earth at 4 feet reached roughly 56°F and that the highest weekly diarrhea mortality occurred in the week with the highest average readings on the 4-foot earth thermometer. Ballard suggested that the cause of epidemic diarrhea would be found to be a soil microbe whose activity depended on local environmental conditions.[82] Dead organic matter in soil or contaminated food and high temperature sustained its growth. The microbe probably produced a toxin which caused the disease in humans.

Newsholme knew Ballard's report very well. In fact, during an epidemic of diarrhea in Brighton in the summer of 1891, he summarized with approval Ballard's conclusions for his Sanitary Committee to explain why the epidemic was taking place and what might be done in response.[83] It is hardly surprising that Newsholme's study a decade later was conceived in similar terms. The two men

---

80 Edward Ballard, "Report to the Local Government Board upon the Causation of the Annual Mortality from 'Diarrhoea,' Which is Observed Principally in the Summer Season of the Year," *Ann. Rep. Med. Off. L.G.B.* 17 (1887–8), B.P.P. 1889 [C-5638], XXXV, 1–127.
81 Ballard summarizes his conclusions in ibid., 1–7.
82 Ibid., 7.
83 Arthur Newsholme [report on mortality from diarrhoea in Brighton], Brighton, Proc. San. Comm. 8 (11 June 1891): 234–47; or Brighton, *Proc. Town Council, Proc. Comm.* (18 June 1891): 22–9.

agreed that summer diarrhea was most prevalent among the lower strata of the urban working class, and that it was favored by loose, porous soils and by high temperature. But Newsholme's discussion of causes was more narrowly focused than Ballard's. He attached particular importance to air temperature and rainfall.[84] By this time Newsholme thought that Ballard's observations with the 4-foot earth thermometer simply recorded the delayed effect of changes in mean air tempera- ture. Diarrheal mortality responded after a week or two to the critical changes in environmental conditions. In this way its occurrence differed from that of rheu- matic fever or diphtheria, which might become epidemic a year or more after the crucial changes in groundwater began. This difference in response time led Newsholme to conclude that while rheumatic fever and diphtheria might be linked to a drying, polluted subsoil, epidemic diarrhea was associated with pollu- tion of the soil surface. He compared the causation of epidemic diarrhea to the growing of grain. Both depended on three things: a seed or specific microbe, summer weather, and a suitable soil. For diarrhea, municipal filth scattered on the ground, especially human and animal excrement and garbage, was the suitable soil. "The fundamental condition favouring epidemic diarrhoea is *an unclean soil, the particulate poison from which infects the air, and is swallowed most commonly with food, especially milk*."[85] The epidemic milieu he imagined was thus like that he had postulated for rheumatic fever and for diphtheria. The difference lay in the location of soil pollution, surface or subsoil. The implications for prevention were obvious, and Newsholme pointed out repeatedly how proper drainage and regular cleansings of streets, yards, and alleys, especially in dry weather when rainwater did not do part of the job, would go far to prevent epidemic diarrhea.[86] In fact he worried lest the acceptance of Ballard's rule would lead municipalities into ac- cepting their high rates of diarrhea mortality as inevitable consequences of climatic change. Newsholme the epidemiologist was never far from Newsholme the practical administrator.

The studies of Newsholme we have been considering fall into a narrow space of time, 1894 to 1900. They represent his attempt to bring recent bacteriological discoveries within the scope of his expansive, eclectic epidemiology. The legacy of Pettenkofer is apparent, but so is Newsholme's inventiveness. The particular solutions he found did not survive very long. By the time, for example, that he published a shortened version of his diphtheria study in a multiauthored textbook, some peers found his suggestions about groundwater, soil air (air present in the soil), and the extracorporeal life of the diphtheria bacillus entirely implausible.[87] Looking back in retirement, Newsholme conceded that some of these efforts had

84 Newsholme, "Study of Epidemic Diarrhoea," 158–66.   85 Ibid., 166.
86 Ibid., 164–5; and Arthur Newsholme, "Epidemic Diarrhoea, Municipal Scavenging, Rainfall, and Temperature," *Public Health* 15 (1902–3): 654–5.
87 See, for example, comments by William H. Park and Charles Bolduan in the same volume in which Newsholme's argument was repeated, "Mortality," in Nuttall and Graham-Smith, eds., *Bacteriology of Diphtheria*, 586. See also the review of this book in *Br. Med. J.* (1908), no. 1: 1050.

been misguided, although he regretted the complete neglect into which climate and groundwater had fallen in studies of epidemics.[88] These investigations of the late nineties are, nevertheless, historically significant. They illustrate Newsholme's resourcefulness, his belief in the power of environment to explain the behavior of human disease in the aggregate, and his determination to make the results of epidemiology practical. In the next three chapters we will investigate the relationship between his administrative activities and his epidemiological investigations. A more effective strategy for dealing with infectious disease emerged from this collaboration.

88 Newsholme, *Fifty Years*, 225, 227, 358.

3

The urban environment and the M.O.H.'s authority

HOUSEHOLDS AND DRAINS

The annual reports of the local medical officers of health and sanitary inspectors reveal a clear picture of slowly improving sanitary conditions. One must admire, and wonder at, the energy and determination of these officials who, in the face of great hostility from all sides (landlords, tenants, slum-owning vestrymen and ratepayers), went about their task with such grim enthusiasm. The number of annual inspections conducted by the local authorities was remarkable, a testimony to Victorian energy.[1]

The greatest success of late Victorian health departments may well have been in the most mundane matters, the enforcing of minimum standards of sanitation in homes, certain businesses, and public spaces. This work was conducted through the periodic visits of Inspectors of Nuisances or Sanitary Inspectors, who came, sometimes unannounced, to see that sanitary regulations were being observed. No other part of the Sanitary Department's work occupied so much staff time. When Newsholme arrived in Brighton, there were more than 20,000 occupied houses in the area of the Sanitary Department's jurisdiction. By the time he left in 1908, that number was nearly 24,000.[2] Early in his career his Department thus had one inspector for every 2,222 inhabited houses. In the middle 1890s this ratio would have placed Brighton about on the middle of the scale of London boroughs, between the Strand at one extreme with one inspector for every 358 inhabited houses and Lambeth at the other with one inspector for every 4,819 inhabited houses.[3] Given these resources, Brighton's Sanitary Department seems nothing short of relentless in its inspections. During 1889, Newsholme's first full year in town, the Department conducted more than 7,000 routine household inspections. As the Department concentrated its efforts on houses in working–class neighborhoods, it seems likely that some houses were visited as often as once a year. In addition to those 7,000 routine visits, the Department conducted that year another

1 A. S. Wohl, "The Housing of the Working Classes in London 1815–1914," in *The History of Working-class Housing: A Symposium,* ed. Stanley D. Chapman (Newton Abbot: David and Charles, 1971), 23.
2 Data from the decennial census reports as cited in Farrant, "The Growth of Brighton and Hove," 29.
3 Wohl, "Housing of the Working Classes," 47.

nearly 2,500 visits to homes following the occurrence of an acute infectious disease. It also made unannounced visits to common lodging houses, 492 of these during the day and 156 at night. Moreover, the inspectors visited certain places of business, primarily those where meat or dairy products were prepared or sold. In 1889, 3,017 of these inspections were of slaughterhouses, 812 of cowsheds, 3,216 of dairies and provisions shops, and 485 of bakehouses.[4]

The focus in this section is on household inspections. Far from declining as newer public health strategies were adopted, the pace of these inspections grew during Newsholme's tenure in Brighton. He would eventually detail five of his Inspectors to devote all their time to this work.[5] In 1907, his last full year as M.O.H., the Department conducted over 13,000 routine inspections of households, nearly twice the number it conducted in 1889, although the number of houses in his jurisdiction had increased only about 20 percent in the interval.[6]

The visit of a Sanitary Inspector had a distinct aura of police authority. The Inspectors wore dark blue uniforms reminiscent of those worn by the police and carried with them a written statement bearing the Town Seal that specified their authority to enter houses and places of business for the purpose of carrying out sanitary inspections.[7] Although an Inspector had the authority to enter premises to conduct inspections, he was to do so with the knowledge and permission of the owner or occupant. On at least one occasion during Newsholme's tenure, the Sanitary Committee reprimanded an Inspector when a middle-class householder wrote complaining that this Inspector had entered his property without his permission.[8] The Inspector's authority was thus limited if very real. If premises were found to be in violation of the sanitary code, the owner or the occupant could receive an oral warning, a written notice, or, in the absence of compliance, a summons to appear in court.

The chief focus of these household inspections, especially in the early years of Newsholme's tenure, was to complete in the private sphere the sanitary revolution begun in the public sphere by the building of the town's interception sewers and the purchase of private water companies. Every year the Department served notices on owners to connect their houses to the sewer system and to fill in their cesspools. Within a decade Newsholme could claim that Brighton was entirely on the water closet system and that the old cesspools had been destroyed. Brighton was then one of only ten large British towns, including the Metropolis, to rely

4 Newsholme, *Ann. Rep.* (Brighton) (1889): 23.
5 Arthur Newsholme, *Special Report on Overcrowding, on the Clearing of Insanitary Areas, and on the Provision of Housing Accommodation by the Town Council* (Brighton: County Borough of Brighton, 1904), 23.
6 Newsholme, *Ann. Rep.* (Brighton) 1907: 31.
7 These written statements were provided following an incident in autumn of 1889 in which a Major F. F. Hallett protested repeatedly the inspection of his cowshed by an Inspector of Nuisances. See Brighton, Proc. San. Comm. 7 (28 Nov. 1889): 127; ibid. (12 Dec. 1889): 151; ibid. (24 Dec. 1889): 162; and ibid. (9 Jan. 1890): 175–6.
8 Brighton, Proc. San. Comm., 10 (31 Aug. 1893): 396, 398–9.

primarily or entirely on water closets.[9] Newsholme was also intent on converting the town from intermittent to constant household service of pure water. He could encourage this change by using his authority under the Brighton Improvement Act, 1884, to insist that water closets had their own supply of piped water. Notices for laying on water to the closet outnumber all others in his early years: 475 in 1888 alone, rising to 943 in 1890.[10] Inspectors insisted that water for flushing the water closet not be drawn from the drinking water cistern. Such an arrangement, Newsholme feared, would allow the house's drinking water to absorb "effluvia from the closet" or sewer gas.[11]

This fear of the airborne products of organic decomposition, a fear widely shared among M.O.H., drove the third element of this household sanitary campaign, the improvement of household drainage. In the first edition of his *Hygiene,* Newsholme repeated the common observation that the entrance into a bedroom of gas from a poorly constructed drain or soil pipe had been known to cause diphtheria, sore throat, and other serious diseases.[12] While M.O.H. for Clapham he reported cases of diphtheria which, in his opinion, had arisen when house drains had been obstructed or when the overflow for the drinking-water cistern had been connected with the soil pipe.[13] Driven by these possibilities, inspectors looked to see that drains were trapped, that soil pipes and house drain traps were ventilated, and that the waste pipes from sinks and bathtubs discharged outside of houses, in the open air over gully traps.[14]

Every year during the late 1880s and the 1890s the Sanitary Department issued hundreds of notices to owners to provide proper traps for their drains, and to modify the way waste water reached the sewers. The inspectors searched drains and soil pipes assiduously for leaks and ordered the relaying of defective drains. In cases of complaints or when infectious disease occurred in a house, existing drains were opened for inspection or were tested by adding a volatile agent, such as peppermint oil. In 1898, for example, 650 household drains were opened for inspection by the Department, and the soil pipes of 136 houses were given the peppermint test for leaks.[15] New or relaid drains and drains in houses where enteric or typhoid fever occurred were subjected to a hydraulic test for leaks and checked for proper gradient and ventilation.[16]

9 Arthur Newsholme, "A Contribution to the Study of Epidemic Diarrhoea," *Public Health,* 12 (1899): 156, 184.

10 Newsholme, *Ann. Rep.* (Brighton) 1888: 11; and ibid. 1890: 20.

11 Newsholme, *Hygiene* (1884), 235.

12 Arthur Newsholme, *Hygiene: A Manual of Personal and Public Health* (London, 1884), 230.

13 Board of Works for the Wandsworth District, Minutes of Proceedings, 23 June 1886: 3; and ibid. 14 Sept. 1887: 3.

14 For current discussions of drainage inspection and of available commercial plumbing equipment, see George Wilson, *A Handbook of Hygiene and Sanitary Science,* 3rd ed. (Philadelphia, 1880), 265–81; and a very similar discussion in Newsholme, *Hygiene* (1884), 227–53.

15 Newsholme, *Ann. Rep.* (Brighton) 1898: 28. For a discussion of how these tests were performed, see A. Wynter Blyth, *A Manual of Public Health* (London, 1890), 192–4.

16 Newsholme, *Ann. Rep.* (Brighton) 1889: 22; and Arthur Newsholme, "An Address on the Spread of Enteric Fever by Means of Sewage-Contaminated Shellfish," *Br. Med. J.* (1896), no. 2: 641.

In reading the *Annual Reports* of the Medical Officer of Health, one is struck today by the persistence of this activity. Each year in Brighton there were thousands of household inspections and, in the early years, hundreds of notices for structural changes and dozens of summonses. Newsholme noted with satisfaction that with each passing year compliance with notices increased and the number of summonses issued declined.[17] By the middle 1890s he was boasting "there is no town which has done more than that in which I live to perfect its system of house sanitation, and each year the proportion of houses which will bear the most rigid tests of modern sanitation is largely increased."[18]

As owners were hounded into compliance and the more serious structural defects were gradually eliminated, Newsholme began to stretch his authority to encourage other household improvements such as the installation of windows in stairways. Such an improvement was desirable in that it would promote ventilation, but it was not mandated, and Newsholme admitted to his professional peers that this demand would be very difficult to enforce, if it were contested.[19]

All this improvement cost money and caused irritation to tenants and landlords. Years later Newsholme was fond of telling a story about his friction with an Alderman who owned much cheap rental property in town and to whom the cost of these structural changes seemed very heavy. This Alderman once brought the M.O.H. his builder's bills and rent receipts for a quarter to prove that he was losing money. "A few months later I met him on the Brighton railway platform," commented Newsholme, introducing the following exchange:

'Hullo, Doctor! Where are you going?'
'On holiday.'
'How long are you going for?'
'A month.'
'I say, Doctor, couldn't you make it six months?'[20]

While this campaign of household inspections had a basis in contemporary disease theory, it also was rooted in standards of housekeeping and decency, in a campaign to teach the working class proper behavior. The inspectors not only scrutinized drainage and ventilation, things for which the landlord was responsible, but they also attempted to exercise some control over housekeeping and domestic behavior. Enforcing standards of housekeeping was problematic to say the least, although the outbreak of infectious disease could provide the occasion for an official review of domestic management and for compulsory action. Consider, as an example, an incident from June 1895. Newsholme reported visiting two houses in response to an outbreak of diphtheria. On his recommendation the Committee voted to require the occupants of the houses to take a series of actions whose

---

17 Newsholme, *Ann. Rep.* (Brighton) 1893: 31–2; and ibid. (1899): 45.
18 Newsholme, "Spread of Enteric Fever," 642.
19 Arthur Newsholme, "The Prevention of Phthisis, with Special Reference to its Notification to the Medical Officer of Health," *Public Health,* 11 (1898–9): 313.
20 Arthur Newsholme, *Fifty Years in Public Health: A Personal Narrative with Comments* (London: George Allen and Unwin, 1935), 154.

precise bearing on the diphtheria cases was rather dubious, even in view of then current disease theory: remove an ash pit, remove an accumulation of rubbish, reduce the number of lodgers, and cease keeping so many cats as to be a nuisance.[21] It is little wonder that these household inspections caused resentment in working-class neighborhoods, where they were concentrated. Newsholme, however, defended these inspections not only for their concrete results but for their less direct influence on working-class domestic behavior. Assessing his first fifteen years in Brighton, he noted with satisfaction that the standard of housekeeping had improved under the steady pressure of these inspections.[22]

Looking back from the vantage point of the 1930s Newsholme asked rhetorically,

Did we overdo it? I think we did in some minor details; but the provision of watertight drains, of flushing cisterns, and of movable dustbins was necessary, and these and other similar improvements rendered life more comfortable, freer from nuisances, and healthier than it would otherwise have been.[23]

Here as in so much else, Newsholme continued to see public health as a force of social amelioration rather than simply as the application of technical knowledge to achieve narrow biological results. His concern for the common good and his confidence in the rightness of middle-class standards of cleanliness and behavior made it easy for him to blur the distinction between the hygienic and the merely proper or decent.

INFANT MORTALITY AND PUBLIC HYGIENE

Newsholme's response to infant mortality while in Brighton has special historical interest for its bearing on two disputes. The first of these is the notorious rivalry between two government departments, the Local Government Board and the Board of Education, for control of infant welfare work during the First World War. The second is a much more recent discussion among historians on the meaning of the infant welfare movement of the turn of the century, in particular whether the reform efforts were really attempts to shift the blame for infant deaths to mothers and to keep married women from seeking employment outside of the home.[24] We will consider both issues in Chapter 11. But notice here that it is possible to find in more routine work at the local level the roots of the positions Newsholme would take, when the issue of infant mortality loomed large in national health policy discussions.

Newsholme's experience in Brighton convinced him that local sanitary authori-

21 Brighton, Proc. San. Comm., 12 (1 June 1895): 384–6.
22 Newsholme, *Special Report on Overcrowding*, 23.   23 Newsholme, *Fifty Years*, 155.
24 The position is argued with particular persistence by Carol Dyhouse, in "Working-Class Mothers and Infant Mortality in England, 1896–1914," in *Biology, Medicine and Society 1840–1940*, ed. Charles Webster (Cambridge: Cambridge Univ. Press, 1981), 73–98.

ties, having begun to deal with infant mortality in their campaigns against epidemic, summer, or infantile diarrhea, had priority for infant welfare work over education authorities and that the former were the natural and proper providers of public services to infants and young children. His own concern with infant mortality began very early in his career, in fact even before he arrived in Brighton. It seems to have been infant mortality's share of total mortality that convinced Newsholme to target it for special attention.[25] While some infant deaths, he believed, were undoubtedly beyond the scope of preventive measures, more than a quarter were due to zymotic or tubercular diseases, and most of these, he believed, might be prevented.[26] Like other early advocates for infant welfare, he soon seized on diarrheal diseases as the chief enemy of infant health. Newsholme recognized, of course, that diarrhea was a symptom, not a disease, and that the mortality registered from epidemic diarrhea probably masked infant deaths caused by a number of conditions, including typhoid fever. But in the late 1880s and early 1890s he was convinced that there must be as well a disease, infant diarrhea, with a specific cause.[27]

Within months of coming to Brighton, in the fall of 1888, he produced a short report on the diarrheal deaths that had taken place from July through September in Brighton that year.[28] This report and several others he produced in Brighton prefigure in significant ways the major studies of infant mortality he undertook between 1910 and 1916 while Medical Officer of the Local Government Board. For this 1888 report the Sanitary Department carefully investigated each reported death attributed to diarrhea. It found that fatal diarrhea was a special problem of the first months of life: Only five of the forty-two deaths occurred after the first year, and fully half occurred under six months of age. Furthermore, this report suggested what all Newsholme's studies of infant mortality concluded: Deaths from infantile diarrhea affected mainly working-class families, particularly those of unskilled workers.[29] Thirty-five of these deaths occurred in a single subdistrict,

---

25 Arthur Newsholme, "On Some Fallacies of Vital Statistics, especially as Applicable to Brighton," Brighton, Proc. San. Comm., 6 (15 Nov. 1888): 216; and Newsholme, *Ann. Rep.* (Brighton), (1889), 8. His interest in the epidemiology of infant diarrhea even precedes his arrival in Brighton. See his report in Board of Works for the Wandsworth District, Minutes of Proceedings, 1 Sept. 1886, 5. For later discussions of this topic, see Arthur Newsholme, "A Contribution to the Study of Epidemic Diarrhoea," *Public Health,* 12 (1899–1900): 139; and Newsholme, *Ann. Rep.* (Brighton) 1897: 12, 35.

26 Newsholme, *Ann. Rep.* (Brighton), 1888, 4–5; Newsholme, *Ann. Rep.* (Brighton), 1889, 9.

27 Newsholme, untitled report on diarrhea, Brighton, Proc. San. Comm., 8 (11 June 1891): 235–6; and ibid., Brighton, *Proc. Town Council, Proc. Comm.* (18 June 1891): 23. Later in his career he became more conscious of the importance of disease labels in the statistics of epidemic diarrhea and argued that much of the apparent reduction in diarrhea mortality was due to a transference of deaths from diarrhea to enteric fever in the G.R.O. statistics. See Newsholme, "Contribution to the Study of Epidemic Diarrhoea," 140–1.

28 Newsholme, *Q. Rep.* (Brighton) 1888, no. 3: 3–4.

29 The registration certificates for the victims recorded exclusively manual occupations for the victims' parents: 2 laborers, 2 painters, 2 plumbers, a bricklayer, a carpenter, a groom, 2 hawkers, 4 servants, a charwoman, 2 single (and presumably indigent) women, etc.

St. Peter's, which had a large, working-class population. Deaths from epidemic diarrhea, Newsholme discovered, almost never occurred in prosperous homes.

In this 1888 report he adopted a model to account for these deaths which is reminiscent of several others he proposed in the nineties and which we have considered in Chapter 2. A specific microbial cause is postulated, but to account for the occurrence of disease in the community, he emphasized environmental factors. In this early report infant feeding received only passing mention.

The chief factor in the production of this disease is putrefying dirt. Whether there is a specific germ causing it is still a moot point. No such germ has been isolated. But allowing the probability of its existence, its active development requires such conditions of uncleanliness, personal and domestic, as exist chiefly among the poorer classes. The contents of imperfectly or infrequently emptied dust-bins, accumulations of foul manure (especially when offal is mixed with the manure), imperfect scavenging of side streets, as well as putrefactive changes in food and milk (and in the feeding bottles used for infants), all seem to aid the conditions under which Diarrhoea thrives.[30]

This model was clearly in the mind of the investigators, who listed for each death the probable local cause of the illness. This column reads like a litany of sanitary sins: "choked and offensive closet," "soakage in yard from W.C. next door," "ventilating pipe close above window," "foul pan in closet," "refuse heaped in yard," "foul yard from fowls," "kitchen requires whitewashing." But mixed in this list of sanitary defects are three entries which show some recognition of the importance of infant feeding: "fed on condensed milk," "fed on condensed milk and water," and "fed on cornflour and a little milk." The key to preventing infant diarrhea, Newsholme concluded, was better sanitation in and around homes and some changes in infant feeding practices.

The next summer he was more specific. On the eve of the season when an outbreak of epidemic diarrhea could be expected, he convinced his Committee to print 20,000 copies, one for almost every house in town, of a pamphlet he had prepared for household distribution on the prevention of this disease.[31] This handbill was reprinted in nearly identical form and distributed to homes each summer for many years. It explained that epidemic diarrhea was caused by a poison that entered the body in tainted food or drink or, less frequently, by being inhaled. Sanitary measures for prevention were listed first: proper drainage and ventilation; cleanliness of rooms, especially kitchens and water closets; and proper disposal of decomposable animal and vegetable material. Householders were urged to notify the Sanitary Department if they did not have an adequate supply of water or if cleanliness did not remove smells. The handbill also gave advice on infant care. It recommended frequent bathing in summer and the use of woolen clothing or a flannel belt next to the skin and warned against exposing children suffering from infectious diseases, including diarrhea, to other children. It urged

30 Newsholme, *Q. Rep.* (Brighton) 1888, no. 3: 3.
31 For a copy of this handbill, see Newsholme, *Ann. Rep.* (Brighton) 1889: 16–18.

that unless a doctor recommended otherwise, infants under eight months should have only milk and that this milk should, if possible be provided by breast-feeding. If other milk had to be used, it should be mixed with one-third dilute lime water or barley water and be boiled before being given to the child. Infant feeding bottles should be washed and scalded daily. The Sanitary Department also made available free of charge a disinfectant, Condy's Fluid, for treating these bottles. Infants were not to be fed pap, that is, bread sops, or starchy patented infant foods.

It was reasonable advice, but advice that placed the responsibility for preventing infant mortality primarily on families. While the Sanitary Department continued to print and to distribute this handbill to households year after year, Newsholme soon recognized the inadequacies of this approach. He complained about "a strong wall of prejudice, ignorance and carelessness" which hampered the Department's modest parental education efforts.[32] In view of his later rivalry with the education authorities it is significant that through the nineties he preferred to leave maternal education to voluntary societies, which held mothers' meetings and sent women into working-class homes to instruct mothers on child care.[33]

More characteristic of Newsholme was his conclusion that individual effort, while necessary, was inadequate. Special municipal services were needed to fight infant diarrhea. He launched his appeal in June of 1891 in a report to the Sanitary Committee.[34] In typical form he arrested his Committee's attention by insisting that while the town's typhoid mortality had been falling steadily over the past decade, its diarrheal mortality had actually risen relative to that of other towns. To explain epidemic diarrhea's occurrence, he summarized for his committee the views of Edward Ballard, whose Report of 1888 we have considered in Chapter 2. Ballard emphasized the roles of filth, especially in and around homes, of dense living arrangements, of high temperature – especially of the soil, and of loose or porous soil. From this review of Ballard's report and from his own experience Newsholme concluded:

The facts enumerated are best explained on the hypothesis that the essential cause of Diarrhoea is some micro-organism not yet identified, which resides ordinarily in the superficial layers of the earth; that this organism is favoured by certain conditions of season, and is dependent for its food and growth on the presence of decomposing organic matter; that in food, especially in milk, this organism finds the necessary nidus and pabulum for its development; and that from food and from the organic putrescent matter of soils or accumulations of refuse, this microorganism can manufacture a *virulent chemical poison,* which is the essential cause of Epidemic Diarrhoea.[35]

32 Arthur Newsholme, "Special Report on the Diarrhoeal Mortality of the Third Quarter of 1895," in Newsholme, *Q. Report* (Brighton) 1895, no. 3: 9.
33 Newsholme, *Q. Rep.* (Brighton) 1888, no. 3: 4; and Newsholme, "Special Report on Diarrhoeal Mortality. . . ," 9.
34 For the following information, see Newsholme, untitled report on epidemic diarrhea, Brighton, Proc San. Comm., 8 (11 June 1891): 234–47.; or ibid., Brighton, *Proc. Town Council, Proc Comm.* (18 June 1891): 22–9. Subsequent citations will be made to the latter, the published edition.
35 Newsholme, untitled report on epidemic diarrhea . . . 1891, 26.

Newsholme concluded that preventing surface pollution of the soil would effectively control epidemic diarrhea. The Corporation needed to see that putrefying organic material did not accumulate on the surface of the ground around houses, just as it had seen that the pollution of the subsoil was reduced by banishing cesspools and, in the process, had reduced the town's typhoid mortality.[36] Accomplishing this goal obviously required changes in working-class behavior. But given the conditions in which many working families had to live, reducing infant diarrhea required also services which only the local authority could provide. The houses of the vast majority of laborers or artisans did not have movable dustbins (garbage cans), and the best that could be hoped for was that rubbish and kitchen wastes would be placed in the fixed ash pits in back yards.[37] But even this measure was seldom employed. Ash pits were often in poor repair, dustmen did not automatically stop at individual houses and had to be called in by family members, and in many small houses whose back yards could be entered only from the house, ash pits had to be emptied by carrying the decomposing refuse through the house. These circumstances provided every encouragement to allow organic waste to collect around houses and the likelihood that this material would be brought into houses on feet or hands, by flies, or as dust where it could "poison food and produce diarrhea."[38]

Newsholme began a campaign to secure better municipal scavenging (garbage collection).[39] His ideal was daily collection of waste from covered metal containers placed in front of every house and more vigorous street cleaning in summer. He had to settle, however, for incremental improvements in household refuse collection: Weekly collection began in the spring of 1892 following a trial the previous spring and then semiweekly collections beginning in 1899. This more vigorous municipal scavenging was assisted by a major capital expenditure undertaken in the 1890s. In 1896 the Corporation received sanction from the Local Government Board to borrow money to construct a municipal dust destructor, or incinerator.[40]

Newsholme was eager to demonstrate the effectiveness of these new measures. In November of 1892 after only a few months of slightly more vigorous scavenging, Newsholme very prematurely announced the success of these new efforts, crediting them with the much lower diarrhea mortality in the third quarter of 1891 over the same period in the preceding year.[41] The naivete of this view was

36 Ibid., 25.   37 For his description of the methods of disposing of this waste, see ibid., 26–27.
38 Ibid., 27.
39 For the following, see Arthur Newsholme, "Letter to Members of the Sanitary Committee, 30 May 1891, Brighton, Proc. San. Comm., 8 (11 June 1891): 233–47; Brighton, Proc. San. Comm., 8 (25 June 1891): 270; Brighton, *Proc. Town Council* (2 April 1892): i–ix; and Newsholme, *Ann. Rep.* (Brighton) 1899: 47–9.
40 See correspondence between the Corporation's officials and the Local Government Board in P.R.O. MH12/12796. The architect's plans for the destructor are in the East Sussex Record Office DB/D16/33 & 34. Brighton was only one of many towns to build an incinerator in these years. Towns usually found that the incinerator both improved municipal cleanliness and saved the town money, Wohl, *Endangered Lives,* 85–6.
41 Newsholme, *Q. Rep.* (Brighton) 1891, no. 3: 4–6.

apparent by 1895 when the diarrhea mortality in Brighton that summer reached a near record high.[42] He was insistent, however, that his strategy was the correct one. He found confirming evidence in the comparative study of diarrhea in the thirty-one largest towns of Britain, which he presented as his Presidential Address to the Society of Medical Officers of Health in 1899, in which he attempted to demonstrate that towns which had the best systems of scavenging and those which relied on water closets rather than on pails or middens had the lowest rates of mortality from epidemic diarrhea.[43] Again in 1902 he argued that the recently instituted semiweekly refuse collection together with frequent summer rains were responsible for the low diarrhea mortality that year.[44]

While Newsholme continued to press for higher standards of municipal scavenging, by the middle nineties he was reassessing his position on epidemic diarrhea, becoming more convinced that epidemic diarrhea, and preventable infant mortality more generally, was a special problem of infant feeding.[45] He noticed, for example, that the incidence of this disease was especially high around six months of age, a time when infants were commonly weaned from breast to bottle. Moreover, bottle-fed babies were much more likely to develop infant diarrhea than were those who were exclusively breast-fed. In Brighton, during the third quarter of 1895, the inspectors found that 43 of 44 (98%) infants under nine months of age who had died from epidemic diarrhea had been bottle-fed. In subsequent years home inquiries about the method of infant feeding for each child who had died of epidemic diarrhea confirmed that most of these young victims had been bottle-fed.[46] As early as 1895 Newsholme was advocating the establishment of a milk depot in Brighton where mothers could purchase sterilized milk in small feeding bottles.[47] But at this time he assumed that this service, like maternal education, would best be provided by private charity rather than by the local authority.

By the end of 1902 Newsholme adopted a bacterial explanation for epidemic diarrhea, and mention of poisonous fumes from drains and ash heaps now disappeared from his discussions. He agreed with the bacteriologist Sheridan Delépine that epidemic diarrhea was caused by the fecal contamination of milk, most likely resulting in the introduction of bacilli of the coli group.[48] But the question of

---

42 Newsholme, "Special Report on the Diarrheal Mortality . . . 1895," 8.
43 Newsholme, "Contribution to the Study of Epidemic Diarrhoea," 155–7.
44 Newsholme, *Ann. Rep.* (Brighton) 1902: 48. This section of the 1902 report was republished as Arthur Newsholme, "Epidemic Diarrhoea, Municipal Scavenging, Rainfall, and Temperature," *Public Health*, 15 (1902–3): 654.
45 For the following argument see Newsholme, "Special Report on Diarrheal Mortality . . . 1895," 8–11.
46 Newsholme, *Ann. Rep.* (Brighton) 1897: 35.
47 Newsholme, *Ann. Rep.* (Brighton), 1895, 21; ibid., 1897: 35.
48 Arthur Newsholme, "Remarks on the Causation of Epidemic Diarrhoea, Introducing the Discussion on Professor Delépine's Paper," *Trans. Epidem. Soc. Lond.*, 22 (1902–3): 34–43. The paper in question is S. Delépine, "The Bearing of Outbreaks of Food Poisoning upon the Etiology of Epidemic Diarrhoea," ibid., 11–33.

how milk became contaminated remained. Delépine suspected that the chief sites of contamination were on the farm and in transit to the consumer. Newsholme found this explanation inadequate. Using the analogy between typhoid fever and epidemic diarrhea, which he had already used productively,[49] and his own inquiries on the milk supply of infants who died of diarrhea in Brighton between 1900 and 1902, he concluded that contamination on the farm or during delivery might cause epidemics of diarrhea but that most cases occurred sporadically and were caused by contamination of milk in the home.[50] Airborne transmission remained important to him with fecal dust and houseflies playing important parts. Ingestion of bacteria in other foods or on fingers also helped explain the occurrence of cases. Newsholme found empirical support for home contamination in the deaths of infants who had not consumed fresh cow's milk and whose cases could not therefore be linked to contamination on the farm or in transit. A study of deaths attributed to diarrhea in Liverpool showed that 20% of the victims had been breast-fed, while his study in Brighton revealed that nearly 10% of the victims of diarrhea were breast-fed and that 44% had been fed on condensed milk, which he assumed was contaminated only after it had been opened.[51]

By this time Newsholme's practical work showed his change of thinking. He revised his circular on how to prevent epidemic diarrhea.[52] While the advice was familiar, the emphasis was very different. Infant feeding now received the most attention and the largest type, and environmental sanitation was reduced to three short, general statements in the lower left corner. By 1896 he had prepared a special pamphlet on infant feeding which was distributed by the local Registrars when a birth was reported, and by 1902 physicians at the Children's Hospital were also distributing copies of a similar pamphlet Newsholme had written.[53] His studies of infant diarrhea in the early twentieth century also reveal his changed views. Beginning in 1903 he systematically gathered information on infant feeding practices, both in families where an infant diarrhea death occurred and among the general population, and he assigned his Assistant Medical Officer to do bacterial counts of samples of fresh and condensed milk.[54] The bacterial studies were inconclusive, but the study of feeding practices gave some striking results. Among the 1,259 babies under one year of age found living during 1903, 1904, and 1905 in 10,308 Brighton homes, 62.3% were fed only at the breast, 7.2% were fed cow's milk only, and 3.1% were fed exclusively condensed milk. But among those infants

49 Newsholme, "Contribution to the Study of Epidemic Diarrhoea," 166–7.
50 Newsholme, "Remarks on the Causation," 37–40. See also Newsholme, *Ann. Rep.* (Brighton) 1902: 49–51.
51 Newsholme, "Remarks on the Causation," 37, 38.
52 For a copy of this circular, see Arthur Newsholme, "The Public Health Aspects of Summer Diarrhoea," *Practitioner*, 69 (1902) 176.
53 Brighton, Proc. San. Comm., 13 (27 Feb. 1896): 299; ibid., 19 (13 March 1902): 123–4; ibid., 22 (25 Jan. 1906): 379.
54 For a summary of the results, see Arthur Newsholme, "Domestic Infection in Relation to Epidemic Diarrhoea," *J. Hygiene*, 6 (1906): 139–48.

who died of diarrhea during their first year of life during these years only 6.5% had been fed exclusively at the breast, 36.0% had been fed only cow's milk, and 30.3% had been fed only condensed milk. Clearly, artificial feeding posed special risks of infant diarrhea.

Despite the importance he began to attach to infant feeding Newsholme resisted making the control of infant diarrhea simply a matter of encouraging breast-feeding or the giving of advice on the preparation of safe formula. The fact that bottle-fed infants in prosperous homes did not contract diarrhea suggested that artificial feeding per se was not the cause of epidemic diarrhea. And the occurrence of fatal diarrhea among breast-fed infants and even among adults in poor homes implicated special conditions in the homes of the poor. Correctly considered, milk, Newsholme argued, was not the cause of diarrhea but rather the vehicle of contagion, just as mosquitoes were the vehicle for malaria and rats for plague.[55] The cause was the ingestion of intestinal organisms. The contamination of milk was a problem of both human behavior and of environmental circumstance.

By the middle nineties Newsholme acknowledged that families had to bear a large share of the responsibility for the contamination of infant food,[56] but he never believed epidemic diarrhea was the product of the failure of motherhood or solely a private matter in which public authority had no responsibility or only an indirect responsibility to provide warnings and advice. The poor faced special risks.[57] They lived in more crowded spaces, in closer proximity to the waste and fecal dust of streets and yards, and they lacked adequate facilities for properly storing and preparing infant food.

Only those who frequently visit the homes of the poor in summer can realize that food can scarcely escape massive foecal infection. There are no pantries; food is stored in cupboards in a living room or bedroom. The sugar used in sweetening milk is often black with flies, which have come from a neighboring dust-bin or manure-heap, or from the liquid stools of a diarrheal patient in a neighboring house. Flies have to be picked out of the half-empty can of condensed milk before its remaining contents can be used for the patient's next meal.[58]

Since many of these circumstances were beyond the control of the poor, the local authority had to bear a large share of the responsibility for controlling diarrhea. Only it could act to provide the basic sanitary services which were needed.

It is important to recognize Newsholme's position here. Just as he tried to balance environmental and behavioral factors in understanding infant diarrhea, he also made the control of infant mortality both a public and a private concern. He never assumed that the prevention of infant mortality and epidemic diarrhea could be reduced to a simple strategy of teaching mothers and future mothers to do

55 Newsholme, "Contribution to the Study of Epidemic Diarrhoea," 167.
56 Newsholme, "Special Report on Diarrheal Mortality. . . ," 10.   57 Ibid.
58 Newsholme, *Ann. Rep.* (Brighton) 1902): 51.

their duty of feeding infants properly. Nor was diarrhea or infant mortality a special problem which could be logically or practically separated from other municipal public health work. This work must be part of an integrated system of preventive medical services supervised locally by the M.O.H. These are positions he consistently held. We will encounter them again, when we consider his career at the Local Government Board, in the studies of infant mortality he directed and in the conflict with the Board of Education.

MEAT INSPECTION AND THE BUTCHERS' REVOLT

In only one area did the Sanitary Department face organized opposition to its inspections. Brighton's butchers were well organized and politically influential.[59] They resented the intrusion of public authority into their trade, and when sufficiently threatened, they were willing to fight. In his conflict with the butchers Newsholme faced a unique challenge to his authority.

The meat trade was a notorious source of nuisances and a special trial to Sanitary Authorities. In Brighton, as in most other towns, animals were slaughtered near the town center.[60] In the late eighties Brighton had 53 private slaughterhouses that prepared meat for 113 butcher shops in town and another 13 in Hove.[61] These slaughterhouses were usually small operations located in courts and alleys adjacent to houses, shops, and even schools. Animals arrived on hoof. They were driven through the streets, where they fouled the roads and pavements and endangered pedestrians. Their confinement in small yards produced noise and the stench of manure and offal that offended neighbors. The accumulating offal and blood attracted rats and sometimes clogged drains.

The Sanitary Department's first concern was to reduce the nuisances associated with slaughtering in densely settled areas. Using the power local authorities possessed to regulate offensive trades such as slaughtering, Brighton had passed bylaws making it unlawful to discharge blood into drains or to allow manure and offal to accumulate on the premises.[62] But enforcement had been lax.[63] Newsholme began by stepping up enforcement of these bylaws. In 1890 consistent with his preference for specialization of function he took responsibility for inspecting premises in which the dairy or meat trades were conducted away from the sanitary

59 For example, the annual dinners of the butchers' trade association were gala affairs attended by the mayor, town councillors and local officials. See accounts in "Brighton Butchers' Association, Annual Dinner," *Sussex Daily News,* 27 Feb. 1896, 7; "Brighton Butchers," ibid., 18 March 1903, 3.
60 For conditions in London, see Wohl, *Endangered Lives,* 84.
61 For Newsholme's descriptions of these slaughterhouses, see Newsholme, *Ann. Rep.* (Brighton), 1889: 24; and Arthur Newsholme, [Report] To the Sanitary Committee, 8 Sept. 1893, Brighton, Proc. San. Comm., 10 (28 Sept. 1893): 428; or ibid., Brighton, *Proc. Town Council, Proc. Comm.,* 5 Oct. 1893: 21. Subsequent citation will be to the latter, the printed version.
62 "Public Health Act, 1875" 38 & 39 Vict., C. 55, sect. 113; Newsholme, "[Report] To the Sanitary Committee," 8 Sept. 1893: 20.
63 For some of the problems of past enforcement, see Newsholme, "[Report] To the Sanitary Committee," 8 Sept. 1893: 20.

inspectors who did the household inspections in particular districts and made one Assistant Inspector responsible for supervising all cowsheds, dairies, slaughterhouses, and butcher shops. His choice, James A. Cuckney, was a very good one.[64] Although he was then a young man and a recently appointed Assistant Inspector, Cuckney knew the meat trade well. His father was a dairy farmer and the superintendent of the cattle market in Lewes, a neighboring Sussex town. The young Cuckney had worked with his father at the market for five years before coming to Brighton to join the police force. After two and a half years as a constable he changed jobs and became an Assistant Inspector of Nuisances. As we shall see, he would prove to be extremely able.

Under this new arrangement inspections were more vigorous and less predictable, and summonses, convictions, and verbal warnings all increased.[65] Newsholme successfully defeated attempts by the Butchers' Association to secure a relaxation of the bylaws prohibiting the discharge of blood into drains, and he eventually convinced the Association to urge its members to contract with private scavengers to remove blood and offal daily.[66] Stricter enforcement through such means brought greater compliance, and through the 1890s complaints of nuisances at slaughterhouses declined.[67]

But as long as slaughtering continued in small private establishments scattered throughout the town, it would be difficult to supervise. Although he did not initiate the movement to establish a public abattoir, that pressure came, as the President of the Butchers' Association described it, "from the cranks on the Council,"[68] Newsholme supported the idea, knowing that it would make supervision easier and more complete.[69] He served on the committee that visited the abattoirs in six other towns and planned the new facility in Brighton.[70] The new abattoir was dedicated on June 29, 1894, by the Mayor, who praised the new facility as an example of the benefits of municipal socialism, but the business of slaughtering at the new facility did not get underway until November.[71] The abattoir, it was hoped, would end the herding of animals through the town's

---

64 For the following information on Cuckney, see ibid., 21–2.

65 Ibid., 21. The Sanitary Committee also called some butchers before it to issue its own warnings. See Brighton, Proc. San. Comm. 7 (24 April 1890): 287–8; ibid., 30 Jan. 1890, 194–5.

66 Brighton, *Proc. Town Council, Proc. Comm.*, 29 Oct. 1891, 20; and Newsholme, *Ann. Rep.* (Brighton), 1891, 8–9; Newsholme, *Ann. Rep.* (Brighton), 1890, 21.

67 See, for example, the rapid decline in the number of convictions for such offenses in Newsholme, "[Report] To the Sanitary Committee, 8 Sept. 1893," 21.

68 J. M. Combridge, at the Thirteenth Annual Dinner of the Brighton and Hove Butchers' Association in "Brighton Butchers," *Sussex Daily News,* 18 March 1903, 3.

69 Newsholme, *Ann. Rep.* (Brighton), 1889, 24. For evidence of his continued support of abattoirs and illustrations of how little slaughtering in Britain changed in the following three and a half decades, see Arthur Newsholme, *Humane Slaughtering and the Public Health: Being the Second Benjamin Ward Richardson Memorial Lecture* (London: The Model Abattoir Society, 1923).

70 Francis J. C. May et al., "[Report] To the Sanitary Committee of the Town Council. Abattoirs," 15 May 1891 in Brighton, *Proc. Town Council, Proc. Comm.,* 4 June 1891: iii–iv.

71 "Opening of the Brighton Abattoir," *Brighton Herald,* 30 June 1894, 3; and Newsholme, *Ann. Rep.* (Brighton), 1894: 37. Council approval of the plans had come as early as the fall of 1891, Brighton, *Proc. Town Council,* 17 September 1891: iii–iv.

streets. Plans called for animals to arrive by rail at the abattoir docks. The new facility would also ensure that the preparation of meat was under constant public supervision. Newsholme made James Cuckney the Superintendent of the Abattoir. Cuckney lived at the abattoir in a house the Corporation provided, adding supervision of the slaughtering and dressing of meat to his other tasks.

While the number of animals slaughtered at the abattoir slowly grew, exceeding 10,000 in 1896 and 20,000 in 1902, the institution did not live up to its promise in the early years.[72] Butchers resisted moving, complaining of the inconvenient location of the abattoir,[73] and dozens who used the abattoir also retained their private slaughterhouses.[74] There were also problems in delivering animals. Neither the Council nor the London, Brighton, and South Coast Railroad was eager to finance the building of docks at the abattoir,[75] and the railroad had a dispute with cattle drovers over the sorting of animals bound for the new facility. The result was that through the nineties most cattle continued to arrive in Brighton at the central station. From there they were driven through the streets to the abattoir, a distance of about three-quarters of a mile. In March 1900 Cuckney reported that although to date a total of 150 trucks of animals had arrived at the abattoir docks, five-sixths of the animals slaughtered there still arrived in the old way, on foot.[76]

The abattoir might be underused, but the Sanitary Department had succeeded in enforcing higher standards of public hygiene on the town's butchers. Nuisances around slaughterhouses were now less common, and an increasing portion of the town's red meat was prepared under public supervision. Butchers complained about the stricter enforcement and closer supervision, and they did not jump at the opportunity to work at the abattoir, but they grudgingly complied with the campaign to abate nuisances. But nuisances were only one of the local authority's hygienic interests in the meat trade. Another was the quality of meat. Brighton had its share of shoddy butchers who bought sick cattle on the cheap and sold their meat in the streets on Saturday night or passed it along to sausage makers and others who could disguise it for resale. It was not only the most disreputable in

72 Newsholme, *Ann. Rep.* (Brighton), 1896, 38; ibid., 1902, 96.
73 See the President's remarks at the annual dinner of the Brighton and Hove Butchers' Association in "Brighton Butchers," *Sussex Daily News,* 18 March 1903, 3.
74 Private slaughterhouses continued to operate in Brighton until well into the twentieth century. The last registration of a new slaughterhouse is recorded to have taken place in 1927, and the last recorded action against a private slaughterhouse occurred in 1935. See Brighton, Register of Slaughter Houses [manuscript], East Sussex Record Office, R/C11/1.
75 Newsholme and the Sanitary Committee had urged the Corporation to negotiate with the London, Brighton, and South Coast Railroad for the delivery of all animals directly to the abattoir and to offer as an incentive for cooperating new unloading facilities at the abattoir at a nominal lease. Arthur Newsholme, letter to the Sanitary Committee 13 Dec. 1894 in Brighton, Proc. San. Comm., 12 (13 Dec. 1894): 125–7; or Brighton, *Proc. Town Council, Proc. Comm.,* 20 Dec. 1894: 20–1; Brighton, Proc. San. Comm., 12 (10 Jan. 1895): 176; or Brighton, *Proc. Town Council, Proc. Comm.,* 17 Jan. 1895: 20. But the Town Council refused to approve this plan, apparently fearing to offer subsidy to a railway company, Brighton, *Proc. Town Council,* 17 Jan. 1895: iii–iv.
76 Brighton, Proc. San. Comm., 17 (8 March 1900): 152; or Brighton, *Proc. Town Council, Proc. Comm.,* 15 March 1900: 16–17.

the trade who engaged in such practices. Some trade leaders also had a hand in this market. The seizure and condemnation of meat was a much more controversial part of the Sanitary Department's agenda. Butchers felt their interests more keenly threatened. The conflict with the butchers came to a head in 1893 and 1894. It nearly ended Cuckney's and Newsholme's careers in Brighton.

The Public Health Act, 1875, empowered Medical Officers of Health and Inspectors of Nuisances to enter premises where meat, fish, poultry, and certain other foods were sold and to seize samples found to be "diseased or unsound or unwholesome or unfit for the food of man."[77] Seized goods were to be taken to a justice, who, if he found that the goods met the preceding criteria could condemn them, order them destroyed, and fine the seller. Justices could also issue warrants to an M.O.H. or to an Inspector to enter a building where there was reason to believe that diseased or unsound meat or certain other food was concealed. Through the Brighton Improvement Act, 1884, the Corporation had secured the extension of these clauses to all food stuffs sold in Brighton for human consumption and had gained the power either to revoke the license of those convicted of selling or having in their possession for sale diseased meat or to remove their premises from the register of slaughterhouses.[78] The law thus provided severe penalties, but the strongest sanctions were seldom invoked. Newsholme in fact found that it was almost impossible to close a registered slaughterhouse.[79]

Enforcement thus had two parts; seizure in town and condemnation before a magistrate. Each posed special problems. Newsholme believed that meat could be properly inspected only at the place where it was slaughtered, so that all internal organs could be inspected.[80] For this reason alone he wanted to see all private slaughterhouses abolished and all slaughtering moved to the public abattoir. But that outcome could not be immediately achieved. In the meantime the Sanitary Department tried to locate diseased meat as best it could. This task fell primarily to Cuckney.[81] In this task he was conscientious, resourceful, even courageous. His experience with police investigation was undoubtedly a help to him. In inspecting cowsheds he found diseased cows, which he later traced to local butcher shops. He learned the ways the shoddy beef trade worked.[82] He learned, for example, that there were a few sources beyond the town's jurisdiction that were responsible for much of Brighton's diseased meat. The market in Haywards Heath was

77 38 & 39 Vict. C.55, sect. 116–19.   78 47 & 48 Vict. C.262, sect. 120 & 121.

79 Arthur Newsholme, testimony, *Report of the Royal Commission Appointed to Inquire into the Administrative Procedures for Controlling Danger to Man through the Use as Food of the Meat and Milk of Tuberculous Animals,* B.P.P. 1898, XLIX: 187–8 & 190.

80 Newsholme, testimony, ibid., 187–8.

81 For Newsholme's report on these activities, see "[Report] To the Sanitary Committee, 8 September 1893," 22.

82 See Newsholme's account of shady trade practices and the ways his Department dealt with them in Newsholme, testimony *Royal Commission on Tuberculosis,* 186–7, 188.

notorious for dealing in questionable cattle, and a pig farmer near Brighton who fed his animals on the offal from Brighton's slaughterhouses pushed many sick animals on to the market. On information supplied by police in neighboring areas Cuckney succeeded in intercepting diseased beef entering town concealed in clothes baskets. He also staged nighttime and early morning raids to catch butchers handling loads of diseased beef. One night he tracked a group of men from farm to butcher shop. They brought with them the carcass of a cow they had dressed on the farm. The cow had died of disease some hours before they had dressed it.

Condemnation and conviction posed even more difficult problems. Proving that meat was diseased or unfit for human consumption was very problematic. The law protected the butcher's interest in his property and placed restrictions on the M.O.H.'s actions.[83] He could not cut into a carcass before seizing it. His determination of its soundness had to be made without dissection. He could only seize a whole carcass and was forbidden to cut off part of it for condemnation. If he seized a carcass, he could then dissect it to further investigate its condition. But if he failed to secure its condemnation, the owner could sue him for damages. Seizures were most frequent and condemnation most uncertain in cases of bovine tuberculosis. Experts disagreed on whether meat from tuberculous cows could be safely eaten. There were physicians, some of them with more experience in public health than Newsholme, who would testify in the defense of butchers.[84] One of these dramatized his testimony for the defense by chewing a piece of the seized meat before the magistrate.

In the early 1890s the major point of contention was how much of a tuberculous carcass should be condemned. Few medical men doubted that tissue containing tubercles was unfit for human consumption. But what about other flesh from the same animal? Was flesh that showed no sign of tuberculosis fit to eat, if it came from a cow that had tuberculosis in other organs? Newsholme wanted to see the entire carcass condemned, if tubercular lesions were found widely in the abdomen and thorax and if the lymphatic glands were involved, regardless of whether muscle tissue were obviously affected.[85] But not all experts agreed. A case Newsholme lost in 1891 highlights the conflict of expert opinion on this issue.[86] Before seizure and dissection, inspection showed tubercles surrounding the ribs, an abscess in the left fore-quarter, and a large abscess in one buttock. Dissection revealed that the carcass was riddled with tubercular masses, abscesses, and caseous glands. Newsholme wanted the entire carcass condemned, but two physicians and two veterinarians testified that since there was no wasting of the flesh, the disease should still be considered local not general, and hence the unaffected portion of the carcass was fit for human consumption. Newsholme countered that using emaciation as the primary criterion of general tuberculosis or as the guideline for condemnation was medically unwarranted. It made as little

---

83 Newsholme, *Ann. Rep.* (Brighton) 1891: 10.   84 Newsholme, *Fifty Years,* 237–8.
85 Newsholme, testimony, *Royal Commission on Tuberculosis,* 186, 190.
86 For discussion of this case, see Newsholme, *Ann. Rep.* (Brighton) 1891: 10–12.

sense as claiming that before the appearance of a general symptom, the rash, smallpox was not contagious. When tuberculosis appeared in many separate organs, it was clear that the bacilli had traveled through the general circulation or the lymphatics. In such a case it would be impossible to say that the tuberculosis bacillus was not also present in other portions of the carcass. In the face of conflicting expert testimony the magistrate compromised, condemning the head and internal organs and returning the four quarters to the owner. Under these circumstances the Sanitary Department was likely to seize only the most obviously diseased meat. Historical evidence suggests that seizures of meat in Brighton in these years were not for trivial or marginal conditions. Meat coming before magistrates was in very poor condition.

An important test of Newsholme's authority as M.O.H. began with a routine seizure on May 2, 1893.[87] Cuckney found part of an emaciated, smelly beef carcass in a sausage maker's shop and the remainder in a butcher shop in North Road. Seizure and investigation led to the conviction of both the butcher and the sausage maker.[88] The significance of this case lay not in the convictions but in the identity of the butcher. John M. Combridge owned three butcher shops in town and was an important member and future president of the Butcher's Association.[89] He had been a member of the Town Council since 1887, and currently he sat on the Sanitary Committee. Unlike many tradesmen who ran afoul of the sanitary authority, Combridge was a formidable opponent. He hired three lawyers, including a Queen's Council, and secured the overturning of his conviction on a technicality.[90] He also saw that there were political consequences of his prosecution. His friends and sympathizers on the Council, particularly the pugnacious solicitor Richard Ballard, criticized the town's officials, called for Cuckney's dismissal and his replacement with a "qualified and experienced" and a "practical" inspector, and blocked the Corporation from retaining counsel to meet the appeal of the convicted sausage maker.[91]

On this occasion Newsholme succeeded in retaining the confidence of his Committee. His forceful defense of his inspectors and his policy on meat inspec-

87 I have described this episode in somewhat greater detail in John M. Eyler, "Policing the Food Trades: Epidemiology, Hygiene, and Public Administration in Edwardian Brighton," in *History of Hygiene: Proceeding of the 12th International Symposium on the Comparative History of Medicine – East and West*, ed. Yosio Kawakita, Shizu Sakai, and Yasuo Otsuka (Tokyo: Ishiyaku EuroAmerican, 1991), 197–201.

88 For evidence and court proceedings, see "Important Meat Prosecution at Brighton," *Brighton Gazette*, 27 May 1893, 6; and "The Tuberculous Cow," ibid., 1 June 1893, 6.

89 For information on Combridge, see *Pike's Brighton & Hove Blue Book*, 1891: 616; and *D. B. Friend & Co.'s Brighton Almanack*, 1894: 22, 24.

90 "Important Meat Prosecution at Brighton," 6; *Brighton Herald*, 22 July 1893, 3; and Brighton. Proc. San. Comm., 10 (13 July 1893): 331; or Brighton, *Proc. Town Council, Proc. Comm.*, 20 July 1893: 25.

91 *Brighton Gazette*, 22 July 1893, 5; *Brighton Herald*, 22 July 1893, 3; and *Brighton Gazette*, 22 July 1893, 5; Brighton, Proc. San. Comm., 10 (8 June 1893): 301; ibid. (27 July 1893): 355; and ibid. (28 Sept. 1893): 426–33. Or see the same text in Brighton, *Proc. Town Council, Proc. Comm.*, 15 June 1893: 23; ibid. 4 Aug. 1893: 25; and ibid. 5 Oct. 1893: 20–3.

tion was accepted by the Sanitary Committee,[92] and it looked as if he had weathered the storm. But that autumn his opponents gained a great advantage when Combridge was elected Chairman of the Sanitary Committee. Another butcher who had been a defense witness at Combridge's trial also sat on the Committee.[93] Unless Newsholme relaxed his enforcement policy, a showdown with his Committee now seemed inevitable. It began on June 13 and 14 of the following year, when Cuckney came to Newsholme with the news that he had found two more emaciated, diseased, beef carcasses in slaughterhouses owned by Combridge.[94] Newsholme seized the carcasses and took them before a magistrate, but in order to protect himself, he also took three allies on the Sanitary Committee, one of them a medical man, to see the carcasses before they were destroyed.[95]

Combridge now resorted to intrigue. He kept a careful distance from formal meetings, but he used his influence in the Committee to block his own prosecution, and his friends on the Council in a long and stormy session kept that body from overturning the Sanitary Committee's action and saw to it that his name and the nature of the offense were not mentioned in the public portion of the meeting.[96] Evidently the other butcher on the Committee maintained that he had seen the carcass and was certain that it was not diseased. In the end the Committee's report was accepted, and a motion of no confidence in the Sanitary Committee brought forward by a disgruntled committee member was defeated. The Council had in effect voted no confidence in its Sanitary Department and seriously undermined the credibility of its health officials.

It looked at first as if the butchers' revolt would succeed, but its architects had not reckoned with the importance that health had acquired in the town's politics. In protest over the Council's action five members of the Sanitary Committee resigned and held interviews with the press.[97] They maintained a discreet silence about details, including Combridge's name, but they complained bitterly about the actions of the Committee and the Council. Brighton's newspapers were sympathetic to the protesting minority.[98] While editorials also did not give details of the alleged wrongdoing at the heart of the controversy, they criticized the secrecy and the lack of dignity of the Council proceedings. It proved impossible

92 Brighton, Proc. San. Comm., 10 (28 Sept. 1893): 426–33; or Brighton, *Proc. Town Council, Proc. Comm.*, 5 Oct. 1893: 20–3

93 This was Christopher Sutton.

94 Brighton, Proc. San. Comm., 11 (28 June 1894): 345; or Brighton, *Proc. Town Council, Proc. Comm.*, 2 July 1894: 18.

95 Newsholme, *Fifty Years*, 156. In this autobiographical account Newsholme mentions no names, but the medical man in question was probably Councillor Turton, F.R.C.S.

96 Brighton, Proc. San. Comm., 11 (28 June 1894): 345; or Brighton, *Proc. Town Council, Proc. Comm.*, 2 July 1894: 18; Brighton, Proc. San. Comm., 11 (30 June 1894): 354–5; Brighton, *Proc. Town Council*, 5 July 1894: iii–v. See also "Brighton Council," *Sussex Daily News*, 6 July 1894, 6; "The Town Council and Condemned Meat: A Secret Sitting," *Brighton Herald*, 7 July 1894, 3; and *Brighton Gazette*, 7 July 1894, 5.

97 *Brighton Gazette*, 12 July 1894, 5.

98 *Sussex Daily News*, 7 July 1894, 7; ibid., 9 July 1894, 4; *Brighton Guardian*, 11 July 1894, 5; and *Brighton Herald*, 14 July 1894, 2.

to control the political damage. Soon the London papers had caught wind of the controversy, and the Local Government Board and the Home Office received letters from Brighton residents calling for an investigation.[99]

Cambridge soon felt himself losing support. While at the next Council meeting his allies mounted a bombastic attack on the tyranny of town officials for harassing an innocent businessman, Cambridge felt that he had no choice but to join the five protesters in submitting his resignation from the Committee.[100] The political tide had turned. A lead editorial in the *Brighton Herald* contended that the issue had become the credibility of the Town Council.[101] In Brighton disgust at Council proceedings and the reflex to protect the town's reputation for health had become potent forces.

The butchers' revolt collapsed by the Council meeting of August 3, about a month after it had begun. All the remaining members of the Sanitary Committee except the second butcher submitted their resignations. The Council dissolved the old Committee and in its place created a new one with some of Newsholme's warmest supporters, including Joseph Ewart, the former mayor and Sanitary Committee chairman and a longtime partisan of Newsholme and of strict enforcement of the sanitary code.[102] Neither of the butchers' henchmen was reelected to the Committee. Thus, belatedly, the Council had backed its M.O.H. and the policy of strict enforcement. The public record makes no mention of Newsholme's actions to defend himself and his policy in his battle with Combridge and associates. As a public official he was barred from direct political activity, but there is no doubt that he lobbied hard for support. Four decades later he observed with quiet satisfaction that "Brighton may claim the distinction of being the only Sanitary Authority whose sanitary officials have been instrumental in ejecting one and securing the election of a new Public Health or Sanitary Committee."[103]

Hereafter in sanitary inspections Newsholme had the full support of the Sanitary Committee, the Town Council, and the Magistrates.[104] For four consecutive years after the butchers' revolt he did not have to contest a single meat seizure before a Magistrate. Trade rebellion had been quelled and public support demonstrated. About the same time he was pleased to observe that the recently issued report of the Royal Commission of Tuberculosis seemed to vindicate the policy of meat inspection and condemnation which Brighton had evolved over the previous few years. He had told that Commission that Brighton's butchers now voluntarily gave up diseased carcasses even though they received no compensa-

99 Newsholme, *Fifty Years*, 157; John George Allen, letter to Local Government Board, 14 July 1894, P.R.O. MH 12/12796. See also reports of appeals for inquiries in *Brighton Gazette*, 12 July 1894, 5; and *Brighton Herald*, 11 Aug. 1894, 3.

100 Brighton, *Proc. Town Council*, 19 July 1894: vii; *Brighton Gazette*, 21 July 1894, 5; and *Brighton Herald*, 21 July 1894, 3.

101 *Brighton Herald*, 21 July 1894, 2.

102 Brighton, *Proc. Town Council*, 3 Aug. 1894: ii, iv–vi, x; and *Sussex Daily News*, 3 Aug. 1894, 4.

103 Newsholme, *Fifty Years*, 157.   104 For the following assessment, see ibid., 157, 238.

tion.[105] Although much trade opposition to the abattoir remained and the animals slaughtered there accounted for only 12 percent of the meat sold in Brighton, and although the abattoir was still not self-supporting, Newsholme believed that public demand would encourage the trade to change. The Sanitary Department might still be reluctant to stamp or mark meat prepared in the abattoir fearing trade opposition, but such meat was beginning to command higher prices, so that some butchers advertised in their shop windows that they sold meat prepared under the constant supervision of the public authority.

While it is undoubtedly true that a Medical Officer of Health had to continually reestablish his authority, this incident was especially important to Newsholme. Sanitary inspections and enforcement inevitably annoyed and financially challenged a wide array of interests, landlords, tenants, shopkeepers, and tradesmen, but this was the only episode during Newsholme's career in Brighton in which the vested interests were so well organized and politically well placed. Newsholme's vindication despite the fact that opponents of his policy had maneuvered themselves into positions of authority over him shows that his policy of selective but strict enforcement of hygienic standards had wide support. In the end, filth and diseased meat had no champions. Growing civic pride and rising standards of public hygiene guaranteed an M.O.H. who was persistent and prudent the essential support he needed in the enforcement of the sanitary code.

HOUSING AND PUBLIC HEALTH

During the twenty years Newsholme was in Brighton the Corporation condemned, purchased, cleared, and supervised the rebuilding of three notorious slum areas (see Illustrations 3.1 and 3.2): the Little St. James's Street Area (A on Illustration 3.2); the Cumberland Place Area, marked B; and the Spa Street Area, marked C. Broad streets and rows of new houses built according to a municipal plan replaced the old houses, narrow streets, and courts. This work was a major undertaking.[106] The Corporation cleared an area in excess of 30,000 square yards and displaced 2,058 people at a net cost (exclusive of new homes) in excess of £71,000.[107] The effort and expense were in fact much greater, because as part of these improvement schemes the Corporation built homes and tenements on vacant land on five streets to the north of these old slums.[108]

Brighton was not in the vanguard of urban renewal. The Corporations of

---

105 For the following, see Newsholme, testimony, *Report of the Royal Commission on Tuberculosis,* 185–6, 188–9.

106 The Little St. James's Street area was now bisected by St. James's Avenue. The Cumberland Place scheme created two new streets, White and Blaker Streets. And Tillstone Street became the focus of the Spa Street project.

107 Newsholme, *Ann. Rep.* (Brighton), 1902, 82; and Arthur Newsholme, *Special Report on Overcrowding, on the Clearing of Insanitary Areas, and on the Provision of Housing Accommodation by the Town Council* (Brighton: County Borough of Brighton, 1904), 14.

108 These streets are Ewart Street, St. Helen's Road, May Road, Elm Grove, and Dewe Road.

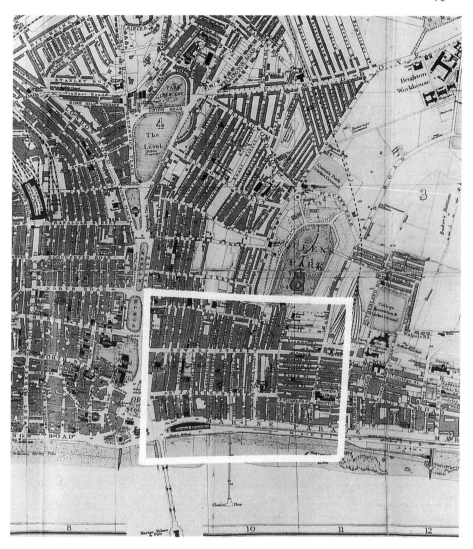

Illustration 3.1. Street plan of Brighton, 1899, showing the area where the improvement schemes were located.

Liverpool, Birmingham, and Glasgow and the Metropolitan Board of Works, for example, had all undertaken large municipal slum clearance projects before 1880.[109] But prior to 1890 few towns had acted. During its first twelve years

109 For a short summary, see Anthony S. Wohl, *Endangered Lives: Public Health in Victorian Britain* (Cambridge, Mass.: Harvard Univ. Press, 1983), 315–17. There is a large historical literature on

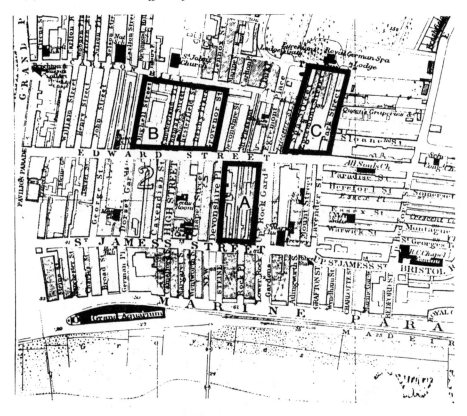

Illustration 3.2. Brighton's improvement schemes begun 1889–98. See Illustration 3.1 for location of this detail.

(1875–87) the Cross Act,[110] the major piece of general legislation permitting this work, was applied by only twelve provincial towns.[111] Brighton Corporation became active in such urban renewal as national interest in the housing questions grew in the late 1880s. Parliament sought to encourage municipal initiative by

slum clearance and housing reform. In the present context see especially Anthony S. Wohl, *The Eternal Slum: Housing and Social Policy in Victorian London* (London: Edward Arnold, 1977); J. A. Yelling, *Slums and Slum Clearance in Victorian London* (London: Allen and Unwin, 1986); Colin G. Pooley, "Housing for the Poorest Poor: Slum-clearance and Rehousing in Liverpool, 1890–1918," *J. Hist. Geography,* 11 (1985) 70–88; Iain C. Taylor, "The Insanitary Housing Question and Tenement Dwellings in Nineteenth-century Liverpool," in *Multi-storey Living: The British Working-Class Experience,* ed. Anthony Sutcliffe (London: Croom Helm, 1974), 41–87; and J. N. Tarn, "Housing in Liverpool and Glasgow: The Growth of Civic Responsibility," *Town Planning J.,* 39 (1968–9), 319–34.

110 "Artizans and Labourers Dwelling Improvement Acts, 1875" 38 & 39 Vict. C. 36
111 Wohl, *Endangered Lives,* 317.

passing the Housing of the Working Classes Act, 1890.[112] This act codified and strengthened existing housing legislation. Part I continued the powers granted under the Cross Act to clear and rebuild whole areas. It was under this authority that Brighton cleared the three areas just mentioned. Part II incorporated the authority given by the Torrens Act[113] to condemn individual houses or areas too small to be dealt with under Part I and to compel their owners to repair them or to tear them down. Part III amended the Shaftesbury Act of 1885, which allowed local authorities to build and operate lodging houses for the working classes.

Responsibility for carrying an improvement scheme to completion fell to other town officials besides the M.O.H., to the Town Clerk and the Borough Surveyor in particular, and to the Sanitary Committee as a whole. But this late Victorian housing legislation made the Medical Officer of Health responsible for initiating slum clearance projects, and it established the threat to the public health, usually measured by high local mortality rates, as the criterion for public action. Medical Officers of Health were often more anxious to employ these powers than their towns were. In 1877, only two years after the Cross Act, Brighton's first M.O.H., R. P. B. Taaffe, recommended the condemnation and destruction of the Cumberland Place and Spa Street areas.[114] While the Sanitary Committee concurred and commissioned the Borough Surveyor to draw up plans for reconstruction, and while the medical press held forth the familiar threat that Brighton would lose its resort trade if it did not do something about its slums,[115] the Town Council refused to act. By the late eighties the political climate had changed. With an outbreak of typhoid fever occurring in the Little St. James's Street area, Newsholme was able to convince his Committee in December 1888 that this area should be cleared and rebuilt.[116] He also started the chain of events that led to the two subsequent improvement schemes by producing studies which demonstrated that crude mortality rates as well as rates for the major infectious diseases and for infant mortality were much higher in these slum areas than in the town as a whole and by arguing that the health of these areas could not be improved by any measures short of replacing the housing stock.[117]

---

112 53 & 54 Vict. C. 70. For a discussion of the terms of the act see Wohl, *Eternal Slum*, 252, and Pooley, 70–1.

113 "Artizans' and Labourers' Dwelling Act, 1868" 31 & 32 Vict. C. 130.

114 Information on this abortive reform effort is found in "Report of the Sanitary Committee 1 Jan 1880" in Medical Officers Annual, Quarterly and Special Reports 1879 to 1894, Sussex Postgraduate Medical Centre. See also Brighton. Proc. San. Comm. 1 (25 Oct. 1877). 89; ibid. (28 Feb. 1878), 120; and ibid. (4 Dec. 1879), 326. The reports of Taaffe and the Sanitary Committee are found in Brighton, Proceedings of Committees, Report Book 4 (26 April 1877), 70–6; ibid. (25 Oct. 1877), 68–9; ibid. (23 Jan. 1878), 93; ibid. (1 Jan. 1880) 222–40; ibid. (22 April 1880), 267.

115 "The Back Slums of Brighton," *Lancet* (1881), no. 2: 432.

116 Newsholme's report is found in Brighton, Proc. San. Comm. 6 (27 Dec. 1888): 255–6. For background information on this incident see ibid. 6 (30 Aug. 1888): 148–50; ibid. 6 (4 Sept. 1888): 154–5; ibid. 6 (26 Oct. 1888): 191–5; Newsholme, *Q. Rep.* (Brighton), 1888, no. 3: 2–4; Brighton, *Proc. Town Council,* 3 Jan. 1889: iii; and *Sussex Daily News,* 10 Nov. 1888, 2; ibid., 31 Oct. 1888, 3: and ibid., 4 Jan. 1889, 3.

117 Brighton, Proc. San. Comm. 7 (28 May 1890); 321–6 or Brighton, *Proc. Town Council, Proc.*

The history of Brighton's improvement schemes has yet to be written, but even the most accessible surviving evidence suggests that its conflicts over these projects echo the local disputes found almost everywhere as slums were cleared. The overt questions were who should build and own the new properties, and what sort of houses should be built and what rents charged? But the more fundamental issue was the goal of municipal housing schemes. Was their purpose to provide the town with better houses or was it to rehouse in decent but affordable housing the same people who were displaced from a cleared area? Brighton Corporation began its improvement schemes with the former aim, giving little thought to the fate of displaced persons. In fact while it was national policy that displaced persons should be rehoused on the cleared area, and while the Local Government Board attempted to hold Brighton to its responsibility to do so, none of those displaced from the Little St. James's Street area could afford to live in the new houses constructed there.[118] Rents for these houses determined by market forces ranged between £40 and £60 per year, whereas displaced families, Newsholme later estimated, could not pay more than 5s or 6s per week or £13 and £15 per year.[119] Responding to pressure from local working-class organizations and certain middle-class reformers, the Sanitary Committee recommended that the Corporation itself build and retain ownership of the houses on the second area to be cleared, the Cumberland Place area, with an eye toward charging lower rents than private enterprise could offer.[120] In the spring of 1896 the Town Council wavered amid a lively controversy, first approving the Sanitary Committee's plan, and then overturning it.[121]

In the end the houses in this second cleared area were also privately built and

    Comm. 5 June 1890: 21–3; and Brighton, Proc. San. Comm. 15 (31 March 1898): 294–303; also Brighton, *Proc. Town Council, Proc. Comm.*, 7 April 1898: 28–32.

118 The Housing of the Working Classes Act, 1890, required the rehousing of displaced persons in improvement schemes undertaken in the City and County of London. It gave the L.G.B. the authority to require this rehousing outside the metropolis. See 53 & 54 Vict. C. 70, sect. 11. For the town's negotiations with the L.G.B. that eventually led to a postponement of its obligation to rehouse those it displaced from the Little St. James's Street site see Newsholme, *Ann. Rep.* (Brighton), 1890, 18; and Brighton, *Proc. Town Council, Proc. Comm.*, 15 May 1890: vii–viii; untitled report by Brighton's Town Clerk, F. J. Tillstone, in Brighton, *Proc. Town Council, Proc. Comm.*, 4 May 1893: 22–3; & F. J. Tillstone, Town Clerk, Brighton, to S. B. Provis, Assistant Secretary, L.G.B., 10 Jan. 1893 and drafts of the modified order dated 10 Jan. 1893 and 7 Feb. 1893 in PRO MH12/12795, L.G.B., Poor Law Union Papers.

119 Newsholme, *Special Report on Overcrowding*, 13, 16.

120 Brighton, Proc. San. Comm. 9 (8 Sept. 1892): 341–2; ibid. 9 (9 Oct. 1892): 408; ibid., 10 (14 Sept. 1893): 408–9; ibid., 12 (13 June 1895): 409–10; ibid. 12 (27 June 1895): 433–5; ibid. 13 (14 Nov. 1895): 155; ibid. 13 (6 Dec. 1895): 182–3; ibid. 13 (13 Dec. 1895): 207–8; and ibid. 13 (19 Dec. 1895): 221–2; ibid. 12 (13 June 1895): 409–10; and "Report of the Sanitary Committee," *Brighton, Proc. Town Council, Proc. Comm.*, 16 Jan. 1896: 1–8.

121 For the Council's action, see Brighton, *Proc. Town Council*, 16 Jan. 1896: v–vii; ibid., 16 Jan. 1896: v–vii; ibid. 5 March 1896: iv–vii; and ibid., 30 April 1896: i–ii. There was a great deal of press coverage of this controversy. See especially descriptions of the public meetings "Brighton's Condemned Area," *Sussex Daily News*, 15 Jan. 1896, 2; and *Brighton Herald*, 18 Jan. 1896, 2; *Brighton Herald*, 18 April 1896, 6; *Brighton Gazette*, 18 April 1896, 4; and *Sussex Daily News*, 28 April 1896, 7; *Brighton Gazette*, 30 April 1896, 4; and *Brighton Herald*, 2 May 1896, 4. *Sussex Daily*

brought rents beyond the means of most working-class families. But the controversy over the Cumberland Place area had made the fate of those displaced from cleared areas a public issue and had demonstrated that there was wide public support for council housing (local authority council housing projects) as the only way to provide decent housing for these families. Brighton's transition to the municipal ownership of working-class housing was made easier by the gift the next year of two pieces of undeveloped land well north of the town center. By 1904 the Corporation had built or was completing 101 houses and tenements on those parcels and rented the properties at 5s to 8s per week, within the means of at least the better paid of those it had displaced.[122] Free land, the absence of old structures that had to be cleared away, and very modest design were all needed to keep rents this low, because the Corporation still insisted that rents charged retire the town's debts for these projects. By the time the Council considered the third and final slum clearance project, the Spa Street Improvement Scheme, public auction of the cleared land and private ownership of the new houses were never seriously considered. Public discussion assumed municipal ownership. The Corporation built and retained ownership of these houses as well. They were larger and more expensive than the houses it had built to the north. But rents might have been even higher had the L.G.B. not forced the Corporation to revise its plans, insisting that the semidetached houses in the scheme were "too ambitious in character and design for persons of the labouring class."[123] While the Sanitary Committee and the Town Council were now committed to building council houses for the working-class families it displaced by municipal projects, they clearly hoped to fill the areas near the town center with larger, more expensive houses and to relegate smaller houses and their poorer residents to the periphery.

Throughout his career Newsholme believed housing was a significant public health problem, and his estimate of its importance grew with his experience. By 1900 he had come to view overcrowding as "the central problem in public health."[124] A quarter century later he wrote that housing was "the most serious social problem of today."[125] Even early in his career he was never content merely to help initiate slum clearance projects. In fact as Brighton's improvement schemes consumed increasing amounts of public attention and municipal resources, he worried that they would exhaust public interest and support. For this reason he began to insist that it was just as important to prevent the formation of slums as it was to clear them away once they developed. By the early nineties he was making frequent use of Part II of the Housing of the Working Classes Act, 1890, to force

News, 6 March 1896, 6; see also the following editorials: *Brighton Gazette,* 18 Jan. 1896, 5; and ibid. 7 March 1896, 5; *Brighton Herald,* 7 March 1896, 4.

122 Brighton, Proc. San. Comm. 21 (9 June 1904): 152–3.

123 See the Borough Surveyor's reports in Brighton, Proc. San. Comm. 20 (1 Dec. 1903): 370–1; and ibid. 20 (10 Dec. 1903): 386.

124 Arthur Newsholme, "Notification of Consumption: Its Pros and Cons. Remarks Introductory to a Discussion on the Prevention of Phthisis," *J. Sanitary Inst.* 21 (1900): 53.

125 Arthur Newsholme, *Ministry of Health* (London and New York: G. P. Putnam's Sons, 1925), 156.

owners to improve or to remove condemned properties.[126] Among the great appeals of this strategy was that its cost fell mainly on owners not on the ratepayers and it permitted the removal of individual properties rather than of whole areas.[127] These condemnations were in addition to the notices served on property owners to remedy defects of drainage or other infringements of the sanitary code. Under the 1890 act the Sanitary Department and its Inspectors looked for gross structural defects and for those features, such as deficient light or ventilation which were believed to make dwellings unhealthy. Even houses that were not structurally unsound might be condemned if they had been built with disregard for the needs of light and air and, in particular, if they failed to provide adequate space in the street and in the backyard for through ventilation.[128]

The rationale for condemning a house that did not have what was regarded as adequate ventilation was the conviction among public health authorities that crowding promoted disease and premature death. In the early nineties Newsholme produced two statistical studies designed to investigate that relationship. The first corrected the demonstration William Farr had offered a generation earlier that there was an exact statistical relationship between general mortality and housing density, the latter measured by the number of persons per unit of land area.[129] In a paper presented to the Statistical Society of London Newsholme showed that the experience of London's Peabody Buildings, sets of philanthropically supported, large block-tenement buildings, did not support Farr's density law.[130] Newsholme found that even though these buildings produced high housing density per acre, the mortality rates for their residents were quite low. The general mortality rate for all residents was slightly below that for London as a whole and their infant mortality much below that of the Metropolis. While Newsholme would eventually recognize and use several criteria of overcrowding,[131] it seemed to him in the early 1890s that a tenement's occupancy per room was the most reliable measure of the hygienic significance of crowding.

In his second study he turned to Brighton's mortality experience. Using then unpublished materials for the 1891 census he produced for his Committee in April

---

126 See, for example, Newsholme's summary for 1893 in Newsholme, *Ann. Rep.* (Brighton), 1893, 35. See also the frequent condemnations in the autumn of 1896 in Brighton, Proc. San. Comm. 14 (27 Aug. 1895): 67–8; ibid. 14 (10 Sept. 1896: 84–7; ibid. 14 (24 Sept. 1896): 99–100; and ibid. 14 (8 Oct. 1896): 116–19.

127 Newsholme, *Ann. Rep.* (Brighton), 1898, 41–3; and ibid. 1896, 35–6.

128 Ibid., 1898, 42–3.

129 For a discussion of this study, see John M. Eyler, *Victorian Social Medicine: the Ideas and Methods of William Farr* (Baltimore: Johns Hopkins Univ. Press, 1979), 143–7.

130 Arthur Newsholme, "The Vital Statistics of Peabody Buildings and other Artisans' and Labourers' Block Dwellings," *J. Statist. Soc. Lond.* 54 (1891): 70–99.

131 He identifies four types in Newsholme, *Special Report on Overcrowding,* 7, 21–2. He sometimes used persons per acre as in Newsholme, *Ann. Rep.* (Brighton), 1894, 8–10. But he also used occupancy figures per room or per house as in Newsholme, *Ann. Rep.* (Brighton), 1902, Appendix II: 3–6; and Arthur Newsholme, "Poverty and Disease, as illustrated by the Course of Typhus Fever and Phthisis in Ireland," *Proc. Roy. Soc. Med.* 1 (1907–8), part 1, Epidemiological Sect.: 23–24.

1892 a study in which he grouped Brighton's ninety-two census numeration districts into eight composite districts according to their general or crude mortality rates.[132] To avoid the fallacies often produced by a comparison of crude rates for dissimilar areas, Newsholme corrected these rates for the presence in certain districts of institutions such as hospitals or workhouses. He also attempted to demonstrate that differences in the age and sex distribution of the districts' populations would not invalidate this comparison. The resulting average mortality rates for the composite districts ranged from a low of 8.7 per 1,000 to a high of 27.99 per 1,000 annually. Some comfort, he claimed, could be found in these figures. Five composite districts, housing 56% of Brighton's population, had average annual mortality rates below 17 per 1,000. The average rate for all five was only 13.72 per 1,000. A sixth district holding 24.6% of Brighton's population had a rate of 18 per 1,000. These were low rates and would stand Brighton in good stead in comparison to any place. On the other hand the death rate of the remaining nearly 20 percent of Brighton's population in the two remaining districts was 25 per 1,000.

Such a result shews that were it not for the incubus of poor, unemployed, or only partially-employed, badly-housed, over-crowded, ill-fed and insufficiently-clad inhabitants of certain districts of the town, Brighton as a whole would be able to shew a general death-rate of surprising lowness.[133]

It seemed then that high crude mortality rates were geographically concentrated and associated with overcrowding. Newsholme found that the rank order of these eight composite districts by average annual mortality was followed closely by their ranking according to the average number of families per occupied house, and it corresponded exactly to the order of districts according to the percentage of tenements containing fewer than five rooms.[134] While in this study he did not attempt to investigate the effect of overcrowding on age-specific mortality rates, he did try to demonstrate the validity of the widely held conviction that over-crowding favored zymotic diseases. In Brighton the mortality registers showed unusually high mortality rates from measles, whooping cough, diarrhea, and tuberculosis in these overcrowded districts.[135] In later, shorter studies, he empha-sized the role that overcrowding played in producing elevated mortality from consumption.[136]

In condemning urban areas for redevelopment and in compelling owners of deteriorating or poorly designed buildings to put them in order or to demolish them, Newsholme was operating within the broad political consensus in Brighton

---

132 For the following discussion, see Arthur Newsholme, "Special Report on the Mortality and Causes of Mortality in Eight Districts of Brighton," Brighton, Proc. San. Comm. 9 (28 April 1892): 158–76; or Brighton, *Proc. Town Council, Proc. Comm.*, 5 May 1892: 19–26. Subsequent citations are to the latter, the published version.

133 Ibid., 22.   134 Ibid., 25.

135 Ibid., 23–4.   136 Newsholme, *Ann. Rep.* (Brighton), 1989, 42.

that found common ground between the twin goals of health and social welfare on the one hand and civic beautification and real estate investment on the other. But when he moved beyond the condemning of properties to represent the needs of the poorest classes in town, he lost this political support and found his efforts frustrated. Newsholme realized that poor housing was much more than a problem of architecture or infrastructure. It was a basic social and economic problem.[137] The town's service economy with its low wages and its high real estate values meant that market value rents were beyond the means of many families. Low wages and high rents encouraged families to take in lodgers. This subletting caused crowding, and it also exacerbated the problem by permitting landlords to charge even higher rents. Working-class families were thus caught in a dangerous spiral of overcrowding and escalating rents. The first batch of council houses was a partial solution, but these houses were too few in number and still beyond the means of the families of many unskilled workers. Furthermore there were the additional needs of the very poor, of the single unskilled laborers, and of a transient population who inhabited the town's common lodging houses. Their problems of finding shelter increased as the town's improvement schemes destroyed many of the town's lodging houses.

The typical Victorian common lodging house was an ordinary house into which the owner packed as many people as he could, charging each a few pennies a night. When the beds and bedrooms were full, lodgers sometimes slept in hallways and even in the kitchen. At midcentury one common lodging house in Brighton at 13/14 Cavendish Street contained twelve beds but was known to house routinely around forty people each night at three pence per head.[138] These houses were regarded with grave suspicion by the respectable classes and came early under public scrutiny. In Brighton the Superintendent of Police was made the inspector of these houses in 1858, and by 1881 the Corporation passed bylaws to regulate them.[139] In Newsholme's day the Sanitary Department licensed and inspected common lodging houses, imposing minimum standards of sanitation and accommodation. It even had the right to make surprise midnight inspections.

When the Cumberland Place Improvement Scheme destroyed fifteen of the town's seventeen registered common lodging houses, displacing 270 people, most Brightonians had no regrets. How many of the displaced lodgers, the *Sussex Daily News* wondered editorially, are residents of Brighton anyway?[140] While most speakers expressed sympathy for the needs of honest, productive working families, they had only contempt for the tramps, vagrants, and ne'er-do-wells who, they alleged, frequented common lodging houses. As Medical Officer of Health, Newsholme's view was different. For four years in a row in his *Annual Reports* and during the Sanitary Committee's deliberations on the Cumberland Place

---

137 Newsholme, "Special Report on the Mortality," 25–6.
138 Kevin Fossey, "Slums and Tenements 1840–1900," in Farrant, Fossey, and Peasgood, *Growth of Brighton*, 54, 56.
139 Ibid., 56.   140 "Housing the People," *Sussex Daily News*, 17 Jan. 1896, 4.

Improvement Scheme, he tried to make the destruction of common lodging houses an issue.[141] He argued that both public health and social control required that these lodging houses should be replaced quickly. The Corporation, Newsholme believed, should construct model lodging houses which could be built according to sound hygienic principles and be under strict public supervision.[142] The success of such houses in Glasgow and London showed that local authorities could even make a fair return on such investment.

Newsholme's position found some support among middle-class reformers and on the Sanitary Committee.[143] Initially the Committee resolved to recommend the building of municipal lodging houses on the Cumberland Place site, and a surviving site plan for the Cumberland Place area includes six 60-foot plots for model common lodging houses.[144] But there was strong opposition from property owners and neighbors.[145] The *Brighton Gazette* observed "Edward Street, which has for so many years been fairly tolerant of Cumberland Place and its contemporary haunts of vice and poverty, is now turning up it [sic] nose at the prospect of a well-regulated, municipally controlled common lodging house. Things must be looking up in Edward Street, and we are glad that it should be so."[146] The Town Council turned a cold eye on the proposal, refusing even to approve the Sanitary Committee's resolution to send a delegation to visit model lodging houses in other towns.[147] The Committee soon reversed itself and removed these lodging houses from its plan. The M.O.H.'s arguments for the health benefits of properly designed lodging houses were no match for the distaste many felt for the residents of such houses and the fear that the value of property in the vicinity would suffer.[148] In the end common lodging houses were included in none of the improvement schemes during Newsholme's tenure at Brighton.

The next year, January 1897, Newsholme approached the Sanitary Committee again with a report on subletting and overcrowding.[149] His recommendations appeared under a comparison of mortality rates which showed that mortality from all causes and from measles, diarrhea, tuberculosis, and from bronchitis and pneumonia was much higher in four of Brighton's wards than in the rest of the

---

141 Newsholme, *Ann. Rep.* (Brighton), 1893, 33; ibid. 1894, 36; ibid. 1895, 35; and ibid. 1896, 36; Brighton, Proc. San. Comm. 7 (3 Oct. 1890): 454–57; and ibid. 12 (16 Jan. 1894): 168–9.
142 Newsholme, *Ann. Rep.* (Brighton), 1893, 33.
143 See, for example, the report of the delegation of ministers and civic leaders which called on the Sanitary Committee in June 1895. Brighton, Proc. San. Comm., 12 (13 June 1895): 409–10.
144 Ibid.; and ibid. 13 (6 Dec. 1895): 182–3. The site plan is dated 1 May 1890 and is housed in the East Sussex Record Office in the collection DB/D13/44.
145 For evidence of opposition to the erection of common lodging houses, see the memorial to the Committee from local residents, Brighton, Proc. San. Comm. 13 (13 Dec. 1895): 209.
146 "Municipal Landlordism," *Brighton Gazette,* 16 Jan. 1896, 4.
147 Brighton, *Proc. Town Council,* 17 Jan. 1895: iii–iv.
148 For a sample of views in the Town Council, see the comments of Councillors Turton and Dunk at the meeting of January 16, 1896 in *Sussex Daily News,* 17 Jan. 1896, 3.
149 The report was presented January 28, Brighton, Proc. San. Comm. 14 (28 Jan. 1897): 239–40. For the text of this untitled report see ibid. 14 (11 Feb. 1897): 251–61 or Brighton, *Proc. Town Council, Proc. Comm.,* 18 Feb. 1897: 23–7. Subsequent citations will be to the latter, the published, version.

town. These diseases were ones known to be associated with dirt and overcrowding. This statistical show was, however, largely gratuitous. He admitted that many factors might cause the high mortality rates in these wards. Furthermore he gave no figures for density or occupancy, and these mortality rates do not enter into the rest of his discussion.

His report undoubtedly grew from administrative frustration, from his inability to deal with the subletting of houses, a practice, he alleged, that was often carried on by nonresident, chief tenants, who could turn a tidy profit. At the time the only way the Sanitary Department could deal with overcrowding caused by subletting was through the complicated and slow process of serving notices for the abatement of nuisances.[150] Enforcement might take several weeks, and compliance need only be momentary. Conditions might return quickly to their former undesirable state. Furthermore overcrowding was hard to detect, especially since the Department's inspections of private houses had to be made before 6:00 P.M. The sanitary inspectors knew that certain houses were overcrowded, but they could not obtain adequate proof. Newsholme presented a table listing sublet houses and giving information on their size, value, rent, and occupants.[151] Some were severely overcrowded. There were, for instance, the six-room house in Southampton Street that housed sixteen people and the seven-room house in Carlton Hill that was home for twenty-two.

Newsholme requested a "prompt stretching out of the arm of the law,"[152] in proposing bylaws allowing him to deal with houses let in lodgings just as he did with common lodging houses. Specifically he asked for authority to register such houses, to impose standards of cleanliness, to limit the number of lodgers, and to make unannounced night visits to enforce compliance.[153] These bylaws would grant the Medical Officer of Health large discretionary powers, for he would have considerable power to determine to which houses the regulations would apply. In order to mitigate objections to this extension of bureaucratic power Newsholme suggested that the bylaws apply only to houses with a rateable value of £26 or less and an occupancy of three or more families.

Although in an early discussion one Town Councillor loudly proclaimed that he knew a local doctor who would refute every statement in Newsholme's report and who branded the "invading" of every £26 house an "abominable thing," the Town Council adopted this proposal and after amendments required by the Local Government Board the bylaws went into effect in May 1898.[154]

Newsholme did not think that such bylaws would solve the problems of overcrowded housing. Greater police powers did not change the economics of the housing market in Brighton. By 1904 he found the opportunity to propose a new public policy. The demand for an investigation following the discovery of a corpse

150 Brighton, *Proc. Town Council,* Proc. Comm., 18 Feb. 1897: 23–4.   151 Ibid., 24–5.
152 Ibid., 24.   153 Ibid., 26–7.
154 *Sussex Daily News,* 19 Feb. 1897, 2; Brighton, *Proc. Town Council,* 17 June 1897: v; and *Brighton Herald,* 19 June 1897, 2; Brighton, *Proc. Town Council,* 17 June 1897: v; and *Brighton Herald,* 19 June 1897, 2.

that had lain undetected for two weeks in a house inhabited by thirty people provided him with a forum to offer an assessment of the town's housing policy and to recommend an unpopular course of action in a substantial report.[155] First, there were grounds for optimism, he claimed. The town's worst housing had been demolished. Furthermore, he argued sanguinely, the need for massive slum clearance was over. The houses the Corporation had recently demolished at such expense were inherently unsuitable. They had been unfit for human habitation from the moment they had been constructed in the eighteenth and early nineteenth centuries. Hereafter if bylaws for new construction and for maintenance were enforced, no new slums would be created.[156] In this he adopted the position of Richard Cross, who twenty years earlier had argued that slum clearance was a one-time task.[157] Individual houses would probably have to be condemned, but when that happened the expense would fall on the property owner, not on the Corporation.

On the other hand the slum clearance work had created additional crowding in poorer neighborhoods. Newsholme estimated that although the census reports showed that the average occupancy per house in the Borough had declined slightly between the censuses of 1891 and 1901, there had been a 7 percent increase in the number of houses inhabited by more than one family in the poorer streets of the town center.[158] Subletting, he repeated, is "a most serious social evil, both from the point of view of health and morals."[159] But the Corporation bore some of the responsibility for subletting, when it destroyed cheap housing and replaced it with homes that commanded much higher rents. "We cannot object to sub-let houses as such, unless we are prepared to provide cottages for families whose total earnings are considerably less than twenty shillings a-week."[160] Since the employment of such laborers was insecure and their wages were low, these families had to live in the town center close to sources of employment.

The Corporation's embarking on construction of council houses created a precedent, Newsholme claimed, which might solve the town's most pressing housing problem.

> If a Town Council embarks in the business of a landlord, it should, I submit, be in the interest of public health, and as this in Brighton is chiefly endangered by the housing conditions of those occupying tenements of two and three rooms, it is for these that intervention is chiefly required.[161]

He proposed that the Corporation buy dilapidated or overcrowded dwellings at market rates. A few of these might be torn down to provide more light and

---

155 Arthur Newsholme, *Special Report on Overcrowding, on the Clearing of Insanitary Areas, and on the Provision of Housing Accommodation by the Town Council* (Brighton: Brighton Corporation, 1904). For the scandal that led to this investigation, see the comments of Councillor Henn in the recorded Council debate, *Sussex Daily News*, 18 Dec. 1903, 2; and Brighton, Proc. San. Comm. 20 (31 Dec. 1903): 409–11.

156 Newsholme, *Special Report on Overcrowding*, 13–15.

157 R. Cross, "Homes for the Poor," *Nineteenth Century*, 15 (1884), 157 in Yelling, 12–13.

158 Newsholme, *Special Report on Overcrowding*, 8–9, 10–11.   159 Ibid., 18.

160 Ibid., 19.   161 Ibid., 18.

ventilation in the street. But the rest could be repaired, converted into small but sanitary tenements, and rented by the Corporation at reasonable rents.[162] The Corporation might, in other words, do for unskilled laborers what it had begun to do for artisans. In doing so it could improve the town plan and promote health, and do so without putting an additional burden on the rates, since he believed even moderate rents could cover costs. The Housing of the Working Classes Act, 1890, authorized local authorities to purchase or construct and to manage lodging houses.[163] In a supplement to his report Newsholme described a similar scheme recently enacted in the Borough of Camberwell that was working smoothly.[164] He also tried to answer objections that had been raised in the past to Corporation purchase of individual houses. If the Corporation would only pay market rates for such property, it would not provide an incentive for owners to neglect their property or provide a windfall to owners of neighboring properties.[165]

The Sanitary Committee had Newsholme's report printed and distributed to each member of the Town Council.[166] After a month's delay it recommended that the M.O.H.'s proposal be adopted on an experimental basis. When the issue finally came before the Town Council on April 7, the Council refused to approve the Committee's recommendation by a margin of twenty-four to sixteen.[167] The proponents repeated Newsholme's arguments. The opponents worried about cost, about creating artificially high prices for slum property, and about creating a precedent. Others questioned Newsholme's knowledge of the slums, blaming house-farmers (tenants speculating in subletting) for overcrowding. Others claimed the Medical Officer of Health needed no additional powers. One critic even accused members of the Sanitary Committee of jobbery, a charge he withdrew under protest.

The Council vote effectively killed Newsholme's proposal, a plan in which he had invested much time, energy, and credibility. He had to content himself with a spurt of house condemnations[168] and with obtaining a stiffening of the bylaws on houses let in lodgings.[169] It was the worst defeat he encountered on a policy issue at Brighton. The incident points out the fragility of the M.O.H.'s influence, especially in housing questions. So long as he worked at removing nuisances, clearing slums, and policing the homes of the poorest residents, his policies received the support of a wide consensus even though they involved considerable capital expense or an extension of the police powers of local officials. When he proposed to move beyond this sphere, the consensus failed.

162 Ibid., 19–20.   163 53 & 54 Vict. C. 70, part III.
164 Newsholme, *Special Report on Overcrowding*, 34–7.   165 Ibid., 19, 20.
166 Brighton, Proc. San. Comm. 21 (25 Feb. 1904): 29.
167 For a summary of the debate in the council chamber see *Sussex Daily News,* 8 April 1904, 2.
168 See, for example, Brighton, Proc. San. Comm. 21 (9 June 1904): 147–51; and ibid. 21 (14 July 1904): 186.
169 The Sanitary Committee recommended this amendment in June, ibid. 21 (9 June 1904): 157. The new bylaws were not adopted until October, ibid. 21 (13 Oct. 1904): 288; and *Sussex Daily News,* 21 Oct. 1904, 3.

4

The municipal hospital and the isolation of acute infectious diseases

THE FACILITIES: SANATORIUM, GRANGE, AND LABORATORY

When Arthur Newsholme took up his post as Brighton's Medical Officer of Health, the town already had a municipal isolation hospital, the Brighton Sanatorium. The Sanitary Committee's intention in appointing a full-time M.O.H. was that the incumbent would also step into the posts of Medical Officer of the Sanatorium and Surgeon to the Police Force when these positions became vacant.[1] The promise of additional income and a more unified health service was soon fulfilled. Six months later the incumbent of the Sanatorium position announced his intention of resigning by Christmas 1888, and Newsholme was appointed in his place at an additional salary of £150 per year.[2] He never held the post with the police force, relinquishing his claim to the job in 1892 in order to secure an increase in his combined salaries from £650 to £800 per year.[3] The loss of the appointment with the police force was not of great moment. But the fact that Newsholme was both M.O.H. and Medical Officer of the Sanatorium was of the utmost importance for his career and for the development of the public health program in Brighton. Over the next fifteen years he would direct the transformation of the institution and its place in the town's social services. From the beginning Newsholme recognized the significance of the second post. In fact, a rumor circulated in the Council for some time after his appointment that he had paid off the previous Medical Officer to secure the latter's resignation.[4]

The fact that it had an isolation hospital in the 1880s placed Brighton in the minority of provincial towns. Although the major sanitary legislation of the past three decades, the Sanitary Act, 1866, and the Public Health Act, 1875, authorized

---

1 "Report of the Sanitary Committee," Brighton, Proc. Comm., Report Book, 6 (22 March 1888): 189–90.
2 "Report of the Sanitary Committee as to the resignation of the Medical Officer of the Sanatorium," ibid., 29 Nov. 1888, 263–4. For the meeting of the Town Council where some Councillors questioned the need for the additional salary see *Sussex Daily News*, 7 Dec. 1888, 3.
3 Brighton, *Proc. Town Council*, 4 Feb. 1892, xix–xx; *Sussex Daily News*, 5 Feb. 1892, 3; *Brighton Gazette*, 6 Feb. 1892, 5; Brighton, Proc. San. Comm., 9 (8 Sept 1892), 340; ibid., 14 Sept. 1892, 355; and *Brighton Gazette*, 10 Sept. 1892, 6.
4 *Sussex Daily News*, 5 Feb. 1892, 3; and *Brighton Gazette*, 6 Feb. 1892, 5.

local authorities to establish these hospitals,[5] and although the central health authority, the Medical Department of the Local Government Board, repeatedly encouraged the building of such facilities and even published model plans,[6] few provincial towns acted before the last decade of the century. As the nineties opened only about 400 of the more than 1,500 provincial sanitary authorities had means to isolate cases of infectious disease, and far fewer had permanent facilities for that purpose.[7] One small authority used as its isolation hospital a converted dog kennel fitted out with five beds. In most places the expense of construction and public fear of pest houses deterred action. A study commissioned by the British Medical Association (B.M.A.) in 1893 found only twenty-eight isolation hospitals in the provinces, and only eleven provided ten or more beds per 10,000 population, the ratio the study took as a safe minimum accommodation.[8] In London much more ample accommodation was available in the institutions of the Metropolitan Asylums Board.[9] But in the provinces the period of large-scale construction of these hospitals began only in the nineties as local authorities adopted the Infectious Disease (Notification) Act, 1889. Between that time and the outbreak of the Great War the scale of infectious disease hospital accommodation grew to rival that of the older voluntary hospital system.

The B.M.A. survey of 1893 reported that the Brighton Sanatorium had a capacity of 110 beds, making it of ample size for Brighton's population. But the figures in that report and the glowing description of the institution by the Chairman of the Brighton Sanitary Committee six years earlier in *The Lancet* are misleading.[10] The isolation hospital Newsholme found was a makeshift affair, and it had never, and probably could have never, accommodated 110 patients at once. Its origins dated from 1879. Under pressure from the Guardians, who resented having to accept smallpox patients who were not paupers simply because there was nowhere in Brighton but the workhouse for their treatment and isolation, the Sanitary Committee had begun planning a permanent isolation hospital.[11] By April 1881 ten acres of land had been acquired and plans for a fifty-bed permanent

---

5   "An Act to amend the Law relating to the Public Health," 29 & 30 Vict. C. 90, sect. 37; and "An Act for consolidating and amending the Acts relating to Public Health in England," 38 & 39 Vict. C. 55, sect. 131–2.

6   See the memoranda issued by successive Medical Officers of the Local Government Board in *Ann. Rep. Med. Off. L.G.B.*, 6 (1876–7): 312–17; ibid. 17 (1887–8): 199–201; and ibid. 24 (1894–5), 195–8.

7   Brian Abel-Smith, *The Hospitals 1800–1948: A Study in Social Administration in England and Wales* (Cambridge, Mass.: Harvard Univ. Press, 1964), 127; Anthony S. Wohl, *Endangered Lives: Public Health in Victorian Britain* (Cambridge, Mass.: Harvard Univ. Press, 1983), 137–9.

8   "An Investigation of infectious hospital accommodation and administration in England," *Br. Med. J.* (1893), no. 1: 185–7.

9   Abel-Smith, *The Hospitals*, 77–82, 119–27; Gwendoline M. Ayers, *England's First State Hospitals and the Metropolitan Asylums Board 1867–1930* (Berkeley and Los Angeles: Univ. of California Press, 1971).

10 Joseph Ewart, "Fever Cases in General Hospitals," *Lancet* (1887), no. 1: 195. Ewart was responding to further criticism of the town's measures to safeguard the health of visitors.

11 For the committee's negotiations with the Guardians, see Brighton, Proc. San. Comm. 1 (29 May 1879): 242–3; ibid. 5 June 1879, 245; ibid. 12 June 1879, 250; ibid. 25 Sept. 1879, 293–4; ibid. 6 Nov. 1879, 312–13.

facility were before the Town Council. But this deliberate planning was cut short by an outbreak of smallpox. In response the Sanitary Committee ordered the Borough Surveyor to build a temporary hospital on the new site as quickly as possible.[12] Three wooden, felt-covered buildings connected by covered open-sided walkways were hastily constructed on concrete piers: two 2-ward pavilions, one for each sex, housing 20 beds each, and a central administration building containing kitchen, storerooms, dispensary, and rooms for matron, nurses, and surgeon.[13] Within a year, the Committee moved to the eastern boundary of the site a prefabricated wooden and corrugated iron building that had just been used in the Brighton Health Congress. It was, in the words of the Medical Officer of the Local Government Board, "a huge, hideous, wooden barn-like structure."[14] However inappropriate as a hospital building, the prefabricated structure was divided into six wards to accommodate cases of scarlet fever and diphtheria which the local voluntary hospitals, first the Sussex County Hospital and then the Children's Hospital, refused to continue admitting.[15] Over the next few years several small service buildings were added, including a disinfection station and in 1890 a steam laundry constructed of brick. Illustration 4.1 shows the hospital as it was when Newsholme became M.O.H. but before the addition of the new laundry.

By the early 1890s, the Corporation's officials reported that the buildings were badly deteriorated and very difficult to heat or clean, and Newsholme complained that infectious cases could not be properly managed in the institution.[16] Servants from the different wards had to enter the kitchen to pick up their patients' food, in the process breaking the required isolation between the services for different groups of diseases. Moreover, there was a serious lack of sleeping accommodation for nurses. As a result some of the nurses had to sleep in the wards, occasionally in the same rooms with patients.

It took more than two years to build a consensus that a new hospital was needed, to clear away legal barriers to the building of a larger facility on the present site, to visit other isolation hospitals and to consult with the Medical Officer of the L.G.B., and to draw up architectural plans.[17] In building its first

---

12 Ibid., 1 (31 May 1881): 526.

13 For a description of the building and modification of the old Sanatorium, see Francis J. C. May and Arthur Newsholme, *A General Description of the History of Isolation Accommodation Provided for the Borough, with a More Detailed Account of the Improved Accommodation Now Provided by the Corporation* (Brighton, 1898), 5, 7.

14 R[ichard] Thorne Thorne, minute to [Alfred] Adrian, 15 Oct. 1895, P.R.O. MH 12/12797.

15 Newsholme offered this explanation at the opening of a new scarlet fever pavilion, "Brighton Sanatorium: New Fever Pavilion Opened," *Brighton Gazette*, 29 Oct. 1903, 3.

16 Francis J. C. May, "Infectious Diseases Hospital," 22 Feb. 1894, in Brighton, *Proc. Town Council, Proc. Comm.*, 2 April 1896, 23; and Arthur Newsholme, report to the Sanitary Committee, 19 May 1892. I have not succeeded in finding a complete copy of this report by Newsholme, but a section of it is reprinted ibid., 2 April 1896, 23. See also Arthur Newsholme, report to the Sanitary Committee 22 Feb. 1894, in *ibid.*, 7 June 1894, 3–5.

17 For the planning of the new institution, see Brighton, Proc. San. Comm., 9 (28 Jan. 1892): 56; and ibid. 11 Feb. 1892, 77; ibid., 9 (9 June 1892): 234–5; Brighton, *Proc. Town Council*, 4 Oct. 1894, v–vi; and *Brighton Herald*, 6 Oct. 1894, [3]. For the legal restrictive covenant governing the use of the

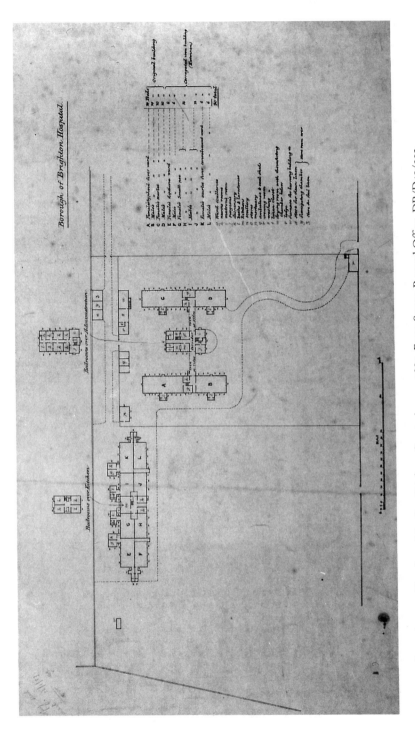

Illustration 4.1. Site plan of the first Brighton Sanatorium, c. 1887. From Sussex Record Office, DB/D41/112.

hospital the Corporation had not needed to seek the approval of the L.G.B., because it had financed the building out of current rates. For this larger and more expensive project, however, it needed a low-cost loan from the Public Works Loan Commission and so was forced to submit its plans to the L.G.B. for its sanction. It took twenty months to get that sanction. It was a frustrating exercise for local officials, a process which illustrates the conflict of purposes found in much that the L.G.B. did in the final years of its existence. On the one hand the Board had responsibility for public health and for a wide range of other local services, and it served as a technical adviser to local authorities in these matters. In this guise its officials encouraged local authorities to provide an increasing range of public services, including the construction of isolation hospitals. But on the other hand the L.G.B. by brief and tradition and under frequent Treasury (formerly "Exchequer") insistence was committed to protecting the interests of local ratepayers, to what Christine Bellamy has called "local possessive pluralism."[18] In trying to guard against local authority incompetence and waste, the Board adopted administrative procedures that created chronic delays, and in dealing with amateur Guardians in the early years of its existence, the Board had used its limited powers of supervision and financial oversight to evolve criteria and standards that local reformers at the turn of the century often found petty, inflexible, and obstructive.

In the process of negotiating the rebuilding of the Brighton Sanatorium, both parties played the game of brinksmanship, at times threatening to let the project die if the other party continued to insist on its demands.[19] In the end a compromise was reached, and the L.G.B. issued its sanction for the loan in June 1896.[20] The Corporation got its loan and a hospital much like the one it had designed for itself at the cost of a lengthy delay. The Board succeeded in securing changes in architectural detail, in getting an agreement that the Corporation would exclude smallpox cases from its new hospital, and in ensuring that there would be ample physical separation between the new facility and the outside world.

Brighton built its new Sanatorium in two stages. Its first loan for £20,500 was used to construct a scarlet fever pavilion, an isolation pavilion, an administration building with living quarters for the staff, a discharge block, and a porter's lodge. By March of 1898 construction was well enough along for the first patients to be

site, see Brighton, Proc. San. Comm., 11 (5 March 1894): 190–1; and *Brighton Herald,* 20 Oct. 1894, [4].

18 Christine Bellamy, *Administering Central–Local Relations, 1871–1919: The Local Government Board and Its Fiscal and Cultural Context* (Manchester: Manchester Univ. Press, 1988), see esp. 11–14, 87–92, 100–2, 141, 233.

19 For the L.G.B. review of the hospital plans and the negotiation that followed, see the correspondence and associated minutes in P.R.O. MH 12/12797 and MH 12/12798. See also Brighton, Proc. San. Comm., 12 (31 Jan. 1895): 205; "Report of Sanitary Committee," in Brighton, *Proc. Town Council, Proc. Comm.,* 4 April 1895, 2 pp; and Brighton, *Proc. Town Council,* 4 April 1895, iv; and Brighton, Proc. San. Comm., 13 (12 Sept. 1895): 76–7.

20 Tillstone to Dalton, 22 May 1896, P.R.O. MH 12/12799; & Adrian to Tillstone, 18 June 1896, ibid.

admitted.[21] The formal dedication was in October, 1898.[22] See Illustrations 4.2 and 4.3. Notice in Illustration 4.3 that the Corporation had allowed space for a very great expansion, more in fact than was ever needed. The second phase, consisting of two large pavilions, was completed between 1902 and 1905.[23] By the time the second of these pavilions opened, the hospital consisted entirely of modern masonry buildings and housed 160 patient beds in four pavilions. See Illustration 4.4. Building the new facility was a major civic undertaking and a source of local pride.[24] The Corporation had taken on debts for construction in excess of £47,000.[25]

The difficult problem of what to do with smallpox cases remained. By the middle nineties smallpox was rarely seen in Brighton. Whole years would pass with no reported cases. Smallpox was considered so rare but threatening that Newsholme reported on every imported case and on any secondary cases that followed. In the late nineties and the opening years of the new century as he grew ever more anxious about the neglect of vaccination and the effects of the Vaccination Act's conscience clause, which permitted parents legally to refuse to have their children vaccinated, these reports grew more thorough, especially in regard to patients' and contacts' vaccination history, and Newsholme used these reports to demonstrate the effectiveness of vaccination in checking the spread of the disease.[26] In an epidemiological study of smallpox in the nineteenth century he published in 1902, Newsholme argued that vaccination had been the major factor causing a reduction in the severity of smallpox epidemics, a lengthening of the period between their occurrence, and a shift in the burden of smallpox mortality from children, the main beneficiaries of compulsory vaccination legislation, to later ages.[27]

In Brighton his policy in combating smallpox was to isolate cases, to revaccinate contacts, to disinfect the sickroom, and to notify the M.O.H. of the district from which the sick had traveled, so that the second local health authority could search for contacts and unnotified cases.[28] Newsholme and the Sanitary Committee were

---

21 Newsholme, *Ann. Rep.* (Brighton), 1897, 52.
22 *Brighton Herald,* 29 Oct. 1898, 3.
23 For a short published account of the new pavilions, see *A Short Description of the Borough Sanatorium Intended for the Use of Delegates* [to the Brighton Sanitary Congress] (Brighton, 1910), 3–4.
24 See, for example, the Mayor's comments at the dedication of a new pavilion in 1903, "Brighton Sanatorium: New Fever Pavilion Opened," *Brighton Gazette,* 29 Oct. 1903, 3.
25 *A Short Description,* 4.
26 See, for example, the table of case histories in the 1902 outbreak and its emphasis on vaccination and revaccination, Newsholme, *Ann. Rep.* (Brighton), 1902, 14–20. For illustrations of his growing anxiety about the antivaccination movement and its effects, see Newsholme, *Ann. Rep.* (Brighton), 1900, 17; ibid., 1901, 18–21; and Brighton, Proc. San. Comm., 19 (13 March 1902): 123.
27 Arthur Newsholme, "The Epidemiology of Small-pox in the Nineteenth Century," *Br. Med. J.* (1902), no. 2: 17–26. Five years earlier Newsholme had recognized that this age shift was taking place, Newsholme, *Ann. Rep.* (Brighton), 1897, 16.
28 See, for example, his actions in 1895, Newsholme, *Ann. Rep.* (Brighton), 1895, 10–11; and Arthur Newsholme, "On a Doubtful Case of Recurrent Small-pox," *Br. Med. J.* (1896), no. 2: 1032.

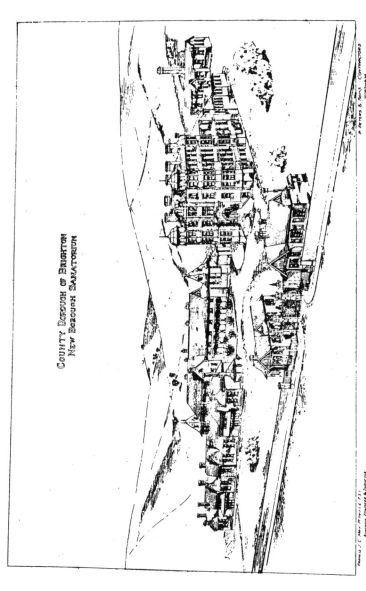

COUNTY BOROUGH OF BRIGHTON
NEW BOROUGH SANATORIUM

BIRDS-EYE VIEW OF NEW SANATORIUM.

Illustration 4.2. First phase of the new Borough Sanatorium. From Newsholme and Francis J. C. May, *A General Description of the History of Isolation Accommodation Provided by the Borough* . . . (Brighton, 1898), 4.

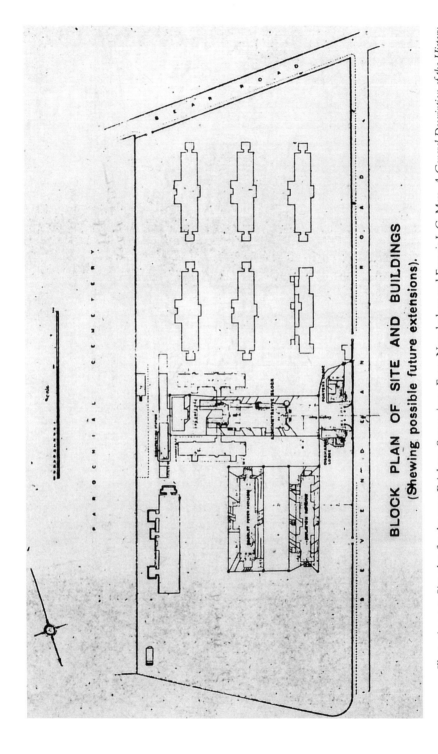

BLOCK PLAN OF SITE AND BUILDINGS
(Shewing possible future extensions).

Illustration 4.3. Site plan for the new Brighton Sanatorium. From Newsholme and Francis J. C. May, *A General Description of the History of Isolation Accommodation Provided by the Borough. . .* (Brighton, 1898), 14.

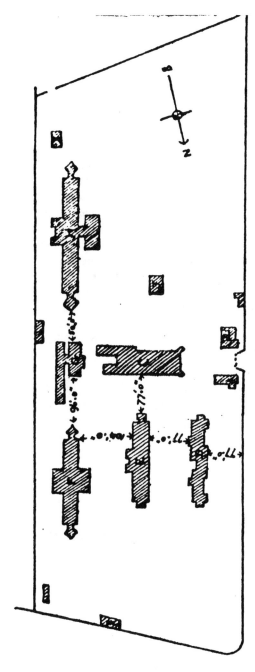

BLOCK PLAN OF ISOLATION HOSPITAL.

A. Discharge rooms. **B.** Porter's lodge. **C.** Administrative building.
D. Isolation pavilion. **E.** Diphtheria pavilion. **F.** Phthisis pavilion.
G. Laundry and disinfecting station. **H.** Scarlet fever pavilion.
I. Mortuary. **JJ.** Shelters for phthisis patients.

Illustration 4.4. Brighton Sanatorium in 1905. From Newsholme and H. C. Lecky, "An Account of the System of Voluntary Notification of Phthisis in Brighton . . . ," *Tuberculosis*, 4 (1906–7): 233.

willing to be quite innovative to make this policy work. At times payments were given to shopkeepers to close their shops for disinfection, and bounties were offered to reluctant contacts to secure their vaccination.[29] The Committee resorted to emergency measures as well. During the serious outbreaks of 1902 and 1903, the Council, with the approval of the L.G.B., temporarily made chicken pox a notifiable disease in the hope of detecting smallpox cases that otherwise might be missed.[30]

For this policy to work the town needed a facility to safely isolate smallpox cases, but the Sanitary Committee was reluctant to spend the sums necessary to maintain a permanent facility for the few cases it could expect year in and year out. Economy argued for treating smallpox cases in the Sanatorium with other cases of infectious disease, but the Corporation had to forfeit this option in order to obtain the L.G.B. sanction to finance the first phase of hospital reconstruction. The L.G.B. insisted that there be at least one half-mile between a hospital where smallpox cases were treated and any inhabited place. Its officials were gravely concerned that the site of the Brighton Sanatorium was within a half mile of the army barracks at Preston, the workhouse, and a number of inhabited streets.[31]

At Newsholme's prompting the Sanitary Committee made a feeble effort to find a site for a smallpox hospital in 1897, but it could find nothing at a price it was willing to pay.[32] The Committee was soon compelled to act by another epidemic. Reports of a serious outbreak in London in late November and early December 1899 induced the Committee and the Sanitary Department to make special preparations.[33] Brighton was spared in late 1899, but during 1901 local medical practitioners asked Newsholme to see a number of suspicious cases of pustular disease.[34] Although no cases of smallpox were officially reported in Brighton in 1901, five suspicious cases and smallpox contacts were admitted to the Sanatorium.[35] When it learned what had been done, the L.G.B. wrote at once condemning this practice and reminding the Corporation of its promise.[36]

29 Brighton, Proc. San. Comm., 19 (3 Feb. 1902): 76; Newsholme, *Ann. Rep.* (Brighton), 1893, 24; and Newsholme's comments on use of petty bribery in a discussion of vagrants and the transmission of smallpox, *Public Health*, 6 (1893–4): 135.

30 Newsholme, *Ann. Rep.* (Brighton), 1902, 20–1; Brighton, Proc. San. Comm., 19 (30 Jan. 1902): 72; ibid., 19 (8 Jan 1903): 434–5; ibid., 20 (29 Jan. 1903): 26; and *Brighton Herald* 18 Jan. 1902, 5.

31 H. F. Parsons, undated minute on Tillstone to Secretary, Local Government Board, 31 Dec. 1894, P.R.O. MH 12/12796.

32 Brighton, Proc. San. Comm., 14 (26 Nov. 1896): 172–3; ibid., 14 (11 March 1897): 307; ibid., 25 March 1897, 326–7; ibid., 27 May 1897, 404–5; ibid., 10 June 1897, 427–8; and ibid., 15 (26 Aug. 1897): 52; and Newsholme, *Ann. Rep.* (Brighton), 1898, 16.

33 The Committee requested that the annual town Christmas party for children be cancelled, it authorized Newsholme to hire an Assistant M.O.H., and it bought some portable shelters for smallpox patients. Brighton, Proc. San. Comm., 17 (28 Nov. 1899): 24–5; Ibid., 30 Nov. 1899, 42–3; ibid., 14 Dec. 1899, 54; and Newsholme, *Ann. Rep.* (Brighton), 1899, 19.

34 Newsholme, *Ann. Rep.* (Brighton), 1901, 18.

35 Newsholme, *Ann. Rep.* (Brighton), 1901, 16, 18, 56. Newsholme also reported on a modified case of smallpox which had been placed in one of the portable shelters on the hospital grounds.

36 Brighton, Proc. San. Comm., 18 (14 Sept. 1901), 382–3.

The L.G.B. urged provincial local authorities to band together to provide joint smallpox hospitals, but in this same year Brighton's Sanitary Committee declined the chance to join with its smaller neighbors in such a project.[37] It decided to proceed alone, purchasing a farm on Fulking Hill near the Devil's Dyke, a favorite natural attraction, to the northwest of town.[38] In the face of protests from neighboring authorities who objected to a smallpox hospital in their neighborhood and warnings that visitors to the Dyke would be perilously close to the deadly contagion,[39] the Committee remodeled the farm buildings and admitted the first acknowledged smallpox patients in 1902.[40] The Fulking Grange, as it was called, consisted simply of a twelve-room farmhouse, which served as the institution's administration building, and a barn, which was modified to provide two smallpox wards accommodating twelve patients.[41] In addition there was a concrete slab on which two portable huts could be erected to shelter four more patients. The facility was very plain and simple. The Corporation brought in a telephone line and added hot-water radiators to the wards. But there was no electricity, and water came only from rainwater cisterns. In fact the Grange functioned simply as an annex to the Sanatorium. For long periods it stood empty, the only permanent staff being a resident caretaker.[42] When smallpox was reported, the wards could be opened and nurses hired or transferred from the Sanatorium in town.

The building of the new Sanatorium offered Newsholme the opportunity to expand the work of the Sanitary Department in two other ways. In June 1897 he requested and received permission to establish a diagnostic laboratory and to appoint an unpaid House Physician for the Sanatorium, who would also serve as Deputy M.O.H.[43] For the remainder of his time in Brighton he had the help of a string of recent medical graduates (some of whom rose to prominence in the public health service) who were then meeting the Medical Council's requirements of six months' practical training for the Diploma in Public Health.[44] They pro-

37 Ibid., 4 Nov. 1901, 419; ibid., 5 Nov. 1901, 420–2; ibid., 19 (18 Dec. 1901): 30.
38 Ibid., 14 Nov. 1901, 443–5; ibid. 19 (28 Nov. 1901): 10; ibid., 12 Dec. 1901, 21–2; and *Sussex Daily News*, 20 Dec. 1901, 3.
39 These protests are recorded in Brighton, Proc. San. Comm., 19 (9 Jan. 1902): 42–5; ibid., 22 Jan. 1902, 53; and ibid. 13 Feb. 1902, 90. Neighboring parishes continued to object to attendants from the farm coming into their jurisdiction to shop. Ibid., 30 Jan. 1902, 73; ibid., 13 Feb. 1902, 91–2.
40 Brighton, Proc. San. Comm., 19 (9 Jan. 1902): 41; ibid. 3 Feb. 1902, 75–6; *Sussex Daily New*, 17 Jan. 1902, 2; and Newsholme, *Ann. Rep.* (Brighton), 1902, 75,
41 For descriptions of the Grange, see "Report of the Sanitary Committee," Brighton, Proc. Comm., Report Books, 11 (28 Nov. 1901): 329–30; Newsholme, *Ann. Rep.* (Brighton), 1902, 75–6.
42 Newsholme, *Ann. Rep.* (Brighton), 1903, 39.
43 Brighton, Proc. San. Comm., 14 (10 June 1897): 420–5.
44 For a discussion of the establishment of the Diploma in Public Health and the training it required, see Roy Acheson, "The British Diploma in Public Health: Birth and Adolescence," in *A History of Education in Public Health: Health That Mocks the Doctors' Rules,* ed. Elizabeth Fee and Roy M. Acheson (Oxford and New York: Oxford Univ. Press, 1991), 44–82, see esp. 76–82. For additional information on the diploma and on the requirement of practical training with an M.O.H., see Porter [Watkins], "English Revolution," 106–50. The Sanitary Committee applied to the Royal College of Physicians and to the Royal College of Surgeons for recognition of the Sanatorium as a site for training in laboratory work for the Diploma in Public Health. Brighton, Proc. San. Comm.,

vided patient care in the periods between Newsholme's daily visits to the Sanatorium and performed laboratory diagnosis; moreover, as we will see, several of them proved to be a great help in Newsholme's research as well.

Newsholme's inspiration for the municipal laboratory may well have come in 1894 at the International Congress on Hygiene and Demography as he listened to William Henry Welch describe the system for the laboratory diagnosis of diphtheria, which the New York City Health Department had just established. Newsholme returned to Brighton and recommended a similar service for his town.[45] By the time the laboratory opened three years later he had already begun to perform some laboratory diagnosis for Sanatorium patients in his home, and in fact the new laboratory began operation using his own microscope.[46] In October 1897 he inaugurated a municipal diagnostic service which offered Widal tests for typhoid fever, throat culture examinations for diphtheria, and sputum examinations for pulmonary tuberculosis.[47] Kits for making the throat swab, or for collecting a specimen of blood or sputum could be obtained from Town Hall. These could be returned to Town Hall at any time; the results of the test would usually be sent to the physician within twenty-four hours. There was no charge for these tests, if the patient were a Brighton resident. In other cases there was a moderate fee, 5s for typhoid or diphtheria and 2s6d for tuberculosis. By 1899 the lab was examining over 2,000 throat cultures per year, and by 1903 that number reached 3,657 plus 338 sputum examinations and 106 Widal tests.[48]

Newsholme was cautious about laboratory diagnosis, holding it to be a useful aid in the diagnosis of doubtful cases but giving primacy to clinical judgment. "In both Diphtheria and Typhoid Fever," he counseled in 1898, "clinical diagnosis must always hold the first place, the aid of bacteriology being required only in cases in which the clinical symptoms are anomalous or dubious."[49] He was also initially cautious about the use of diphtheria antitoxin. In 1894 he warned about unguarded optimism, reminding his readers about the unfortunate results of Koch's therapeutic use of tuberculin.[50] However, by the following year he had begun

15 (9 Dec. 1897): 166. It is clear that Newsholme and the Committee regarded the position as a stepping-stone to a career in public health. See Newsholme's comments in requesting a title change for the House Physician and his report that three former officeholders have gotten good jobs, ibid., 18 (8 Aug. 1901): 337–8. He later recalled several of these in Newsholme, *Last 30 Years*, 274.

45 Arthur Newsholme "Report as to the Buda-Pesth International Congress of Hygiene and Demography," *Q. Rep.* (Brighton), 1894, no. 3: 8–9.

46 The Committee did not resolve to buy its own until the end of 1898. Brighton, Proc. San. Comm., 16 (22 Dec. 1898): 119. The new laboratory opened in the Municipal Technical School and moved to the Administration Building of the new Sanatorium when that building was finished.

47 Arthur Newsholme, "Facilities for Bacteriological Diagnosis Offered by the Brighton Town Council," in Newsholme, *Q. Rep.* (Brighton), 1898, no. 1: 11–17.

48 Newsholme, *Ann. Rep.* (Brighton), 1899, 60; and ibid. 1903, 37. For the use of the laboratory in its first six months see Newsholme, *Q. Rep.* (Brighton), 1898, no. 1: 8–9.

49 Newsholme, "Facilities for Bacteriological Diagnosis," 12–13. See also his views a few years later in Arthur Newsholme, "Address on Possible Medical Extensions of Public Health Work," *J. State Med.* 9 (1901): 542.

50 Newsholme, "Report as to the Buda-Pesth," 10.

administering antitoxin to Sanatorium patients suffering with severe cases of diphtheria.[51] Within three years the Sanitary Department was maintaining a supply of antitoxin for the use of local practitioners,[52] and by 1901 he was urging medical practitioners to administer at least a small dose of diphtheria antitoxin in all cases of sore throat where an exudate was visible and to do so without delay, not even waiting for the results of the throat culture.[53] His experience quickly overcame his skepticism.

The Sanitary Department found other uses for the laboratory. It soon began to make regular bacteriological and chemical tests of the water from taps and from each of the sources of the town's water supply.[54] It occasionally diagnosed animal disease as well. In the first months the new facility was in operation, the ever-alert Inspector Cuckney carried some blood from a suspicious-looking hide at the abattoir to the laboratory on a piece of broken glass.[55] Newsholme found the blood swarming with anthrax bacilli. The diseased animal was traced to a farm where an unnotified outbreak of anthrax was occurring.

MANAGEMENT AND OUTCOME

The Brighton Sanatorium was a sturdy specimen of what Edwardian medical opinion demanded of an isolation hospital.[56] It had a perimeter wall, a strictly limited visiting policy, and a decentralized architectural plan. It consistently segregated infectious cases within the institution, and it maintained strict discipline of patients and staff. The Medical Officer had absolute authority in the daily operations of the institution. In his absence, which of necessity was for long periods of time, the work of the nurses and servants was overseen in the old institution by the Matron and in the new by the House Physician and Deputy Medical Officer of Health. Newsholme established his control over the institution from the outset. Within a year of becoming Medical Officer of the Sanatorium, he had the Matron called before the Sanitary Committee to answer charges of irregularities in dispensing drugs and insubordination.[57] The Matron and her husband, the Steward, soon resigned, and the Committee rewrote the job description of the

51 Newsholme, *Ann. Rep.* (Brighton), 1895, 45–6.
52 Arthur Newsholme, "Directions for Obtaining Materials for Cultural Examination from Cases of Diphtheria," in Newsholme, *Q. Rep.* (Brighton), 1898, no. 1: 16.
53 Arthur Newsholme, draft of circular to medical practitioners, in Brighton, Proc. San. Comm., 18 (8 Aug. 1901): 339.
54 Newsholme, *Ann. Rep.* (Brighton), 1897, [3]; and ibid., 1902, 74.
55 Newsholme, *Q. Rep.* (Brighton), 1898, no. 1: 10; and Newsholme, *Fifty Years,* 235.
56 For a concise statement of the principles on which these hospitals were to operate, see A. Wynter Blyth, *A Manual of Public Health* (London, 1890), 557–65. See also the discussion of a paper by E. W. Goddall, especially the comments of Dr. Willoughby in *Lancet* (1900), no. 1: 1208–9. A set of Sanatorium rules and lists of duties of the staff, rules which evidently predate September 1890, is housed in the Sussex Postgraduate Medical Centre, *Brighton Sanatorium: Duties of the Medical Officer of the Sanatorium, Duties of the Steward, Duties of the Matron, Duties of the Nurses* (Brighton, n.d.).
57 Brighton, Proc. San. Comm., 7 (31 Oct. 1889): 93, 95–6.

Matron making her subordination to the Medical Officer more explicit and replacing the Steward with a Head Porter.[58] The new Matron, Miss C. Ratcliffe, seems to have been capable and submissive. She remained at the Sanatorium for as long as Newsholme was Medical Officer.

The work of the Sanatorium was performed by a staff whose size depended on the patient census. At the old Sanatorium staff size varied typically between twenty and thirty-five, of whom about half were nurses.[59] At the new facility the numbers increased, as the new facility provided accommodation both for more patients and for a larger resident staff.[60] The institution's labor costs jumped accordingly. In the last days at the old Sanatorium wages paid to resident nurses and servants totaled between £400 and £500 annually, but in the second full year at the new hospital that figure exceeded £1200.[61]

The Sanatorium was by far the single largest item in the Sanitary Committee's budget. This is true even when the cost of the construction loans is not included.[62] But these institutions were not only expensive; they were inefficient as well. An isolation hospital needed to be large enough to meet the anticipated demands of any epidemic and to be managed so that it was ready to use on short notice. But an institution of that size was bound to have many of its beds standing empty much of the time. This was certainly the case in Brighton. The British Medical Association survey of isolation hospitals reported that for the years 1889–91 each bed in the Brighton Sanatorium was occupied on average by 2.4 patients per year.[63] Patients' stays at the Sanatorium were quite long, between four and five weeks,[64] but even allowing for a lengthy stay each time a bed was occupied, one must conclude beds were often empty. Conditions in this regard were not much different at the new facility. After the second phase of construction, that is, after 1905, the Brighton Sanatorium's 160 beds could have accommodated at maximum capacity over 8,000 patient weeks of care per year. We find, however, that the

58 Ibid., 30 Aug. 1890, 417–18. Handbills announcing the new positions and describing the duties of each are preserved in the Sussex Postgraduate Medical Centre, Francis J. Tillstone, *Sanatorium or Borough Hospital for Infectious Cases: Duties of the Matron* (Brighton, 1890); and Francis J. Tillstone, *Sanatorium or Borough Hospital for Infectious Cases: Duties of Head Porter* (Brighton, 1890). For the appointment of the new Matron, see Brighton, Proc. San. Comm., 7 (25 Sept. 1890): 447–8.

59 Arthur Newsholme, *Borough Sanatorium, 1889, To the Members of the Sanitary Committee* (Brighton, 1890), 5. A copy of this published report is found in the Sussex Postgraduate Medical Centre. See also Newsholme, *Ann. Rep.* (Brighton), 1897, 53.

60 The Administration Building of the new hospital had six bedrooms for servants, twelve single and two double bedrooms for day nurses, four single bedrooms for night nurses, and single bedrooms for resident physician and matron. In addition there were separate sitting rooms for physician, matron, nurses, and servants. May and Newsholme, *General Description,* 15.

61 Newsholme, *Ann. Rep.* (Brighton), 1898, 51; and ibid., 1901, 57.

62 See, for example, "Estimate of General District Rate for Service of Half-year Commencing 1 Jan. 1899," in Brighton, *Proc. Town Council,* 28 Oct. 1898.

63 "Investigation of infectious hospital accommodation," 186.

64 Figures are not available for the earlier years, but there is no evidence that institutional policy on length of stay changed significantly over this period. For figures on admissions and weeks of treatment, see the series of reports Newsholme, *Ann. Rep.* (Brighton), 1903, 38; ibid., 1904, 68; ibid., 1905, 54; ibid., 1906, 26; ibid., 1907, 24.

Sanatorium Admissions

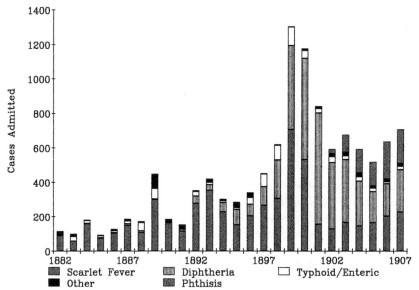

Illustration 4.5. Admissions to the Brighton Sanatorium, 1882–1907. Compiled from Brighton Corporation, Medical Officer of Health, *Annual Reports on the Health, Sanitary Condition, &c. of the Borough of Brighton.*

annual average number of patient weeks spent in the institution for the years 1903–7 was 3,348, and the maximum (1907) was only 4,102.[65]

Discussions of averages, however, fail to convey how the institution functioned. As Illustration 4.5 shows, the numbers accommodated each year in the institution were anything but steady. There is an upward trend through the 1890s, but the outstanding feature of this chart is the great fluctuation in admissions from year to year. Such differences were even more pronounced within a single year. Consider 1892 for example. The biweekly institutional census shows that the number of patients in the institution varied that year between ten and seventy.[66] With seventy cases of acute infectious disease the institutional staff was very busy, and the old facility was probably stretched to near capacity. To cope with such fluctuations in use, Newsholme regularly hired extra staff and then laid them off. There were thus periods of intense activity in the institution. Newsholme encountered one of these as soon as he became Medical Officer of the Sanatorium.[67] Epidemics of scarlet fever and measles occurred that year, and the institution was soon crowded with young cases, sometimes four and five from the same family. To meet the

65 Ibid., 1903, 38; ibid., 1904, 68; ibid., 1905, 54; ibid., 1907, 26; and ibid., 1907, 24.
66 Ibid., 1892, 20.   67 Ibid., 1889, 15.

crisis two temporary shelters were set up on the hospital grounds next to the pavilions which themselves had been constructed as temporary wards. The institution's staff was probably busiest during 1899, 1900, and 1901. These years saw admissions peak. To complicate matters those were also years when the institution was making the transition to its new facility.

Newsholme began his efforts to transform the place of the municipal hospital in the town's health policy with the issue of patient fees. When he became Medical Officer, the Sanitary Committee charged patients or their families for treatment received in the Sanatorium.[68] Adult, working-class residents were charged 10s per week and children under age ten 5s. For pauper cases the Sanitary Committee billed the Guardians 15s and 7s6d respectively. For the very few patients of means who found their way into the Sanatorium in the early days of the institution the fee scale was 21s per week for a ward bed or two to three guineas for private rooms. In these years the Committee typically spent between 20s and 30s per patient per week to operate the institution.[69] The fees charged to working-class residents, in other words, did not cover the full cost of their care. But even at these rates the Committee had trouble collecting its fees. During 1889 and 1890 the Committee could collect only 39 percent of what it had assessed nonpauper families. Newsholme estimated that the weekly income of Sanatorium patients' families was usually below 25s per week, and that they could not be expected to pay such fees for several weeks on end. However, the Committee had apparently believed that it was proper to insist that working families pay for treatment according to their means, although it was prepared to reduce or even to waive charges on appeal.

In December 1891 Newsholme offered a new perspective and recommended a policy change. He suggested abolishing fees for working-class residents, arguing that while the patient received benefit from hospitalization, the main benefactor was the community, since a source of infection had been removed from its midst.[70] Free treatment in the isolation hospital would encourage earlier and more universal admission of infectious disease among the working class, and it would reduce the chance and the cost of having to contend with secondary cases in the same households. Regarded from either a financial or a public health perspective, care in the municipal hospital should be viewed as a basic preventive service whose use should be encouraged not deterred. Soon Newsholme would begin measuring his success by the percentage of notified cases which were admitted to the isolation hospital. As he frequently did when trying to convince the Committee and the Council to make a major policy change, he collected information on what other towns were doing and favorable testimony from other Medical Officers of Health

---

68 For a description of this rate structure, see Arthur Newsholme "[Report] To the Sanitary Committee," 7 Dec. 1891, in Brighton, *Proc. Town Council, Proc. Comm.,* 14 Dec. 1891, 1.

69 Newsholme, *Ann. Rep.* (Brighton), 1893, 39.

70 Newsholme, [Report] in Brighton, *Proc. Town Council, Proc. Comm.,* 14 Dec. 1891, 2–3.

to append to his report. The Town Council accepted the proposal retaining fees only for visitors, paupers, and patients requiring a private room or special services.[71] Hereafter residents of Brighton received treatment in the municipal hospital free of charge and without civil disability. It is doubtful that the Councillors and Aldermen believed that they were creating an important precedent in making this change. There was no discussion in the Council of principles. The change seemed to most a matter of efficiency. It helped that no great financial loss threatened. The Committee usually did not collect annually as much as £200 in fees from nonpauper residents. Newsholme encouraged this pragmatic view of the change, arguing soon after that the increase in fees from paying patients more than made up for the loss of income from working-class residents.[72]

The Sanitary Committee did hope to attract paying patients to its new Sanatorium. It had in mind children from boarding schools and visitors living in hotels or boarding houses. The new facility offered special private accommodation: six rooms in its Isolation Pavilion and two rooms in an annex to the scarlet fever pavilion.[73] The Committee attempted to make the institution more attractive by permitting paying patients to be attended by their own physician, and it offered accommodation for an accompanying family member in the Administration Building. It sought to publicize the new institution among the more comfortable classes by encouraging medical practitioners, school principals, and owners of hotels and boarding houses to visit.

In succeeding years paying patients were occasionally admitted from the town's hotels and schools, and the Committee proved willing to make special arrangements with the managers of local nursing homes who wished to have standing agreements for transferring infectious cases.[74] As many as forty-one paying patients were treated in the Sanatorium in 1900, paying fees that year of more than £420.[75] But that unusually large number represented only 3 percent of the patient census that year. In most years paying patients numbered fewer than twenty. The majority of the Sanatorium patients continued to be drawn from the working classes of Brighton. To this majority were added a few paupers and working-class patients sent by neighboring towns or parishes and soldiers from the Preston Barracks. The presence of a few paying patients did little to alter the character of the institution.

A municipal isolation hospital was understood as part of a town's defense system against infectious disease. By the late nineteenth century the law gave local

71 Brighton, *Proc. Town Council*, 14 Dec. 1891, vii.
72 Newsholme, *Ann. Rep.* (Brighton), 1893, 39.
73 For the following information on these facilities for private patients, see May and Newsholme, *General Description*, 21. For the fee schedule for private patients at the new Sanatorium, see Brighton, Proc. San. Comm., 16 (20 Oct. 1898): 55–6.
74 Brighton, Proc. San. Comm., 16 (10 Nov. 1898): 76; ibid. 24 Nov. 1898, 91–2; ibid. 17 (12 July 1900): 307; and Newsholme, *Ann. Rep.* (Brighton), 1907, 24.
75 Newsholme, *Ann. Rep.* (Brighton), 1900, 85.

authorities broad powers to protect the public from the perceived risks posed by infected objects and persons.[76] A local authority might prosecute anyone who knowingly gave, sold, or rented objects or property which had been exposed to infection and not subsequently disinfected. It also could prosecute those who knowingly exposed others to infection by appearing in public, riding in a public conveyance without informing the driver of their condition, or leaving their home without disinfecting it or informing the owner of their condition so that the owner could have the property disinfected.

Under Newsholme's administration the Sanitary Department made regular use of these powers, and with the town's adoption of Infectious Disease (Notification) Act, 1889, it was much easier to trace infected persons and objects. The Department's regular visits to notified cases usually concluded with a final inspection to determine that the premises had been properly disinfected and that bedding and other porous objects from the sickroom were steam disinfected at the Sanatorium.[77]

When the Committee learned of cases which had been concealed from the authorities it sometimes prosecuted the head of the household and ordered a thorough disinfection of the house including the stripping of wallpaper from all walls, the washing of all walls and woodwork, and the disinfection of all clothing and bedding in the borough facility.[78] In other instances it ordered a frightened parent, usually the mother, to appear before the Sanitary Committee or the Town Clerk to be "severely reprimanded" for negligence in household isolation.[79] In the pamphlet the Department circulated to thousands of households every summer on the prevention of diarrhea it warned parents that children must be kept isolated during illness and convalescence and gave as the periods of required isolation: six weeks for scarlet fever, three weeks for measles, and two weeks for whooping cough.[80] Especially in the early 1890s after the adoption of compulsory notification, the Brighton Corporation undertook a string of prosecutions of adults for appearing in public while ill or for taking their sick children with them in the streets or on trains.[81] But after a decade of vigorous enforcement Newsholme realized that the real danger to the public health in diseases like scarlet fever and diphtheria lay not in the occasional concealed case but in the many mild cases

76 For the following provisions, see Public Health Act, 1875, 38 & 39 Vict. C. 55, sect. 120–9; Infectious Disease (Prevention) Act, 1890, 53 & 54 Vict. C. 34, sect. 5–7 & 12; and Brighton Improvement Act, 1884, 47 & 48 Vict. C. 262, sect. 56–8 & 64.

77 The Corporation was responsible for damage to the objects it disinfected, although it was seldom forced to pay such damages. In 1900 after it paid £7 10s 0d to a Madame Lambert for damages to her clothing, the Corporate adopted Infectious Disease (Prevention) Act, 1890, 53 & 54 Vict. C. 34, sect. 6 to protect itself from such damage claims in the future. Brighton, Proc. San. Comm., 17 (8 March 1900): 159; ibid., 29 March 1900, 173–4; ibid. 11 April 1900, 198–200; and Brighton, *Proc. Town Council,* 19 April 1900, vi.

78 See, for example, the case of the Richens family in Brighton, Proc. San. Comm., 17 (25 Jan. 1900): 99, and ibid. 1 Feb. 1900, 106.

79 Ibid., 8 (13 Nov. 1890): 17–18; and ibid., 9 (26 May 1892): 218.

80 For a copy of this pamphlet, see Newsholme, *Ann. Rep.* (Brighton), 1889, 17–18.

81 Ibid., 1891, 7; ibid. 1892, 10; Brighton, Proc. San. Comm., 9 (8 Sept. 1892): 348–9; and ibid. 10 (25 May 1893): 287.

which escaped attention, because the parent did not think them serious enough to call a doctor, or because the doctor was lazy or incompetent.[82] We will consider the issue of mild or misdiagnosed cases further in Chapter 5.

Mild or undiagnosed cases were a special problem for the town's elementary schools. These institutions were perfect places to spread the common infectious diseases, bringing together daily, as they did, one-seventh of the town's population, often under crowded conditions.[83] In the first decade of the twentieth century as one measure of controlling infection, Newsholme urged that children under that age of five, the ages when morbidity and case fatality of some of the most common infectious diseases was highest, be barred from elementary schools.[84] The more immediate problem, however, was dealing with cases of infectious disease which appeared in the classroom. The Sanitary Authority had the power to close schools, when outbreaks of infectious disease struck, and to temporarily bar individual infected children.[85] On Newsholme's recommendation the Sanitary Committee periodically closed schools to control outbreaks of diphtheria and measles.[86] But this was a drastic measure, one which the town's officials preferred to avoid. If infection were to be effectively controlled in the schools, individual cases had to be detected early in their course, before they could infect others. This was a stiff order in the absence of medical examination of schoolchildren or, in Newsholme's first years in Brighton, of compulsory notification of infectious disease. Nor would the Sanitary Committee later make Newsholme's task easier by agreeing to his request to add measles to the schedule of diseases notifiable in Brighton under the Infectious Disease (Notification) Act, 1889.[87]

Newsholme, like a number of other Medical Officers of Health, resorted to a series of voluntary agreements with teachers and school authorities. During the nineties he notified schools of households in which infected children lived and

82 Arthur Newsholme, *The Role of 'Missed' Cases in the Spread of Infectious Diseases* (London and Manchester: Sherratt and Hughes, 1904); and Arthur Newsholme "Address on the Possible Medical Extensions of Public Health Work," *J. State Med.*, 9 (1901): 541.

83 Newsholme, *Ann. Rep.* (Brighton), 1889, 18.

84 Arthur Newsholme, "The Lower Limit of Age for School Attendance: A Plea for the Exclusion of Children under Five Years of Age from Public Elementary Schools," *Public Health,* 14 (1901–2): 570–83; Arthur Newsholme, "The Lower Limit of Age for School Attendance," *Practitioner,* 79 (1907): 593–607.

85 See, for example, the L.G.B. instructions in George Buchanan, "Memorandum on School-Closure and Exclusion from School of Particular Scholars, as Means for Controlling Spread of Infectious Disease," *Ann. Rep. Med. Off. L.G.B.,* 13 (1883–4): 90–5; "Memorandum on the Circumstances under Which the Closing of Public Elementary Schools or the Exclusion therefrom of Particular Children May Be Required in Order to Prevent the Spread of Disease," ibid., 20 (1890–1): 213–17; and Richard Thorne Thorne, "Memorandum, Prepared in the Medical Department, on the Circumstances under Which the Closing of Public Elementary Schools or the Exclusion Therefrom of Particular Children May Be Required in Order to Prevent the Spread of Disease," ibid., 26 (1896–7): 148–52.

86 Brighton, *Proc. San. Comm.,* 7 (1 Oct. 1890): 451–2; ibid., 9 (3 Oct. 1892): 384–6; ibid., 10 (8 Dec. 1892): 54–5; ibid., 18 (13 Dec. 1900): 37–8; Newsholme, *Ann. Rep.* (Brighton), 1896, 20; and ibid., 1898, 22.

87 Brighton, *Proc. San. Comm.,* 10 (22 Feb. 1893): 167; and Arthur Newsholme "To the Sanitary Committee [special report of measles epidemic, 1892]," ibid., 186–202.

specified a length of time the sick child and any other children in the house should be kept from attending.[88] Teachers agreed to comply with the M.O.H.'s request and further to provide him with a weekly list of suspicious absences from school, so that the Sanitary Department could investigate. This agreement, however, put the school authorities in a bind, since it lowered their average attendance figures. Attendance figures were important to schools, because they helped determine the size of a school's Treasury grant. Efforts to keep enrollments up led schools to adopt practices that Newsholme deplored, such as sending a child from the school to call at the home of an absent classmate to learn why the latter was not attending and the use of penny bribes to coax sick or convalescent children back to school on the day of an official visit.[89] The way was cleared for smoother cooperation between schools and the Sanitary Department when the Board of Education agreed to count absent pupils, certified by the M.O.H. as suffering from an infectious disease, as equivalent to attendances for purposes of the grant. To encourage prompt notification, Newsholme certified each child's absence only from the day on which he received notice of the child's illness from the local school authorities.[90]

In the community at large recognized cases could be confronted directly and isolated. Armed with an order from a Justice of the Peace, an M.O.H. could compulsorily take a person suffering from an infectious disease to the Sanatorium and hold that patient there, provided that the sick were without a proper home or that effective isolation at home were impossible.[91] Newsholme occasionally used these compulsory powers, but their use was time consuming and unpopular.[92] He wisely sought instead voluntary admission. The abolition of fees at the Sanatorium removed one disincentive. Local pride in the new Sanatorium and favorable press attention may also have helped soften parental opposition. But it was probably the visit of the inspector following the notification of the case that was most im-

88 Newsholme, *Ann. Rep.* (Brighton), 1889, 18–19; Newsholme, [special report . . . measles], 193–5; Brighton, Proc. San. Comm., 10 (29 Dec. 1892): 76; ibid., 15 (14 Oct. 1897): 104; and Arthur Newsholme "A National System of Notification and Registration of Sickness," *J. Roy. Statist. Soc. Lond.*, 59 (1896): 35.

89 Arthur Newsholme, "The Bearing of School-Attendance upon the Spread of Infectious Disease," *Trans. Sanitary Inst.*, 11 (1890): 106.

90 Newsholme, *Ann. Rep.* (Brighton), 1897, 28–9; and Arthur Newsholme, in "A Discussion on the Means of Preventing the Spread of Infection in Elementary Schools," *Br. Med. J.* (1899), no. 2: 590.

91 Public Health Act, 1875, 38 & 39 Vict. C. 55, sect. 124–5; and Infectious Disease (Prevention) Act, 1890, 53 & 54 Vict. C. 34, sect. 12. For a very useful discussion of the issue of compulsory powers in public health, which notes as exceptional the little public opposition which compulsory notification and isolation generated, see Dorothy Porter and Roy Porter, "The Enforcement of Health: The British Debate," in *AIDS: The Burdens of History*, ed. Elizabeth Fee and Daniel M. Fox (Berkeley: Univ. of California Press, 1988), 97–120, esp. 107–8.

92 In December 1890 and against the parents' wishes Newsholme took a child suffering with scarlet fever to the Sanatorium, Brighton, Proc. San. Comm., 8 (11 Dec. 1890): 49. Actions like these sometimes brought protests. See the episode in the autumn of 1898 in which the Sanitary Committee steadfastly backed their M.O.H. in the face of protests from the Regency Ward Ratepayers Association, ibid., 15 (8 Sept. 1898): 474–75; and ibid., 16 (13 Oct. 1898): 44.

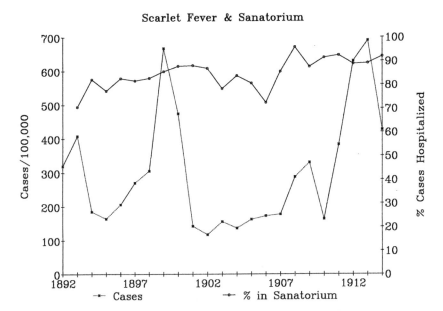

Illustration 4.6. Scarlet fever and sanatorium isolation in Brighton, 1892–1914. Compiled from Brighton Corporation, Medical Officer of Health, *Annual Reports on the Health, Sanitary Condition, &c. of the Borough of Brighton.*

portant. By emphasizing the dangers and the inconvenience of keeping the sick child at home, the inspector could frequently secure voluntary hospitalization.

Illustration 4.5 has been drawn to illustrate the mix of diseases the isolation hospital admitted. Cases of smallpox, measles, chicken pox, epidemic or summer diarrhea, whooping cough, puerperal fever, and erysipelas sometimes appeared in the institution.[93] Typhoid or enteric fever cases were admitted every year, and, as we shall see in Chapter 6, after admissions for phthisis or pulmonary tuberculosis began in 1902, the number of cases of that disease treated every year grew steadily. But two diseases, scarlet fever and diphtheria, dominate the institution's records. These two diseases could account for more than 90 percent of admissions to the Sanatorium in years such as 1899, when epidemics of both occurred in Brighton.[94] Given the prominence of these two diseases it comes as no surprise then to learn that, before the admission of tuberculosis cases, most patients were children. In the absence of specific therapy other than diphtheria antitoxin, patients stayed in the hospital a long time. In the first years of the twentieth century, average stays

93 The admission of erysipelas was considered an exceptional and particularly dangerous action, so that Newsholme asked for special permission from the Sanitary Committee. Ibid., 21 (10 March 1904): 42–4.
94 Newsholme, *Ann. Rep.* (Brighton), 1899, 64.

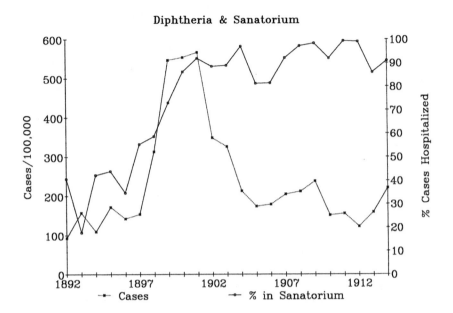

Illustration 4.7. Diphtheria and sanatorium isolation in Brighton, 1892–1914. Compiled from Brighton Corporation, Medical Officer of Health, *Annual Reports on the Health, Sanitary Condition, &c. of the Borough of Brighton.*

for all admissions were between four and a half and five weeks, while for scarlet fever it was even longer, between five and six weeks.[95]

Newsholme was especially anxious to hospitalize cases of scarlet fever, diphtheria, and typhoid fever. As Illustrations 4.6 to 4.8 show the Department had considerable success. Within three years of the beginning of compulsory notification of infectious disease, 82% of notified cases of scarlet fever were admitted to the isolation hospital. With the exception of only three years, every year for the remainder of Newsholme's tenure in Brighton between 80% and 90% of scarlet fever cases were hospitalized. For the sixteen years 1891 through 1907 the average annual rate of institutional confinement of notified cases was 81.1%. For the other two major diseases the average rates of confinement for the period were lower: 67.1% for diphtheria and 50.8% for typhoid or enteric fever, but those averages include the very low confinement rates in the first years after notification began and before the new Sanatorium opened. After 1900 the hospital admitted more than 80% of notified cases of diphtheria every year, and an annual average of 63% of notified typhoid cases entered the institution in the first eight years of the new century.

95 Figures were not published for all years, but see this series of reports, Newsholme, *Ann. Rep.* (Brighton), 1903, 38; ibid. 1904, 68; ibid., 1905, 54; ibid., 1906, 26; ibid. 1907, 24.

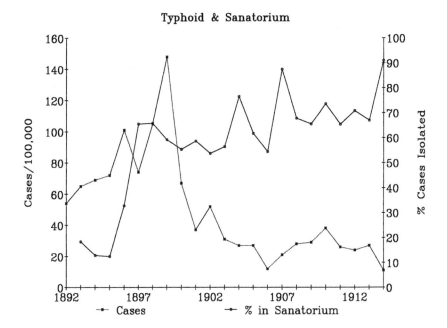

Typhoid & Sanatorium

Illustration 4.8. Typhoid and sanatorium isolation in Brighton, 1892–1914. Compiled from Brighton Corporation, Medical Officer of Health, *Annual Reports on the Health, Sanitary Condition, &c. of the Borough of Brighton.*

This is a remarkable record, especially for scarlet fever. Before 1900 only two of the thirty-three largest towns of England and Wales, Birmingham and Huddersfield, institutionally isolated a higher percentage of their cases of scarlet fever.[96] These rates are testimony to the vigor of local health programs, and to the fact that the emphasis in public health work was beginning to change. Treatment and other personal services now occupied much of the Sanitary Department's attention and a large chunk of its budget. These figures also suggest that by the turn of the century the municipal isolation hospital was beginning to reach quite far up the social scale for patients. It seems that in Brighton after 1890 most scarlet fever cases and after 1900 most diphtheria cases occurring in poor and artisan families were removed to the isolation hospital.

It is, of course, possible that these isolation figures are inflated, because notification was working much less well than contemporaries believed, and many cases of infectious disease were not reported. But available evidence does not support the idea of widespread, deliberate violation of the law. As we shall see, some diseases, scarlet fever in particular, frequently were not reported, because the disease was

96 C. Killick Millard, "The Influence of Hospital Isolation in Scarlet Fever," *Public Health,* 13 (1900–1): 493.

poorly understood and was often misdiagnosed. But given the limitations of medical knowledge, Newsholme and his Department must have institutionalized nearly every known case of notifiable disease which did not occur in a middle-class house, where it was assumed isolation could be properly conducted under the supervision of a private physician.

As the Sanitary Department put increasing pressure on families to send their sick members to the Sanatorium, the results of treatment in the institution became a more pressing issue. The anecdotal evidence of satisfaction with the institution is mixed. On the one hand the records of the Sanitary Committee contain several letters of thanks for the way in which the staff of the Sanitary Department conducted itself and for the care received in the institution. The following one of 1899 may stand as an example. It was addressed to Newsholme and came from the proprietor of a boarding house who seems as anxious about business as about the sick family member.

Last Friday week I had the misfortune to have my little girl stricken down with Scarlet Fever which was at once notified by Dr. Whittle. My object in writing to you is to express my gratitude to your staff of Officers for the kind consideration with which they treated me and for the thoughtful manner in which they studied my convenience in removing the little sufferer. So admirable were all the arrangements carried out that as far as I know no one in the house or in the square knew of the removal. The same courtesy and consideration was also shown by the Sanitary officials who came to disinfect the room and in removing and returning the disinfected bedding. . . . May I also trouble you to convey my best thanks to the Matron at the Sanatorium and to the Nurses for their kindness[,] for my little one writes that everybody there is so kind to her and that she is as happy as possible. In conclusion allow me to say how proud I am that the Sanitary Committee has made such excellent arrangements for the reception of such cases; and that it will be in no grudging spirit that I shall pay my rates in future.[97]

But there is contrary evidence as well. Young patients usually leave no mark in the written record, but one child, Wilfred Stevens, who had been confined with scarlet fever, voted with his feet. Newsholme reported that on July 5, 1899, young Stevens had "escaped."[98] The prolonged separation from family (one 12-year-old suffering from scarlet fever spent a total of ninety-seven days in the institution), [99] the isolation procedures themselves, and the measures taken to render patients noninfectious must have been terrifying to some patients. Parents occasionally complained about the treatment their children received. H. S. Baker wrote to the Committee twice in February and March 1900 complaining of his child's condi-

97 W. D. Cooke to Newsholme, 2 May 1899 in Brighton, Proc. San. Comm., 16 (11 May 1899): 284–5.
98 Ibid., 13 July 1899, 350.
99 Arthur Newsholme, "Protracted and Recrudescent Infection in Diphtheria and Scarlet Fever," *Med.-Chir. Trans.* 87 (1904): 561–3. The same text was published in *Public Health,* 16 (1903–4): 700–1. Future citations will be to *Med.-Chir. Trans.*

tion on discharge from the institution.[100] The Committee interviewed Newsholme, a Sanatorium nurse, and a private physician, decided that the problems the parent complained of had developed after the child left the institution, and refused to admit liability. In at least two other instances, however, the Corporation paid damages to the parents of children who had been scalded in the Sanatorium.[101] Serious burns were not confined to patients. In March 1902 a nurse's clothing caught fire at the Sanatorium, and she died within four days.[102]

Accidents such as these must have happened in every hospital where crude heating devices and steamers were used in the wards. A more essential criterion for judging isolation hospitals was their success in preventing the spread of the lethal infections they contained. Cross-infection was the curse of these institutions. In fact one cynical Edwardian definition of an isolation hospital was a "place where a patient goes in with one infectious disease and catches all the rest."[103] Textbooks of the period acknowledge that "post-scarlatinal diphtheria" was a special hazard of hospital treatment.[104] Brighton Sanatorium took special precautions to prevent cross-infection. Not only were patients with different infections physically separated, but nursing services were also divided so that the same nurse did not attend patients with different diseases. Unlike some isolation hospitals where the same towel, wash cloth, or tongue depressor went round the entire ward in the morning, as early as 1890 the nurses in Brighton were instructed in simple means to prevent contact infection.[105] They were to disinfect patients' excreta immediately; they were to boil the instruments used to examine throats or noses and to burn cotton or linen used to absorb nasal discharge, and they were instructed to carefully wash their hands after coming into contact with patients and especially before eating. The regimen outlined here was not as strict as those that would be recommended within fifteen years, and, of course, we do not know how faithfully such rules were followed, but these instructions do show an awareness of the risk of contact infection, and they acknowledge that the hospital staff had a large role in its causation.

But cross-infection still took place. In one instance four cases of scarlet fever broke out in the diphtheria ward in 1902, when a child apparently suffering from

100 Brighton, Proc. San. Comm., 17 (22 Feb. 1900): 142–3; and ibid., 8 March 1900, 157–8.
101 Ibid., 16 (8 Dec. 1898): 108; ibid., 22 Dec. 1898, 121; ibid., 19 (13 March 1902): 125 and ibid., 10 July 1902): 248.
102 Ibid., 19 (18 March 1902): 127.
103 A. Mearns Fraser, "Is the Hospital Isolation of Scarlet Fever Worth While?" *Public Health,* 16 (1903–4): 211.
104 F. Foord Caiger, "Scarlet Fever," in *A System of Medicine,* ed. Thomas Clifford Allbutt, 2 vols. (London and New York: Macmillan, 1900), 2: 159–60.
105 "Borough of Brighton, Brighton Sanatorium" (Brighton, n.d.) pp. 4–6. Duties of the Nurses, and Precautionary Instructions to Nurses, a printed handbill probably written by Newsholme before September 1890 in the collection of the Sussex Postgraduate Medical Centre. For recollections of ward practices in an unnamed large midland fever hospital which promoted cross infection, see William Scatterty, "Hospital Isolation," *Public Health,* 17 (1904–5): 361.

both infections was placed in the ward.[106] In 1908 a mother complained that her daughter contracted both scarlet fever and ringworm while in the institution.[107] And nurses and other Sanatorium employees sometimes caught patients' diseases.[108] Newsholme believed that his own severe case of typhoid fever, which kept him away from his post for nearly four months in 1896, may have been contracted during a postmortem examination he conducted at the Sanatorium.[109]

The limitations of personal freedom that isolation required and the burns, head lice, ringworm, and secondary infection that occasionally accompanied confinement might have been grimly accepted as the necessary cost of protecting the community from infection, if it could have been demonstrated that the chains of infection in the community stopped at the isolation hospital. But by the middle nineties public health workers were growing anxious on that score. The crux of the matter was the regular occurrence of what were called return cases – that is, cases which appeared in a home to which a patient had recently been discharged from the isolation hospital after treatment for the same disease. While Medical Officers of Health had known about return cases for some time, public indignation in the middle nineties forced professional soul searching. In 1894, on receiving a complaint from the Beckenham Urban Authority, the Local Government Board conducted an investigation of return cases allegedly caused by mismanagement at the Bromley and Beckenham Joint Hospital.[110] Two years later a family sued the Mayor and Corporation of Birmingham and succeeded in collecting damages for several return cases, one of them fatal.[111] The Brighton Sanitary Committee, like other local authorities, worried about their own vulnerability to such suits and tried to limit their liability.[112]

Return cases occurred most frequently with scarlet fever and diphtheria. Isolation hospitals adjusted their practices in an attempt to rid patients of infection

106 Newsholme, "Protracted and Recrudescent Infection," 569.
107 Mrs. M. Gray, to the Sanitary Committee, 21 Jan. 1908 in Brighton, *Proc. San. Comm.*, 24 (30 Jan. 1908): 217–18.
108 See, for example, Newsholme, *Ann. Rep.* (Brighton), 1895, 44; ibid. 1898, 47; and ibid. 1902, 75.
109 Ibid., 1896, 3. Newsholme discussed his case in Arthur Newsholme, "An Address on the Spread of Enteric Fever by Means of Sewerage-Contaminated Shellfish," *Br. Med. J.* (1896), no. 2: 639. He could not be certain how he was exposed, because he had served as a consultant for two suspect cases of typhoid fever about the same time. For the administrative record of his sick leave, see Brighton, *Proc. San. Comm.*, 13 (9 Jan 1896): 238; ibid. 30 April 1896, 357; and ibid., 14 May 1896, 393.
110 T. W. Thompson, "Report on Re-invasion by Scarlatina of Households to Which Persons from the Bromley and Beckenham Joint Hospital Had Returned on Their Recovery from That Disease," *Ann. Rep. Med. Off. L.G.B.*, 24 (1894–5): 103–4. See also T. W. Thompson, "Considerations in Respect to 'Return' Cases of Scarlatina," *Trans. Epidem. Soc. Lond.*, n.s. 15 (1995–96): 1–16.
111 The case was *Keegan v. The Mayor and Corporation of Birmingham*, 1896. For M.O.H. discussion of the case see *Public Health*, 8 (1895–6): 244–5; J. Wright Mason, "Secondary and Return Cases of Scarlatina," ibid., 10 (1897–8): 221; and C. Killick Millard, "The Etiology of 'Return Cases' of Scarlet Fever," *Br. Med. J.* (1898), no. 2: 614.
112 Brighton, *Proc. San. Comm.*, 13 (30 April 1896): 371–2. For this concern in other towns, see "Isolation Hospitals," *Lancet* (1901), no. 1: 413; and ibid. (1903), no. 2: 499.

before discharge. Periods of confinement were lengthened, for scarlet fever especially. By the late nineties average confinements for scarlet fever were between 39 and 65 days, and one authority recommended that they be increased to between 56 and 91 days.[113] Hospitals also began to segregate more carefully acute from convalescent cases and to combat infection on the bodies of patients by the use of chemical disinfectants in throats, ears, and noses, especially in septic cases, that is, in cases having chronic discharges. To remove any last trace of infection before the patient left the institution hospitals also instituted "bathing out" procedures, such as those in Brighton we will describe shortly.[114]

Brighton had its share of return cases. Newsholme discussed them in his *Annual Reports*, and in 1904 he published a detailed clinical and epidemiological study of the return cases of scarlet fever and diphtheria which had occurred in connection with Sanatorium practice during the last ten years.[115] In his early years Newsholme had not insisted that acute and convalescent cases be segregated, but before long he saw to it that the acute and convalescent cases were kept on opposite sides of a six-foot-tall partition which divided the large iron pavilion down the middle.[116] Newsholme was among the earliest isolation hospital medical officers to go a step further and to segregate septic from ordinary cases of scarlet fever as well as convalescent from acute cases.[117] The institution staff began to attack the septic discharges from ears, noses, and throats with formalin, lysol, and iodine irrigation. It also instituted a bathing-out procedure in which the patient was bathed, given clean clothing, and put in a separate room three days before discharge. The patient left the institution through the discharge lodge, where another bath was administered and clean clothes from home were provided.[118]

As throat culture techniques were employed with increasing frequency in the late 1890s, it was possible to reduce the risk of return cases of diphtheria. But there was no similar help for scarlet fever. Although streptococci had been isolated from scarlet fever cases, and although a few researchers believed that these bacteria were the cause of the disease, the etiology of scarlet fever and the methods for distinguishing the strains of streptococci were not worked out until the mid-twenties.[119] In the meantime most physicians could not believe that an organism

---

113 These practices and recommendations are summarized in Mason, "Secondary and Return Cases," 220–1.

114 For a discussion of the bathing-out procedure in Birmingham, see Millard, "Etiology of 'Return Cases," 616.

115 Newsholme, *Ann. Rep.* (Brighton), 1895, 44; ibid., 1901, 25, 31–2; ibid., 1905, 17–18; and Newsholme, "Protracted and Recrudescent Infection," 549–93.

116 Newsholme, "Protracted and Recrudescent Infection," 556, 561.

117 Newsholme, *Ann. Rep.* (Brighton), 1901, 25.

118 For the bathing-out procedure in Brighton, see ibid. See also Newsholme, "Protracted and Recrudescent Infection," 551, 555.

119 For a concise summary of the development of knowledge of scarlet fever, see Arthur L. Bloomfield, *A Bibliography of Internal Medicine: Communicable Diseases* (Chicago: Univ. of Chicago Press, 1958): 108–26. Emmanuel Klein and associates at the L.G.B. isolated streptococci in culture from patients and argued that they were the cause of the disease, see *Ann. Rep. Med. Off. L.G.B.*, 26 (1896–7): 263–6; ibid., 27 (1897–8): 326–34; ibid., 28 (1898–9): 480–97; ibid., 29 (1899–1900): 385–457; and ibid., 30 (1900–1): 353–404. Klein's collaborator had even discussed the implications

as common as the streptococcus could be responsible for a disease such as scarlet fever, and isolation hospitals at the turn of the century made no regular attempts to culture this organism from patients' throats. Scarlet fever continued to be diagnosed from symptoms alone, especially from the characteristic rash which usually was followed by peeling skin. There was no way to tell when a patient was no longer infective. In the past physicians suspected that the peeling skin was the primary vehicle of contagion and advised that the patient remain in isolation until the skin had ceased to peel. Acting on the same hypothesis they also recommended that the bodies of scarlet fever patients be coated with a mixture of olive oil and phenol to control cross-infection in hospital wards.[120] By the nineties flaking skin received less attention, and mild or atypical cases, the ones that escaped detection, were being blamed more often for spreading the disease.[121] But that realization was of little practical help without a more certain method of detecting cases. More important was that fact that no one knew how or whether scarlet fever was related to other cases which shared some of its symptoms: sore throat, headache, malaise, but were without its characteristic rash. In retrospect we can see that medical officers at the turn of the century knew of only a small percentage of the streptococcal infection in their community. In such circumstances a policy of controlling scarlet fever by isolating only overt cases was doomed to fail.

Isolation hospitals were most vulnerable to criticism in their management of scarlet fever, and at the opening of the century a prolonged debate erupted when voices within the medical community claimed that these hospitals were worse than useless for controlling scarlet fever.[122] Such critics claimed that not only did these hospitals not reduce the mortality or the morbidity from scarlet fever in the community they served, but that by aggregating cases they produced a "hospitalized" strain of scarlet fever contagion that was more virulent, more infective, and more likely to cause return cases than the contagion usually found in the community. I have argued elsewhere that although the ensuing debate was conducted in terms of efficiency, at least some of the critics attacked the hospitals because they believed that the use of these institutions constituted an intolerable use of public authority to control the individual, and because the policy of isolation represented a turning away from the established preventive strategies: sanitation and environ-

---

of this research for the control of return cases; see Mervyn H. Gordon, "The Cause of Return Cases of Scarlet Fever," *Br. Med. J.* (1902), no. 2: 445–46.

120 See, for example, Arthur Newsholme, *Hygiene: A Manual of Personal and Public Health* (London, 1884): 366.

121 Blyth, *Manual*, 380; and Newsholme, *Role of 'Missed' Cases*.

122 For representative criticisms, see Edward Dean Merriott, "Scarlet Fever – The Case against Hospital Isolation," *Sanitary Record*, n.s. 25 (1900): 118–19; Edward Dean Merriott, "The Passing of the Isolation Hospital," ibid., n.s. 26 (1900): 71, 85, 124, 157–8, 175–6, 199–200; C. Killick Millard, "The Influence of Hospital Isolation in Scarlet Fever: An Appeal to Statistics," *Public Health*, 13 (1900–1): 462–3; and C. Killick Millard, "The Hospital Isolation of Scarlet Fever: Some Points of Uncertainty," ibid., 14 (1901–2): 285–94.

mental hygiene.[123] The profession rose in defense of the hospitals, attacking the critics' arguments and statistics as shoddy and deceptive and touting the institutions as the only defense against a serious disease.

Newsholme was one of the isolation hospital's most vocal defenders. During the early 1890s his examination of broad statistical trends had convinced him that institutional isolation for scarlet fever was helpful. Based on the timing of past epidemics, he had expected an epidemic of scarlet fever in Brighton in 1888 and 1889. When mortality from the disease did not increase during those years (he still did not have information on the number of cases), he gave credit to hospital isolation.[124] While he continued to attribute the steady decline in scarlet fever mortality to the Sanatorium, with each passing year after the notification of infectious disease went into effect, he grew more certain that the decline in mortality was due in large measure to the fact that cases were growing milder and that severe cases, which in the past would have entered the mortality records as scarlet fever, were now notified as diphtheria.[125] Still he maintained that universal isolation was the proper policy for the disease.

This was not a well-founded conclusion, as Newsholme came to recognize. The public controversy provided the occasion for more reasoned consideration. Like many of the hospital's defenders, he found it easier to attack the critics' statistical arguments than to demonstrate the hospital's utility. In his criticism he emphasized that since scarlet fever's case fatality was falling steadily, it was not safe to estimate a community's morbidity from its recorded mortality rates as the critics had done for the period before notification began, and that the critics had failed to acknowledge that scarlet fever occurred in wavelike patterns.[126] The effect of isolation in two towns which isolated very different percentages of cases could only be fairly tested if it could be shown that the towns were in a similar phase of their epidemic cycle. The critics had failed to do this; in fact they had compared periods of maximum occurrence in one town with minimum occurrence in others to prove their point.

Hospital defenders like Newsholme could subject the critics' demonstrations to withering analysis, but this analysis did not prove that the hospitals were effective in controlling scarlet fever. A direct demonstration was needed. Although Newsholme offered a loose descriptive analysis of scarlet fever statistics from major cities on both side of the Atlantic,[127] he pinned his hopes on two demonstrations that

123 John M. Eyler, "Scarlet Fever and Confinement: The Edwardian Debate over Isolation Hospitals," *Bull. Hist. Med.* 61 (1987): 1–24.
124 Newsholme, *Ann. Rep.* (Brighton), 1890, 12–13.
125 See the evolution of Newsholme's position on this point in ibid., 1892, 10; ibid., 1894, 21–3; ibid., 1895, 12–13; and ibid., 1899, 23–4.
126 Arthur Newsholme, "The Utility of Isolation Hospitals in Diminishing the Spread of Scarlet Fever. Considered from an Epidemiological Standpoint," *J. Hygiene,* 1 (1901): 148; and Arthur Newsholme, "The Epidemiology of Scarlet Fever in Relation to the Utility of Isolation Hospitals," *Trans. Epidem. Soc. Lond.,* n.s. 20 (1900–1): 59.
127 Newsholme, "Epidemiology of Scarlet Fever," 49–58.

I.—*Cases removed to Hospital.*

	Attack-rate among those living in the same Family, and aged		Attack-rate among those living in the same House, and aged	
	Under 20.	Over 20.	Under 20.	Over 20.
First Period ...	33·5	3·1	29·0	2.2
Second ,, ...	30·9	5·5	27·4	3·7
Both Periods ...	32·5	4·1	28·5	2·8

II.—*Cases treated at Home.*

First Period ...	47·9	3·8	45·3	2·9
Second ,, ...	56·0	6·7	50·0	5·9
Both Periods ...	51·1	5·1	47·2	4·1

Illustration 4.9. Newsholme's calculation of the attack rate for scarlet fever per 1,000 among nonimmunes in Brighton. From Newsholme, "Epidemiology of Scarlet Fever in Relation to the Utility of Isolation Hospitals," *Trans. Epidem. Soc. Lond.*, n.s. 20 (1900–1): 65.

early institutionalization reduced the rate of secondary infection in Brighton. In the first he compared the experiences of households in which the first case of scarlet fever was removed to the Sanatorium with those in which the first case was nursed at home.[128] The 511 first cases removed to the isolation hospital before a second case appeared were followed by 32 cases in the same household, yielding as Newsholme calculated a secondary infection rate of 6.2%. That figure dropped to 3.1%, if one excluded, as Newsholme thought one should, any secondary case that appeared more than seven days after the removal of the first case, because cases appearing that late were probably caused by some other source than the hospitalized case. By contrast the 71 cases nursed at home had caused 23 subsidiary cases, a rate of 32.1%. Newsholme ruled out of hand another 31 subsidiary cases in households where the first case was sent to the Sanatorium at the same time or after the secondary cases. In these last instances, he argued, isolation had not been properly conducted, and so the secondary cases would not be attributed to the

128 Newsholme, *Ann. Rep.* (Brighton), 1900, 18–20; and Newsholme, "Epidemiology of Scarlet Fever," 61–4.

influence of the Sanatorium. It was not an elegant or very convincing demonstration. Among other deficiencies it was unaware of the number of susceptible patients who were at risk in the two groups of households. Newsholme introduced it rather tentatively "as indicating lines of useful record, than as justifying very dogmatic conclusions."[129]

His second demonstration was more sophisticated.[130] For the period 1899 to 1900 he calculated the rate at which subsidiary cases occurred among the nonimmune in the patient's family and among those families living in the same house. He separated his figures for two periods. During the first Brighton's morbidity rate for scarlet fever was increasing, and during the second it was decreasing. He also divided the subsidiary cases into two groups by age. The number of immunes in the household was determined during the household visits which followed notification of the disease. For several years family members had been asked during these visits whether they had previously had scarlet fever. Given the problems of diagnosing the disease, the unreliability of human memory, and the intimidating presence of the Inspector or the M.O.H. there is reason to question the accuracy of that return. This approach does show, however, that Newsholme was trying to define more carefully the population actually at risk. Illustration 4.9 represents the attack rates calculated in this way. The calculation was based on a total of 744 houses, 444 in the first period and 300 in the second. Except for the uncertainty of determining who was actually nonimmune, this is a much more satisfactory demonstration of the hospital's value in halting the spread of scarlet fever. It seemed that for children, especially, hospital isolation was of value in preventing transmission.

Newsholme repeated this demonstration for each of the following two years.[131] In 1901 and 1902 the number of reported cases of scarlet fever was much lower than it had been in 1899 and 1900, so for each repetition of this demonstration he used combined figures for each year since 1899. However, with each subsequent annual calculation the isolation hospital's advantage slipped away. We do not have the figures for individual years, but as the number of cases in 1901 and 1902 was so much smaller than in the first two years, we must conclude that the experience of 1901 and 1902 was not very comforting to the friends of hospital isolation. By 1903 Newsholme permitted this line of investigation to drop quietly.

He grew irritated at critics who demanded proof that hospital isolation was stamping out scarlet fever. That was an impossible demand. What hospital isolation could reasonably be expected to do was to reduce the severity of epidemics, in turn making them more manageable and less socially and economically disruptive; to lengthen the interepidemic period, and to delay the age at which children

---

129 Newsholme, "Epidemiology of Scarlet Fever," 61.
130 Newsholme, *Ann. Rep.* (Brighton), 1900, 20–1; Newsholme, "Epidemiology of Scarlet Fever," 64–6.
131 Newsholme, *Ann. Rep.* (Brighton), 1901, 23–4; and ibid., 1902, 22–3.

contract scarlet fever in this way rendering cases less severe.[132] Newsholme was convinced that the hospital was having this effect, although he could not prove it satisfactorily.

Where statistics failed, Newsholme resorted to special pleading. The preventive advantages of hospital isolation were not more obvious because the hospitalized and the home-treated cases were not alike.[133] Home-treated cases were most often from prosperous homes where there were ample means to properly isolate the sick person. Hospital cases usually came from poor homes where lack of space and overcrowding were common. Since mild cases escaped detection and other cases were sometimes not reported or isolated promptly, second and third patients were frequently infected before the mechanism of hospital isolation could be brought into play. The isolation hospital was the only known preventive measure for scarlet fever and diphtheria. For typhus isolation hospitals had almost become unnecessary, and if smallpox vaccination were universal, they would be unnecessary for that disease as well. "Until better means or supplemental means, the results of fuller knowledge of the natural history of scarlet fever, are devised, it is our obvious duty to persevere with the best known means of preventing the spread of this disease. . . . It would therefore constitute a sin against knowledge to abstain from preventive action in these directions."[134] In an analogy that became a favorite among the hospitals' defenders, he compared the isolation hospital to the fire brigade. No one was audacious enough to call for the abolition of the fire brigade simply because there were still fires.[135]

As an administrator he was alarmed by the criticism of the isolation hospitals. "Anything tending to undermine the confidence of the public in their efficiency is much to be deprecated, as it is only by the active cooperation of all concerned that the full efficiency of these measures can be ensured."[136] For the city fathers of Brighton he argued,

The question arises whether the town obtains, under the circumstances of the extreme mildness of the present type of the disease, a sufficient return for the large sum of money spent in isolating patients suffering from it in the Borough Sanatorium. For Brighton there can be but one answer to this question. It is of 'the utmost importance' for its reputation that every infectious case, which cannot be efficiently isolated at home, shall be treated in the Sanatorium.[137]

There was something to the complaint of one critic of isolation who accused his opponents of abandoning statistics and clinging instead to theory.[138] The town

132 Newsholme, "Utility of Isolation Hospitals," 149–52; and Newsholme, "Epidemiology of Scarlet Fever," 50–1, 60–1, 68–9.
133 Newsholme, *Ann. Rep.* (Brighton), 1901, 24.
134 Newsholme, "Utility of Isolation Hospitals," 150.
135 Ibid. For the use of this analogy elsewhere, see "Isolation Hospitals," *Lancet* (1901), no. 1: 413.
136 Newsholme, "Epidemiology of Scarlet Fever," 61.
137 Newsholme, *Ann. Rep.* (Brighton), 1900, 17–18.
138 A. Mearns Fraser, "Is the Hospital Isolation of Scarlet Fever Worth While?" *Public Health,* 16 (1903–4): 214–15.

and its Medical Officer of Health had invested too much money and too large a
share of a professional reputation in the success of the isolation hospital to
repudiate or even substantially modify its use for even one of the important
notifiable diseases. Isolation must be working even though that fact could not be
effectively demonstrated. Illustration 4.6 shows the number of notified cases in
Brighton and the percentage of these isolated in the Sanatorium. It is easy to see
how in the early and middle 1890s Newsholme might have an easy confidence
that hospital isolation was bringing the disease under control. The epidemic of
1898–1900 seriously eroded that complacency, but Newsholme could still argue
that institutional isolation reduced the rate of secondary infection.

The critics' assaults and scarlet fever's intractable morbidity rate in spite of a
high rate of isolation forced a gradual reevaluation. The defenders of hospital
isolation for scarlet fever now began to emphasize the economic and social
advantages of institutional isolation.[139] When the first case in a household was
taken to the isolation hospital, other children in the family might continue to
attend school, and other family members could remain employed at jobs from
which they would be barred if a case of scarlet fever were being nursed at home.
When the Local Government Board finally answered the calls of professional
societies and mounted an official investigation of the use of isolation hospitals for
scarlet fever, Newsholme was Medical Officer of the Board.[140] In his introduction
he endorsed the report's use of social and economic convenience in defense of the
hospitals.[141] He also acknowledged that isolation policy had sometimes been
misguided, as when wholesale isolation of cases had led to crowding in isolation
hospitals and precautions against cross-infection had been lax, and he suggested
that local authorities might experiment with more flexible isolation policies and
shorter periods of confinement. By the 1920s after he had left public office and
the etiology of scarlet fever was better known, Newsholme recognized that a
generation earlier the need for institutional isolation of scarlet fever had been
exaggerated.[142] Isolation hospitals had not controlled the disease, but, he argued,
they had proven valuable as treatment centers and had saved many lives.

The debate over the use of isolation hospitals for scarlet fever reminds us how
limited the knowledge of some infectious diseases was at the turn of the century.
The episode also reveals how quickly universal isolation for the major notifiable

139 Edward Walford, "The Influence of Hospital Isolation upon Scarlet Fever in Cardiff," *Public
Health,* 16 (1903–4): 685–6; and John C. Thresh, "The Utility of Isolation Hospitals," *Lancet*
(1906), no. 1: 1060.
140 The British Medical Association's Section on State Medicine and the Metropolitan Asylums Board
had both called on the L.G.B. to mount an investigation. *Lancet* (1904), no. 2: 315–16, 634–5; *Br.
Med. J.* (1905), no. 2: 636; and *Lancet,* (1908), no. 1: 42. See also James Wheatly, "The Desirability
of an Inquiry into the Effect of Hospital Isolation of Scarlet Fever, and the Form an Inquiry
Should Take," *Public Health,* 16 (1903–4): 355–9.
141 Arthur Newsholme, "Introduction," in H. Franklin Parsons, *Report on Isolation Hospitals, Supplement to Ann. Rep. Med. Off. L.G.B.,* 40 (1910–11): iv–vi.
142 Arthur Newsholme, *The Elements of Vital Statistics in Their Bearing on Social and Public Health
Problems* (London: George Allen and Unwin, 1923): 433–4; and Newsholme, *Fifty Years,* 183.

diseases had become a goal of the more active local authorities. This debate was narrowly focused. While some of the hospital critics wanted to halt future construction and close existing hospitals, the discussion of the hospitals' value centered on scarlet fever, the disease where their effectiveness was most in question. The critics would have won even fewer sympathetic ears, if they had questioned the value of these hospitals for typhoid fever, diphtheria, and smallpox. As events transpired, the debate seems to have had no effect on the establishment of these hospitals, although it forced the institutions to modify their practices and to adopt greater precautions against cross-infection.[143] The debate had an effect on Newsholme as well. The extensive study of return cases he undertook in its wake made him aware of the importance of asymptomatic and convalescent carriers.[144] His awareness of that possibility was first alerted by studies of milk-borne epidemics of scarlet fever he had investigated in the recent past. We consider those studies, among other topics, in the next chapter.

143 Eyler, "Scarlet Fever and Confinement," 21–4.
144 Newsholme, "Protracted and Recrudescent Infection," 557–8, 560–1, 580–3.

5

The epidemiology of infected food and the limits of sanitary jurisdiction

TYPHOID FEVER AND OYSTERS

By the middle nineties Brighton had done everything that had been thought necessary to conquer typhoid fever. It had built main intercepting sewers to divert sewage from the sea front. It had required owners to connect their houses to this system and to fill in their cesspools. Its Sanitary Department mounted an energetic inspection program to see that household drainage was properly installed and maintained. The town also provided pure water as a municipal service. Furthermore, it acted to prevent direct interpersonal transmission by requiring and closely supervising notification, isolation, and disinfection. Why then had the decline in the incidence and mortality from typhoid leveled off, leaving the town with a substantial endemic typhoid problem? Newsholme began to suspect that while the town had solved most of its old sanitary problems, some previously unappreciated factor continued to spread the contagion.[1] Careful inquiry following notification indicated that after one excluded cases that had been acquired outside Brighton and cases for which there was a known source of infection, between 30 and 40 percent of notified cases were unaccounted for during these years.[2]

In March 1894 Newsholme announced to the Sanitary Committee that he had found the cause of such unexplained cases.[3] His postnotification investigation in an outbreak of eleven cases led him to conclude that the only likely cause of at least five, and perhaps as many as eight, of these cases was the consumption of sewage-contaminated oysters. Newsholme believed that he was the first British

---

1 Arthur Newsholme, "An Address on the Spread of Enteric Fever by Means of Sewage-Contaminated Shellfish," *Br. Med. J.* (1896), no. 2: 640. The same text was also published as Arthur Newsholme "The Spread of Enteric Fever by Means of Sewage Contaminated Shell-Fish,' " *J. Sanitary Inst.*, 17 (1896): 391–2. Subsequent citations will be to the version in *Br. Med. J.*

2 Newsholme, *Ann. Rep.* (Brighton), 1897, 24. This section of Newsholme's report was republished as Arthur Newsholme, "Memorandum as to the Connection between the Consumption of Shell-fish Contaminated by Sewage and Infectious Disease," *Public Health*, 10 (1897–8): 423.

3 Arthur Newsholme, "Special Report on an Outbreak of Enteric Fever Apparently Caused by Eating Oysters," Brighton, Proc. San. Comm., 11 (29 March 1894): 233–42.

author to trace typhoid cases to sewage-contaminated shellfish since Charles Cameron of Dublin first suggested, largely on the basis of the analogy to transmission by water and milk, this possibility at the British Medical Association meeting in 1880.[4] He was certainly in the vanguard of renewed interest in this topic, and he would prove a major impetus behind the demand by local authorities for new measures to deal with this threat to public health.[5]

Most of the oysters sold in Brighton came from two suppliers in the neighboring coastal community of Southwick, who planted young French oysters in the estuary of the River Adur at Shoreham near the sewerage outlets of Southwick and Shoreham. When Newsholme unofficially inspected those beds in March 1894, he found that before going to market the oysters were moved to storage ponds built on the mud of the river's north shore, 150 yards downstream from the main Southwick sewerage outfall and even closer to several smaller sewerage outlets.[6] "At the time of my visit a black stream of sewage was trickling down this mud bank and rats were disporting themselves on its margin. The smell was most offensive."[7] Twice a day at high tide a fresh wave of highly contaminated water washed over the ponds, displacing the water brought by the previous high tide.

The conditions in which these oysters lived were certainly revolting, but how could Newsholme be sure that such conditions caused typhoid in Brighton? Linking these oysters with typhoid cases was difficult. There was much circumstantial evidence, but important links in the chain of evidence were missing.[8] He could show that most of the oysters sold in Brighton were grown and stored in water that was highly contaminated with sewage. The typhoid bacillus was probably present in the sewage. This conclusion followed from the fact that typhoid was endemic in the areas served by the sewers which discharged their untreated effluent close to the oyster beds. The high case fatality rates from typhoid fever in the populations using these sewers suggested that many cases were unreported, suggesting in turn that the water in those oyster beds must be even more highly contaminated with typhoid organisms than one might otherwise expect. Recent

4 Arthur Newsholme, "The Spread of Enteric Fever and Other Forms of Illness by Sewage-Polluted Shellfish," *Br. Med. J.* (1903), no. 2: 295. Cameron's paper is summarized in the report of the B.M.A. meeting in *Br. Med. J.* (1880), no. 2: 471.

5 Soon after Newsholme's initial report several clinicians were led by their experience in practice to suspect the same mode of transmission. See, for example, Sir William Broadbent, "A Note on the Transmission of the Infection of Typhoid Fever by Oysters," *Br. Med. J.* (1895), no. 1: 61; and Sir Peter Eade, "Typhoid Fever and Oysters and Other Mollusks," ibid., 121–2. Within a few years other M.O.H. were attributing typhoid outbreaks to oyster eating.

6 This description is derived from Newsholme, "Special Report . . . Oysters," 238–9; and H. Timbrell Bulstrode, "Report on an Inquiry into the Conditions under Which Oysters, and Certain Other Edible Mollusks are Cultivated and Stored along the Coast of England and Wales," *Report and Papers on the Cultivation and Storage of Oysters and Certain Other Mollusks in Relation to the Occurrence of Disease in Man, Suppl. Ann. Rep. Med. Off. L.G.B.*, 24 (1894–5): 72–4.

7 Newsholme, "Special Report . . . Oysters," 238.

8 For a concise statement of his argument, see Newsholme, *Ann. Rep.* (Brighton), 1897, 23; or Newsholme, "Memorandum . . . Shell-fish," 423. See also Newsholme, "Address . . . Shellfish," 640–4.

studies by bacteriologists had shown that the typhoid bacillus could remain viable in salt water for a considerable length of time and that the organism could be recovered from oysters which had been kept in water very highly contaminated with this bacterium.[9] Given the environment in which they were raised the Southwick oysters might be expected to harbor the typhoid organism. Finally Newsholme's visit to each home where a typhoid case had been reported showed that in many cases where other sources of infection could be discounted, the patient had eaten oysters or other shellfish a week or two before becoming sick. Frequently the sick person was the only one in the household to have eaten the oysters.

Suggestive evidence, certainly, but hardly conclusive. Three major links were missing. First, although he twice collected samples of the water and mud from the storage ponds for analysis by bacteriologists, his consultants failed to culture the typhoid organism from his samples, although they reported finding plenty of fecal organisms. Second, he could not prove that the oysters which any of his cases had eaten had come from the suspect source. Other oysters were sold in town. Third, since he did not know how many people ate the Shoreham oysters, he could not compare the attack rates of people who did to those who did not consume these oysters. The latter evidence would have helped answer the objection that not everyone who ate oysters contracted typhoid, and it would have reduced the risk of falsely attributing the disease to a food which many people consumed.

Newsholme's argument of necessity was made by a process of exclusion. When no other source of contagion could be found, the patient or his family were asked whether the sick person had eaten shellfish in the last two weeks. It was not surprising that with such a popular food the answer was often yes. The problem with arguments by exclusion is, of course, that not all alternatives may have been considered. In the 1890s Newsholme had no way of knowing that an important means for spreading typhoid would soon be recognized. The earliest explicit statement of the importance of the healthy or convalescent carrier in the epidemiology of typhoid fever was no earlier than 1903 and 1904 in connection with the work undertaken at German typhoid stations at Koch's suggestion, and the results of this research were not publicized in Britain before 1908.[10] With the benefit of

---

9 E. Klein, "Report by Dr. Klein on his Bacteriological Researches," in *Report and Papers on the Cultivation*, 116–20. The use of bacteriological methods to assess water purity was itself contested ground in the 1890s, and Klein's work in this case can be seen as developing from the disputes among experts at the Metropolitan Water Commission of 1892–3. See Christopher Hamlin, "Politics and Germ Theories in Victorian Britain: The Metropolitan Water Commissions of 1867–9 and 1892–3," in *Government and Expertise: Specialists, Administrators and Professionals, 1860–1919*, ed. Roy MacLeod (Cambridge: Cambridge Univ. Press, 1988), 121–7; and Christopher Hamlin, *A Science of Impurity: Water Analysis in Nineteenth Century Britain* (Berkeley and Los Angeles: Univ. of California Press, 1990), 284–92.

10 Alexander Ledingham and J.C.G. Ledingham, "Typhoid Carriers," *Br. Med. J.* (1908), no. 1: 15–17; George Dean, "A Typhoid Carrier of Twenty-nine Years' Standing," ibid., 562–3; J.C.G. Ledingham, "The Typhoid Carrier Problem, with Some Experiments on Immunity in Carriers," ibid., no. 2: 1173–5. See also editorial comment in ibid., no. 1: 584–5, 701–3, 1129–31. See also the

hindsight we can see that some of the cases of typhoid fever Newsholme could not account for and some he attributed to shellfish consumption were probably those caused by contact with a carrier. Suggestive of the problem is the fact that using his approach Newsholme could not identify a probable cause for almost 25 percent of Brighton's cases. There were no sanitary defects in the house. There was no evidence to implicate contaminated water or milk. And there was no history of oyster eating.

He realized that his evidence was circumstantial, but he argued that "circumstantial facts which may from a mathematical standpoint be extremely weak, become strong when each link in the chain of evidence is visible."[11] Here, as in so much else he did, Newsholme acted as an administrator for whom suggestive epidemiological evidence was as valuable as conclusive demonstration. Historical interest in this episode lies not only in Newsholme's rough and ready epidemiology but also in his use of that knowledge. The risk to public health posed by sewage-contaminated shellfish was one area where local authorities seized the initiative in identifying a new public health problem and in demanding new means for meeting it. Newsholme became convinced that sewage-contaminated shellfish were a serious threat to the public health and that these shellfish should be kept off of the market. In regular sections in his annual reports, in special reports to the Sanitary Committee, and in papers to medical audiences, he presented the accumulating weight of circumstantial evidence and tried to convince his colleagues and his local authority of the necessity for public action.[12]

But direct action was impossible. Except in the case of milk, Medical Officers of Health had no authority to inspect food produced outside their jurisdictions. Newsholme did not at first consider seeking changes in the law. In his first report to the Sanitary Committee Newsholme suggested that the Committee had two alternatives: to publicize the fact that these oysters were dangerous and hope that the public would stop buying them, or to keep his report from the public and try to persuade the oyster growers to move their beds to safer water.[13] The Committee opted for the second choice.[14]

The choice involved the Committee in a frustrating and unsuccessful campaign, one that reveals some of the most basic limitations of local sanitary authority at

more thorough analysis of J.C.G. Ledingham, "Report on the Enteric Fever 'Carrier': Being a Review of the Current Knowledge of This Subject," *Ann. Rep. Med. Off. L.G.B.*, 39 (1909–10), Appendix B: 246–84; J.C.G. Ledingham and J. A. Arkwright, *The Carrier Problem in Infectious Diseases* (London: Edward Arnold, 1912), 5–135.

11 Newsholme, "Address . . . Shellfish," 640.
12 As an example of Newsholme's continuing interest in this subject, see his special report in Newsholme, *Ann. Rep.* (Brighton), 1902, 36–46.
13 Newsholme, "Special Report . . . Oysters," 240.
14 For information on the Committee's activities during 1894 to secure changes in sewage disposal and oyster cultivation, see Brighton, Proc. San. Comm., 11 (29 March 1894): 242; ibid., 26 April 1894, 272; ibid., 13 Sept. 1894, 433; ibid. 12 (11 Oct. 1894): 22–3; ibid., 15 Nov. 1894, 80; ibid., 29 Nov. 1894, 105–6; ibid., 13 Dec. 1894, 134–7. Newsholme also published an account of the town's efforts to secure these changes: See Newsholme, "Memorandum . . . Shell-fish," 423–4 in Newsholme, *Ann. Rep.* (Brighton), 1897, 24–5.

the turn of the century. The Brighton Sanitary Committee first contacted the New Shoreham Port Sanitary Authority and the Rural Sanitary Authority of the Steying Union about the oyster beds in their districts. These negotiations resulted only in a temporary closing of the beds for "cleaning." They were soon in use again. Brighton appealed for help to the L.G.B. Newsholme conferred with the Board's Assistant Medical Officer, William Henry Power, and Brighton's M.P. arranged a meeting of a delegation from the Town Council with the Board's Parliamentary Secretary. Although the Parliamentary Secretary "regarded the site where the oyster ponds were now placed as an open sewer, and absolutely unfit for its present use," the Board offered little hope of an immediate remedy.[15] Special legislation would be needed to permit local authorities to inspect food produced outside their jurisdiction, and that would probably take three years to accomplish. In the meantime the Board suggested that Brighton seize and attempt to condemn individual lots of oysters. Given the trouble that health authorities had experienced in condemning tubercular meat when the lesions were obvious, the prospects of success in attempting to condemn oysters that looked perfectly sound were very dim. While the appeals to the L.G.B. were fruitless in the short run, Brighton's complaints did pique the interest of the Board's Medical Department, which assigned one of its inspectors to undertake a major investigation of oyster cultivation and disease.[16]

It seemed then as if new legal powers were necessary. Brighton's officials turned first to private legislation. The Town's M.P. introduced a bill in the Commons destined to become the Brighton Corporation Act, 1896.[17] Section 33 of this bill would have empowered Brighton's M.O.H. to inspect places inside or outside the town's boundaries where food was prepared for sale in the town, and it gave the Corporation authority to prohibit the sale in its jurisdiction of food that its M.O.H. found likely to cause disease.[18] The bill's authors had seriously underestimated the opposition these provisions would raise. Individuals as well as neighboring local authorities wrote to protest this attempt to extend the town's jurisdiction, and the Sussex Law Society objected that such a broad expansion of powers should only be acquired by general legislation.[19] When Brighton's Town Clerk

15 See the report of the delegation that met with the L.G.B.'s Parliamentary Secretary 7 Dec. 1894 in Brighton, Proc. San. Comm., 12 (13 Dec. 1894): 134–7; and Newsholme, "Memorandum . . . Shell-fish," 424.
16 Bulstrode, "Report on an Inquiry."
17 Gt. Brit., *Local and Personal Acts,* 59 & 60 Vict., C. 137.
18 A printed version of the original form of this bill is found in P.R.O., MH 12/12797 "Brighton Improvements."
19 For reaction in the press, see "Brighton 'Improvements' Bill," *Sussex Daily News,* 16 Jan. 1896, 4; and letters to the editor, ibid., 23 Jan, 6; & 24 Jan. 1896, 2. For the opposition of neighboring local authorities, see the following in P.R.O., MH 12/12798: H. Endicott (Town Clerk, Hove) to Sir Hugh Owen (Secretary, L.G.B.) 29 Jan. 1896; F. Merrifield (Town Clerk, West Sussex County) to F. J. Tillstone (Town Clerk, Brighton) 21 Feb. 1896; and F. Merrifield to President, Local Government Board, 23 March 1896. For opposition from Shoreham, see Brighton, Proc. San. Comm., 12 (11 Oct. 1894): 22–3; and Arthur Newsholme, *Fifty Years in Public Health: A Personal Narrative with Comments* (London: George Allen and Unwin, 1935), 211.

proposed to limit Section 33 to shellfish from sewage-contaminated water, the Fisheries Division of the Board of Trade and the Kent and Essex Sea Fisheries District objected strenuously.[20] By the spring of 1896 the bill's opponents had made their views widely known, and the Police and Sanitary Regulations Committee of the House of Commons threw out several clauses, including Clause 33, on constitutional grounds.[21] Newsholme was bitterly disappointed and blamed the Local Government Board for failing to support the bill.[22]

The town's officials next attempted to pressure the L.G.B. to sponsor general legislation. It prepared a petition to the L.G.B. to this effect and collected the endorsement of twenty-seven of the thirty-three largest towns plus the London Port Sanitary Authority.[23] The petition may in fact not have been necessary. The L.G.B. was becoming convinced that the conditions local authorities were complaining of were a hazard to public health and that new legislation was needed. The Board's own recent study of oyster cultivation showed that conditions like those Brighton complained of were common on the British coast.[24] Within a year of the appearance of this report one of the Board's inspectors confirmed the conclusion of an M.O.H. from Essex that a typhoid outbreak in October 1897 was caused by the eating of sewage-contaminated oysters.[25] The L.G.B. drafted a bill giving the local authorities the power to inspect oyster cultivation outside their districts. But during the summer of 1899 strong opposition to this legislation from the fishing industry made itself felt in the House of Lords. The Lord's Select Committee heard testimony from medical officers of the L.G.B. and from local officials, including Newsholme, who described the hazards posed by the present methods of cultivation. The Committee acknowledged that some overseeing was necessary, but it proposed to give authority to the local district fisheries committee rather than to the local health authority. This change so weakened the bill that its sponsors abandoned it.[26]

20 F. J. Tillstone to F. Merrifield, 22 Feb. 1896, in P.R.O. MH 12/12798; T.H.W. Pelham (Assistant Secretary, Harbour Department) to Secretary, Local Government Board, 14 March 1896 forwarding letter from Herbert W. Gibson (Committee for the Kent and Essex Sea Fisheries District) 11 March 1896, in ibid. For a copy of the revised section see "New Clause 33, page 23" in ibid.

21 "The Brighton Corporation's Bill," *Times*, 5 June 1896, 3; and "Brighton Corporation Bill," *Brighton Gazette*, 6 June 1896, 4.

22 Newsholme, "Address . . . Shellfish," 644. An unnamed L.G.B. official penned a note with a news clipping of Newsholme's remarks reading "Another *opinion* of the *Brighton Authorities* – Local Government Board wrong again. Why do they not consult the Brighton Town Council before deciding matters of importance to the country?" See undated news clipping in P.R.O. MH 12/12799.

23 The Council approved the Sanitary Committee's draft of this petition on 15 April 1897, *Sussex Daily News*, 16 April 1897, 2; and Newsholme, "Spread of Enteric Fever," 296.

24 Bulstrode, "Report on an Inquiry."

25 George S. Buchanan, "Report upon the Occurrence of Certain Cases of Enteric Fever in Six Sanitary Districts of East Essex and Suffolk, and upon Oysters in relation thereto," *Ann. Rep. Med. Off. L.G.B.*, 27 (1897–8): 47–64.

26 "Report from the Select Committee of the House of Lords on the Oysters Bill together with Proceedings of the Committee and Minutes of Evidence," *House of Lords Sessional Papers*, 1899, [172], X. See also "Oysters Bill," *Times*, 1 Aug. 1899, 10.

Up to this point the force for Brighton's campaign against contaminated oysters had come from Newsholme and a few members of the Sanitary Committee. Other members of the Council, including the Chairman of the Sanitary Committee, did not take the matter too seriously and enjoyed joking with their M.O.H. about his oyster fad.[27] But in May 1899, while the Oyster Bill was still in the House of Lords, a local tragedy changed the political climate. A member of the Sanitary Committee, one of those who enjoyed ribbing the M.O.H. about his little fad, gave a fashionable dinner party for the town's notables.

> The supper was an oyster and champagne feast. Care had been exercised to obtain the oysters from a known safe source; but they ran short, and others were sent for from 'round the corner.' Within the next sixteen days three cases of enteric fever were notified from guests of this supper party. One of them, my chairman, was my patient in the Fever Hospital; and no further opposition to my shell-fish recommendations was experienced in Brighton.[28]

Typhoid killed one guest, a member of the Town Council.[29] This grim demonstration of the hazards of contaminated oysters followed by the Lords' emasculation of the Oyster Bill made the Committee willing to try publicity, the alternative strategy Newsholme had suggested five years earlier. Soon placards with the following message appeared on the sea front.[30]

> The public are warned against eating oysters, mussels and cockles derived from sewage polluted sources.
> Serious illness is frequently caused by neglect of this precaution.
>
> (signed) Arthur Newsholme,
> Medical Officer of Health[31]

The Sanitary Department gave no guidance to the public in how to tell whether oysters had been derived from such a source. No wonder that fishmongers complained that their trade was being ruined and asked repeatedly that the signs be taken down, and no wonder that the signs were frequently defaced, or that sneering voices accused the Council of being grandmotherly.[32] But the town's health authorities refused to bend, and the signs remained on the beach year after

---

27 Newsholme, *Fifty Years*, 211.   28 Ibid., 211–12.
29 See Newsholme's report on the incident in Brighton, Proc. San. Comm., 16 (29 June 1899): 334–6.
30 By a sizable margin the Town Council approved the Committee's proposal for these placards, *Brighton Herald*, 5 Aug. 1899, 8; and Brighton, Proc. San. Comm., 16 (27 July 1899): 366.
31 Newsholme, *Ann. Rep.* (Brighton), 1899, 69. This is a revised version of the original text. The first version confused the issue by referring to the closed season for oysters. The revision was made within a month of the original passage. Brighton, Proc. San. Comm., 16 (24 Aug. 1899), 401.
32 Ibid., 28 Sept. 1899, 441; ibid., 17 (12 July 1900), 306; ibid., 16 (28 Sept. 1899), 439; ibid., 17 (14 Nov. 1899), 21; ibid. 22 (28 Sept. 1905), 252; ibid. 23 (11 Oct. 1906), 180; and *Sussex Daily News*, 21 Aug. 1899, 4. The critics often claimed that the problem was merely one of protecting the public from spoiled fish. See, for example, the Council debate over the posting of these signs. *Sussex Daily News*, 5 Aug. 1899, 3. See also Councillor Jarvis's discussion in a later Council debate, *Brighton Gazette*, 20 Oct. 1906, 8. The oyster growers wrote protesting these signs and using similar arguments in Brighton, Proc. San. Comm., 16 (24 Aug. 1899): 400–1.

Typhoid/Enteric Fever

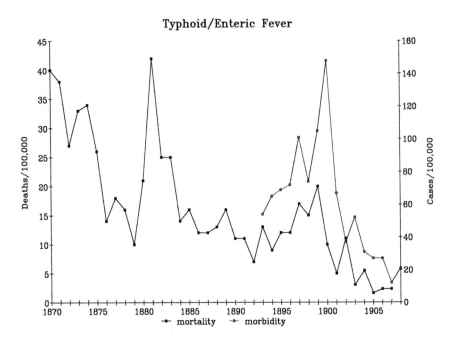

Illustration 5.1. Mortality from typhoid fever in Brighton, 1870–1907. Compiled from Brighton Corporation, Medical Officer of Health, *Annual Reports on the Health, Sanitary Condition, &c. of the Borough of Brighton.*

year. Newsholme was convinced that the signs were having a beneficial effect on the town's morbidity and mortality rates.[33] As Illustration 5.1 shows, Brighton's typhoid morbidity and mortality rates both began to drop again around 1900. In the twenties Newsholme continued to give credit for this decline to the discovery that contaminated shellfish spread typhoid, although by this time he also recognized that carriers probably played a role in the town's experience with this disease.[34]

Buoyed by the assurance that they were finally having an effect in their own jurisdiction Brighton's officials continued the campaign against sewage-contaminated shellfish beyond the town's boundaries. The Town Council continued to press for general legislation permitting an M.O.H. to supervise the production of food sold within his jurisdiction.[35] The town's officials also addressed the problem of sewage pollution of coastal waters. Newsholme sought to pressure

---

33 See his report in Ibid., 17 (11 Jan 1900): 73–7 reprinted in Newsholme, *Ann. Rep.* (Brighton), 1899, 20–1.

34 Arthur Newsholme, *Public Health and Insurance: American Addresses* (Baltimore: Johns Hopkins Univ. Press, 1920): 17.

35 See, for example, Brighton, Proc. San. Comm., 17 (11 Jan. 1900): 75–7; ibid., 20 (11 Feb. 1903): 41–6; Newsholme, *Ann. Rep.* (Brighton), 1899, 21; and ibid., 1902, 45–6.

Brighton's neighbors to abate their sewage nuisance, and he took his case for reform to the Royal Commission on Sewage Disposal and expressed pleasure with the Commission's conclusion that contaminated shellfish constituted a significant public health problem demanding a remedy.[36] Finally Brighton tried to institute trade pressure to keep contaminated shellfish off the market. It forwarded to the London Fishmonger's Company copies of Newsholme's reports on typhoid cases traced to shellfish consumption and the results of the microscopic analysis Newsholme had arranged for Emanuel Klein at the Local Government Board to perform on oysters from Southwick. The Fishmonger's Company first announced that it would no longer permit the sale in London of oysters from one of these producers, and within months it pledged to sell only oysters from uncontaminated sources and called on local authorities to inform it of oyster beds known to be polluted.[37] It is quite clear that the initiative in this matter was in the hands of local authorities rather than with the central authority in London. A persistent M.O.H. who had the support of his Committee could play a significant role in framing a public health issue. The episode illustrates some of the legal obstacles to the control of certain health risks, but it also shows that local authorities had nonstatutory remedies they might use.

SCARLET FEVER AND MILK

Just as the failure of sanitation to eliminate typhoid fever led Newsholme to seek another source of infection, the profession's gradual realization that hospital isolation was not controlling scarlet fever encouraged him to study the disease from a new perspective and to rethink his strategy of prevention. There is another similarity between Newsholme's work with typhoid fever and his efforts with scarlet fever we are about to discuss. From the beginning of his career, he knew that transmission by milk had been suggested for both diseases. By 1881 at least fifteen outbreaks of scarlet fever had been attributed to milk in Britain.[38] Newsholme knew of these reports, and in the 1884 edition of his *Hygiene* he discussed the possibility of transmitting the disease from a milker's family to the dairy's

---

36 The Sanitary Committee forwarded copies of Newsholme's report on conditions in Shoreham harbor in December 1903 to the New Shoreham Port Sanitary Authority and to the Sussex Sea Fisheries District, Brighton, Proc. San. Comm., 20 (31 Dec. 1903): 415. For Newsholme's report see ibid., 412–14. For his testimony to the Royal Commission, see *Fourth Report of the Commissioners Appointed to Inquire and Report What Methods of Treating and Disposing of Sewage (Including Any Liquid from Any Factory or Manufacturing Process) May Properly be Adopted. Pollution of Tidal Waters with Special Reference to Contamination of Shell-Fish,* vol. 2, B.P.P. 1904, XXXVII, Cd. 1884, questions 17537–662. For Newsholme's summary of the Commission's recommendations on this problem, see Brighton, Proc. San. Comm., 21 (11 Feb. 1904): 9–12.
37 See the letter of J. Wrench Towse for the Company to Newsholme 12 Jan. 1903 in Newsholme, *Ann. Rep.* (Brighton), 1902, 42. See also Brighton, Proc. San. Comm., 20 (29 Jan. 1903): 20. For the Fishmongers' announcement and the Committee's response, see ibid., 8 Oct. 1903, 314–15. The report in question is in Newsholme, *Ann. Rep.* (Brighton), 1902, 37–46.
38 Ernest Hart, "The Influence of Milk in Spreading Zymotic Disease," *Trans. Int. Med. Congress,* 7th session, 5 vols. (London, 1881), IV, 528–39.

customers.[39] But almost without exception that information had no effect on Newsholme's administration before 1900.[40]

By 1900, however, faced with doubts about the efficacy of isolation with scarlet fever, Newsholme began to consider seriously that milk might be playing an important role. Having once begun to consider this possibility, he detected four milk-borne scarlet fever epidemics in six years. It seems highly probable, therefore, that in previous years other milk-borne outbreaks went undetected. Nineteenth-century British towns were particularly vulnerable to such outbreaks, because the milk supply was not pasteurized.[41] Physicians and public health officials recognized, of course, that heating milk could kill pathogenic microbes living in it, but they were reluctant to recommend this method to control infection, because they feared that the process would rob milk of its nutritive value or make it less digestible to infants. A lengthy discussion of this topic in *The Lancet* in these years illustrates how poorly nutrition was understood and how reluctant physicians were to endorse what seemed to be the altering of a basic, natural food.[42] The exchange of letters was initiated by Clements Dukes, the Physician to Rugby School and authority on diseases of children. Dukes was convinced that boiled milk caused infantile scurvy and rickets and cited cases in his experience where a sickly child began to thrive when taken off heated milk and given pure, unboiled milk. In this climate of opinion it is hardly surprising that pasteurization or boiling of milk played almost no role in the response to these epidemics.[43] Brighton's milk supply was produced close to home, delivered in raw form and, in the absence of refrigeration, consumed soon after production.

As noted in Chapter 4 in these years the cause of scarlet fever was unknown and the relation of scarlet fever to cases of severe sore throat without the characteristic rash was also uncertain. Furthermore, not only was the boundary between scarlet fever and other illnesses producing some of the same symptoms unclear, it was not at all obvious when a milk-borne epidemic had begun. Cases of scarlet fever occurred year in and year out. Under these circumstances it might appear rather surprising that Newsholme was able to piece together an administrative apparatus that allowed him to detect early and to respond quickly to a milk-borne outbreak. The secret behind Newsholme's success lay in the use he made of the postnotification household visits and of an informal working relationship he

---

39 Arthur Newsholme, *Hygiene: A Manual of Personal and Public Health* (London, 1884): 366.

40 That exception came in 1890 when he hospitalized the child of a milker on a farm that supplied milk to Brighton. Since no scarlet fever cases were reported among the customers of the dairy supplying this milk, it is impossible to know how Newsholme would then have responded to a milk-borne epidemic. See Brighton, Proc. San. Comm., 8 (11 Dec. 1890): 50–1.

41 For the London milk supply, see M. W. Beaver, "Population, Infant Mortality and Milk," *Population Studies*, 27 (1973): 251–2.

42 *Lancet*, 1901, no. 1: 1859–60; ibid., 1901, no. 2: 49–51, 101–3, 169–70, 227–8, 536–8; ibid., 1902, no. 1: 1358, 1561–2; ibid., 1903, no. 1: 331, 398.

43 The one exception is a private recommendation Newsholme made to medical practitioners that they advise their patients temporarily to boil their milk until it was clear what was causing a string of suspicious sore throats. Newsholme, *Ann. Rep.* (Brighton), 1906, 49.

formed with the local milk trade. His studies of the milk-borne scarlet fever epidemics offer another demonstration that Newsholme's epidemiological research grew out of practical administrative problems of disease prevention and that the results of that research might influence not only his preventive policy but also his understanding of disease.

The four milk-borne epidemics in question occurred in January 1900, November and December 1901, July 1905, and October 1906.[44] Since I have discussed these outbreaks and Newsholme's study of them in detail elsewhere, I limit my comments here to the more important changes in administration and understanding that accompanied them.[45] In dealing with these epidemics Newsholme faced two basic problems: first, detecting that a milk-borne epidemic had begun, and second, finding the source of the infection. The former would have been nearly impossible without notification and the visit to the home of the sick that followed notification. As we have seen, Brighton adopted the Infectious Diseases (Notification) Act, 1889, in 1891. In 1900 Newsholme began to ask regularly during the postnotification visit the source of the family's milk supply. When a series of scarlet fever cases closely spaced in time occurred among the customers of one dairy, Newsholme had reason to suspect that the milk might be infected. So sensitive did the Sanitary Department become to this possibility that in the third epidemic, the small outbreak of July 1905, Newsholme's current deputy, Thomas Barrett Heggs, was able to determine that milk was spreading scarlet fever contagion and to pinpoint its source after only six cases had been registered.[46]

Once he was convinced that a dairy's milk was spreading disease, Newsholme had the option of banning the sale of all milk from that dairy.[47] But such an action would certainly be unpopular with the dairy trade and with farmers, and furthermore, such sweeping action seemed unnecessary. If, as seemed probable, the milk was being infected at a single source, a more discriminating policy should be possible. But locating the source of infection could be difficult. Brighton's dairies bought their milk from several farms and traditionally had mixed the milk before sale or delivery. Even in the first decade of this century this local distribution network could be complicated. The dairy that sold the infected milk in 1905, for example, bought its supply from thirteen farms and distributed it through five shops and thirty-three home delivery routes. To complicate matters further, each of those milk carriers called on each house three times a day and might supply

---

44 For his accounts of these outbreaks, see Newsholme, *Ann. Rep.* (Brighton), 1900, 22–7; ibid., 1905, 18–21; ibid., 1906. 48–63; Arthur Newsholme, "On an Outbreak of Sore Throats and of Scarlet Fever Caused by Infected Milk," *J. Hygiene,* 2 (1902): 150–69; and Arthur Newsholme, "On an Outbreak of Scarlet Fever and Scarlatinal Sore Throat Due to Infected Milk," *Public Health,* 19 (1906–7): 756–72. The latter is a reprinting of the report in his *Annual Report* for 1906. These outbreaks are also discussed in the manuscript proceedings of the Sanitary Committee.

45 For a more complete account, see John M. Eyler, "The Epidemiology of Milk-borne Scarlet Fever: The Case of Edwardian Brighton," *Am. J. Public Health,* 76 (1986): 573–84.

46 Newsholme, *Ann. Rep.* (Brighton), 1905, 18.

47 Infectious Disease (Prevention) Act, 1890, 53 & 54 Vict., C. 34, sect. 4.

milk from different sources each time. Newsholme's experience with the first epidemic in January 1900 led him to suspect that when milk was contaminated, the infection occurred on the farm rather than in transit or in handling by the vendor, and, as we will see, his experience in later epidemics confirmed this suspicion.[48] Hereafter, when he had reason to believe that a dairy's milk was spreading scarlet fever, he directed his attention to conditions on the farms supplying the dairy.

His solution to the dilemma of how to keep infected milk off the market without putting an unnecessary burden on the milk trade was to urge local dairies to make two changes in the way they conducted their business: to refrain from mixing milk from different suppliers and to keep careful records of which milk was distributed by individual shops or carriers. He first made this suggestion informally to the town's milk vendors following the epidemic of 1900. Because the manager of the dairy which supplied the infected milk in the 1905 epidemic had followed Newsholme's suggestion, the Sanitary Department could quickly find the source of infection, although that dairy's milk came from thirteen farms. Illustration 5.2 is Newsholme's table showing how six cases were sufficient to implicate Farm "A," although milk from seven farms was supplied to the six households in twelve deliveries over a four-day period. Only Farm "A" had supplied all six households. This success in early detection and intervention encouraged Newsholme to be bolder. In a printed letter to all dairies in November 1905 he made explicit what had merely been implied before, their cooperation would help protect their business.[49] He reminded them of his authority to ban the sale of milk that was spreading disease and of the authority he had under private legislation[50] to require each of them to supply him with a list of their customers. He also pointed out that should he conduct a house-to-house investigation of the health of a dairy's customers, their business was likely to suffer. But, he promised, if milk supplies were properly earmarked and remained unmixed, in the event that milk from one farm became infected it should be possible with the aid of company records to identify the source and to suspend only the sale of the milk from a particular farm. That could all be accomplished without public notice or much inconvenience to the seller. In short, armed with much more sweeping powers, the M.O.H. was able to secure the cooperation of local dairies in an informal scheme which permitted prompt and selective intervention.

A similar strategy was employed in dealing with the source of infection on the farm. An M.O.H. could ban the sale of milk from a farm under the terms of the

48 In the epidemic of 1900 suspicion fell on one farm which sold milk to three dairies among whose customers scarlet fever cases began appearing around the same time. Eyler, "Epidemiology of Milk-borne Scarlet Fever," 576.

49 "The Importance of Being Able to Identify the Exact Source of Milk Supply," in Newsholme, *Ann. Rep.* (Brighton), 1905, 20–21. The letter is reprinted in ibid., 1906, 62–3 and in Newsholme, "On an Outbreak of Scarlet Fever," 771–2.

50 Brighton Improvement Act, 1884, 47 & 48 Vict., C. 262, sect. 55.

ANALYSIS OF THE SOURCE OF THE DAIRY MILK SUPPLIED TO THE FIRST SIX CASES OF SCARLET FEVER.

Initials of Farm whose milk was delivered on

CASE.	No. of MILK CARRIER	July 8th.	July 9th.	July 10th.	July 11th.	
1. (Onset 12th)	No. 21	A	C	A	D	1st round.
		B	B	B	B	2nd round.
		A	C	A	D	3rd round.
2. (Onset 12th)	No. 16	D	B	E	F	1st round.
		B and A	B and A	B and A	B and A	2nd round.
		A	A	A	A	3rd round.
3. (Onset 13th)	No. 3	E	B	F	A	1st round.
		B	B	B	B	2nd round.
		D or C	D or C	D or C	D or C	3rd round.
4. (Onset 11th or 12th)	No. 12	E	A	E	D	1st round.
		B	B	B	B	2nd round.
		D or C	D or C	D or C	D or C	3rd round.
5. (Onset 13th)	No. 19	D	G	E	A	1st round.
		D or C	D or C	D or C	D or C	2nd round.
6. (Onset 12th)	No. 24	A	A	A	A	1st round.
		D or C	D or C	D or C	D or C	2nd round.

Illustration 5.2. Milk-borne scarlet fever: Newsholme's reconstruction of the chain of infection in July 1905. From Newsholme, *Ann. Rep.* (Brighton), 1905, 19.

Infectious Disease (Prevention) Act, 1890.[51] But this legal process was slow and cumbersome, and Newsholme wanted to get the suspect milk off the market at once. He resorted instead to an informal purchase agreement with the farmer that permitted the Sanitary Department to buy and destroy the milk while the exact source of its contamination was found and removed. He used this approach in 1900 and again in 1905 and 1906.[52] But experience during the first epidemic demonstrated to him that it was necessary to have in addition the leverage which threat of enforcement of the Infectious Disease (Prevention) Act offered. In the first epidemic the farmer agreed to sell his milk to the Department but resisted cooperating in other ways, in removing his cows from their shed, for example, so the shed could be disinfected. Newsholme had to begin the enforcement process by getting an order from a Justice of the Peace authorizing him to make a formal inspection of the farm and then by seeking a notice from the Sanitary Committee. Only on the brink of having his milk banned from Brighton did the farmer cooperate with the Department. Hereafter Newsholme obtained the purchase agreement as soon as the disease registration and milk sale records implicated a farm's milk, but he soon thereafter began the process of legally prohibiting the sale of the milk by at least conducting the formal inspection under an order from a Justice of the Peace. In the future farmers cooperated fully with the Department's efforts.[53] The Sanitary Department clearly held the upper hand in dealing with farmers in the later epidemics. Its advantage can be seen in the rates of compensation it offered farmers, one shilling per gallon in 1900, but only four pence per gallon in later epidemics.[54]

While the infected milk was kept off the market, Newsholme tried to identify the specific source of infection. He paid particular attention to human sources and examined the farm laborers and their families in search of scarlet fever cases and convalescents. In the 1900 and 1905 epidemics he thought that he could reconstruct how the milk had become infected. In the first instance a child suffering from scarlet fever had been brought from Hove on December 11, 1899, to be nursed through the illness in a house only 200 yards from the farm whose milk became infected. There was regular contact between the farm staff and the house, because the farm supplied milk to the household. When Newsholme examined the farmhands on January 25, he found one milker suffering from peeling skin on his hands, feet, and thighs and learned that this man had been absent from work with what was described as a sore throat, a high fever, and a severe cold. Newsholme considered this man to be a scarlet fever convalescent, and, even though he lived outside the town, sent him to the Brighton Sanatorium and ordered his house disinfected.[55] During the 1905 epidemic Newsholme's deputy

51 53 & 54 Vict. C. 34, sect. 4.
52 Eyler, "Epidemiology of Milk-borne Scarlet Fever," 576, 577, 578.
53 See, for example, the extent of the farmer's cooperation in 1906 in ibid., 578.
54 Newsholme, *Ann. Rep.* (Brighton), 1900, 25; ibid., 1906, 50; and Brighton, Proc. San. Comm., 22 (19 July 1905): 166.
55 Newsholme, *Ann. Rep.* (Brighton), 1900, 25–6, 26–7.

found an ongoing scarlet fever epidemic among the farm employees and their families about which the Brighton authorities hitherto had known nothing, since the farm was located beyond municipal boundaries. The first farm case seems to have been infected at the village school in West Dean, where a scarlet fever epidemic was in progress, and it preceded by several days the first case among the families who consumed this farm's milk in Brighton.[56] The search for infected persons was followed by standard preventive measures. In the epidemics of 1900, 1905, and 1906, the sick and convalescent were sent to isolation hospitals, members of their families were temporarily barred from contact with cattle, and the homes of the sick as well as farm buildings were disinfected.

Newsholme was aware, of course, that there was another possible source of infection. Milk-borne scarlet fever contagium might have its origin in cattle. He knew that in 1885 William H. Power and Emanuel Klein at the Local Government Board claimed to have traced an outbreak of human scarlet fever through milk to diseased cattle on a farm in Hendon and found the streptococci to be the responsible organism.[57] Klein's hypothesis received an unsympathetic reception in the scientific and public health community, and that skepticism continued into the early twentieth century.[58] But the possibility that a cattle infection might be responsible for human cases did receive some notice during the investigations of these epidemics in Brighton. The formal inspection of the farms in the outbreaks of 1905 and 1906 was conducted by a panel of experts: M.O.H. from the jurisdiction in which the farm was located and from each town in which the milk was sold, and by veterinarians. By the 1906 epidemic the visiting team of inspectors had expanded to include three M.O.H., two veterinarians, and the Superintendent of the Brighton Abattoir, each of whom visited the farm several times. The veterinarian who examined the cattle in 1905 thought the herd was healthy. He did notice a scabby ulcer on one cow's teat. Cultures were made, but streptococci were not found.[59] The following year the veterinarians concluded, apparently on physical examination alone, that the herd supplying the infected milk showed no sign of the Hendon cow disease. Two cows did have ulcers on their udders, but no attempt was made this year to culture streptococci from these lesions, and the investigators' attention remained firmly fixed on human sources of infection.[60] The negative results of these perfunctory investigations served further to discredit the theory of bovine origin of milk-borne scarlet fever.

56 Ibid., 1905, 19–20.
57 For the work of Klein and Power, see *Ann. Rep. Med. Off. L.G.B.*, 15 (1885); 73–89, 90–9; "On the Relationship between Milk-scarlatina in the Human Subject, and Disease in the Cow," *Practitioner*, 37 (1886): 61–80, 143–60. For a recent discussion of the history of research on these outbreaks, see Leonard G. Wilson, "The Historical Riddle of Milk-Borne Scarlet Fever," *Bull. Hist. Med.*, 60 (1986): 321–42.
58 A. Wynter Blyth, *A Manual of Public Health* (London, 1890), 391–4; Harold Swithinbank and George Newman, *Bacteriology of Milk* (London: John Murray, 1903), 282–9.
59 Newsholme, *Ann. Rep.* (Brighton), 1905, 20; and Brighton, Proc. San. Comm., 22 (19 July 1905): 166.
60 Newsholme, *Ann. Rep.* (Brighton), 1906, 59, 61.

Streptococci received even less attention in the investigation of human cases. Early in the 1906 outbreak, when two recent scarlet fever cases among the customers of one dairy made Newsholme wonder whether the dairy's milk might be infected, the Sanitary Department received two throat swabs from a local medical practitioner who suspected diphtheria. These proved negative for the diphtheria bacillus, but, Newsholme reasoned, they might be from scarlet fever cases, since the two diseases often resemble each other in the early stages. Rather than trying to culture streptococci from these throats, Newsholme contacted the manager of the dairy whose milk he had begun to suspect to learn if it supplied milk to the houses from which the throat swabs came.[61] Similar inattention to the relevance of bacteriological findings in scarlet fever can be found in the early stages of the 1901 epidemic when Newsholme received three throat swabs from a practitioner. When these produced cultures of streptococci, Newsholme notified the practitioner of the fact but did not regard this result as justification for intervention or further investigation. Even in retrospect, when he recognized that these cases belonged to the epidemic, he was not prepared to recognize such bacteriological evidence as critical.[62] It was epidemiological not bacteriological evidence that caused Newsholme to conclude that these cases of sore throat were part of the 1901 epidemic.

During the outbreak of 1900 and especially in the 1905 epidemic, the Brighton Sanitary Department responded promptly and effectively. Its task was made easier by the fact that in those two outbreaks the cases had clearly marked symptoms and were readily diagnosed as scarlet fever. In the outbreaks of 1901 and 1906, however, many cases suffered from severe sore throats but did not exhibit the characteristic scarlet fever rash. Since the cause of scarlet fever was unknown and health authorities were little interested in the presence of streptococci, the significance of such sore throats to the health of the community went unappreciated. In fact while scarlet fever was a notifiable disease, sore throat was not. Thus the M.O.H. had no official way of knowing the incidence of the latter.

The epidemic of 1901 can be put down as an administrative failure for Newsholme. In fact it was six weeks old before he recognized that it was going on, and he acted too late to have had any effect on its course. However, his retrospective investigation was very significant conceptually for it demonstrated that cases of severe sore throat and scarlet fever might be related, and that future study and prevention action must take both types of cases into account.[63] Newsholme was belatedly alerted to the outbreak on December 9, when three cases of scarlet fever were registered, and all three were found to obtain their milk from the same dairy. The notification records showed that three other recent cases also consumed milk

---

61 Ibid., 1906, 49.   62 Newsholme, "On an Outbreak of Sore Throats," 151–2.
63 For a more complete discussion of this epidemic, see Eyler, "Epidemiology of Milk-borne Scarlet Fever," 580–1. It is significant that Newsholme made no mention of this outbreak in the usual administrative records, Brighton, Proc. San. Comm. or Newsholme, *Ann. Rep.* (Brighton). He instead published his investigation as a scientific paper, Newsholme, "Outbreak of Sore Throats."

from the same dairy. This dairy supplied milk from two farms, and it had not followed Newsholme's suggestion of recording which milk was supplied to individual households. Only a chance circumstance permitted Newsholme to implicate a particular farm. One of the notified cases occurred in the home of a fussy customer who, fearing adulteration of his milk in transit, had arranged for its delivery direct from the farm in a padlocked can. Since it was unlikely that the milk from both farms was infected simultaneously, Newsholme concluded that the infection must have originated on the farm that filled that locked can. When he visited the farm, however, he found no cases of scarlet fever. Cases of sore throat had occurred in three farm families, and he arranged to have members of these households temporarily removed from cattle-tending chores.

Having been alerted to the milk-borne epidemic, Newsholme was able to recognize that in October and November there had been outbreaks of illness in two boarding schools which he believed were caused by the drinking of this same milk. He had missed these outbreaks earlier, because they had consisted primarily of severe sore throat. During the course of these outbreaks Newsholme had been consulted by the school physicians on particularly severe sore throats or on doubtful diagnoses of scarlet fever. Illustration 5.3 is Newsholme's reconstruction of the outbreak, showing the date of onset of cases of both scarlet fever and sore throat. Group C consists of the cases notified in town. Group B is a school outbreak which Newsholme believed consisted of one case of sore throat acquired by drinking the suspect milk at home and seventeen secondary cases acquired in the school. It was from three of these cases of severe sore throat that the municipal laboratory cultured streptococci.[64] Group A is the other school outbreak consisting of one case of scarlet fever and five cases of sore throat.

Newsholme was puzzled by the fact that during the 1901 epidemic, cases appeared over a long period of time and assumed different clinical forms. As Illustration 5.3 shows, he reasoned that the milk must have been infected several times over a six-week period. He suggested that there had been at least three contaminations, each responsible for a group of cases of slightly different types. The incidence of cases in the exposed population also seemed remarkably low. Excluding secondary cases there were only sixteen cases of scarlet fever and sore throat attributable to the milk supply. Milk, it appeared, might carry a small amount of infectious material over a long period of time. Most significant was the fact that the same milk supply had caused cases of both scarlet fever and sore throats without the scarlet fever rash. Since he believed that he was dealing with only one infection, not two, Newsholme concluded that "infected milk may carry the scarlatinal contagium in such an attenuated form or in such a minute amount that it is not capable of causing all the phenomena of scarlet fever."[65] In other words such anomalous sore throats were scarlatinal – produced by the scarlet fever contagium but in weaker or attenuated form. The implications for disease

64 Newsholme, "Outbreak of Sore Throats," 151–2.   65 Ibid., 165.

(1). As to Dates of Onset of Cases.

Cases on P.'s farm	Group A	Group B	Group C		Cases on P.'s farm	Group A	Group B	Group C
	(Oct. 29)	Oct. 29				Nov. 13...		
Oct. 30						Nov. 18		
Nov. 2		Secondarily infected cases				Nov. 16		
(?) ,, 4		Nov. 4				(scarlet fever)		
		,, 5				Nov. 18	Nov. 18	
	Nov. 6	,, 6 ⎫					(scarlet fever)	
		,, 6 ⎬			Nov. 30			
		,, 8					Dec. 2 (do.)	
		,, 9 ⎫					,, 3 ,,	
		,, 9 ⎪					,, 4 ⎫ ,,	
		,, 9 ⎬					,, 4 ⎬ ,,	
		,, 9 ⎭					,, 5 ,,	
		,, 10					,, 6 ,,	
(?) Nov. 11		,, 11					,, 6 ,,	
		,, 12 ⎫					(in another sanitary district)	
		,, 12 ⎪						
		,, 12 ⎬						
		,, 12 ⎭						

Illustration 5.3. Milk-borne scarlet fever: Newsholme's attempt to link cases of scarlet fever to antecedent cases on the farm. From Newsholme, "Outbreak of Sore Throats and of Scarlet Fever caused by Infected Milk, *J. Hygiene,* 2 (1902): 162.

prevention were important. He now recognized that any efforts to control scarlet fever must be cognizant of cases of sore throat as well as of scarlet fever. The epidemic of 1901 made Newsholme particularly aware of the danger that such cases among milkers could pose to the community. Scarlatinal sore throats should be made notifiable.[66]

Newsholme applied the lessons of the 1901 epidemic when cases of scarlet fever and of severe sore throat began to appear among the customers of one dairy in 1906. His epidemiological study of the 1901 outbreak encouraged him to associate the two types of cases together, although he knew the cause of neither. The 1906 outbreak was the largest of the four he dealt with in Brighton. It was also one of the two for which he could not identify a likely human source on the farm. Without a first case at the point of origin, Newsholme was forced to weigh more carefully the circumstantial evidence linking the epidemic to milk from one farm. In trying to do this he produced his most elaborate study on a milk-borne epidemic.[67]

66 Ibid., 168.
67 Newsholme, *Ann. Rep.* (Brighton), 1906, 48–63. This report was republished as Newsholme, "On an Outbreak of Scarlet Fever."

He first began to suspect a particular dairy's milk when two cases of scarlet fever were registered among its customers on one day, and on the following day he received from a medical practitioner the two throat swabs, which proved negative for diphtheria and from which he did not try to cultivate streptococci. He soon discovered these swabs also came from homes served by the same dairy. Sore throat remained an unnotifiable condition, so he privately asked medical practitioners to notify him of cases of sore throats they saw in their practice, and he advised them to recommend to their patients the temporary boiling of milk. From local doctors he would eventually learn of 99 cases of sore throat among the customers of this dairy. After the outbreak was well advanced and rumors were abroad that milk from that dairy was spreading disease, he felt justified in undertaking a house-to-house survey of the dairy's customers. In this survey his Sanitary Inspectors learned of another 104 such cases.

Newsholme began the usual preventive measures quite early in the outbreak, after 12 cases of scarlet fever had been registered and he had learned privately of 31 cases of sore throat.[68] Since the usual investigations on the suspected farm turned up no definite source of the milk's infection, he resorted to more elaborate arguments and less direct evidence to implicate the milk from a particular farm. Two features of the epidemic suggested to him that this was indeed a milk-borne epidemic. First, personal infection seems highly unlikely, since cases appeared close to each other in time but not necessarily in place. Second, the outbreak had a very explosive onset and the incubation period of cases appeared to be short, as one would expect if the unknown agent of scarlet fever lived in milk producing its "poison."[69] The explosive nature of the epidemic can be seen in Illustration 5.4 in which Newsholme represented monthly morbidity rates for scarlet fever and scarlatinal sore throat among the customers of Dairy A, the dairy suspected of supplying infected milk, and among all other residents of Brighton. This explosive onset can be seen even more clearly in the daily records of the onset of new cases.[70] The morbidity figures for October 1906, plotted in Illustration 5.4, strongly implicated Dairy A's milk. Newsholme reported that among its customers there were 5 cases of scarlet fever and 28 cases of scarlatinal sore throat per 100 families. In the rest of Brighton there were only 0.06 cases of scarlet fever and 0.10 cases of scarlatinal sore throat per 100 families. The comparison was highly suggestive if not entirely fair. Family size differed, so the numbers at risk per 100 families in each group might differ somewhat. More important, however, is the fact that the Sanitary Department had systematically tried to discover cases of sore throat among Dairy A's customers, but it had not tried to do the same among other households.

68 Brighton, Proc. San. Comm., 23 (17 Oct. 1906): 186–9.
69 Newsholme, *Ann. Rep.* (Brighton), 48; or Newsholme, "On an Outbreak of Scarlet Fever," 756–7. This discussion of the characteristics of milkborne epidemics should be compared with a more comprehensive one to which Newsholme did not refer in Swithinbank and Newman, *Bacteriology of Milk*, 262–78.
70 Newsholme, *Ann. Rep.* (Brighton), 1906, bar graph between 50 and 51.

FIGURE II.

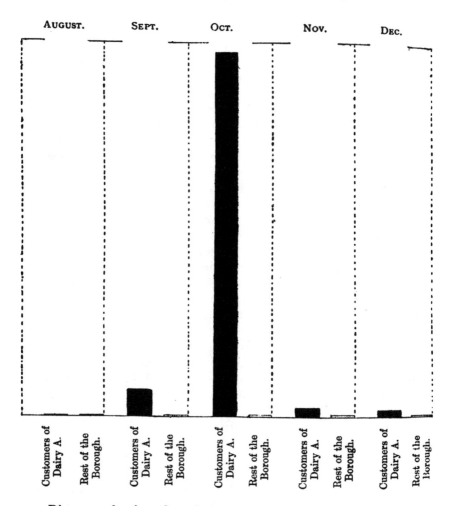

Diagram showing the relative incidence of Scarlet Fever and Scarlatinal Sore Throat in every 100 houses.

(*a*) Among customers of A.'s Dairy.

(*b*) In the rest of the Borough.

Illustration 5.4. Milk-borne scarlet fever: comparing the incidence of scarlet fever and scarlatinal sore throat in those consuming suspect milk with the rest of the population of Brighton, 1906. From Newsholme, *Ann. Rep.* (Brighton), 1906, 54; or Newsholme, "Outbreak of Scarlet Fever and Scarlatinal Sore Throat due to Infected Milk," *Public Health*, 19 (1906–7): 762.

Newsholme suspected that the milk had been infected on the farm again rather than in transit or during subsequent handling. In support of this view he pointed out that cases appeared in the routes of different milk carriers. He was able to implicate milk from a particular farm, labeled "B" in Illustrations 5.5 and 5.6, through a chance circumstance and by the use of the distribution records kept by the dairy. The chance element was a repetition of the circumstance of 1901 when cases occurred among those who drank milk which arrived direct from the farm in a padlocked can.[71] In this case the customer was a boarding school out of town, whose experience in the epidemic strongly suggested that the milk was the vehicle of contagion. The cases in the school, labeled "Z" in Illustration 5.6, began at the same time as cases appeared in town among families who drank the same milk, although the school was separated from the town by a considerable distance. Only students who drank raw milk got sick. Living arrangements of the students and the careful isolation of the first case suggested that the disease was not spread person-to-person at the school.

The milk distribution records of the dairy provided a more uncertain picture. In this case the dairy bought milk from two farms, "B" and "T." Some of the milk from farm B was also sold to another dairy, labeled "U." Illustration 5.5 shows how Newsholme demonstrated the distribution of scarlet fever cases according to the source of the family's milk. This reconstruction was based on the information initially supplied by the dairy's manager, and it pointed clearly to the milk from Farm B. Unfortunately the manager later admitted that the supplies had not been kept as carefully separated as this reconstruction suggests. Milk from farm T had occasionally been distributed on routes normally supplied with milk from farm B. This admission weakened considerably the force of Newsholme's demonstration. He was convinced, however, that he had correctly identified the source of the epidemic. He pointed to the fact that the new cases stopped appearing when the suspected milk was destroyed.

Newsholme's studies of milk-borne scarlet fever outbreaks and his administrative responses to these epidemics demonstrate the limitations under which public health officials worked before the role of the streptococcus in scarlet fever and in some sore throats was understood. Diagnosis could be difficult and uncertain. For that reason it might be difficult to administer isolation or to do adequate disease surveillance. Most sobering was the gradual recognition that cases which did not present the classic signs of scarlet fever and for which notification was not required might harbor the contagium of scarlet fever. In the absence of pasteurization milk-borne epidemics could be controlled only if the health authorities were able to determine quickly that a supply of milk was causing illness and to respond effectively. Using compulsory notification of scarlet fever cases and occasional voluntary notification of sore throat, as well as the voluntary earmarking of milk supplies, Newsholme devised a practical system of disease surveillance. His

71 For a discussion of the outbreak at this school, see ibid., 58–9, 56; or Newsholme, "On an Outbreak of Scarlet Fever," 767–8, 764.

DISTRIBUTION OF CASES OF SCARLET FEVER AND SORE THROAT ACCORDING TO SOURCE OF MILK SUPPLY.*

	Milk Supplies.					Total Cases.
	B. B.	B. B. (occasionally T.)	B. T.	U. (i.e. B. in part).	T. T.	
1st List of Cases ...	5	0	11	1	0	17
2nd „ „ „ ...	13	0	15	5	0	33
3rd „ „ „ ...	34	9	54	5	0	102

51

Illustration 5.5. Milk-borne scarlet fever: distribution of scarlet fever cases according to the milk supply, 1906. From Newsholme, *Ann. Rep.* (Brighton), 1906, 57; or Newsholme, "Outbreak of Scarlet Fever and Scarlatinal Sore Throat due to Infected Milk," *Public Health,* 19 (1906–7): 765.

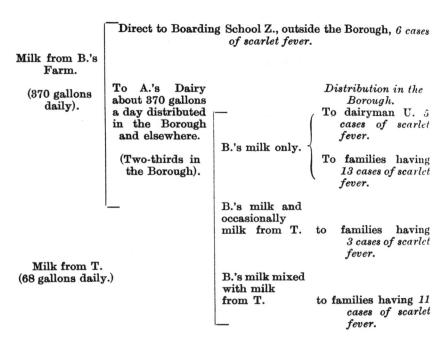

Illustration 5.6. Milk-borne scarlet fever: tracing infection through the milk supply, 1906. From Newsholme, *Ann. Rep.* (Brighton), 1906, 58; or Newsholme, "Outbreak of Scarlet Fever and Scarlatinal Sore Throat due to Infected Milk," *Public Health,* 19 (1906–7): 766.

epidemiological studies of these epidemics developed from the same administrative measures. These epidemiological investigations in turn confirmed suspicions that some cases of sore throat and scarlet fever were related and suggested that the prevailing strategy of combating scarlet fever by notifying and isolating only cases with all the classics signs of scarlet fever was flawed.

6

Tuberculosis: Public policy and epidemiology

No other aspect of Newsholme's activities in Brighton gave him as much personal satisfaction or added so significantly to his professional reputation as his work with tuberculosis. His success in Brighton in constructing a comprehensive preventive strategy brought him attention outside the world of public health administration and helped win him the Medical Officership of the Local Government Board. In turn the use he made in Whitehall of this local experience offers historians a good example of the influence of municipal experiments on the nation's health policy. In retrospect it is easy to find a logic in the successive administrative changes that created Brighton's tuberculosis policy. But the historical evidence suggests that Newsholme began his work against tuberculosis with no master plan. Rather, we find that over a period of nearly two decades a policy slowly emerged in response to administrative experience and changing medical ideas. In this process we find operating at two levels an interplay between epidemiological studies on the one hand and his policy recommendations on the other. At the local level, through case finding and efforts to trace infection through the community as he had done for scarlet fever, his epidemiology helped shape his policy. On a grander scale of explanation, however, his policy experience helped determine the design and the outcome of his epidemiological studies. The former work won him nearly universal respect from his professional peers. Although he put great stock in the second class of investigations, and although they were influential in some quarters, these studies, pursued so vigorously over a number of years, involved him in protracted and bitter controversy and failed to convince even some of his friends.

The lack of a clear strategy for preventing tuberculosis when Newsholme arrived in Brighton was due in part to the confusion surrounding this common and costly disease. It was not that Medical Officers of Health like Newsholme were slow to accept Koch's discovery of the tuberculosis bacillus. Newsholme's earliest writings show that he had done this within months of Koch's first publication on this topic.[1] It is rather that the occurrence of pulmonary tuberculosis in

---

1 Newsholme, *Hygiene* (1884), 354–5.

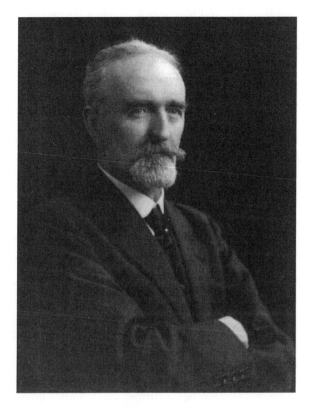

Illustration 6.1. Arthur Newsholme as he was at the Local Government Board.
From Newsholme, *Last Thirty Years in Public Health*, frontispiece.

the community seemed much too complex to be explained on a simple contagionist model. It was well known that exposure to the tuberculosis bacillus was
very common. Half the adults undergoing postmortem examinations in hospitals,
Newsholme explained, had healed tuberculosis lesions.[2] They had been infected
but had not developed overt disease. Furthermore, there were important differences in the occurrence of tuberculosis among the trades and occupations and
between the better housed and those who inhabited the poorest and most crowded
dwellings. Early in his career Newsholme thought that these differences suggested
that although tuberculosis was a contagious disease, its occurrence could be
adequately explained only by recourse to nonspecific, environmental factors. It
was a conclusion similar to the one we have seen him reach in his studies of
rheumatic fever and diphtheria. His discussions of tuberculosis preserve a place for
factors such as dampness and subsoil moisture, sedentary occupations, the "habit-

2 Arthur Newsholme, *The Prevention of Tuberculosis* (New York: E. P. Dutton, 1908), 62, 161.

ual breathing of rebreathed air," and dark dwellings much longer than those he provided for any other disease.[3]

It is hardly surprising, then, to find that early in his career Newsholme hoped that environmental reforms already underweigh would do much to reduce the toll of tuberculosis in lives. Thus in 1889 when Brighton's slum clearance program was just beginning, Newsholme could claim "the problem of the Housing of the Poor involves in its solution also the material reduction, if not the practical extinction, of some forms of tubercular disease."[4] He predicted that "if we can succeed in opening up courts and alleys in which no proper circulation of air occurs; in preventing overcrowding in single rooms; and in insisting that every house shall be free from damp and provided with through ventilation" the mortality from pulmonary tuberculosis would fall to the level of that for scarlet fever.[5] Tuberculosis, Newsholme observed, occurred in certain houses at a rate much higher than one might expect by chance.[6] In fact it seemed to "cling" to certain houses.[7] But early in his career he is rather ambivalent in his explanations of how poor housing influenced tuberculosis. Was the foul air of crowded rooms a predisposing cause of tuberculosis, an environment encouraging the saprophytic life of the tuberculosis bacillus, or the vehicle for contagion? Newsholme considered this question and concluded that from a practical point of view its answer did not matter.[8]

At this time Newsholme believed that the tuberculosis organism was transmitted primarily in dried sputum as dust and through milk and meat from tubercular cows.[9] The emphasis on dried sputum was commonplace among his peers. In fact it was only in the early years of the new century that the role played by droplet infection was prominently discussed in the British public health literature.[10] In dried sputum the tuberculosis organism was believed open to attack by those sanitary panaceas, fresh air and sunlight, which slum clearance promised to provide. Even though neither policy was initiated primarily to prevent tuberculosis, the Sanitary Department's recent action against poor housing and its energetic attack on defective household drainage should be understood as part of the initial phase of a community effort to control this dread disease.

3 See for the persistent use of these factors over nearly two decades, Newsholme, *Hygiene* (1884), 355; Arthur Newsholme, "The Prevention of Phthisis, with Special Reference to Its Notification to the Medical Officer of Health," *Public Health* 11 (1898–9): 312; Arthur Newsholme, "The Influence of Soil on the Prevalence of Pulmonary Phthisis," *Practitioner,* 66 (1901): 206–13; and Newsholme, *Prevention of Tuberculosis,* 62, 161.

4 Newsholme, *Ann. Rep.* (Brighton), 1889, 13.   5 Ibid., 1890, 9.

6 Newsholme, "Prevention of Phthisis," 312.

7 Newsholme's comments in "A Discussion on the Prevention and Remedial Treatment of Tuberculosis," *Br. Med. J.* (1899), no. 2: 1158.

8 Newsholme, "Prevention of Phthisis," 312.

9 Newsholme, *Ann. Rep.* (Brighton), 1890, 9; ibid. 1893, 20; and ibid. 1894, 15.

10 See, for example, Alfred Hillier, "The Prospect of Extinguishing Tuberculosis. Based on the Researches of Koch, Flügge, Frankel, Niven, and Others," *Public Health,* 15 (1902–3): 304–8, 312. See also "British Congress on Tuberculosis," *Br. Med. J.* (1901), no. 2: 324.

The Sanitary Department directed special attention to those houses in which tuberculosis cases had occurred. Before tuberculosis was made notifiable, the M.O.H. could learn officially only of fatal cases. Beginning in 1892 Newsholme sent a Sanitary Department employee to the local registrar of births, deaths, and marriages every Monday morning to collect a list of the names and addresses of those dying from pulmonary tuberculosis during the previous week. Each address was then visited, ostensibly to make a sanitary inspection and to correct sanitary defects. But the Department also collected information about the case: its duration and nature, other cases in the same family, the occupation of the deceased, previous residences during the fatal illness, and the family's milk supply.[11] Newsholme took advantage of this opportunity to encourage careful cleaning and disinfection of the sickroom in order to reduce the family's continued exposure to contagion and to protect the next tenants of the house. At first he acted cautiously, acknowledging a reluctance to cause public alarm and probably recognizing as well the need to avoid conflict with private practitioners attending some of these families.[12] In the first few years he strongly urged disinfection only in those instances where the family doctor also suggested it. But by middecade the Department had begun to act more boldly, sending a letter to the head of each household in which a death from phthisis had occurred.[13] The letter recommended that the floor, ceiling, and durable articles from the sickroom be washed, that the wallpaper be stripped and burned, and that movable articles in the room be exposed to strong sunlight for several hours. The Department made chemical disinfectant available free of charge but stated that its use was unnecessary if objects were kept wet during cleaning and handling. Within a day or two a Sanitary Inspector called to see whether the cleaning and disinfection had been performed. The Department did not have authority to compel this action, but this more aggressive encouragement resulted in a tripling between 1895 and 1896 of the number of houses disinfected after the death of a consumptive patient.[14] By the end of 1898 the Sanitary Department had secured the cleaning of 573 of such houses.

In these years Newsholme was also active against the other major recognized means of transmitting tuberculosis, through the meat and milk of tubercular cattle. As we saw in Chapter 3, after a short but intense controversy, the Sanitary Department gained by the end of 1894 the uncontested authority to keep tubercular meat off the market. It proved to be much more difficult, however, to prevent the transmission of bovine tuberculosis through milk. Newsholme had given evidence before the second Royal Commission of Tuberculosis, 1898, and he worked to publicize its findings and conclusions, in particular the evidence that

11 For a copy of the form which would later be used to collect this information, see Newsholme, "Prevention of Phthisis," 321.
12 Newsholme, *Ann. Rep.* (Brighton), 1893, 21.
13 Newsholme, "Prevention of Phthisis," 320; and Arthur Newsholme and H. C. Lecky, "An Account of the System of Voluntary Notification of Phthisis in Brighton, and of the Treatment and Training of Patients in Its Isolation Hospital," *Tuberculosis,* 4 (1906–7): 231–2.
14 Newsholme, "Prevention of Phthisis," 320.

tuberculosis could be acquired by drinking the milk of cows suffering from tuberculosis of the udder.[15] Working through the Sanitary Committee he was able to secure a resolution from the Town Council calling on the Local Government Board to introduce legislation enacting the Commission's recommendations.[16]

He also worked to drum up support from within the medical profession.[17] In March 1897 he led a discussion of tuberculosis and the milk supply at the Brighton and Sussex Medical Chirurgical Society that resulted in a resolution urging medical practitioners to advise their patients to drink milk only from tuberculin-tested cows.[18] To dramatize the issue, Newsholme brought to the meeting the udder of a cow suffering from extensive tuberculosis that had been supplying milk for the Brighton market. He also convinced the Sanitary Committee to allow him to modify the milk contract for the Sanatorium to require the tuberculin testing of all cows supplying milk to the institution and to recommend officially to the Poor Law Guardians and to the managing committees of the Sussex County Hospital and the Children's Hospital that they do the same.[19]

But freeing the town's milk supply of bovine tuberculosis proved to be very difficult. Commercial dairies did not follow the town's lead as Newsholme had hoped, and neither certified nor pasteurized milk was widely available during his tenure in Brighton. The same trade opposition and jurisdictional jealousies that made it difficult to prohibit the sale of milk or shellfish likely to carry acute infectious diseases such as scarlet fever or typhoid fever, hampered the efforts of local authorities to free their milk supply of bovine tuberculosis. The Board of Agriculture's revised Dairies, Cowshed and Milkshops Order of 1899 forbade the mixing or sale for human consumption of milk from cows with tuberculosis of the udder, but this order was completely unsatisfactory in Newsholme's opinion in failing to give to Medical Officers of Health the authority to inspect herds outside of their jurisdiction.[20] Newsholme campaigned for and the Corporation eventually succeeded in acquiring private legislation which granted the M.O.H. of Brighton that authority.[21]

15 Arthur Newsholme, testimony, *Report of the Royal Commission Appointed to Inquire into the Administrative Procedures for Controlling Danger to Man through the Use as Food of the Meat and Milk of Tuberculous Animals,* 1898, XLIX, pp. 185–91. For his summary of the Commission's findings, see Newsholme, *Ann. Rep.* (Brighton), 1900, 58–61; and "Report of Sanitary Committee," Brighton, *Proc. Town Council, Proc. Comm.* 7 July 1898, 1–6. The latter report had first been presented to the Sanitary Committee on May 26 and deferred until June 30, Brighton, Proc. San. Comm., 15 (26 May 1898), 368; ibid., 9 June 1898, 387; and ibid., 30 June 1898, 405.

16 Brighton, *Proc. Town Council,* 7 July 1898, iii. See also Newsholme, *Ann. Rep.* (Brighton), 1898, 24.

17 Arthur Newsholme, "Tuberculosis in Relation to Milk Supply," *Public Health,* 66 (1901): 675–83; and Arthur Newsholme, "Tuberculosis in Relation to Milk Supply," *Proc. Brighton and Sussex Medico-Chirurgical Society,* 1897: 83–9.

18 Newsholme, *Ann. Rep.* (Brighton), 1900, 59.

19 Brighton, Proc. San. Comm., 16 (13 Oct. 1898): 35–9; or Brighton, *Proc. Town Council, Proc. Comm.,* 20 Oct. 1898, 19–20. For the new terms of the contract, see Newsholme, *Ann. Rep.* (Brighton), 1899, 32–3.

20 For Newsholme's comments on this order, see ibid., 1900, 61–2.

21 Brighton Corporation Act, 1901, Gt. Britain, *Local and Personal Acts,* 1 Ed. VII, C. 224, Sect. 51. As he frequently did when lobbying for policy changes, he surveyed other towns for their experience with similar private legislation. See Newsholme, *Ann. Rep.* (Brighton), 1900, 62–4.

On the eve of his departure from Brighton, Newsholme began what might have developed into a system of microscopic surveillance of the Brighton milk supply. He got permission to collect samples from milk vendors for analysis by the Lister Institute, and he then attempted to locate the diseased cows which had supplied the infected samples.[22] Although he left for Whitehall before he could pursue this line of investigation further, the initial results showed that the town's milk supply was heavily contaminated with the tuberculosis organism, and this initial screening should have ended any complacency on that score.

Nearly forty years later, when he was writing his autobiography, Newsholme recognized that at the end of the nineteenth century British authorities had overestimated the role of infected milk and meat and undervalued direct interpersonal infection in tuberculosis.[23] It was the experience of visiting homes after a death from tuberculosis that caused Newsholme to change his mind. He found that the recent fatal case, the one he had come to investigate, was often not the first in the family's recent history. This was true even in middle-class houses where there was no crowding and where sanitation was impeccable. He once told a medical audience about the case of Mrs. X, who died at age thirty-one after suffering from pulmonary tuberculosis for several years.[24] Upon investigation he found that Mrs. X's daughter had died five months earlier of tubercular meningitis, and that her two servants, whose duties included washing her handkerchiefs and sweeping out the sickroom daily, both died of pulmonary tuberculosis, one before, the other after their mistress. Even Mrs. X's own sister, who came to help nurse the invalid, left town with a "bad cough." Patients who took no precautions to protect others were likely to transmit their cases to those around them. The orderliness, space, and comfort of a middle-class life were, in themselves, no protection.

Beginning with his *Annual Report* for 1894, Newsholme's discussions of tuberculosis began to summarize instances in which a string of cases occurred in a household, often following a chronic case in a parent or sibling.[25] By the time he wrote his comprehensive monograph on tuberculosis, he had developed a set of tables to summarize these sometimes complicated family histories. Illustration 6.2 reproduces the one he prepared for Florence S., who entered the Brighton Sanatorium in September 1906 at age twenty-four. This sort of evidence soon convinced him that interpersonal infection, most often in the home, was the most important source of new cases. But demonstrating the truth of this proposition was difficult. He once asked his Assistant Medical Officer to investigate thoroughly

22 Brighton, Proc. San. Comm., 23 (27 June 1907): 452–3; ibid. 24 (12 Sept 1907): 57; ibid. 24 (24 Oct. 1907): 107–9; and ibid. 24 (12 Dec. 1907): 166–70.

23 Arthur Newsholme, *Fifty Years in Public Health: A Personal Narrative with Comments* (London: George Allen and Unwin, 1935), 237, 241–2.

24 Arthur Newsholme, "An Introductory Address on the Relation of the Medical Practitioner to Preventive Measures against Tuberculosis," *Lancet* (1904), no. 1: 282–3. For further details of this episode in which Mrs. X is now called Mrs. F, see Newsholme, *Ann. Rep.* (Brighton), 1902, 66.

25 Newsholme, *Ann. Rep.* (Brighton), 1894, 16.

Domestic Influences.	Age.	Year.	Extra-domestic Influences.
Has been exposed to domestic infection probably from early childhood.	o	1882	
Father, a waiter, died, æt. 45, of phthisis.	8	1890	After the father's death in 1890, the mother began a small laundry, and the patient and her two sisters have helped in it. The patient is chiefly engaged at needlework.
A brother, æt. 15, died of phthisis.	11	1893	
A sister died of phthisis . .	12	1894	
Mother died, æt. 48, of phthisis .	16	1898	
First noticed enlarged cervical glands. Axillary glands soon afterwards inflamed and suppurated for two years.			
A brother died, æt. 28, of phthisis .	17	1899	
A brother, æt. 34, died of phthisis.	21	1903	
A sister, then aged 27, was notified as phthisis in June 1903. Tub. bac. present. Was in sanatorium Aug.–Sept. 1903. Is now (Dec. 1906) quite well.	21	1903	
Cough developed a few weeks before admission to sanatorium. Tub. bac. found. Cervical glands still large and indurated, axillary glands the same.	24	1906	

Illustration 6.2. Tuberculosis: a patient's probable sources of infection (Florence S's). From Newsholme, *Prevention of Tuberculosis*, 67.

and attempt to trace all possible sources of infection in 100 consecutive tuberculosis cases seen at the Sanatorium. Although every effort was made to locate the source of infection, no such source could be located in 25 of these cases.[26] In only 32 was Newsholme confident he could identify the source. Nevertheless, although conclusive statistical evidence could not be found, Newsholme was confident in his conclusion that direct interpersonal contagion, mainly from sputum, was the most important factor in the causation of pulmonary tuberculosis.

In 1905, drawing on his experience with the local system of notification he helped originate, he observed

26 Newsholme, *Prevention of Tuberculosis*, 71–2.

Having investigated nearly 1,600 voluntarily notified cases of phthisis, as well as a much larger number of fatal cases of phthisis, from a public health standpoint, I do not conceive it to be possible that any physician having personally done similar work could fail to realize to the full extent the infectivity of this disease, when exposure to infection is protracted and the dosage of infection is great: a state of matters which is the common domestic lot of most of the working classes, when tubercular infection attacks a member of the household. The evidence convincing one as to this does not lend itself to statistical statement, and when stated in print it may not be convincing; but the steady succession of cases in infected households at intervals of one or two years, or longer, the intercurrent destruction of children by tubercular meningitis or 'broncho-pneumonia' while their parents are suffering from chronic phthisis, and other similar evidence, can leave no doubts in the minds of those who come into continuous contact with the actual facts.[27]

If infected people were the most likely source of new cases of tuberculosis, then it seemed that the focus of preventive work had to change from things – milk and meat, crowded and poorly ventilated houses, sickroom artifacts – to persons – those afflicted with tuberculosis and those who lived with them. In addresses, articles, and in his official reports, Newsholme began to argue for an active tuberculosis campaign aimed at controlling interpersonal transmission.[28] In doing this he tried to strike a balance. To fight complacency, ignorance, and fatalism, he emphasized that tuberculosis was contagious and that there was a real danger of contracting the disease from exposure to the sputum of a pulmonary case. On the other hand he tried to avoid alarm and the ostracism of the sick by stressing that tuberculosis was infectious in a different degree than smallpox or typhoid. Almost everyone had had some exposure to the tuberculosis bacillus, but only a few people contracted the disease. Whereas some people concluded from this latter observation that the crucial factors in determining who contracted tuberculosis were innate or acquired differences in resistance, Newsholme continued to stress the role of prolonged exposure. Tuberculosis was not highly contagious, but it was a disease where contagion might be sustained for long periods. Just as a city might suffer little damage from a siege, if the siege were lifted soon, Newsholme argued that the healthy occupants of a house need not contract tuberculosis from a pulmonary case in their midst, if simple precautions were begun early and consistently observed thereafter.[29]

To see that these precautionary measures were known and observed the local health authority would have to know who suffered from tuberculosis. The simplest

27 Arthur Newsholme, "The Relative Importance of the Constituent Factors Involved in the Control of Pulmonary Tuberculosis," *Trans. Epidem. Soc. Lond.*, n.s. 25 (1905–06): 70, reprinted in Newsholme, *Fifty Years*, 245–6.
28 See, for example, Newsholme, "Prevention of Tuberculosis"; and Newsholme, "Notification of Consumption."
29 For Newsholme's use of this analogy, see Newsholme, "Prevention of Tuberculosis," 311. Newsholme liked this section so well he reprinted part of it in his autobiography: Newsholme, *Fifty Years*, 246.

way to have gathered this information would have been to add tuberculosis to the list of notifiable diseases under the permissive legislation of 1889 or the compulsory legislation of 1899.[30] While there was some support for this approach, most public health officials opposed it, and it was contrary to official policy. During the 1890s in fact the Local Government Board had a standard letter of refusal it sent to local authorities who asked whether they might add tuberculosis to the list of reportable diseases in their jurisdiction.[31] Health officials realized that patients and their families would suffer unduly if the ordinary measures of quarantine and debarment from school, from public transport, and from some forms of employment that often followed notification were applied in a chronic disease like tuberculosis which might last months or even years and which afflicted many in their working and child-rearing years. As late as 1898 Sir Richard Thorne Thorne insisted that local authorities promised no constructive action following notification which would justify the risks and the inconvenience that notification of tuberculosis would entail.[32]

Other health officials feared that notification would lead to ostracism and discrimination of those with tuberculosis and to the concealment of cases.[33] They also warned that notification of pulmonary tuberculosis represented an extension of state authority which neither the medical profession nor the public would tolerate. "To compel every medical man to notify every suspected case of consumption, and to treat the house in which the case occurred as if it contained small-pox or typhoid fever would be simply outrageous," and, warned R. Sydney Marsden, M.O.H. of Birkenhead, "the people of this country would not tolerate being overruled as the citizens of New York [City, where compulsory notification of tuberculosis had been established in 1897] were by the Health Department."[34]

Newsholme probably preferred a system of compulsory notification of phthisis, pulmonary tuberculosis, but he was pragmatic. He recognized that compulsory notification would arouse opposition, but he hoped that a system of voluntary notification would be acceptable to medical practitioners who could choose which cases, if any, they would notify; he also hoped that a system of notification independent of the one for the acute infectious disease would give the Health Department flexibility in dealing with cases which would minimize the opposition of patients and their families. He became, accordingly, an early champion of voluntary notification. He secured a resolution in its favor from the provincial branch of the Society of Medical

---

30 The legislation in question is the Infectious Disease (Notification) Act, 1889 [52 & 53 Vict., C. 72] and the Infectious Disease (Notification) Extension Act, 1899 [62 & 63 Vict., C. 8].

31 This letter is reproduced in Newsholme, "Prevention of Tuberculosis," 314.

32 Sir R. Thorne Thorne, "The Administrative Control of Tuberculosis. The Harben Lectures for 1898," *Public Health*, 11 (1898–9): 204–5.

33 See, for example, the comments of C. A. Heron and Shirley Murphy in the discussion of the paper: Newsholme, "Prevention of Tuberculosis," 324–5. Newsholme also summarized some of these arguments in Newsholme, *Fifty Years*, 246.

34 Marsden's comments are found in the discussion of Arthur Newsholme, "Notification of Consumption: Its Pros and Cons. Remarks Introductory to a Discussion on the Prevention of Phthisis," *J. Sanitary Inst.*, 21 (1900): 57, 58.

Officers of Health in 1893 and another from the parent body six years later, but he failed to carry the Sanitary Institute with him in 1900.[35]

Newsholme evidently believed that if enough incentives were offered to doctors and to tuberculosis patients, notification would slowly gain acceptance. In rough outline, this is what happened in Brighton. The town became the first in England to implement a system of voluntary notification for pulmonary tuberculosis, although James Niven, then M.O.H. of Oldam, had suggested such a system as early as 1893, and although Manchester soon followed Brighton in establishing a voluntary system.[36] In Brighton voluntary notification was introduced in stages. The Sanitary Department first learned of active cases as a by-product of offering free sputum examinations for medical practitioners. The new municipal laboratory began offering these examinations in December 1897. The results of the examination were made available to the practitioner, but no official action followed a positive sputum examination. The public health authority gained information and perhaps some goodwill but not the power to intervene. Newsholme was soon stressing the need for early diagnosis in tuberculosis and recommending that patients who have a persistent cough be given a sputum examination even if they showed no other signs of tuberculosis.[37] A growing consensus on that point and the beginning of a formal notification system help account for the sharp rise in the number of medical practitioners availing themselves of this municipal laboratory service in the early years of the new century.[38]

In January of 1899 Newsholme began the process of securing the voluntary notification of cases of pulmonary tuberculosis. In Brighton, as he would later do at the L.G.B., he worked cautiously, beginning with those cases whose notification, he believed, would cause the least objection, and moving gradually to other types of cases. On January 12 he obtained the Sanitary Committee's permission to send a circular letter to all medical practitioners in public institutions and in the poor law medical service, asking them voluntarily to notify any cases of pulmonary tuberculosis they encountered in their practices.[39] The letter accompanied a card of printed instructions for the patient, which the Department's inspectors would leave when they visited the infected dwelling. Sixty-eight cases were notified under these terms during the next seven months.[40]

35 *Public Health*, 5 (1892–3): 362; ibid. 11 (1898–9): 322, 325; and *J. Sanitary Inst.*, 21 (1900): 61.

36 Arthur Newsholme's comments in the Section of Public Health at the seventeenth annual meeting of the British Medical Association, "A Discussion on the Administrative Prevention of Tuberculosis," *Br. Med. J.* (1902), no. 2: 439; Arthur Newsholme, "The Voluntary Notification of Phthisis in Brighton: Including a Comparison of Results with Those Obtained in Other Towns," *J. Roy. Sanitary Inst.*, 28 (1907): 26–7; and Arthur Newsholme "Address on Possible Medical Extensions of Public Health Work," *J. State Med.*, 9 (1901): 539.

37 Arthur Newsholme, *The Role of "Missed" Cases in the Spread of Infectious Diseases* (London and Manchester: Sherratt and Hughes, 1904): 6.

38 For a table of summary statistics, see Arthur Newsholme, "The Voluntary Notification of Phthisis in Brighton," *J. Roy. Sanitary Inst.*, 28 (1907): 35.

39 Brighton, Proc. San. Comm., 16 (12 Jan. 1899): 134. Newsholme, *Ann. Rep.* (Brighton), 1899, 33–4.

40 Newsholme and Lecky, "Account of the System," 226.

Charity and pauper cases were a safe place to begin. No objection to their notification was anticipated, and none was recorded. After seven months, in August 1899, Newsholme approached the Sanitary Committee again asking permission to seek voluntary notification of cases among the working classes seen in private practice.[41] He promised to send his letter inviting voluntary notification and his card of patient advice only to those medical practitioners known to have a practice among the poor. As an incentive for cooperation he convinced the Sanitary Committee to conduct a six-month trial in which it offered physicians who notified a case of pulmonary tuberculosis the same fee they received for notifying any of the compulsorily notifiable infectious diseases. Physicians in private practice would receive 2s6d and those in the public medical service would receive 1s. for each such notification. In addressing the practitioner, he was careful to appeal to public spirit and to emphasize the separation between public health measures and the practice of medicine.

I beg therefore to invite you to co-operate with me in notifying cases of Phthisis occurring in your practice, where in your opinion public good can be achieved by such notification. I may remind you that even though in the individual case under your care no further precautions and no sanitary improvements are required, the official knowledge of your case may direct my attention to "infected areas," and possibly be the means of facilitating important sanitary reforms.

There will, I need hardly say, be no official interference, as the result of the notification, with your patient, either at home or in connection with his occupation, the steps taken being confined to a sanitary inspection of the house and giving a copy of the card to the patient or a responsible relative.[42]

This separation, of prevention from treatment and of public from private medicine, is one he would later strive to break down, and, as we shall see, his experience with tuberculosis would provide some of his most compelling reasons for doing so.

The first notification for a fee was received on September 11, 1899, and by the end of the year the Committee had paid for forty-four.[43] In the following April, after the six-month trial of paying for voluntary notification had passed, Newsholme took the final step in implementing his plan by gaining permission to invite notification from all practitioners and to offer the notification fee on a permanent basis.[44] It had thus taken about fifteen months to establish a system of voluntary notification. The implementation seems to have occurred smoothly, without serious objection. As may be seen in Illustration 6.3, a table Newsholme prepared toward the end of 1906, which summarizes the tuberculosis work in

41 Brighton, Proc. San. Comm., 16 (10 Aug. 1899): 385. For a copy of Newsholme's report on the first nine months of voluntary notification, see Newsholme, "Notification of Consumption," 50–2.

42 Newsholme, *Q. Rep.* (Brighton), 1899, no. 2: 11.

43 Newsholme, *Ann. Rep.* (Brighton), 1899, 34.

44 Brighton, Proc. San. Comm., 17 (26 April 1900): 216–17.

Particulars of Cases of Phthisis notified in Brighton.

Year	Number of Cases notified for first time	Number of Cases re-notified	Total number of Deaths from Phthisis in Brighton	Population	Cases treated at Sanatorium outside Brighton	Brighton Sanatorium: New cases	Brighton Sanatorium: Re-admissions	Notified Cases: Left Brighton	Notified Cases: Changed address and lost	Notified Cases: Deaths of notified Cases	Notified Cases: Wrong address given	Cases living and under observation, Sept. 30th, 1906	Notified Cases in which death was not certified as Phthisis	Specimens of Sputum examined: From Doctors in Brighton	Specimens of Sputum examined: For Sanatorium
1897	…	…	…	…	…	…	…	…	…	…	…	…	…	⎱ 21 for fourteen m'ths	…
1898	…	…	…	…	…	…	…	…	…	…	…	…	…	⎰	…
1899	111	2	180	123,327	…	…	…	6	43	57	7	…	…	47	…
1900	105	4	173	124,148	…	…	…	15	21	58	2	9	…	86	…
1901	153	9	164	123,478	6	…	…	22	42	62	4	23	4	125	…
1902	224	52	174	124,539	…	25	…	29	38	107	7	43	5	146	23
1903	316	82	182	125,405	…	96	3	22	69	112	9	104	5	227	111
1904	363	85	174	126,286	…	131	6	32	95	117	11	108	5	284	188
1905	308	102	172	127,183	…	130	7	31	57	82	3	135	3	279	104
1906 to Sept. 30	313	91	126	128,095	…	146	25	10	19	36	3	245	1	422 (to Oct. 11th)	196 (to Oct. 11th)
Total	1893		1345			534	41	167	384	631		667	23	1637	622

Deaths of cases notified in a given year and dying in that or a subsequent year.

Year notified	Died 1899	1900	1901	1902	1903	1904	1905	1906	Remainder uncertain in
1899	23	15	1	1	1				1
1900		24	20	2	5	3			2
1901			35	16	6	3	1		1
1902				53	35	10	8		4
1903					62	30	16		17
1904						62	38		28
1905							51		36
1906									
Total	23	39	56	72	109	108	120		89

Illustration 6.3. Tuberculosis work in Brighton, 1897–1906. From Newsholme, "The Voluntary Notification of Phthisis in Brighton . . .", *Journal of the Sanitary Institute*, 28 (1907): 35.

[*For Discussion on this Paper, see page 40.*]

Brighton, notifications soon exceeded 300 a year. Newsholme estimated, rather generously perhaps, that by the end of that year around 80 percent of new cases of pulmonary tuberculosis were being notified.[45]

In Brighton voluntary notification for pulmonary tuberculosis operated mainly among the working classes. In his *Annual Report* for 1902 Newsholme published the occupations of the 224 persons, 121 men and 103 women, notified that year.[46] While it is notoriously difficult to determine class boundaries precisely from self-assigned returns of occupations, it is clear that propertied families were conspicuously absent from this list. Most men were unskilled laborers and tradesmen; married women, domestic servants, and dressmakers head the list for women. Newsholme found that only rarely did the families of notified cases have incomes above £2 per week.[47] Medical practitioners in Brighton chose not to notify cases among middle- and upper-class families, and Newsholme acquiesced in that decision. He explained, apparently forgetting the case of Mrs. X, that "those of higher social status are not so likely to be the cause of infection to others" as working-class families who live and work in crowded quarters where casual habits of coughing and spitting are so dangerous.[48] And all concerned realized that the middle and upper classes would object strongly to the actions the Sanitary Department took in working-class homes following notification.[49]

With the advent of voluntary notification the system of home visitation could be greatly expanded to include active cases. After each voluntary notification the Assistant Medical Officer visited the address to interview the patient. In some instances the patient was also asked to go see Newsholme at his office in Town Hall. Information was collected: on the duration of the case, on previous addresses and occupations, on possible sources of infection, on other cases in the family, and on the sanitary condition of the house.[50] The Assistant Medical Officer instructed the patient in how to avoid infecting others and left a printed card of advice.[51] Most of the tenets of the new campaign against tuberculosis made themselves felt in this set of instructions: the belief that dried sputum posed the greatest danger, the faith in the principles of open-air treatment (fresh air, good nutrition, and rest), the appeal to patient self-interest – the patient would be the greatest beneficiary from the control of sputum, and the efforts to incite protective action while allaying panic in those who had to live with the consumptive.

45 Arthur Newsholme, "The Voluntary Notification of Phthisis in Brighton: Including a Comparison of Results with Those Obtained in Other Towns," *J. Roy. Sanitary Inst.*, 28 (1907): 29.
46 Newsholme, *Ann. Rep.* (Brighton), 1902, 67–78.
47 Newsholme and Lecky, "Account of the System," 236.
48 Arthur Newsholme, "Four and a Half Years' Experience of the Voluntary Notification of Pulmonary Tuberculosis," *J. Sanitary Inst.*, 24 (1903): 256–7.
49 The most complete accounts of actions taken after notification are Newsholme, "Four and a Half Years' Experience," 254–5; Newsholme, *Ann. Rep.* (Brighton), 1905, 35–6.
50 For a copy of the form on which this information was recorded, see Newsholme and Lecky, "Account of the System," 239–41.
51 For a copy of this card, see Newsholme, *Ann. Rep.* (Brighton), 1899, 35. This text is also found in Newsholme, "Prevention of Phthisis," 317.

Teaching responsible expectoration became the fundamental principle of prevention. To encourage cooperation the Sanitary Department began offering free of charge to poor patients disposable tissues, Japanese paper handkerchiefs as they were then commonly called, and pocket spittoons. A Sanitary Inspector visited each notified case periodically, at least once a quarter, to reinforce the hygienic creed.[52] The Department also began a campaign against public spitting, posting warning signs in pubs, music halls, and workshops, at cab stands, in tram waiting rooms, and on the sea front.[53] Newsholme would have liked to have taken stronger action, but he found little sympathy for it. The railway companies were reluctant to accept his posters, and while the police agreed to warn cabmen and "loafers" against spitting, they refused to extend this policy to the general public.[54] Spitting in public was never outlawed except on the Corporation trams.

At the time of notification the patient's house was given a sanitary inspection, and notices were served to remedy structural or hygienic defects. Newsholme found that with a consumptive patient in the house the Department had more leverage in securing compliance.[55] Cleansing and disinfection were often also recommended. The Sanitary Department also visited the place of employment of notified cases, although in the guise of a general sanitary inspection and without any reference to the notified case.[56] We do not know how discreet the Sanitary Inspectors were in those visits and whether they were able to guarantee the confidentiality of the notified case. No complaints have been recorded. On his quarterly visits to the patient's house, the Sanitary Inspector inquired into the health of the patient and of other family members. If suspicious complaints in other family members were reported, the Inspector made a referral to a doctor, if the family had one, or to the Outpatient Department of the Sussex County Hospital. This policy stretched Newsholme's promise to medical practitioners of noninterference with notified cases, and it presaged a redirecting of health department efforts from environmental to personal services.

Since notification was voluntary, and the Sanitary Committee paid practitioners for each notification, Newsholme was selective. He did not accept all notifications, arguing that the Committee should pay only for those notifications that were administratively, not just statistically, useful. He refused, for example, to accept notification of moribund patients or notifications offered on condition that no Sanitary Department visit be made. In print he explained that the notification of such cases had little public health value.[57] Off the record he told one of Beatrice

---

52 Newsholme and Lecky, "Account of the System," 231.
53 For a copy of these notices, see Newsholme, *Ann. Rep.* (Brighton), 1905, 36; and Newsholme, "Discussion of Administrative Prevention," 439.
54 Brighton, Proc. San. Comm., 19 (10 July 1902): 245; ibid., 19 (29 May 1902): 196; ibid., 21 (10 Nov. 1904): 313; ibid., 22 (8 June 1905): 127–8; ibid., 23 (10 May 1906): 44; ibid., 23 (31 May 1906): 63–4; ibid., 23 (10 May 1906): 44; and ibid., 23 (31 May 1906): 63–4.
55 Newsholme, "Four and a Half Years' Experience," 254.
56 "A discussion on the Administrative Prevention of Tuberculosis," *Br. Med. J.* (1903), no. 2: 440; and Newsholme, *Ann. Rep.* (Brighton), 1905, 36.
57 Newsholme, "Voluntary Notification of Phthisis," 26.

Webb's staff researchers more bluntly that when he paid 2s6d for a notification, he expected something in return.[58] The question soon arose whether a practitioner should receive a fee for notifying a case which had already been notified. This problem was raised again when notification was established for the nation. Newsholme argued consistently that such duplicate notifications were useful, especially in tracing poor consumptives who often moved without notifying the health authority, and he argued in favor of paying for subsequent notifications.[59] He worried that new tenants would move into the dwelling before it had been properly cleaned and disinfected. When the Department learned that a notified case had moved, it undertook to disinfect the former residence: spraying formalin in rooms, stripping and white-washing walls, and disinfecting fabric with saturated steam.[60]

By the opening of the new century, notification of phthisis remained controversial among public health officials who worried about infringements with the liberty of the patient and feared that patients would be reluctant to consult practitioners who notified cases.[61] But the successful working of voluntary notification in Brighton and in several other towns caused many health officers to change their minds. Three years after the Congress of the Sanitary Institute had failed to pass Newsholme's resolution favoring notification of pulmonary tuberculosis, a resolution that would have left up to the local authority the decision whether that notification should be compulsory or voluntary,[62] it heard another paper by Newsholme on the system of voluntary notification in Brighton. Now, in 1903, most members who participated in the discussion claimed that voluntary notification was not enough, and a resolution was passed favoring "systematic notification," a term Clifford Allbutt had recommended to replace the more repugnant title "compulsory notification."[63] Allbutt claimed "he had never come across anyone, whether in the wage-earning or middle or upper classes, who had raised any serious objection to the notification." Ironically Newsholme found himself in the position of defending voluntary notification by demonstrating that in Brighton it had achieved nearly as good results as compulsory notification had produced in New York City and better results than had been achieved in Sheffield, where compulsory notification had been adopted in 1904.[64] Illustration 6.4 shows a table Newsholme prepared in 1907 comparing for New York City,

58 Minutes of interview with Newsholme, 22 Dec. 1906, in Sidney and Beatrice Webb, Local Government Collection, vol. 335, British Library of Political and Economic Science, London School of Economics. These papers will hereafter be cited as Webb, Local Government Collection.
59 Newsholme, *Ann. Rep.* (Brighton), 1900, 57–7.
60 Ibid., 1902, 53; Newsholme and Lecky, "Account of the System," 232 and; Arthur Newsholme, "Public Health Authorities in Relation to the Struggle against Tuberculosis in England," *J. Hygiene*, 3 (1903): 455–6.
61 See, for example, the comments of the President of the Society of Medical Officers of Health in the discussion of Alfred Hillier's paper "The Prospect of Extinguishing Tuberculosis," *Public Health*, 15 (1902–3): 319.
62 *J. Sanitary Inst.*, 21 (1900): 61.   63 Ibid., 24 (1903): 275, 278–9, 281, 285, 187.
64 Newsholme, "Voluntary Notification of Phthisis," 26–9.

YEAR	NEW YORK (Compulsory notification, from 1898) No. of cases notified			BRIGHTON (Voluntary notification) No. of cases notified			MANCHESTER (Voluntary notification) No. of cases notified			LIVERPOOL (Voluntary notification) No. of cases notified			SHEFFIELD (Voluntary notification to 1904, Compulsory notification 1904-05) No. of cases notified		
	No. of new cases of phthisis notified.	per 100,000 of population	per 100 deaths from phthisis	No. of new cases of phthisis notified.	per 100,000 of population	per 100 deaths from phthisis	No. of new cases of phthisis notified.	per 100,000 of population	per 100 deaths from phthisis	No. of cases of phthisis notified.	per 100,000 of population	per 100 deaths from phthisis	No. of new cases of phthisis notified.	per 100,000 of population	per 100 deaths from phthisis
1894	*4,166	231	90	...	...	...	...	...	...	...	...	...	...	...	...
1895	*5,824	312	112	...	...	...	...	...	...	...	...	...	...	...	...
1896	*8,334	436	167	...	...	...	...	...	...	...	...	...	...	...	...
1897	*9,735	502	201	...	...	...	...	...	...	...	...	...	...	...	...
1898	8,559	432	173	111[1]	91	61	425[5]	78	38	...	...	...	...	...	...
1899	8,012	399	153	105	85	61	1,573	289	133	...	...	...	29[7]	8	6
1900	7,203	352	137	153	124	93	1,339	245	118	...	...	...	309	83	58
1901	9,130	436	175	224	179	128	1,275	231	112	1,797[6]	283	139	282	74	49
1902	9,645	451	197	316	253	174	1,357	245	113	2,199	318	163	326	78	66
1903	11,089	505	211	363	288	209	1,202	216	109	1,874	262	149	519	122	91
1904	13,813	596	251	308	243	179	1,406	223	142	1,709	237	116	826	191	154
1905	15,036	629	265	327[2]	326[3]	252[4]	...	...	...	1,861	252	150	741	170	152
1906	...	...	...	...	...	...	...	...	...	...	...	...	...	...	...

* No statement as to duplicate certificates. After 1897 all duplicates are omitted. Voluntary notification 1894-97, compulsory afterwards.

1 Notification began Jan. 7th, 1899. 2 To October 13th. 3 Estimated to end of year. 4 To October 13th.

5 Notification began September 11th.

6 Notification began February 14th, 1903.

7 Notification one month during 1899.

Illustration 6.4. Pulmonary tuberculosis: notification and mortality in five towns. From Newsholme, "The Voluntary Notification of Phthisis in Brighton . . . ," *Journal of the Sanitary Institute*, 28 (1907): 33.

Brighton, Manchester, Liverpool, and Sheffield new cases notified each year and annual rates of notification per 100,000 population and per 100 deaths from phthisis. Newsholme was proud of the fact that his results with voluntary notification of phthisis were better than those of any other British town.[65] He attributed this success to the incentive to notify provided by treatment offered at municipal expense.

The last of these services, the municipal treatment of tuberculosis, has yet to be considered. Newsholme began his campaign to secure it after the London meeting of the British Congress on Tuberculosis in July 1901.[66] He had been a member of the municipal delegation to the Congress, and afterward he successfully lobbied the Sanitary Committee to appoint a subcommittee to consider the Congress's emphasis on sanatorium treatment.[67] He led the Sanatorium Subcommittee's deliberations by preparing a substantial report explaining the principles of the open-air treatment, summarizing the present state and scale of sanatorium care in England, and recommending a specific course of action for Brighton.[68] The sanatorium, he argued, offered cure, isolation, and patient education. At this time he predicted that one-third of early cases would be cured and another third would be greatly improved by a short stay in a properly conducted institution. While it was thus in the interest of both the patient and the community that sanatorium treatment be widely available, private enterprise, charity, and working-class self-help were incapable of providing adequate tuberculosis institutions. A great many of the afflicted spent their last days in the workhouse infirmary, and many more suffered in poverty at home, refusing any association with Poor Law institutions.

Local authorities, Newsholme reported, were just beginning to interest themselves in this problem. A public sanatorium had recently been built at Kendal in Westmoreland with the joint support of the County Council and seven local authorities with substantial help from private subscriptions. A similar joint venture was planned for Gloucestershire, Somerset, and Wiltshire. As yet no urban sanitary authority had built its own sanatorium, although Sheffield had resolved to do so.

Newsholme concluded,

I assume that Brighton will not allow itself to lag behind other towns in the attempt to cope with this most fatal disease. We have been to the fore in adopting measures of notification of the disease and of improved sanitary arrangements. It now remains to give those already attacked by it the best possible prospects of recovery and to prevent the

65 He made this argument again in his testimony before the Royal Commission on the Poor Laws B.P.P., 1909, [Cd. 5068], XLIV, 156.

66 For accounts of the Congress, see "British Congress on Tuberculosis," *Br. Med. J.* (1901), no. 2: 205–17, 313–24.

67 The Congress had resolved that "the provision of sanatoria is an indispensable part of the means necessary for the diminution of tuberculosis," ibid. 324. For the appointment of the subcommittee, see Brighton, Proc. San. Comm., 18 (14 Nov. 1901), 440.

68 The report is dated 1 January 1902 and is reprinted in Newsholme, *Ann. Rep.* (Brighton), 1901, 40–52. It is the source for the information contained in the following two paragraphs. This report was also republished as Arthur Newsholme, "Local Authorities and Sanatoria for Consumption," *Practitioner*, 68 (1902): 79–83.

immense pecuniary loss to the town, resulting from the lingering illness and death of so many wage-earners.[69]

The Local Government Board had recently assured the Sanitary Committee that the Corporation could build its own sanatorium for tuberculosis under authority of Section 131 of the Public Health Act, 1875.[70] Newsholme estimated construction would cost between £200 and £300 per bed, and he reported that the annual operating expenses at Kendal were £78 per bed.[71] A new separate institution for tuberculosis would thus be an expensive undertaking. As an immediate and temporary measure, he recommended that the Corporation subscribe to a private sanatorium so that it could reserve a number of beds for patients from Brighton. He also recommended that the Town Council negotiate with the Board of Guardians with a view toward erecting a separate joint sanatorium for advanced consumptives so that poor consumptives could receive care free of Poor Law taint.

The Town Council decided to maintain three patients at a private sanatorium and made the Sanitary Committee, assisted by Newsholme and the physicians at the County Hospital and Children's Hospital, responsible for selecting the patients.[72] In April an agreement was reached with the Stourfield Park Sanatorium in Bournemouth, and by the end of the year the Sanitary Committee had sent six tuberculosis patients to be treated in this sanatorium at Corporation expense.[73]

Then in mid-July of 1902, after only two and a half months of this experiment, Newsholme got permission to try another which he had not even mentioned in his earlier report on sanatorium care. He asked for and received permission to admit patients with pulmonary tuberculosis to the Brighton Sanatorium, the borough isolation hospital, accommodating these patients in the Isolation Pavilion in an empty four-bed ward intended for typhoid fever patients.[74] This experiment was carried on for six months with twenty-five tuberculosis patients receiving treatment.[75] During these months the Committee continued to send patients to the Stourfield Park Sanatorium. The following January, at Newsholme's request, Brighton discontinued sending patients to this private sanatorium and increased the number of tuberculosis beds in the Brighton Sanatorium from four to ten, committing two of the three wards in the Isolation Pavilion to tuberculosis.[76] This provision for the care of pulmonary tuberculosis was now considered a permanent, not a temporary or experimental, municipal function.

69 Newsholme, *Ann. Rep.* (Brighton), 1901, 50–1.
70 Brighton, Proc. San. Comm., 19 (12 Dec. 1901), 23.
71 Newsholme, *Ann. Rep.* (Brighton), 1901, 50.
72 *Sussex Daily News,* 7 Feb. 1902, 3.
73 Brighton, Proc. San. Comm., 19 (24 April 1902): 168–9; and ibid., 29 May 1902, 198. The committee had first planned to send its patients to the Swiss Villa Sanatorium in Dorset, ibid., 13 March 1902, 124. For information on these cases and their treatment, see Newsholme, *Ann. Rep.* (Brighton), 1902, 56–7.
74 Brighton, Proc. San. Comm., 19 (10 July 1902), 241–2; or Brighton, *Proc. Town Council, Proc. Committees,* (17 July 1902), 16–17.
75 Information on each of these cases is found in Newsholme, *Ann. Rep.* (Brighton), 1902, 60–3.
76 Brighton, Proc. San. Comm., 20 (29 Jan. 1903), 19.

It is easy in retrospect to find important precedents in these developments. The municipal isolation hospital was now used for a new type of patient, a patient with a chronic not an acute disease, a patient thought to be mildly contagious to others who came willingly, ignoring the risks of cross-infection known to exist in such institutions. Furthermore, in offering sanatorium treatment for tuberculosis, the Corporation expanded enormously the scale of medical treatment it was willing to provide at municipal expense. The latter is especially significant in view of the fact that no formal restrictions were placed on the social class of the tuberculosis patients eligible for municipally financed care. Newsholme would later find important precedents in the public provision of treatment for tuberculosis. But at the time of its initiation in Brighton his arguments in its favor were entirely pragmatic.[77] Some patients would be cured; others would have their productive working lives extended; and all would leave the institution less likely to serve as foci of infection to others. Furthermore, while the patient was in the Sanatorium, the Sanitary Department would see that the dwelling was disinfected, and during the patient's absence his family would have a respite from exposure to infection. The Corporation could provide proper open-air treatment and hygienic training more economically in its own isolation hospital than it could obtain by contract with a private institution. The Brighton Sanatorium currently had space for tuberculosis. Furthermore, another phase of the new Sanatorium was nearing completion, so that soon there might well be even more space for tuberculosis.

Brighton's Councillors and Aldermen also did not seem to believe they were breaking new ground in state medicine or creating precedents in social policy. In fact, despite Newsholme's immense pride in the treatment of tuberculosis provided by the local authority, such treatment was begun with little public attention and no recorded resistance. Consider for example the initial decision to admit tuberculosis patients to the borough Sanatorium. In July 1902 when Newsholme asked for permission to admit such patients, he requested only a three-month trial period.[78] The Committee not only granted his request but went even further by opening its Sanatorium's doors for twice as long as he had requested. When the proposal came before the Town Council a week later, there was not a bit of opposition, and approval was granted without discussion.[79] Compare this response to the lengthy and often acrimonious Council discussion when housing was the issue. Preventing tuberculosis was either an issue without local opponents, or the specific matter being considered here, the admissions policy of the borough Sanatorium, was considered so arcane that it was best left firmly in the hands of the Sanitary Committee and its Medical Officer of Health.

It is difficult to tell how conscious of precedents Newsholme was at this time.

77 For Newsholme's initial arguments for this treatment, see his letters to the Sanitary Committee, Brighton, Proc. San. Comm., 19 (10 July 1902), 241–2: and ibid., 20 (29 Jan. 1903), 15–19. For published statements, see Newsholme, "Four and a Half Years," 256; and Newsholme and Lecky, "Account of the System," 227.

78 Brighton, Proc. San. Comm., 19 (10 July 1902), 241–2.   79 *Brighton Herald,* 19 July 1902, 2.

He may well have been intent merely on filling out his local preventive program and come to realize that the Sanatorium could play an important part. He may have found additional significance in this policy innovation only later, after the social reforms of the New Liberals had begun. Or he may already have begun to think that treatment as well as sanitation ought to be provided by the local health authority. In any event it seems likely that certain administrative needs also influenced him. By the turn of the century, beds in isolation hospitals for acute infectious diseases stood empty for extended periods.[80] Empty beds might be defended as reserves necessary to meet the demands of epidemics, but expensive, underused institutions invite criticism. A more stable patient base would certainly make it easier to justify the current maintenance costs and recent capital expenses of reconstructing the Brighton Sanatorium and to maintain a trained institutional staff.[81] New patients might not only be accommodated, but they might also help to justify the institution. For this purpose tuberculosis patients were ideal. They existed in nearly unlimited supply. They were currently receiving increasingly public attention. They were not thought to pose a great danger to other patients or to staff. And they could be dismissed on rather short notice if beds were needed to deal with an epidemic of acute infectious disease. He may well have wondered whether a separate tuberculosis institution might jeopardize his goal of uniting all public health services under his authority. His appointment as Medical Officer of the Brighton Sanatorium was independent of his appointment as the town's Medical Officer of Health, and, as we have seen, he did not receive the former appointment as a matter of course. In the unlikely event that the Corporation should choose to build a separate institution for the treatment of tuberculosis as some local authorities were considering doing, he could not be assured of having authority over the new institution. Since he was beginning to view sanatorium treatment of tuberculosis as the linchpin of any program to deal with that disease, Newsholme probably was unwilling to risk losing control of municipally funded treatment.

An unexpected event allowed Newsholme to expand his program of sanatorium treatment. In November 1903 Philip Hedgcock, who had made a fortune in real estate and building in and around Brighton, died, leaving a large legacy to the mayor and town council for charitable purposes.[82] The first use of this money was the award in July 1904 of £2,000 to the Sussex County Hospital for rebuilding a surgical ward for women.[83] In late September 1904 Newsholme boldly applied for

---

80 This fact is pointed out by both Newsholme and James Beatty of Manchester in "A Discussion on the Administrative Prevention of Tuberculosis," *Br. Med. J.* (1902), no. 2: 440, 441.

81 Newsholme uses this reasoning in a carefully argued report to the Sanitary and General Purposes Committees dated 15 March 1905, Brighton, Proc. San. Comm., 22 (30 March 1905), 20–1, 25. See also Newsholme and Lecky, "Account of the System," 233.

82 *Brighton Herald*, 19 Dec. 1903, 5 and *Sussex Daily News*, 18 Dec. 1903, 2. Newsholme occasionally spelled Hedgcock erroneously as Hedgecock. He later explained that the bequest totaled £80,000, Arthur Newsholme, interview, 22 December 1906, Webb, Local Government Collection, vol. 335.

83 *Brighton Herald*, 9 July 1904, 2.

the income of £20,000 of the Hedgcock Bequest to permit the maintenance of an entire pavilion of the Brighton Sanatorium for the care of pulmonary tuberculosis.[84] In making this request he repeated his standard defense of a public tuberculosis policy, and he estimated the costs of providing care in a thirty-bed facility, emphasizing that capital expenses of using one of the new pavilions of the Borough Sanatorium would be minimal, and suggesting that private funds might also be sought to help support the work. He also predicted that with such institutional care available the number of tuberculosis cases in Brighton would drop, so that in ten or twelve years the need for tuberculosis accommodation would be much smaller. He proposed that ten beds be reserved as at present for one-month stays by working people. Another ten beds would be used to treat early cases for three-month periods with a view to effecting a cure. The final ten beds would be reserved for advanced cases. These cases would stay longer, for indefinite periods.

His proposal was withdrawn without coming to a vote at the Council meeting of October 20. Critics feared that free treatment would attract consumptives to Brighton and tarnish the town's reputation for health.[85] Over the next year Newsholme lobbied for his idea and added a two-year residency requirement for eligibility for sanatorium treatment.[86] In this revised form the proposal received the support of the Sanitary and the General Purposes Committees, who worked out details for a scheme in early 1906, and the Town Council approved the plan without objection on April 5.[87] The Sanitary Committee was granted the interest on £20,000 of the Hedgcock Bequest for a ten-year period to help support the municipal treatment of tuberculosis in the Borough Sanatorium.[88]

To put the enlarged treatment plan into operation Newsholme rearranged the Sanatorium, moving the tuberculosis patients into the new diphtheria pavilion, which had been completed the previous year in the second phase of rebuilding.[89] The diphtheria cases in turn were moved into the older pavilion which the scarlet fever cases vacated when they moved into the second new pavilion. The Hedgcock Bequest did not support quite so grand a scheme as Newsholme had

84 I have not found his report of 22 Sept. 1904, but he explains that his report to the Sanitary and General Purposes Committees of 15 March 1905 repeats and brings that earlier report up to date. Information on his request is found in the latter report, Brighton, Proc. San. Comm., 22 (30 March 1905), 11–31.

85 For accounts of this Town Council meeting, see *Brighton Herald*, 22 Oct. 1904, 6; and *Sussex Daily News*, 21 Oct. 1904, 3.

86 Brighton, Proc. San. Comm., 22 (30 March 1905), 25, 27, 28–31.

87 For an example of the negotiations on details, see Brighton, Proc. San. Comm., 22 (22 Feb. 1906), 12; for the Council's approval see *Brighton Gazette*, 7 April 1906, 8.

88 Newsholme and Lecky, "Account of the System," 227.

89 The change in plans for the new pavilions can be understood by comparing Brighton, *Minutes of Town Council*, 21 Nov. 1901, iv–vi; Francis J. C. May and Arthur Newsholme, *A General Description . . . of the History of Isolation Accommodation Provided for the Borough, with a More Detailed Account of the Improved Accommodation Now Provided by the Corporation* (Brighton, 1898), 13; Newsholme and Lecky, "Account of the System," 233; and Brighton Sanitary Congress, *A Short Description of the Borough Sanatorium* ([Brighton], 1910), 3 & 4.

outlined. In 1907, the first full year the Hedgcock funds were available to support this work, Newsholme maintained tuberculosis wards with twenty-five beds.[90] Ten were for the patients the Corporation had already committed itself to supporting from municipal funds. These were usually, although not necessarily, working men and women who were treated free of charge in the Sanatorium for a month. Twelve beds were supported by the income from the Hedgcock bequest. These beds were intended for working-class patients who were unable to pay for their own care, and among them were advanced cases who would be treated longer than the municipal patients, the period of treatment being determined by the nature of the individual cases.[91] The last three beds were pay beds whose use cannot be determined exactly from existing records.

There were always more applicants for admission than could be accommodated. Newsholme was primarily responsible for making the selection. He called each candidate to his office in Town Hall for an examination and an interview.[92] His choice was dictated primarily by social goals.[93] He preferred patients with dependents and those likely to infect others. In practical terms this meant that young adults with families, more often fathers than mothers, especially those who worked in crowded factories or workshops were given top priority. Children, older persons, and those without families had lower priority. Family income was not a major factor in the selection. Newsholme reasoned that although families with incomes of 35s per week had much more comfortable lives than those living on 25s, when tuberculosis struck, the former needed sanatorium care as much as the latter. Paupers were a special category. Those who were deemed curable were accepted in the Sanatorium. Others were sent to the Workhouse Infirmary. By 1906 Newsholme did not believe that the stage of the disease was a very important factor in selecting patients. Since most patients could only stay four to six weeks, there was seldom hope of cure. He told a medical readership that "the possibility of permanent benefit or cure, obviously is the factor of least importance in deciding as to the admission of patients to our sanatorium," and he held that the primary function of institutionalization was patient training.[94]

Newsholme's assessment now sounded quite different from what it had been when he had begun campaigning for municipal treatment of tuberculosis. In 1901 he had told the Sanitary Committee that curing patients was one of the three goals of tuberculosis sanatoria, and, convinced by the claims of sanatorium managers, had declared that in a properly conducted institution "in a very considerable proportion of cases cure is secured."[95] He did acknowledge at this time that hope

90 Newsholme, "Voluntary Notification," 31.
91 See also Newsholme and Lecky, "Account of the System," 228.
92 Beatrice Webb's researcher reported witnessing one of these occasions, interview with Arthur Newsholme, 22 Dec. 1906, Webb, Local Government Collection, vol. 335.
93 Newsholme explained his criteria in Newsholme and Lecky, "Account of the System," 235–7; and in Newsholme, "Public Health Authorities," 460.
94 Newsholme and Lecky, "Account of the System," 235.
95 Newsholme, report to the Sanitary Committee in Newsholme, *Ann. Rep.* (Brighton), 1901, 41.

of cure was brighter with early cases, but his reports of the results of the first cases treated at the Stourfield Park Sanatorium and in the Brighton Sanatorium were optimistic, almost glowing.[96] Of the six patients sent to the private sanatorium during 1902 two, both early cases, were discharged apparently cured, three left improved, and one, an advanced case, was reported "very slightly improved." Weight gain in institutionalized patients was one of the major signs of improvement, and Newsholme's reports listed for each case the amount of weight gained. Of the twenty-five tuberculosis patients admitted to the Brighton Sanatorium before the end of 1902, four were declared cured or almost well; ten were discharged greatly or much improved, and only four were reported slightly or not improved. However, by March of the next year, experience called such initial optimism into question. Of the six patients sent to Bournemouth for treatment, one had already died and two others had experienced a return of their coughs. Three of the first twenty-five patients treated in the Brighton Sanatorium had already died, one of them in the institution; five had relapsed but remained at home, and three others had already been admitted to another institution for tuberculosis.[97]

Newsholme was soon declaring that most cases entering the Brighton Sanatorium were too advanced for there to be hope of a cure and that purpose of institutionalization was, and by implication always had been, not cure of the individual but protection of the community by teaching patients to manage their sputum responsibly.[98] The lessons in hygiene practiced in the institution, he insisted, had an impact on patient behavior that no amount of teaching by the Sanitary Inspector in the home could match. While Newsholme claimed that patients admitted to the Sanatorium were informed that their cure in the institution was unlikely,[99] the size of the applicant pool suggests that patients and their families did not share that vision of the purpose of institutionalization. It is scarcely credible that so many would have applied had they viewed the month in the Sanatorium primarily as an educational opportunity.

By 1905 Newsholme believed that the tuberculosis program he had helped design had two great gaps. The first was a need for more complete information on cases. Within a year or two he thought it might be time to consider introducing compulsory notification of tuberculosis in Brighton.[100] He justified compulsory notification now, because he believed that the Corporation at last offered enough services to the sick to make notification not only acceptable but attractive. The scale of municipal activity in tuberculosis had, in fact, grown significantly. In 1907 the Sanitary Department had 667 notified cases under observation, four cases for each tuberculosis death, and 52 percent of these notified cases had already spent at

96 Newsholme, *Ann. Rep.* (Brighton), 1902, 56–7, 58, 60–1. See also Newsholme's report to the Sanitary Committee, Brighton, Proc. San. Comm., 20 (29 Jan. 1903), 17.
97 Newsholme, *Ann. Rep.* (Brighton), 1902, 56–7, 60–3.
98 See for example, ibid., 1905, 36; Newsholme, "Voluntary Notification," 30.
99 Newsholme, "Four and a Half Years'," 257.
100 Newsholme, *Ann. Rep.* (Brighton), 1905, 38.

least one month in the Sanatorium and been drilled in the means of protecting others from infection.[101] Newsholme had become convinced that sanatorium care was the feature of Brighton's program that made the whole scheme work. Its presence was the reason why Brighton had achieved better results with voluntary notification than Sheffield had with compulsory notification.[102] Notification of tuberculosis could be expected to work only if local authorities were prepared to offer something in return. It is perhaps for this reason that Newsholme did not discourage the hope of cure in the institution even though he was coming to realize that in many cases that hope was an illusion.

The second gap was inadequate accommodation for advanced cases. Like other public health authorities, he was coming to regard these advanced cases as the greatest threat to the community.[103] The issue here was neither cure nor even education but rather separation of the sick from the well. The Workhouse Infirmary was frequently the last refuge of the dying consumptive. About 20 percent of deaths from pulmonary tuberculosis in Brighton occurred in the Workhouse Infirmary. His recommendation that the Corporation and the Poor Law Guardians cooperate to provide institutional accommodation for advanced cases that was free of the stigma and disabilities of the Poor Law was never heeded during his career. But his preoccupation with the role that advanced cases played in spreading the infection had a strong influence on the epidemiological studies of tuberculosis he undertook in these years.

EPIDEMIOLOGY

Newsholme's first paper on the epidemiology of tuberculosis, a brief presentation to the Brussels meeting of the International Congress on Hygiene and Demography in September 1903,[104] was prepared only fourteen months after he had gained permission to admit a few tuberculosis patients to the Brighton Sanatorium on an experimental basis. This rather unexceptional summary of what British local authorities were beginning to do to combat the disease suggests, nonetheless, how quickly his mind was changing at this time. The body of his published paper, what he probably told the Congress, indicates that he viewed the recent accelerating decline in tuberculosis mortality as the unintended result of local authority initiatives in sanitation and general public health work and of favorable economic changes. His conclusions in the body of the paper were broad, inclusive, and

---

101 Newsholme, "Voluntary Notification," 32.
102 Newsholme, "Voluntary Notification," 26, 32, 34; and Newsholme and Lecky, "Account of the System," 237.
103 For the following observations, see Newsholme, *Ann. Rep.* (Brighton), 1905, 36–7. For the growing concern for the sanatorium care of advanced cases, see Hillier, "Prospect," 303–4.
104 Arthur Newsholme, "Public Health Authorities in Relation to the Struggle against Tuberculosis in England," *J. Hygiene*, 3 (1903): 446–67. This paper was first presented to the thirteenth International Congress of Hygiene and Demography, Brussels, 1903 and may also be found in its *Compte Rendu*. Subsequent citation will be to the former version.

conciliatory. It was unnecessary, he held, to decide whether conscious public policy or the unconscious effects of economic change were responsible for the progress that had been made. Measures undertaken for one purpose had sometimes served another as well. For the future it made sense both to increase the resistance of individuals to tuberculosis infection and to prevent such infection from taking place.[105]

It was only in the postscript which apparently was added just before the paper went to press that Newsholme mentioned institutionalizing the sick.[106] We can see in this postscript the effects of his recent interest in institutional care and his hope to harness some of the resources of the Poor Law to find acceptable accommodation for patients in advanced stages of the disease. In this postscript he began by casting doubt on a statement Robert Koch had made at the London meeting of the British Congress on Tuberculosis two years before. Koch had asserted that the singularly rapid decline of tuberculosis in Britain was due to the fact that Britain had more tuberculosis sanatoriums than any other nation. In Newsholme's opinion it was obvious that Britain's special institutions for tuberculosis were simply too few in number and too recent in origin to have exercised such an influence. He wondered, however, whether Koch might be correct in a more general way, if one were to consider not only institutional confinement in special sanatoriums but also confinement provided by other institutions, particularly by those of the Poor Law. In this early publication Newsholme could offer only two bits of suggestive evidence. First, using mortality data and information supplied by the Guardians, he estimated that in the three years ending October 1, 1901, that 18 percent of phthisis cases in Brighton had been confined to the workhouse at an advanced stage of the disease during a significant part of the period when they were most likely to infect others. Second, he showed by way of a graph that the decline in pauperism in England and Wales during the second half of the nineteenth century was due almost entirely to a reduction in outdoor relief, that is, assistance given outside of institutions. What this trend meant was that paupers, many of whom were sick, were increasingly likely to be confined in a workhouse or a workhouse infirmary. The recent past seemed to vindicate the emphasis he placed on institutional confinement as a strategy of preventing tuberculosis.

What was only implied in the postscript of 1903 was made explicit in the series of papers he published between 1905 and 1908.[107] Of these the most statistically

105 Newsholme, "Public Health Authorities," 450, 461.
106 Ibid., 461–5.
107 "A Study of the Relation between the Treatment of Tubercular Patients in General Institutions and the Reduction in the Death-Rate from Tuberculosis," *Rapports, Congrès International de la Tuberculose* (Paris, 1905), 5: 413–37; "The Relative Importance of the Constituent Factors involved in the Control of Pulmonary Tuberculosis," *Trans. Epidem. Soc. Lond.*, n.s. 25 (1905–6): 31–112; "An Inquiry into the Principal Causes of the Reduction in the Death-Rate from Phthisis during the Last Forty Years, with Special Reference to the Segregation of Phthisical Patients in General Institutions," *J. Hygiene*, 6 (1906): 304–84; "Poverty and Disease, as Illustrated by the Course of Typhus Fever and Phthisis in Ireland," *Proc. Roy. Soc. Med.*, I (1908), Epidemiological Sect., pt. 1:

complete and critical was his eighty-page 1906 article in the *Journal of Hygiene*.[108] The most accessible version and the one which probably had the greatest influence among a wider audience of public health and social workers was his lecture to the Washington meeting of the International Congress on Tuberculosis in 1908.[109] His tuberculosis monograph republished the later versions of his argument and suggestions.[110] These are a remarkable series of publications. Seldom had he worked as doggedly on an epidemiological project with such an apparent purpose. While these studies recognize that many forces were at work in the decline of pulmonary tuberculosis, one factor, he believed, was critical, and that was the isolation of the sick.

These studies used an approach like the one Newsholme had used to study rheumatic fever and diphtheria in the middle nineties, the compiling of statistics for very large population groups, whole nations or their capital cities, and the search for apparent associations between mortality trends and suspect environmental forces. In making these comparisons Newsholme drew special attention to the exceptions to the rule that everywhere the disease was in decline. While mortality from phthisis was declining in England and Wales, in Scotland, in the United States, and in Germany, it had not fallen the same way in France, and in Ireland and Norway it had actually increased. Pointing to such exceptions, he argued that the improved standard of living most Western nations were experiencing cannot have been the major force in lowering the death rate from phthisis. See Illustrations 6.5 to 6.7. In 1906, for example, he calculated the following correlation coefficients for wheat prices, an established proxy for cost of living, and the mortality from phthisis.[111]

England and Wales	(1866–1902)	+.90
Scotland	(1868–1902)	+.87
Ireland	(1866–1902)	−.80
Prussia	(1877–1901)	+.55
Paris	(1866–1902)	+.31

1–44; "The Causes of the Past Decline in Tuberculosis and the Light Thrown by History on Preventive Measures for the Immediate Future," *Trans., Sixth International Congress on Tuberculosis* (Washington, D.C., 1908), Suppl. *A Series of Public Lectures,* 80–109. Newsholme saw that his results were made known to broader audiences. Newsholme, "Causes of the Past Decline," was republished under the same title in *Charities,* 21 (1908–9), 206–29. Hereafter citation to this work will be to the version published in *Charities* unless otherwise noted. Newsholme, "Inquiry into the Principal Causes," was incorporated with a few changes into Newsholme, *Prevention of Tuberculosis,* 205–97.
108 Newsholme, "Inquiry into the Principal Causes."
109 Newsholme, "Causes of the Past Decline." This lecture is often said to have been widely influential in the American tuberculosis movement. See Walter I. Trattner, *From Poor Law to Welfare State: A History of Social Welfare in America,* 2nd ed. (New York: Free Press, 1979), 125.
110 Newsholme, *Prevention of Tuberculosis.*
111 Newsholme, "Inquiry into the Principal Causes," 335.

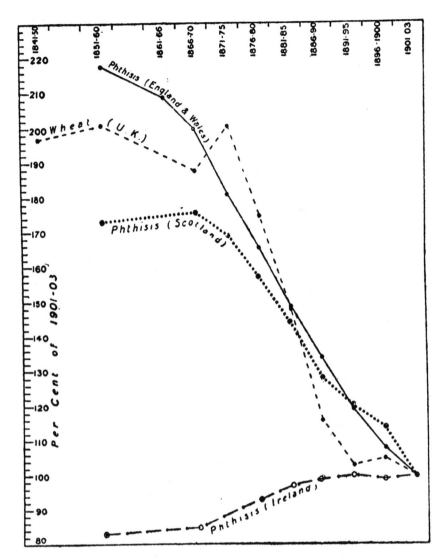

Illustration 6.5. Newsholme's curves for mortality from pulmonary tuberculosis and for the price of wheat in the United Kingdom. From Newsholme, *Prevention of Tuberculosis*, 233.

In some nations, he argued, the improvement in the standard of living had been closely and positively associated with a decline in mortality. In others it had been weakly associated. And in a few there had been a strong negative correlation.

Since both his interest and information were greatest for Britain, Newsholme

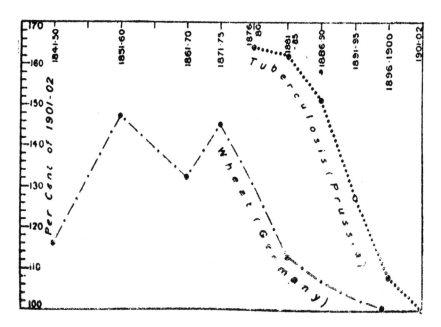

Illustration 6.6. Newsholme's curves for mortality from pulmonary tuberculosis and for the price of wheat in Prussia. From Newsholme, *Prevention of Tuberculosis*, 234.

found Ireland to be a critical instance. It is the example he used most often to demonstrate that living conditions could improve without there being a fall in the death rate from pulmonary tuberculosis and that similar socioeconomic forces could produce very different effects on phthisis within the British Isles. Despite Ireland's great poverty, wages had increased in Ireland. In fact, wages for Irish agricultural laborers had increased faster since 1860 than had the wages of their English counterparts, while the cost of living in Ireland had fallen.[112] More significant, given the known pathology of the disease, was information on housing collected by the Registrar-General of Ireland which Newsholme reproduced in his studies.[113] These data suggested that there had been a substantial improvement in the housing stock in Ireland in the very decades when the mortality from pulmonary tuberculosis was increasing. The same report by the Irish Registrar-General provided Newsholme with a table on the most crowded tenements in the

112 For the following discussion, see Newsholme, "Poverty and Disease," 22–4; Newsholme, "Causes of the Past Decline," 220; Newsholme, "Inquiry into the Principal Causes," 331, 338; and Newsholme, "Relative Importance of the Constituent Factors," 55.
113 Newsholme, "Causes of the Past Decline," 220; and Newsholme, *Prevention of Tuberculosis*, 226–7. More complete figures are presented without the chart in Newsholme, "Inquiry into the Principal Causes," 325.

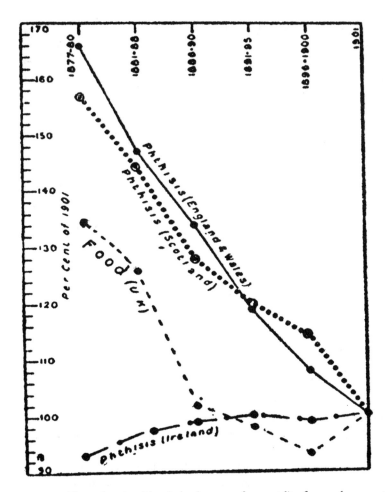

Illustration 6.7. Newsholme's curves for mortality from pulmonary tuberculosis and for the price of food in the United Kingdom. From Newsholme, *Prevention of Tuberculosis*, 237.

largest British cities based on the censuses of 1901.[114] See Illustration 6.8. Newsholme interpreted these figures in the following way.

Thus in Glasgow, which has twenty-six times as large a proportion of one-roomed tenement dwellings as Belfast, and fifty-two times as many persons in its one-roomed tenements with five or more occupants, the death-rate from phthisis instead of being higher is forty-three per cent lower than that of Belfast. This does not imply that in a given town the death-rate from phthisis is not higher in the smaller and more overcrowded tenements. Abundant statistics show this to be the case. But it is clear from the above table that size of

114 Newsholme, "Poverty and Disease," 24; and Newsholme, "Causes of the Past Decline," 218.

	Number of One-roomed Tenements Per Cent of Total Dwellings or Tenements.	Number of One-roomed Tenements having Five or more Occupants each in every 100 Tenements of all Classes.	Number of Persons in One-roomed Tenements with Five or more Occupants in every 100 of the Total Population.	Average Death-rate from Phthisis, per 100,000 living, in the Three Years 1900-1-2.
Dublin	36.70	8.69	10.61	329
Belfast	1.00	0.09	0.10	313
London	14.66	0.57	0.70	171
Liverpool	6.14	0.22	0.24	190
Manchester	1.90	0.04	0.05	208
Edinburgh	16.98	1.80	2.33	164
Glasgow	26.11	4.28	5.24	177

Illustration 6.8. Newsholme's figures for overcrowding and the mortality of pulmonary tuberculosis in seven towns. From Newsholme, "The Causes of the Past Decline in Tuberculosis . . . ," *Charities*, 21 (1908–9): 218.

dwellings or even degree of overcrowding may be overshadowed by the effect of other influences. . . .[115]

Newsholme did not attempt to rule out the possibility that the dwellers of the most crowded tenements in both cities might have similarly high phthisis mortalities or that the lower mortality for Glaslgow might be due to the more favorable conditions of the rest of the town's population. He did not, for example, compare the phthisis mortality rates for the one-room tenement dwellers with the rest of the population in each city.

Newsholme also attempted to use the differences between urban and rural mortality rates to suggest that general living conditions alone did not determine tuberculosis mortality.[116] Urban congestion ought to favor mortality from phthisis, but in most Western nations phthisis had declined in spite of substantial urbanization. Furthermore while death rates from phthisis were usually still higher in urban than in rural districts, phthisis was often found to be declining faster in the urban areas. Other forces, it seemed, were working powerfully enough to overcome the adverse effects of urbanization.

Using information from the English Registrar-General's reports, Newsholme constructed the table shown in Illustration 6.9, which provided for selected urban and rural districts of England and Wales mortality rates for phthisis and for all causes for males and females separately.[117] This table demonstrated the familiar fact

115 Newsholme, "Causes of the Past Decline," 217.
116 For the following discussion, see Newsholme, "Inquiry into the Principal Causes," 321–3.
117 This table is reproduced from Newsholme, "Relative Importance of the Constituent Factors," 47. '

ENGLAND AND WALES.
Selected Urban and Rural Counties of the Registrar-General,
1898 to 1902.

	Corrected Death-Rates per 1,000 of Population.			
—	**Males.**		**Females.**	
	All Causes.	Phthisis.	All Causes.	Phthisis.
Urban Counties ...	20.6	1.69	17.9	1.13
Rural „	15.1	1.26	13.6	1.09

	Proportional Figures (Rural Rate=100).			
—	**Males.**		**Females.**	
	All Causes.	Phthisis.	All Causes.	Phthisis.
Urban Counties ...	137	134	132	104
Rural „	100	100	100	100

Illustration 6.9. Corrected male and female death rates for pulmonary tuberculosis for select urban and rural counties. From Newsholme, "Relative Importance of the Constituent Factors Involved in the Control of Pulmonary Tuberculosis," *Trans. Epidem. Soc. Lond.*, n.s. 25 (1905–6): 47.

that the urban counties of England did have an excess mortality from both phthisis and from all causes of death. It also allowed Newsholme to make two other contentions: first, that differences in population density were not the key to understanding the epidemiology of phthisis, and second, that the decline of phthisis was not governed by the same forces that were driving down the general death rates. The argument in both cases rested on the comparison of sex-specific rates. The forces which were producing the fall in general mortality were acting on both sexes about equally. But this was not the case with tuberculosis. Because

He brought this comparison up to date as subsequent reports appeared from the Registrar-General, and in these later versions Newsholme compared phthisis mortality to the mortality from all causes other than phthisis. See Newsholme, "Inquiry into the Principal Causes," 323; and Newsholme, "Causes of the Past Decline," 217.

Newsholme contended that the deleterious effects of aggregation of the population in towns should also be gender-neutral, he interpreted these figures as demonstrating that the hazards of town life did not consist primarily in reducing human resistance to disease but in increasing the chances of infection. Men, he argued, were more frequently exposed to tuberculosis in towns than women were.[118] He also took these differences in mortality by gender as added evidence that economic change was not the primary force in the decline of tuberculosis. If it were, the two sexes should have benefited more equally.

Newsholme also used tables such as this one to suggest that the sanitary reforms, which he was sure had helped suppress the general mortality rate, were not the dominant force at work in the decline of phthisis. Once again, he argued, such a force should not have affected sex-specific mortality rates so differently. Occasionally he attempted more direct demonstrations. In his 1905 paper to the International Congress on Tuberculosis he drew attention to the fact that in the decades between 1851–60 and 1880–90 the average annual phthisis death rate had fallen much faster in Chichester (44%), a town without sewers, than in Ely, a drained town, (20.5%) and nearly as fast as in another sewered town, Salisbury (50.6%).[119]

Newsholme recognized that such local comparisons of phthisis mortality could be seriously biased by unrecognized differences in the composition of local populations, and he began to seek other means to demonstrate that phthisis was responding to special forces other than those affecting the general death rates.[120] He found, for example, that average annual mortalities between 1881–5 and 1901–3 had fallen faster for phthisis than for all causes of death other than phthisis in most European nations. In England phthisis mortality had fallen faster than had the mortality from other causes in each age group from birth to age seventy-five between the periods 1861–70 and 1896–1900. The difference in the rate of decline was greatest in the working years of life. Once again Norway and Ireland were exceptions.

Such statistical demonstrations proved, to Newsholme's satisfaction at least, that while a population would undoubtedly be healthier and safer from phthisis, if it were better fed, better housed, and provided with better sanitary facilities, the undisputed improvement during recent decades in these features of life was insufficient to explain the behavior of the death rate from phthisis in western nations. For a more adequate explanation of these mortality trends he returned to the suggestions found in his postscript of 1903, in particular to the possibility of a connection between pauperism and the death rate from phthisis.

His key arguments depended on the trends in poor relief and phthisis mortality in the British Isles since the 1860s. The curves in Illustrations 6.10 to 6.12 suggested that phthisis mortality in the United Kingdom was strongly correlated

118 Newsholme, "Study of the Relation between the Treatment of Tuberculosis Patients," 425–6; and Newsholme, "Relative Importance of the Constituent Factors," 48–9.
119 Newsholme, "Study of the Relation between the Treatment of Tubercular Patients," 422–3.
120 For the following comparisons, see Newsholme, "Inquiry into the Principal Causes," 318.

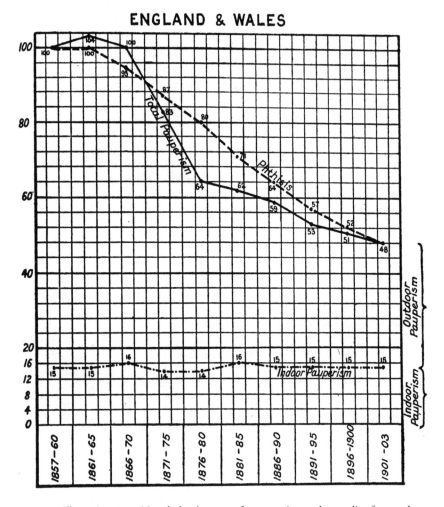

Illustration 6.10. Newsholme's curves for pauperism and mortality from pulmonary tuberculosis in England and Wales. From Newsholme, *Prevention of Tuberculosis*, 245.

with the total amount of pauperism. Newsholme computed the following correlation coefficients for those series:[121]

England and Wales	(1866–1903)	+.89
Scotland	(1868–1902)	+.90
Ireland	(1866–1902)	+.83

121 Ibid., 350.

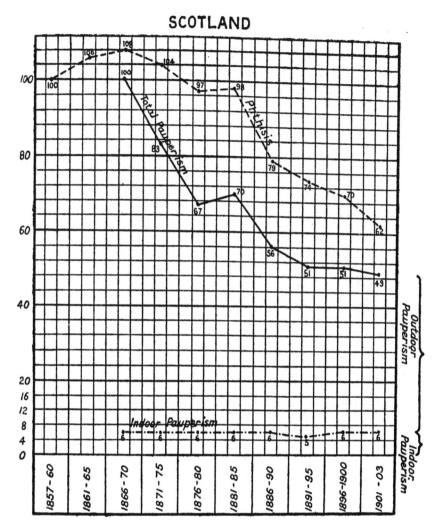

Illustration 6.11. Newsholme's curves for pauperism and mortality from pulmonary tuberculosis in Scotland. From Newsholme, *Prevention of Tuberculosis*, 247.

Newsholme insisted that such strong correlations did not prove, after all, that standard of living, as indicated by the level of pauperism, was the key element determining the mortality for phthisis.[122] Pauperism was too complex a phenomenon for such a simple inference to be drawn. As he explained:

122 For the following discussion, see ibid., 344–5; and Newsholme, "Causes of the Past Decline," 221–2.

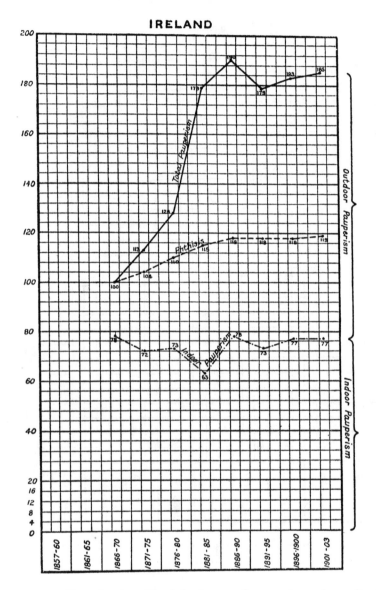

Illustration 6.12. Newsholme's curves for pauperism and mortality from pulmonary tuberculosis in Ireland. From Newsholme, *Prevention of Tuberculosis*, 248.

In each of these countries, pauperism comprises enough phthisiogenetic influences to make its figures vary closely with the figures of phthisis. This does not necessarily show that the variations in pauperism explain the variations in the death rate from phthisis. Within the bundle of phenomena which constitute pauperism such an explanation may be found; but until we ascertain which individual element or elements of the bundle contain the explanation, to explain the figures of phthisis by those of pauperism is for any practical purpose to explain a complex *ignotum* by a yet more complex *ignotius*.[123]

Newsholme interpreted the curves like those in Illustrations 6.10 to 6.12 as indicating the changing chances that advanced cases of phthisis, the type of cases most likely to be impoverished by their disease and the cases he believed most likely to infect others, were to be confined in institutions and the effects of that confinement. It was now clear, he believed, why Ireland represented an exception when one considered the relationship of standard of living and phthisis mortality. Only in Ireland had the likelihood of a pauper's being confined to an institution declined over the past half century, and only in Ireland had mortality due to phthisis increased in the same decades. When he computed correlation coefficients for the time series representing the ratio of indoor (institutionalized) paupers to total paupers and for the death rate for phthisis, he found an even stronger (although negative) correlation than he had found between total pauperism and phthisis mortality.[124]

England and Wales	(1866–1903)	−.94
Scotland	(1868–1902)	−.91
Ireland	(1866–1903)	−.85

This ratio of indoor paupers to total paupers Newsholme called a "segregation ratio." It was the first and most common of several ratios he used to attempting to demonstrate that institutionalization had been the prime element in the decline of phthisis.[125] He also used at various times these segregation ratios: (institutional deaths from phthisis : total deaths from phthisis); (institutional deaths from all causes : total deaths from all causes); and (cases of phthisis institutionally treated : total deaths from phthisis). Newsholme recognized that these ratios were only proxies for what he needed to know, and that was the portion of total illness caused by pulmonary tuberculosis that had been confined in institutions. The correct segregation ratio would be (days of phthisis sickness spent in institutions : days of phthisis sickness in the whole population). But the amount of phthisis in the British populations was unknown. Strictly speaking, the different segregation ratios measured different things, but, Newsholme maintained, the tests he had made using different ratios for the same population in the same years had given similar, although not identical, results.[126]

Newsholme also sought to represent the relationship between phthisis mortality and his segregation ratios in graphic form by plotting logarithmic curves for each series. Such curves represented rates of change in segregation ratios and phthisis

123 Newsholme, "Causes of the Past Decline," 222.
124 Newsholme, "Inquiry into the Principal Causes," 367.
125 Newsholme, He employed this ratio in each of his publications in this series from 1905 to 1908, although he did not label it as such in the first. Newsholme, "Study of the Relation between the Treatment of Tubercular Patients," 419–20.
126 Newsholme, "Inquiry into the Principal Causes," 356–7.

mortality. See Illustrations 6.13 and 6.14. Notice that in this case different segregation ratios did yield somewhat different curves for the same population.

To make institutional segregation a more plausible determinant of phthisis mortality, Newsholme also gathered information on the practices of individual parishes, the local administrative units of the Poor Law. Some of this information was unquantifiable. Guardians reported that in recent decades inmates of English workhouses were increasingly likely to be sick, and that phthisis was a common cause of admission to the institution.[127] Some parishes provided separate accommodation for phthisis patients, but most did not. Newsholme argued, however, that even in the general ward of a workhouse or workhouse infirmary, a patient with advanced phthisis would be less likely to infect others than he would be in the typical homes of impoverished families.

The responses from parishes did allow him to frame some additional quantitative arguments. He could, he thought, explain the surprising result of the contrast of Ely's and Chichester's death rates from phthisis.[128] In Ely, the town with a municipal drainage system and a high death rate from pulmonary tuberculosis, he found that only 1.6 percent of registered deaths from phthisis had occurred in the workhouse in 1861–5, and that percentage had risen to only 2.7 in 1886–90. The much more rapid decline of deaths from phthisis in Chichester had taken place in the absence of drainage, but in circumstances where 12.2 percent of phthisis deaths between 1861 and 1865 and 24.7 percent between 1886 and 1890 took place in the workhouse.

More significant for his case was information he was able to secure on the period of confinement of sick paupers in select parishes. During 1897 average stays in workhouse infirmaries from which he could gain information varied between 48 and 97 days.[129] He reasoned that cases of phthisis were likely to be kept longer than average in the institution. For three parishes, Kensington, Sheffield, and Brighton, he acquired information on the confinement of phthisis patients. In these parishes the workhouse or its infirmary seemed to confine a significant portion of the phthisis in the community. In the Sheffield Infirmary the average confinement of phthisis cases was 311 days in 1904, and in the Brighton Workhouse the average stay for phthisis in the years 1897–1905 was 221 days. In Kensington one-third and in Brighton one-fifth of all deaths from phthisis occurred in Poor Law institutions.[130] Periods of institutional confinement of that length and for that percentage of all advanced cases, Newsholme reasoned, might be expected to exert a significant influence on the epidemiology of the disease. He offered a hypothetical calculation as demonstration.[131] If one assumed that the nation had confined its pauper consumptives as Brighton had, and assumed also

127 Ibid., 368–9.
128 Newsholme, "Study of the Relation between the Treatment of Tubercular Patients," 430.
129 For the following, see Newsholme, "Inquiry into the Principal Causes," 369.
130 Newsholme, "Relative Importance of the Constituent Factors," 88–91.
131 Newsholme, "Inquiry into the Principal Causes," 370–1; and Newsholme, "Causes of the Past Decline," 223–4.

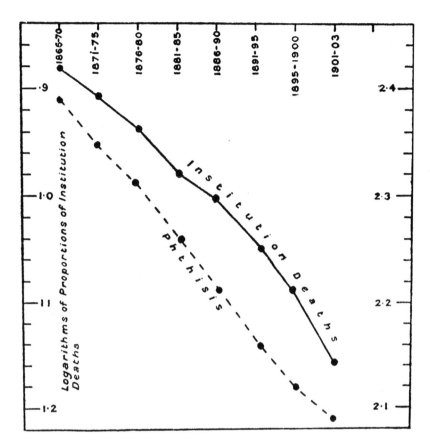

Illustration 6.13. Newsholme's logarithmic curves for mortality from pulmonary tuberculosis and for one of his segregation ratios. From Newsholme, *Prevention of Tuberculosis*, 271.

that the period of infectiousness in phthisis was three years, then one-fifth of all cases in England and Wales would have spent one-ninth of their infectious period in a Poor Law institution. Assuming likewise that personal infection is the major cause of new phthisis cases and that there is a direct relationship between the total number of days of unconfined phthisis and the amount of infectious material in the community, Newsholme estimated that the phthisis mortality rate in England and Wales should have declined 2 percent each year. In point of fact since 1871 it had declined annually somewhat under 2 percent. The results, he believed, confirmed the hypothesized mechanism for the decline in the phthisis death rate.

In two papers he offered another rhetorical calculation.[132] He tried to show that in both Brighton and Berlin there had been a direct relationship between the

132 Newsholme, "Study of the Relation between the Treatment of Tubercular Patients," 428–9, 432–3; and Newsholme, "Relative Importance of the Constituent Factors," 93–5.

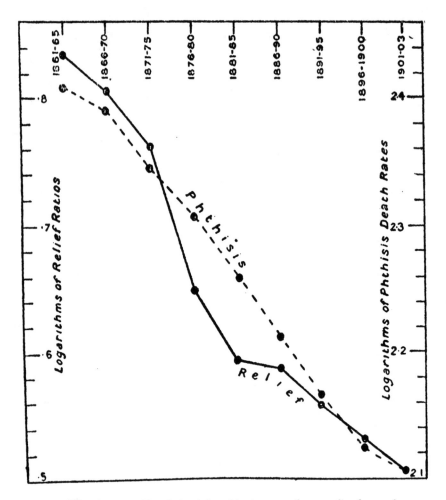

Illustration 6.14. Newsholme's logarithmic curves for mortality from pulmonary tuberculosis and for another of his segregation ratios. From Newsholme, *Prevention of Tuberculosis, 278.*

decline in the death rate from phthisis and the percentage of deaths from the disease which took place in institutions. He did this by using segregation ratios to calculate a series of mortality figures which closely approximated the observed series for phthisis. It was an old device in public health literature. William Farr had made good use of it in the mid-Victorian decades in computing what he called statistical laws.[133] But it was not very effective in this case; under criticism

133 John M. Eyler, *Victorian Social Medicine: The Ideas and Methods of William Farr* (Baltimore and London: Johns Hopkins Univ. Press, 1979): 34, 108–22, 130–3, 143–8.

Newsholme abandoned it and relied thereafter on displaying similarity of rates of change by plotting logarithmic curves.[134]

Newsholme was, of course, not arguing that Poor Law institutions were peculiarly suited to aid in the reduction of phthisis, except that in Britain during the nineteenth century they had been the most widely available institutions for the reception of advanced cases. As Illustrations 6.15 and 6.16 show, he also attempted to assess the role which confinement in hospitals and asylums may have played.

The final element in Newsholme's case was analogies drawn to other diseases. These appear quite late in his presentations on this problem. In his Presidential Address to the Epidemiological Section of the Royal Society of Medicine in October 1907, he attempted to show that the history of typhus in Ireland confirmed the importance of institutional segregation to control infection. Irish Poor Law policy, he argued, had not only permitted the increase in phthisis mortality by discouraging the confinement of chronic cases, but it had helped control typhus by encouraging the admission to the workhouse of acute diseases.[135] By the following year he had added the decline of leprosy in Norway to his argument.[136] In the early nineteenth century Norway had very few leper asylums and a high incidence of the disease, but during the second half of the century increased use of such asylums had been associated with a marked decline in the disease. These analogies were not nearly as fully developed as his statistical studies of phthisis, especially in Britain. Newsholme apparently intended them as only suggestive of the value of isolation.

Newsholme was certainly aware that he was dealing with a very complex problem. The epidemiology of a chronic infectious disease was extremely difficult.

The problem is one in which inferences to be valid must be drawn with considerable caution. The conditions determining the successful invasion even of an individual with an infectious disease are highly complex. They depend not merely on the life-history and modes of activity of the infecting organism but also on the far more complex processes of the person attacked. . . . The complexity of the problem is still greater when we come to consider the conditions which determine the spread of an infectious disease in a community; for in addition to the problems of individual cases, further complexities arise from the economical and other vital processes of the body corporate. The communal complexities are greater in the case of diseases with protracted incubation than in the case of diseases in which infection and onset follow in rapid succession.[137]

It was possible, perhaps even likely, that many factors had acted beneficially in the reduction of phthisis. "There is scarcely any factor which has been advocated

134 Newsholme in these two publications arrived at different calculated series from the same data for Brighton. Using the method he says he used, I have been unable to confirm either one for Brighton, although I can do so for Berlin. A hint about the criticism he had received is found in Newsholme, "Relative Importance of the Constituent Factors," 94.

135 Newsholme, "Poverty and Disease," esp. 31–7.

136 Newsholme, *Prevention of Tuberculosis*, 259, 263–5; and Newsholme, "Causes of the Past Decline," 213–15.

137 Newsholme, "Inquiry into the Principal Causes," 3–7.

TABLE LXII.—ENGLAND AND WALES

Percentage of Total Deaths in Public Institutions

Years.	Workhouses and Workhouse Infirmaries.	Hospitals.	Lunatic Asylums.	Total Institutions.	Death-rate per 1000 of Population from Phthisis.
1869–70 . .	5·7	1·9	0·7	8·3	2·45 (1866–70)
1871–75 . .	...	...	...	8·8	2·22
1876–80 . .	6·3	2·4	0·9	9·6	2·04
1881–85 . .	6·6	2·9	1·0	10·5	1·83
1886–90 . .	6·7	3·4	1·1	11·2	1·64
1891–95 . .	7·2	3·9	1·1	12·2	1·46
1896–1900 . .	7·7	4·6	1·4	13·7	1·32
1901–03 . .	8·5	5·9	1·8	16·2	1·23

Illustration 6.15. Newsholme's table for institutional confinement and mortality from pulmonary tuberculosis in England and Wales. From Newsholme, *Prevention of Tuberculosis*, 270.

seriously as predominant in the control of tuberculosis which would not be admitted generally as at least influential in this direction."[138] But he concluded that no other factor he could identify had shown such a consistent relationship to the decline in the death rate from pulmonary tuberculosis as the segregation ratio. "Institutional segregation, notably of advanced cases, is the most powerful single means available for controlling phthisis."[139]

Newsholme's papers on the decline of pulmonary tuberculosis are ambitious, resourceful, and suggestive, but limitations are also very noticeable. In fact, his analysis received some sharp criticism from his colleagues.[140] Newsholme's approach depended on a number of assumptions, some of which were open to question. His international comparisons, for example, assumed that phthisis mortality must respond in the same way, to the same forces, in roughly the same time frame in all nations considered. This assumption was probably most questionable for those nations where mortality trends seemed to run counter to the trends in other nations, in Norway and Ireland especially. We will return to this point

138 Newsholme, "Relative Importance of the Constituent Factors," 32.
139 Ibid., 111. See also Newsholme, "Inquiry into the Principal Causes," 375; and Newsholme, "Causes of the Past Decline," 227.
140 See, for example, the discussion of his presentation to the Epidemiological Society of London in Newsholme, "Relative Importance of the Constituent Factors," 112–31. Note in particular the comments of Niven, Murphy, Ransom, and Beevor.

TABLE LXIII.—LONDON

Percentage of Total Deaths in Public Institutions

Years.	Workhouses and Workhouse Infirmaries.	Public, Lunatic, and Imbecile Asylums.	M. A. B. Hospitals.	Other Hospitals.	Total Institutions.	Death-rate per 1000 of Population from Phthisis.
1852–55 . .	9·6	0·7	...	...	16·7	...
1856–60 . .	9·0	0·6	...	...	16·3	...
1861–65 . .	9·0	0·4	...	...	16·2	2·80
1866–70 . .	9·1	0·5	...	...	16·3	2·86
1871–75 . .	9·8	0·5	...	...	17·3	2·51
1876–80 . .	11·3	0·4	...	...	18·6	2·40
1881–85 . .	12·3	0·4	...	...	20·5	2·11
1886–90 . .	11·8	1·9	0·7	8·7	23·1	1·88
1891–95 . .	13·3	2·0	2·0	9·4	26·7	1·87
1896–1900 .	14·8	2·1	2·1	10·2	29·2	1·80
1901–03 . .	17·7	2·8	2·2	12·2	34·7	1·65 (1901–04)

Illustration 6.16. Newsholme's table for institutional confinement and mortality from pulmonary tuberculosis in London. Newsholme, *Prevention of Tuberculosis,* 270.

momentarily. Newsholme's argument also assumed that there had not been changes in the virulence or in the infectivity of pulmonary tuberculosis over the period he was considering. This assumption is particularly interesting in view of the demands that Newsholme and other defenders of the isolation hospitals had made of critics of the institutional isolation of scarlet fever. As we have seen, the hospital defenders insisted that the critics recognize not only that the virulence of scarlet fever was declining but also that it exhibited wavelike patterns of incidence over time and that different towns might be at a different place on the epidemic wave at any particular time. When challenged on this point, Newsholme freely conceded that he assumed that the contagion of phthisis was the same in the whole period and in all nations he considered.[141] There was, he claimed, neither pathological nor clinical evidence that such differences existed, and he argued that the cyclical variations known in some acute infectious diseases such as scarlet fever were unknown in tuberculosis. He dealt rather sarcastically with this objection by suggesting that it was tantamount to claiming that diseases died out naturally, which was only another way of saying that we did not understand the factors that suppressed them.[142]

141 Newsholme, "Inquiry into the Principal Causes," 310–11.
142 Newsholme, "Poverty and Disease," 26–8; and Newsholme, "Causes of the Past Decline," 206.

Newsholme's use of segregation ratios as proxies for the actual portion of illness treated in institutions was also very problematic. This was particularly the case with the ratio he used most frequently for British statistics, the ratio of indoor paupers to all paupers. We have seen that Newsholme demonstrated a close connection between the level of pauperism in Britain and the mortality from phthisis. However, he found himself in the awkward position of having to argue that this connection was so close that pauperism could serve as a proxy for phthisis,[143] while at the same time trying to argue against inferring that pauperism was a major contributing factor to phthisis mortality. His defense of the latter position was rather unconvincing, especially for a very poor nation like Ireland.

Newsholme recognized that as a special case in his argument, Ireland deserved special attention, and he eventually prepared a substantial paper on phthisis and typhus in Ireland.[144] This paper gave detailed information on the great epidemics of typhus and on the increase in phthisis mortality, and it described in more detail than his previous papers had done the history of the Irish Poor Law, but it failed to remove some of the most critical questions remaining from his earlier papers. First of all, was Ireland really a special case as far as phthisis mortality was concerned? The reported increase for Ireland was actually quite modest. Newsholme's own statistics showed that between 1861 and 1890 the crude death rate for phthisis in Ireland had increased between 2 and 5 percent per five-year period, that is, an average annual rate of about seven-tenths of 1 percent.[145] Between 1890 and 1903 phthisis mortality had been almost stable in Ireland. Knowing the difficulties of providing adequate medical attention to a very poor rural population and knowing that vital registration began in Ireland only in the 1860s, it seems quite likely that at least some of the recorded increase may have been due to improvements in access to medical attention, in diagnosis, and in registration. While Newsholme admitted that the data he had to work with contained flaws, he minimized the dangers of using them, and he did not address the problem we have just raised.[146] In fact he claimed that the most likely source of error in early-nineteenth-century mortality returns for phthisis was the erroneous diagnosis of other fatal diseases as phthisis. The net effect of this systematic error, he claimed, was to understate the amount phthisis mortality had increased in Ireland. But suspicions that Ireland may not have been so special a case are heightened by figures Newsholme compiled a few years later, while he was at the Local Government Board.[147] These figures showed that, during the first decade of the twentieth century, phthisis mortality had fallen faster in Ireland than in England and Wales and as fast as in Scotland.

A related problem concerns Newsholme's handling of the cost of living. If the

143 Newsholme, "Inquiry into the Principal Causes," 355.
144 Newsholme, "Poverty and Disease."
145 Newsholme, "Relative Importance of the Constituent Factors," 45.
146 Newsholme, "Poverty and Disease," 21–2 fn; and Newsholme, "Relative Importance of the Constituent Factors," 31–2. His most complete discussion of the accuracy of the statistics of tuberculosis has somewhat wider implications. See Newsholme, *Prevention of Tuberculosis,* 22–34.
147 [Arthur Newsholme], "Memorandum on Tuberculosis," 17 July 1911, in Newsholme Papers,

Irish mortality trend were not taken at face value, then Newsholme should not have dismissed so readily the apparent correlations between the economic trends he considered and phthisis mortality. The slope of Ireland's phthisis mortality curve was the primary reason to decide against food prices as determinants of phthisis mortality. Newsholme had in fact very little information on nutrition. In discussing Ireland, for example, he used only one set of values for wheat prices and for the cost of a family's food, and these were values for the whole of the United Kingdom.[148] (See Illustrations 6.5 and 6.7.) His argument throughout assumed that each nation of the United Kingdom had shared equally in these trends in consumer prices. More detailed price figures may not have been available, but Newsholme did not address this problem in his method or warn his readers that food costs in Ireland may not have been correctly indicated by these statistics.

It is also possible that Newsholme did not understand precisely the Irish Poor Law statistics he used. At the Royal Commission on the Poor Laws the Bishop of Ross persistently questioned Newsholme on his use of Irish data.[149] The Irish prelate pointed out that the figures for outdoor relief Newsholme had used in his papers on tuberculosis were for aid in money and food only. In Ireland, unlike in England, "outdoor" medical relief (provided in dispensaries or in the homes of the poor) was nonpauperizing and so did not appear in the Poor Law records. He also pointed out that existing statistics showed that Ireland institutionalized more patients in proportion to its amount of poverty than either England or Scotland. By the time Newsholme appeared before the Royal Commission, he realized that Irish Poor Law statistics posed some difficulties for his theory, and he tried to explain this apparent problem.[150] As Newsholme's figures showed, a higher percentage of the Irish population was resident in Poor Law Institutions and a higher proportion of deaths occurred in Ireland's institutions than in England's.[151] One might expect then that phthisis mortality in Ireland would be falling rather than increasing.

Newsholme accounted for this anomaly by referring to the composition of the Irish population and the manner in which segregation took place in Irish workhouses. Surprisingly it is only at this time that Newsholme considered the effect of Ireland's very high rates of out-migration. He argued that Ireland's high rates of birth and out-migration meant that the age structure of the Irish population was different from the population of the rest of the British Isles. One of the consequences of Ireland's peculiar age structure was that a smaller portion of the Irish

London School of Hygiene and Tropical Medicine. Hereafter cited as Newsholme Papers. This memorandum was clearly composed at the Local Government Board while the National Insurance Bill was under consideration, but I have not succeeded in finding it at the Public Record Office.

148 Newsholme, "Relative Importance of the Constituent Factors," 52–6; Newsholme, "Inquiry into the Principal Causes," 329–37; and Newsholme, "Causes of the Past Decline," 218–19.

149 *Royal Commission of the Poor Laws and Relief of Distress, B.P.P.* 1909, XXXVII, Cd. 4499, 171.

150 For the following discussion, see Newsholme, "Inquiry into the Principal Causes," 375–82. See also Newsholme, "Relative Importance of the Constituent Factors," 55–6.

151 Newsholme, "Relative Importance of the Constituent Factors," 71, 72.

population lived at ages when phthisis mortality was likely to occur and a larger portion lived at ages when pauperism most likely took place. The differences in risk of phthisis and of pauperism in Ireland, Newsholme reasoned, would mean that fewer of Ireland's indoor paupers suffered from phthisis. In addition, official investigations of Irish workhouses, Newsholme claimed, suggested that isolation of phthisis cases in Irish institutions worked less effectively than in England. Periods of confinement were shorter; hygienic standards were lower, and phthisis patients were not as effectively separated from other inmates in Irish institutions. Such reasons, Newsholme believed, explained why institutional segregation had not exerted a greater influence in Ireland.

Newsholme's conclusions for Ireland were plausible, but they depended on a large number of unverifiable assumptions. The other special case in his analysis, Norway, got almost no detailed analysis or investigation. In fact, Newsholme's data for most foreign nations were very sparse, and he had almost no way to test their validity or to investigate special circumstances which might influence the foreign mortality returns.

Problems with Newsholme's argument, such as the ones we have just considered, do not, of course, mean that Newsholme's conclusions were wrong, but they raise doubts about the certainty of his results. A fair reading of his papers on the epidemiology of tuberculosis demonstrates that while they are among his most ambitious and certainly among the ones with the greatest bearing on national policy, they were, from a critical or methodological point of view, not his strongest. Even some of his colleagues who admired his investigations of this problem were skeptical of the role he assigned to the workhouse in the historic decline of tuberculosis.[152] In his retirement Newsholme continued to insist that institutional confinement had been an important factor in the historic decline of tuberculosis and continued to be skeptical that improved nutrition alone could explain the decline, but now he acknowledged that the causes of tuberculosis's retreat were probably multiple and very complex, and he recognized that other factors – improved cleanliness and personal habits, better nutrition, earlier diagnosis, and better treatment – had probably all contributed.[153]

These studies by Newsholme between 1905 and 1908 illustrate how closely his epidemiological studies were related to his administrative work and policy concerns. His recent experience with sanatorium treatment in Brighton and his observations of phthisis among paupers in the Brighton workhouse encouraged him to frame his epidemiological studies as he did. His conclusions in turn buttressed the policy recommendations he soon made in Whitehall. Newsholme's

152 Even Newsholme's coeditors of the *Journal of Hygiene* were skeptical of this conclusion, while they agreed to publish the long article by Newsholme, "Inquiry into the Principal Causes," in 1906. See J. S. Haldane to Newsholme, 13 June 1906 in Newsholme Papers, FA: D1(4). See also Arthur Ransome to Newsholme, 31 Oct. 1906, ibid.

153 Arthur Newsholme, "Housing and Tuberculosis," [notes for a lecture, 22 Oct. 1937], Newsholme Papers; and Newsholme, *The Elements*, rev. ed., 452–62, esp. 460–2.

writing in these years suggests that these epidemiological studies were intended to demonstrate not only the role that isolation had played in the decline of phthisis, but in a more fundamental way to demonstrate the primacy of infection in the epidemiology of pulmonary tuberculosis, and on a practical level to suggest that Poor Law institutions might serve public health purposes. While granting the serious objections that might be raised to using Poor Law institutions in any community tuberculosis program Newsholme pointed out that these institutions were the most numerous and universal of the potential sites for the treatment of tuberculosis. In his 1906 paper he argued that given the complexity, scale, and cost of a national tuberculosis campaign, it was essential to determine which measures promised the greatest yield on the investment and particularly which could be begun without "the delay and expense involved in creating a new service."[154] The need to remake Poor Law institutions so that they would be acceptable to the working poor became a recurring theme in Newsholme's remarks on tuberculosis. We consider this topic further in Chapter 9.

In making his case in these epidemiological studies for the primacy of infection, Newsholme faced two sets of opponents who, from very different points of view, insisted that variations in human resistance were responsible for changes in phthisis mortality. On the one hand were more traditional sanitarians, who believed that environmental improvement increased resistance to constitutional diseases like tuberculosis, and on the other were hereditarians, who believed that resistance and susceptibility were inherent and inherited. We have seen how he answered the former by trying to demonstrate that phthisis mortality had not receded merely in step with general mortality as a consequence of the sanitary movement. It had in fact declined much faster. The analogies he drew between the history of phthisis in Britain and the history of other diseases should be understood in this context. The history of typhus and leprosy showed that diseases could be controlled by the isolation of human patients. If he were merely intent on demonstrating the value of isolation, he might have stopped there. But in the same section of one paper, Newsholme goes on to discuss typhoid fever, bubonic plague, malaria, yellow fever, Malta fever (brucellosis), and rabies.[155] To none of these diseases had the resistance of the human species increased, nor had the control of any, with the possible exception of typhoid, been achieved by general sanitation. These diseases were controlled by preventing a specific link in the chain of infection.

In these studies of phthisis Newsholme also tried to forestall objections from hereditarians. For example, he answered those who might account for the increased phthisis mortality in Ireland by assuming that the Irish population was degenerating.[156] Ireland's corrected birth rates, he found, had increased in the very decades that its phthisis mortality rate was also increasing. Such increased fertility, Newsholme reasoned, was unlikely in a population that was allegedly degenerat-

154 Newsholme, "Inquiry into the Principal Causes," 305.
155 Newsholme, "Causes of the Past Decline," 210–12.
156 For the following discussion, see Newsholme, "Poverty and Disease," 29–31.

ing. Furthermore if the degeneration of the population in Ireland were to be explained by the emigration abroad of the fittest stock, then the Irish living in other lands, in America for example, should have noticeably lower phthisis mortality than the Irish in Ireland. But the phthisis mortality rates, properly corrected for differences in age and sex, which Charles V. Chapin had collected, showed that the Irish living in Providence, Rhode Island, suffered even higher mortality from phthisis than the Irish in Ireland. Selective immigration, Newsholme asserted, should in fact have the opposite effect from what the hereditarians alleged. The emigrants leaving Ireland were often from the poorest families. The effect of that emigration should have been to eliminate the weakest stock, leaving in Ireland a population whose fitness was increased as a result.

Perhaps the best indication of the centrality of infection to Newsholme's analysis is the blistering criticism given his epidemiological studies of tuberculosis by Karl Pearson, who acknowledged that it was over the role of infection that he had his greatest differences with Newsholme.[157] Pearson, then Professor of Applied Mathematics at University College, London, and soon to become Galton Professor of Eugenics, was also studying trends in tuberculosis mortality, and he despaired at the notice Newsholme's *Prevention of Tuberculosis* was receiving.[158] It was, Pearson wrote, a "thoroughly unsatisfactory book"; the sections on the decline of phthisis were "purely fallacious; their only service can be to arouse the medical profession to the crying need for an efficient medico-statistical logic."[159] The methodological weaknesses in his studies left Newsholme open to Pearson's wilting statistical criticism. The Medical Officer of Health, Pearson claimed, committed the classic statistical error of confusing correlation with causation. Pearson computed correlation coefficients for phthisis mortality and for either expenditure on the Royal Navy or for Canadian exports that were nearly as high as Newsholme had computed for phthisis mortality and his segregation ratios.[160] He claimed that Newsholme could have chosen equally well the price of bananas or the sale of newspapers.

While the disputes between Newsholme and Pearson were conducted in statistical terms, their hostility toward each other was rooted in irreconcilible differences over social policy. Newsholme had by this time moved to his new post at the L.G.B. and was helping implement a national tuberculosis policy which Pearson abhorred. As we will see in Chapter 9, Newsholme drew upon his experience in Brighton and these studies of tuberculosis to support his policy

157 Karl Pearson, *Fight against Tuberculosis and the Death Rate from Phthisis* (London: Dulau & Co., 1911), 8; and Karl Pearson, *Tuberculosis, Hereditary, and Environment* (London: Dulau & Co., 1912): 21–4.

158 For introductions to Pearson's career and statistical approach, see Donald A. MacKenzie, *Statistics in Britain 1865–1930: The Social Construction of Scientific Knowledge* (Edinburgh: Edinburgh University Press, 1981), 73–93; Daniel J. Kevles, *In the Name of Eugenics: Genetics and the Uses of Human Heredity* (New York: Alfred A. Knopf, 1985), 20–40.

159 Pearson, *Fight against Tuberculosis*, 17, 12.

160 Ibid., 10–12.

recommendations. Although not denying that the tuberculosis bacillus was responsible for tuberculosis, Pearson was attempting to prove that natural selection was responsible for decline of phthisis. In his view, action by public authorities to prevent tuberculosis was a waste of public money promising dire consequences to the nation. Pearson identified three periods in the mortality history of England and Wales during the nineteenth century: 1835–66, 1867–91, and 1892–1910. By fitting straight lines to the mortality curves, Pearson described rates of change for general mortality and phthisis mortality in these three periods. The fall in phthisis mortality, although initially faster than the fall in general mortality, was retarded in each successive period. In the third period the slope of the curve for phthisis was nearly horizontal. Pearson interpreted this result as an indication that the fall in tuberculosis had been retarded in the very years that the tuberculosis movement was most active. Was not the shape of the curve for phthisis, Pearson asked, "precisely what we should anticipate, if we attribute the change in death-rate to the natural increase of immunity due to a selective death-rate acting on a community with varying grades of hereditary immunity?"[161]

Pearson frankly assumed the existence of a "tuberculous stock," although he conceded that it was difficult to characterize exactly.[162] The Eugenics Laboratory had collected family histories of tuberculosis, from which Pearson computed figures for the correlation of phthisis in parent and child (.40 to .60) and in husband and wife (.20 to .30). The former, he claimed, showed that the "tubercular diathesis," was inherited at the same rate as other inherited traits such as stature or eye color.[163] The latter was similar to correlations for other physical characteristics in marriage partners, such as length of forearm, eye color, "truthfulness," or "reserve," that Pearson held to be the result of sexual selection.

This is not the place to analyze Pearson's studies of tuberculosis except to notice that he could be every bit as willing to make generous assumptions and to correct weak data as Newsholme had been and every bit as intent on influencing public policy.[164] "Natural selection," Pearson claimed, "may have done more for racial health in this matter than medical science."[165] "Without placing ourselves in the dogmatic position of asserting that every ill works to ultimate good, may we not believe that in this case human suffering has been for the benefit of the race?"[166] The good of the race and of the nation demanded that natural selection not be impeded by public action and that the danger posed by the breeding of tubercular

161 Pearson, *Tuberculosis, Hereditary, and Environment*, 32.
162 Ibid., 12–13, 15.
163 For the following discussion, see ibid., 7–21; and Karl Pearson, *A First Study of the Statistics of Pulmonary Tuberculosis* (London: Dulau & Co., 1907), 10–15.
164 Recently the weakness of Pearson's data in these studies has been noticed by historians. See F. B. Smith, *The Retreat of Tuberculosis 1850–1950* (London, New York, Sydney: Croom Helm, 1988), 39. In the case of the correlation of phthisis in parent and child Pearson was very generous in allowing for the number of children of tubercular parents who had not yet developed phthisis but who would do so in the future.
165 Pearson, *Fight against Tuberculosis*, 35.
166 Pearson, *Tuberculosis, Hereditary and Environment*, 42.

stocks be recognized. "The fertility of stocks tainted with pulmonary tuberculosis" Pearson tried to prove, was at least as high as the fertility of other human stock, and was "markedly greater in artisan tuberculous stocks than in any class of brain workers."[167] The marriage of those who carried the tuberculosis trait but did not exhibit its symptoms he considered "the gravest source of danger to the community" and medical advice that such persons could safely marry "an antisocial disregard for national eugenics."[168]

Pearson was a frequent critic of public health policy.[169] But his studies of tuberculosis and his criticism of Newsholme's findings had particular policy relevance. The success of the tuberculosis movement in influencing national policy and in gaining access to the public purse ignited his ire. He accused the tuberculosis activists of misstatement and exaggeration, of approaching the public under false pretenses, and of siphoning off for "leper houses" an immense amount of money which could be put to much better use elsewhere.[170] The national policy's emphasis on environmental reform and publically financed treatment was an anathema.

No one can study the pedigrees of pathological states, insanity, mental defect, albinism, & c., collected by our Laboratory, without being struck by the large proportion of tuberculous members – occasionally the tuberculous man is a brilliant member of our race – but the bulk of the tuberculous belong to stocks which we want *ab initio* to discourage. Everything which tends to check the multiplication of the unfit, to emphasize the fertility of the physically and mentally healthy, will *pro tanto* aid Nature's method of reducing the phthisical death-rate. That is what the Eugenist proclaims as the "better thing to do," and £1,500,000 spent in encouraging healthy parentage would do more than the establishment of a sanatorium in every township.[171]

The £1.5 million and the label "leper houses" were both references to the provision funds from the Exchequer under the Finance Act of 1911 for the construction of tuberculosis sanatoriums. We will consider that issue in Chapter 9.

Pearson's criticism should be understood as another round in a long series of eugenics attacks on public health programs. Such programs were not only wasteful, the critics alleged, but they threatened the future health and fitness of the nation. By the opening of the twentieth century the public health community had considerable influence in public policy, and it was sufficiently well organized and entrenched to resist most challenges from the eugenicists.[172] But given Pearson's scientific authority and his academic position, his criticisms demanded special attention. Newsholme took the opportunity to respond in his next major epide-

167 Pearson, *First Study of Statistics,* 19–21, 25.
168 Ibid., 21, 15.
169 As an example see Karl Pearson, *Eugenics and Public Health* (London: Dulau & Co., 1912).
170 Pearson, *Fight against Tuberculosis,* 3–4; and Karl Pearson, *Tuberculosis, Hereditary and Environment,* 32–44.
171 Pearson, *Tuberculosis, Hereditary and Environment,* 46.
172 See, for example, the discussion in Dorothy Porter, " 'Enemies of the Race': Biologism, Environmentalism, and Public Health in Edwardian England," *Victorian Studies,* 34 (1991): 159–74.

miological project, his studies of infant and child mortality. We will consider that subject in Chapter 11. But his major counteroffensive came once he left public life, in a series of addresses and in a new edition of his textbook, *Vital Statistics.* That topic we will consider in Chapter 12. Finally we should notice that he already had framed a more general response to eugenics in the course of his discussions of poverty and disease. That is a subject we consider in the next chapter.

PART II

Newsholme at the Local Government Board

7

Poverty, fitness, and the Poor Law

POVERTY, EVOLUTION, AND CHARACTER

Some months ago an intelligent clergyman expressed surprise that with so many doctors there was any disease left. I made the obvious retort that it was even more surprising that with so many clergymen, sinners still abounded. The two cases are of course only comparable in so far as sin and disease are both caused by aberrations from the path of duty over which the individual or the community could exercise control.[1]

During his years in Brighton Newsholme had risen to prominence in his profession. He had developed a reputation as an active and able administrator. In 1907 Edward Cox Seaton, Medical Officer of Health for Surrey County Council and lecturer at St. Thomas's Hospital Medical School, described the work of Brighton's Health Department in glowing terms and called the Brighton system a model for other local authorities to emulate.[2] He emphasized especially Brighton's achievement in housing, its success in establishing an effective, comprehensive, tuberculosis program, and the care and economy in administration. Newsholme had proven to be a prolific writer as well as a successful administrator. By the time he left Brighton, he had published six books and at least four later editions of these, some ninety articles and chapters, two dozen annual reports, and numerous quarterly and occasional reports. His works were distinguished for their mastery of epidemiology, and he was without question one of the nation's leaders in the field.

Ample recognition by his peers followed.[3] He was chosen the Royal College of Physicians' Milroy Lecturer in 1895; he presented on the occasion his study of rheumatic fever. Three years later he became a Fellow of the College. He was a

1 Arthur Newsholme, "An Address on the Spread of Enteric Fever by Means of Sewage-Contaminated Shellfish," *Br. Med. J.* (1896), no. 2: 639.
2 See discussion of Arthur Newsholme, "The Voluntary Notification of Phthisis in Brighton: Including a Comparison of Results with Those Obtained in Other Towns," *J. Roy. Sanitary Inst.*, 28 (1907): 40–1.
3 His professional accomplishments and offices are best found enumerated in his obituaries. See in particular *Br. Med. J.* (1943), no. 1: 680–1; *Lancet* (1943), no. 1: 696; *Nature*, 151 (1943): 635–6; *St. Thomas's Hospital Gazette*, 41 (1943): 92.

very active member of the Society of Medical Officers of Health, serving on its Council and twice as the editor of its journal, *Public Health* (1892–6, and 1906–8).[4] He served a term as president of the Society (1900–1) and in 1907 terms as President of the Royal Society of Medicine's Section of Epidemiology and of the British Medical Association's Section of State Medicine. He was also a member of the Statistical Committee of the Imperial Cancer Research Fund and served regularly as an examiner for the Diploma in Public Health at London University and at Oxford and Cambridge. In 1901 he helped found and for some years served as coeditor of the *Journal of Hygiene*. This recognition was not only honorific. Brighton Town Council's estimate of Newsholme's worth grew with his professional accomplishments, and it proved only too willing to grant the increases in salary he requested – first from £650 to £800 in 1892 and then to £1,000 per year in 1899.[5]

He also came to the attention of people with a very different interest in his career. Beatrice Webb, the Fabian socialist, was one of these. She was then working on the Royal Commission on the Poor Laws. Her assistant traveled to Brighton to interview Newsholme in his office on December 22, 1906, and reported extensively on the tuberculosis work in Brighton. The report of the interview stressed the high priority Newsholme attached to finding adequate institutional treatment of the disease, free from Poor Law taint, and to the need for unifying under one authority all local health functions. These answers met responsive ears in the Webb household. The report of the interview includes an assessment of Newsholme, "very able and enthusiastic."[6] The Webbs believed they had found an ally. They soon began their campaign to draw him into their circle of reforming professionals and civil servants and to elicit his help in their campaign to dismantle the Poor Law and to remake British social policy.

During Newsholme's last years at Brighton the condition of the poor captured public attention in ways it had not done for more than half a century. In these years Britain rethought established attitudes toward poverty and destitution, formed new political alliances, and began the process of building the welfare state.[7] Both national

---

4 The offer came from the founder in May 1892. A. Wynter Blyth to Arthur Newsholme, 5 May 1892, Newsholme Papers, London School of Hygiene and Tropical Medicine FA: D1 (4). Hereafter cited simply as Newsholme Papers.
5 Brighton, *Proc. Town Council, Proc. Comm.*, 4 Feb 1892, xix–xx; and ibid., 2 March 1899, 38–40.
6 Minutes of interview with Newsholme, 22 Dec. 1906, Webb, Local Government Collection, vol. 335.
7 For very useful discussions of these developments, see Bentley B. Gilbert, *The Evolution of National Insurance in Great Britain: The Origins of the Welfare State* (London: Michael Joseph, 1966); G. R. Searle, *The Quest for National Efficiency: A Study in British Politics and Political Thought, 1899–1914* (Oxford: Basil Blackwell, 1971); E. P. Hennock, *British Social Reform and German Precedents: The Case of Social Insurance 1880–1914* (Oxford: Clarendon Press, 1987); Gertrude Himmelfarb, *The Idea of Poverty: England in the Early Industrial Age* (New York: Alfred A. Knopf, 1984); and Bernard Semmel, *Imperialism and Social Reform: English Social-Imperial Thought 1895–1914* (Cambridge, Mass.: Harvard Univ. Press, 1960).

anxiety and political opportunism drove the process. The anxieties began in the 1880s in the face of high unemployment, labor agitation, and an accumulating mass of social investigation which documented the squalid and brutal conditions in which the lowest strata of the urban working classes lived and worked. The discomfort waxed as Britain's economic and military preeminence waned and was intensified by Germany's military buildup. The sense of unease was transformed into a crisis and a time of soul searching by Britain's poor showing in the Boer War (1899–1902). The war disclosed incompetence, inefficiency, and corruption in high places and was a profound national embarrassment. In response spokesmen in the press and in both major political parties demanded changes to promote "national efficiency." The leaders of this broad and influential movement looked enviously at Germany's system of higher education, its science-based industries, its disciplined and productive labor force, and its system of social insurance, and in response they proposed dozens of schemes for national renewal. The immediate postwar mood was both exhilarating and terrifying. "The war and its aftermath turned imperialism inward and directed its energy, its violence, and its intolerance back onto England."[8]

Perhaps the most troubling disclosures during the war came from urban recruiting stations. It was reported that of 11,000 men who had been examined at recruiting stations in Manchester, 8,000 were rejected as unfit for service, and 2,000 of the remaining 3,000 were accepted for service only in the militia.[9] For a nation that was being forced to think of its people as a national resource on whose condition the fate of the empire rested, such revelations of stunted growth and chronic disability were shocking. Was the race growing too puny to rule a great empire? The experience of the war seemed to many confirmation of those hereditarian views which saw in urban slums signs of racial deterioration and in the falling birth rate of the upper classes impending catastrophe. Edwardian governments were forced to investigate. The Royal Commission on Physical Training in Scotland (1902)[10] and the Interdepartmental Committee on Physical Deterioration (1903–4)[11] were the more immediate official responses to the crisis. The Royal Commission on the Poor Law and Relief of Distress (1905–9),[12] a more extensive investigation of the condition of the laboring poor and of the state's response to destitution, reflected some of the same national concerns. The first two inquiries documented that there was indeed much ill health and disability among the urban working classes. They also served as contests for conflicting environmental and hereditarian explanations for pauperism and associated disease and disability. In these deliberations the testimony of medical and public health experts was crucial in undermining a simple hereditarian explanation and in

8 Gilbert, *Evolution of National Insurance*, 61.   9 Searle, *National Efficiency*, 60.
10 B.P.P. 1903, XXX, [Cd. 1507] & [Cd. 1508].   11 B.P.P. 1904, XXXII, [Cd. 2175] & [Cd. 2210].
12 This commission published separate reports of England and Wales, Scotland, and Ireland and thirty-six volumes of evidence. For the reports for England and Wales, see *Report of the Royal Commission on the Poor Laws and Relief of Distress*, B.P.P. 1909, XXXVII, Cd. 4499.

helping to build the case for state efforts to improve the lot of the unskilled laboring classes.[13]

Although he did not testify before either the Royal Commission on Physical Training in Scotland or the Interdepartmental Committee on Physical Deterioration, Newsholme took part in these public discussions of health and national prowess. First, during the war he helped publicize the failures of the war effort by calling attention to the squandering of human life that was occurring in South Africa.[14] Using figures gleaned from the army's own meager reports, he demonstrated the terrible losses from preventable diseases among the troops and in the crowded civilian concentration camps. In keeping with the spirit of the national alarm, he emphasized the inefficiencies current practices fostered.

An efficient army is required. Disease and fighting contribute to diminish the forces and produce inefficiency in the proportion of 38 to 22 or 19 to 11. What proportion do the respective weights of armaments and hygienic necessaries (including food, blankets, and other clothing, and arrangements for boiling or filtering water) bear to each other? Is the amount allowed for hygienic necessaries anything near the proportion indicated by their relative importance as a means of preventing inefficiency of the army? One mule would carry sufficient filtering apparatus . . . for 100 men.[15]

Second, and more characteristically, he tried to reassure his colleagues and uneasy public officials that efforts to prevent disease and to save lives did not lead to racial degeneration. In other words public health work was the solution to and not the cause of the national crisis in personal fitness. We find him arguing this case in a series of addresses and articles between 1903 and 1909. But in fact Newsholme had anticipated by at least a decade the objections to extended preventive services which might be raised on hereditarian grounds. In doing so Newsholme was grappling with an intellectual dilemma faced by many radicals and progressives of his generation, a dilemma that is exposed more systematically in the works of the New Liberals, the academics and journalists on the left flank of Liberalism in the years preceding the Great War. British thinkers of this generation were profoundly impressed with Darwin's synthesis, and many sought to apply evolutionary notions to society. But for those like the New Liberals who favored collective solutions to social problems and a more active role for the state, appeals to biological evolution were very problematic. On the one hand biological evolution seemed to affirm the idea of progress and to demonstrate that its laws were susceptible to human understanding.

13 For a good short discussion of the evidence presented at these investigations, see J. M. Winter, *The Great War and the British People* (Cambridge, Mass.: Harvard Univ. Press, 1986), 10–18. See also G. R. Searle, *Eugenics and Politics in Britain 1900–1914* (Leyden: Noordhoff International Publishing, 1976), pp. 20–4.

14 Newsholme was the author of a series of reports and editorials, among them: "The Waste of Life and Efficiency in South Africa," *Br. Med. J.* (1901), no. 1:; 165–6; "The Rates of Mortality in the Concentration Camps in South Africa," ibid, no. 2: 1418–20; "The Concentration Camps in South Africa," ibid., 1423–4. Newsholme claimed authorship of these pieces in Newsholme, *Fifty Years,* 368. See also "Bills of Mortality in South Africa," *Br. Med. J.* (1901), no. 1: 160–2, 221–2.

15 "Waste of Life and Efficiency," 166.

It also might be employed to encourage readers to think of the community as an organism whose parts were interdependent and acted together for the benefit of the collective. But on the other hand natural selection was already commonly used to justify individualism, competition, and laissez-faire economics. To put it crudely, the problem for the New Liberals was to have Darwin without Spencer.[16]

Newsholme was keenly aware of the phenomena that led his contemporaries to hereditarian explanations of social problems. Like many others, he worried about changes in the patterns of human fertility. In these years he produced both a technical article for the Statistical Society of London, in which he and his former assistant T.H.C. Stevenson employed corrected birth rates to accurately measure changes in fertility patterns, and a semipopular short book, in which he discussed the social significance of these changes.[17] Like many contemporaries he worried about the racial and strategic implications of the British upper classes' declining birth rates. While that rate declined, that of other classes at home remained unchanged, and abroad other nations and races had much higher birth rates.[18] These anxieties, however, did not lead Newsholme to conclude that the nation's problems could be traced to racial degeneration among the poorest classes or to the latter outbreeding their betters.

Even before the Boer War he tried to demonstrate to his colleagues how biological evolution and conscious ameliorative efforts could be reconciled. In passages that echo Thomas Henry Huxley's Romanes Lecture, Newsholme argued that, with the evolution of human intelligence and the cooperation which organized society made possible, the action of natural selection had been modified.[19] The human collective

16 On the use of biological evolution by the New Liberals, see Michael Freeden, *The New Liberalism: An Ideology of Social Reform* (Oxford: Clarendon Press, 1978), 76–116; Stefan Collini, *Liberalism and Sociology: L. T. Hobhouse and Political Argument in England 1880–1914* (Cambridge: Cambridge Univ. Press, 1979), 147–208; Peter Clarke, *Liberals and Social Democrats* (Cambridge: Cambridge Univ. Press, 1978), 148–51. On the New Liberals' role in the Liberal Party, see also George L. Bernstein, *Liberalism and Liberal Politics in Edwardian England* (Boston: Allen and Unwin, 1986), 96–100. For further discussion of this issue, see John M. Eyler, "The Sick Poor and the State: Arthur Newsholme on Poverty, Disease and Responsibility," in *Framing Disease: Studies in Cultural History*, ed. Charles E. Rosenberg and Janet Golden (New Brunswick, N.J.: Rutgers Univ. Press, 1992), 284–9 also reprinted in *Doctors, Politics and Society: Historical Essays*, ed. Dorothy Porter and Roy Porter (Amsterdam: Rodopi, 1993), 198–203.

17 Arthur Newsholme and T.H.C. Stevenson, "The Decline of Human Fertility in the United Kingdom and Other Countries as Shown by Corrected Birth-Rates," *J. Statist. Soc. Lond.*, 69 (1906): 34–87; Arthur Newsholme, *The Declining Birth-Rate: Its National and International Significance* (London, New York: Cassell & Co., 1911).

18 Arthur Newsholme, "The Influence of Civilization upon the Survival of the Fittest," *Annual Report of the Brighton and Sussex Natural History and Philosophical Society*, 1893–4, 10–12; Newsholme, *Declining Birth-Rate*, 57–58; Arthur Newsholme, "The Control of Conception," in *Sexual Problems of To-day*, ed. Mary Scharlieb (London: Williams & Norgate, 1924), 152–3; Arthur Newsholme, "Some Public Health Aspects of 'Birth Control,' " in *Medical Views on Birth Control*, ed. James Marchant (London: Martin Hopkinson & Co., 1926), 132.

19 For the following argument, see Newsholme, "Influence of Civilization," 6–8; Arthur Newsholme, "An Address on Social Evolution and Public Health," *Lancet* (1904), no. 2: 1331–2. See also Thomas Henry Huxley, "Evolution and Ethics" [The Romanes Lecture, 1893] in *Evolution and Ethics and Other Essays* (New York: D. Appleton & Co., 1899), 46–86.

had learned to interpose itself between the individual and the brute forces of nature. There was no better example of this than the work of medical practitioners who "prevent the death of multitudes of weaklings and thus apparently check the operation of natural selection."[20] This change was not to be feared. Nor must it result in physical decline, because fitness for survival should be understood as a relative not an absolute quality. Fitness was nothing other than the ratio of individual strength to environmental strain. For that reason it could be increased either by raising the strength of the individual or by reducing the strain imposed by the environment. The progress of civilization had been marked by increases in personal fitness brought about by conscious efforts to reduce environmental strain. In other words the force of the struggle for survival had been progressively transferred from the individual to the group. Recently the state had begun to act to protect whole groups, and civilization had reached a collectivist stage. "Once the State had intervened by limiting the hours of labour of women and children and by forbidding them from undertaking certain kinds of labour, the sluice gates were opened and it only became a question of time as to how soon State Socialism on a gigantic scale should replace the strict Individualism of the older economists."[21]

Newsholme challenged the alarmist statements about racial degeneration heard so often after the Boer War. In a column in the *Manchester Guardian's* series on National Physical Training he argued that such claims were groundless. No one doubted that the poor were in worse health and physique than the more well-to-do, but there was no evidence that individual classes were degenerating. Much evidence suggested that the standard of health of each stratum of society was improving, although infant mortality was still shockingly high and there was still much preventable disease and premature death.[22] Newsholme rejected the hereditarian assumption that fitness or other socially desirable qualities were class characteristics.[23] One's current status in society depended as much on opportunity as on inherent qualities.

Even the greatest ability may fail through lack of favoring circumstances; and it is impossible to say how many mute inglorious Miltons may have failed to be discovered. The fact that the poorest are lowest in the social scale cannot be used as a completely satisfactory argument that – as proved by selection – they are the poorest stock.[24]

Using evidence presented to the Royal Commission on Physical Training in Scotland and to the Interdepartmental Committee on Physical Deterioration, Newsholme challenged the claim that there was clear evidence of physical degeneration among the urban poor, and he argued that the smaller stature and more

20 Newsholme, "Influence of Civilization," 6.   21 Ibid., 7.
22 Arthur Newsholme, "National Physical Training: Is the Nation Physically Degenerating?" *Manchester Guardian*, 27 May 1903, 12. This piece was republished as Arthur Newsholme, "Our Premises Challenged," in *National Physical Training: An Open Debate*, ed. J. B. Atkins (London: Isbister, 1904), 101–16.
23 Newsholme, *Declining Birth-Rate*, 44, 49–52; Newsholme, "Public Health Aspects," 145–6.
24 Newsholme, *Declining Birth-Rate*, 52–53.

frequent physical disability among the urban poor could be explained much more adequately as the result of poor nurture than of hereditary deterioration.[25] Over the next few years, as we shall see, he tried to turn whatever evidence he could find to the task of discrediting the claim that hereditary defects explained the condition of the urban poor. Even when he shared a concern of the hereditarian alarmists, as in the case of the falling birth rates of upper- and middle-class families, Newsholme preferred an environmental to a hereditarian assessment. What troubled him about the trends in the nation's birth rates was not that the most unfit were outbreeding the more fit, but that those who could best afford to provide their children with the nurturing they needed were having fewer children than those who reared children in very unfavorable circumstances.[26]

Even if one did not accept a eugenic analysis for the condition of the urban poor, the disease and disability which school authorities and army recruiters observed among the poor demanded explanation. The first impulse of an M.O.H. of Newsholme's generation when faced with disease and destitution in the slums was to argue that disease caused pauperism. By the late nineteenth century this had become the traditional public health position, the contention that had helped launch the sanitary movement of the 1840s. It had been, after all, the discovery that many charges against the poor rates were produced by illness, illness which his medical advisers assured him was preventable, that first drew Edwin Chadwick's attention to disease.[27] Arguing, as Chadwick and his associates did, that preventing disease saved public money as well as human suffering served to broaden the appeal of public health reform and made intervention more tolerable to generations who favored laissez-faire economics and government retrenchment. Sanitary reform would not only prevent disease, but indirectly and economically it would help solve the problem of dependency without compromising individual responsibility or challenging personal liberty.

The discussions of national efficiency and physical fitness following the Boer War provoked Medical Officers of Health to reemphasize the pauperizing force of disease and the necessity of environmental reform and preventive medicine for controlling both destitution and disease. In summarizing for fellow M.O.H. the evidence the Poor Law Commission had collected, Newsholme pointed out that 30 percent of paupers were sick and 50 percent of the poor rate went to relieve sickness; he also offered estimates of the economic cost to the nation of diseases like tuberculosis and typhoid fever.[28] These losses should remind public health workers of their intellectual roots.

25 Arthur Newsholme, "Alleged Physical Degeneration in Towns," *Public Health*, 17 (1904–5): 293–5; Arthur Newsholme, "Physical Inspection," *J. Roy. Sanitary Inst.*, 26 (1905): 67; and Newsholme, *Declining Birth-Rate*, 49–50.
26 Newsholme, "Control of Conception," 154.
27 S. E. Finer, *The Life and Times of Sir Edwin Chadwick* (London: Methuen, 1952), 147–49, 154–63, 209–29.
28 For the following estimates, see Arthur Newsholme, "Some Conditions of Social Efficiency in Relation to Local Public Administration," *Public Health*, 22 (1908–9): 406, 408.

We need to learn again the lessons taught to our parents by Southwood Smith, Chadwick, and their co-workers, that one of the chief causes of poverty is disease, and that extended public health administration must continue to be a chief means of removing destitution from our midst.[29]

These findings should also demonstrate that public health work was efficient. They showed that

by combined efforts on the part of the community the total mass of poverty and sickness can be decreased, and that such efforts are not mere unproductive expressions of altruism. They represent, in fact, the best investment that the community can make. . . . Health is always cheaper than disease, and without an efficient state of health progress in other social concerns is being constantly impeded.[30]

However, Newsholme was not blind to the force of economic privation. Like many Medical Officers of Health he had come to realize early in his career that poor nutrition, overcrowding, and poor clothing placed barriers on what he could hope to do in improving the health of children.[31] He was also quick to recognize the significance of contemporary studies of poverty. Within months of the appearance of Rowntree's *Poverty: A Study of Town Life*, Newsholme had absorbed the lessons of this influential study of poverty in York and was trying to convert his medical colleagues to a more modern view.[32] He explained the definition of the poverty line and the use Rowntree had made of it to divide York's population into social classes according to their ability to purchase the minimum necessities for maintaining physical efficiency. Although Rowntree's poverty line was calculated on the purchase of the cheapest articles and a standard of comfort comparable to that of able-bodied paupers, his study reached the remarkable conclusion that in relatively prosperous times and using these very strict criteria of minimum physical needs 28 percent of York's population lived below the poverty line. Newsholme sympathetically described the self-denial and the desperate penny-pinching required of families of unskilled laborers. "The family must never spend a penny on 'bus, or railway, or on newspapers; they must write no letters; they can join no sick club [prepaid health plan]; if there is illness the parish doctor must be called in – and he will only attend when the father is out of work." There could be no luxuries like beer or tobacco. In harder times the family's only alternative to parish relief was to reduce further an inadequate diet. "To give the father sufficient food, wife and children go short."[33]

Significantly, Rowntree also had found that over the years the family of a typical unskilled laborer cycled above and below the poverty line as its needs and earning capacity changed. Discoveries such as these were encouraging Liberals to think of

29 Ibid., 404–5.   30 Ibid., 408.
31 See his explanation to his committee in his second year on the job. Newsholme, *Q. Rep.* (Brighton), 1889, no. 3: 1.
32 B. Seebohm Rowntree, *Poverty: A Study of Town Life* (London: Macmillan & Co., 1901); and Arthur Newsholme "Poverty in Town Life," *Practitioner*, 69 (1902): 682–94.
33 Newsholme, "Poverty in Town Life," 690.

poverty as an economic rather than a moral problem. The economist John A. Hobson probably stated the case better than anyone else: Poverty was the result of economic and legal systems that denied opportunities and cheapened the value of labor, a condition that could not be eliminated as long as there was a surplus of labor and the standard of living, that is, the minimum the laborer insisted in gaining in return for his labor, remained so low.[34]

Medical Officers of Health were not nearly so bold in economic or political reasoning, but the same climate of opinion that gave a hearing to Hobson's radical proposals for the reform of British institutions encouraged M.O.H. to think more carefully about the physiological effects of privation. The Medical Officer of Health for Manchester, James Niven, came to recognize that trade cycles and the system of casual labor were important causes of both poverty and disease in his town.[35] Newsholme also was learning to reason in economic terms about poverty and disease. The investigations of the Royal Commission on the Poor Law, he claimed, demonstrated the "extravagant parsimony" involved in the current system of outdoor relief for widows with children. Not only did the meager stipend not provide enough for adequate nutrition or shelter, but it actually exacerbated the problem of poverty by encouraging the widow to enter the labor force at the earliest opportunity and at the lowest wages, thus depressing the wages of other workers.[36]

Newsholme sometimes reversed the usual equation that disease caused poverty and concluded that poverty was a cause of disease. Usually he described the force of economic privation acting indirectly through ignorance, crowding, and uncleanliness.[37] But in a few instances, such as in his study of the epidemiology of typhus and pulmonary tuberculosis in Ireland, he gave poverty a more direct, physiological role, suggesting that the cruel privations in Ireland's history not only facilitated the transmission of disease but also increased its case fatality.[38]

To say that poverty caused disease did not negate the more ordinary formulation that disease caused poverty. The two views were not, in his opinion, contradictory. He tried to explain himself with a metaphor.

The conditions of poverty in a community exposed to typhus, as to phthisis, may be compared with the dryness of timber exposed to the onset of fire. The poorer and the more over-crowded the population, the drier and the more densely aggregated the timber,

---

34 For Hobson's views on this point, see J. A. Hobson, *The Crisis in Liberalism: New Issues of Democracy* (London: P. S. King, 1909): 159–75; and J. A. Hobson, *Problems of Poverty: An Inquiry into the Industrial Condition of the Poor*, 8th ed. (London: Methuen, 1913): 171–82. For a fine analysis of the remaking of Liberal social thought represented by Hobson's work, see Michael Freeden, *The New Liberalism: An Ideology of Social Reform* (Oxford: Clarendon Press, 1978).

35 James Niven, "Poverty and Disease," *Proc. Roy. Soc. Med.*, 3, pt. 2 (1910), Epidemiological Sect., 4–11.

36 Newsholme, "Conditions of Social Efficiency," 406.

37 Arthur Newsholme, "A Discussion on the Co-ordination of the Public Medical Services," *Br. Med. J.* (1907), no. 2: 656–7.

38 Arthur Newsholme, "Poverty and Disease, as Illustrated by the Course of Typhus Fever and Phthisis in Ireland," *Proc. Roy. Soc. Med.*, 1, pt. 1 (1908), Epidemiological Sect., 2–4, 10–14.

the more extensive will be the epidemic or the conflagration produced by infection or flame.[39]

In a town free from fire or in a population free from infection, there might be time to increase resistance to fire or illness. But when fire was in the vicinity or infectious disease epidemic in the community, the only practicable policy was to combat the spread of fire or infection. With the exception of vaccination for smallpox, other means of increasing human resistance to disease worked too slowly and uncertainly to be relied on in a crisis.

In a figure of speech that was becoming a commonplace, Newsholme often described poverty and disease as forming a vicious circle with one producing the other.[40] Just as one might break a circle at any point, one might attack either poverty or disease. The decision was mainly one of expedience. In the present state of knowledge the most efficient approach, the strategy likely to yield the quickest and most certain return, was to prevent disease, knowing that this action would also help reduce poverty.[41] In such discussions he grew fond of comparing contemporary solutions for poverty to medical treatment of the past.

The treatment of poverty has historically shown the same confusion between symptom and disease as appeared in earlier times in medicine and illustrates as clearly as medical history the mischief and the hindrance to real progress which are caused by adopting an empirical treatment of symptoms instead of a scientific treatment of disease.[42]

Poverty, Newsholme was recognizing more fully, was a complicated human condition having economic, behavioral, and biological components. In this and in his advocacy of state intervention as a moral imperative he was in step with the New Liberals. But there were important differences between his views and theirs. Not only was Newsholme quicker than New Liberals like Hobson to see the dangers that lay in eugenic solutions to social problems, but he differed in his assessment of individual responsibility. If we take Hobson again as an example, we find a scheme in which economic and legislative remedies dominated. Self-help and moral transformation were impossible remedies for the problems of poverty as long as the struggle for existence consumed all the energy of slum dwellers.[43] Security of employment and a higher standard of living, Hobson insisted, had to precede any hope of civilizing the poorest classes. Similarly, while temperance might be good advice on the personal level, permitting individual workers to better themselves, it was no solution to the social problems of poverty. If all

39 Ibid., 4.
40 Arthur Newsholme, "The Causes of the Past Decline in Tuberculosis: And the Light Thrown by History on Preventive Measures for the Immediate Future," *Charities*, 21 (1908–9): 222; and Newsholme, "Conditions of Social Efficiency," 406. For uses of the same image by other authors we have already cited, see Niven, "Poverty and Disease," 10; and Hobson, *Crisis*, 161.
41 Newsholme, "Discussion on the Co-ordination," 657.
42 Arthur Newsholme, "An Address on Social Evolution and Public Health," *Lancet* (1904), no. 2: 1334. He made use of this analogy again in Newsholme, "Conditions of Social Efficiency," 409.
43 Hobson, *Problems of Poverty*, 175.

workers gave up their beer, the most likely result would be a drop in their wages by just the amount they formerly spent on beer unless some essential expense replaced the beer.[44] For Hobson the state might have moral purposes, but these could not be achieved by the moral transformation of the individual.

It is here that Newsholme's differences from the new strains of liberalism are most obvious. Newsholme believed that changes in human behavior, moral reforms in his terms, were essential, if the most difficult public health problems of his age were to be solved. Consider briefly just one such problem, alcoholism. Newsholme was a strong advocate of temperance, troubled that those living near the poverty line spent, by some estimates, as much as 25 percent of their earnings on drink.[45] As a public official he blamed alcoholic indulgence for national inefficiency, crime, disease, and poverty, and as an epidemiologist he tried to demonstrate statistically those effects.[46] Its pernicious effects were not only physiological and social but economic as well. Increased expenditure on drink, he believed, had diminished the benefits of economic growth.[47] Consistent with his environmental, reformist posture and his propensity to see social and medical problems forming vicious circles, he recognized that social and economic conditions, such as poor housing and a monotonous diet, as well as social custom, fatigue, and chronic pain encouraged drinking.[48] "The pinch of poverty leads many to drunkenness."[49]

But all excessive drinking and other irresponsible behavior could not be blamed on the environment. In the slums one often came on a home which was "an oasis of cleanliness and sweetness in a desert of dirt and neglect. The structural condition of the house is no better than that of the neighboring houses but the character of the inmates has impressed itself upon the house."[50] Not all poor parents led drunken lives, squandering their resources and neglecting their children. Part of the condition of the poor must be the result of choices made individually by the poor. Those who wanted to conquer poverty or disease must see that responsible behavior was taught and encouraged. Even sanitary inspectors making their rounds should be part of the moral campaign. They should think of themselves as "home missionaries to the poor and helpless" who by promoting "cleanliness and self-

44 Ibid., 178–9.   45 Newsholme, "Social Evolution," 1336.
46 Arthur Newsholme, "The Possible Association of the Consumption of Alcohol with Excessive Mortality from Cancer," *Br. Med. J.* (1903), no. 2: 1529–31; Arthur Newsholme, "Alcohol and Public Health," in *The Drink Problem in its Medico-Sociological Aspects,* ed. T. N. Kelynack (London: Methuen & Co., [1907]) pp. 122–51; Arthur Newsholme, "The Influence of the Drinking of Alcoholic Beverages on the National Health," in *Alcohol and the Human Body,* ed. Victory Horsley and Mary D. Sturge, 5th ed. (London: Macmillan & Co., 1915), pp. 317–26; and Arthur Newsholme, *Second Report on Infant and Child Mortality, Suppl. Ann. Rep. Med. Off. L.G.B.,* 42 (1912–13): 78–82.
47 Arthur Newsholme "Alleged Physical Degeneration in Towns," *Public Health,* 17 (1904–5): 300.
48 Newsholme, "Conditions of Social Efficiency," 406; and Arthur Newsholme, *Public Health and Insurance: American Addresses* (Baltimore: Johns Hopkins Univ. Press, 1920): 149–50.
49 Arthur Newsholme, "Special Report on the Mortality and Causes of Mortality in Eight Districts in Brighton," Brighton, *Proc. Town Council,* 5 May 1892, 26.
50 Newsholme, "Social Evolution," 1333.

respect" and the "decencies of family life" made "moral and social improvement" possible.[51]

Newsholme's insistence that moral reform be part of the remedies to the health and social problems of his age can be seen as a survival of his Methodist upbringing and a reflection of conventional, middle-class, Victorian mores. But it was more than that. The reformation of character and of individual will provided him with a way to reconcile his belief in Darwinian evolution with his liberal faith in progress, amelioration, and liberty. Moral reform, in other words, allowed him to reconcile his politics with his science. Newsholme followed Huxley in arguing that a process of moral evolution had paralleled human biological and social evolution.[52] The evolution of altruism and self-denial for the good of others created a new moral environment. The effects during the past century could be traced in efforts to protect the weak from the exploitation of the strong through such collective actions as the abolition of the slave trade, the passage of factory legislation, public efforts to end cruelty to animals and to children, and the calls to abolish the double standard in sexual conduct. This new moral environment substituted cooperation for competition. It provided the incentive for the group to protect its members and to raise their fitness for survival by lessening the strain imposed by the environment.

In this new moral environment new ethical standards had been created; these standards provided the most basic reason for rejecting crude eugenic solutions to public health problems. A civilized nation could no longer, for example, allow a disease like tuberculosis to run unchecked in the expectation that the good of the race or herd would be served.

The logical alternative [to preventive work] is to kill off the susceptible stock or, as has been suggested, to allow them to infect their susceptible brethren and together with them perish of their disease. Such proposals have only to be stated in their crude terms in order to be apprehended and reprehended as an unsocial negation of civilization.[53]

Reverting to natural selection to solve human problems, he argued a decade later, threatened civilization. "To think otherwise is the secret behind German aggression; to act otherwise is to revert to barbarism. Man has definitely replaced natural by rational selection, and will, I have no doubt, to a steadily increasing extent replace competition by cooperation."[54]

The human capacity to act purposefully, collectively, and altruistically permitted humans in modern societies to escape the tyranny of natural selection. In a Liberal state, the sort of state Newsholme of course assumed in these discussions, much of the force for right conduct had to come from within. Behavior which threatened

51 Arthur Newsholme, "The Duties and Difficulties of Sanitary Inspectors," *Sanitary Record*, n.s. 10 (1888–9): 412.
52 For the following, see Newsholme, "Influence of Civilization," 7–8; Newsholme, "Social Evolution," 1334; and Newsholme, *Health Problems*, 98–9, 118–19, 182–3.
53 Arthur Newsholme, *The Prevention of Tuberculosis* (New York: E. P. Dutton & Co., 1908), 189.
54 Newsholme, *Public Health and Insurance*, 165.

the social order – crime, drunkenness, and vice – Newsholme described as survivals of earlier and less civilized ages. This formulation reduced the fundamental problems of ethical conduct to a simple dynamic between coexisting human impulses: the primitive and selfish on the one hand and the more evolved and altruistic on the other.[55] The state could do some things to tip the balance in favor of civilization and ethical conduct. It could ensure that public assistance encouraged rather than discouraged responsible behavior.[56] It might have to use compulsion against "those who do not evolve in response to the advancing tide of morality."[57] Ultimately, however, in a free and progressive society citizens had to learn to act responsibly.

Newsholme was aware that this was a very tall order, one which placed greater demands on the poor than on the more comfortably off. "Sometimes I think that those to whom a farthing is a rare coin do not realize effectively the demands on character which are made by a life in which every farthing counts." But those oases of "cleanliness and sweetness" in deserts of "dirt and neglect" proved, to his satisfaction at least, that

the necessary sacrifices can be made and made cheerfully. The constant self-denial which they entail cannot conceivably be improvised. It must result from the possession of habits both of conduct and of mind. Life without such habits in conditions which hourly call for them is not only miserable for the individual but also mischievous to the community. And yet how small a part of our national educational system is devoted to the training of character, which is, I take it, the resultant of habits of mind and conduct.[58]

These demands on character must be made and satisfied. Newsholme saw no other ways in which human welfare, liberty, and evolution could be reconciled.

THE POOR LAW, THE WEBBS, AND A UNIFIED MEDICAL SERVICE

When Newsholme left Brighton, Sidney and Beatrice Webb were engaged in their strategy of permeation, hoping to exert so decisive an influence on key members of the government and the civil service that they could lead the Liberal government to bring about a revolution in social policy.[59] Sidney had made a start in local government using his position on the London County Council to secure the municipalization of public services. The Poor Law was a next logical target.

---

55 Newsholme, *Health Problems,* 118–19, 182–4.   56 Newsholme, "Social Evolution," 1334–5.

57 Newsholme, *Health Problems,* 119. These measures might include such acts as the garnishing of wages of those who did not support their children. Newsholme, "Social Evolution," 1336; Newsholme, "Conditions of Social Efficiency," 405; and Newsholme, "National Physical Training," 12.

58 Newsholme, "Social Evolution," 1333.

59 There is a vast historical literature on the political activities of the Webbs during these years. For brief discussions of their policy of permeation and its failure, see Norman MacKenzie, "Introduction," in *The Letters of Sidney and Beatrice Webb* (Cambridge: Cambridge Univ. Press, 1978), II: ix–x; A. M. McBriar, *An Edwardian Mixed Doubles: The Bosanquets versus the Webbs. A Study in British Social Policy 1890–1929* (Oxford: Clarendon Press, 1987), 21–2, 23–4, 32; Gilbert, *Evolution of National Insurance,* 66–81; Bernard Semmel, *Imperialism and Social Reform,* 64–72.

In its treatment of sick paupers it was particularly vulnerable, and Beatrice Webb's recognition of this fact led her to seize the work of local health department as a model for public services after the breakup of the Poor Law and to change her tactics on the Poor Law Commission.[60]

In listening to the evidence brought by the C.O.S. [Charity Organization Society] members in favour of restricting medical relief to the technically destitute, it suddenly flashed across my mind that what we had to do was to adopt the exactly contrary attitude, and make medical inspection and medical treatment compulsory on all sick persons – to treat illness, in fact, as a public nuisance to be suppressed in the interests of the community. At once, I began to cross-examine on this assumption, bringing out the existing conflict between the poor law and public health authorities, and making the unfortunate poor law witnesses say that they were in favour of the public health attitude![61]

She set out at once to find support among Medical Officers of Health. She turned for advice to Dr. George F. McCleary, a member of the Fabian Society, and M.O.H. of Hamstead, and George Newman, then M.O.H. of Finsburg, who, like McCleary, was known for infant welfare work. She soon initiated a private investigation of the relation of Poor Law medical relief to public health work, seeking facts and supporting testimony from Medical Officers of Health. With Sidney's help she drafted a letter, which she planned to mail to 600 M.O.H.[62] The letter ostensibly solicited a copy of the M.O.H.'s last report, and any other information the recipient would care to send which would help her understand the views of the M.O.H., but the letter was aggressively partisan and calculated to identify M.O.H. who were likely to be useful to the Webbs.[63]

It has been pointed out to me that the free (and even compulsory) treatment of certain diseases is undermining the Poor Law principle of restricting Medical Relief to such persons as are technically destitute. The extension of this work from fevers to phthisis, and from Isolation Hospitals to Health Visiting, the Prevention of Infantile Mortality and Milk Depots, is criticized as virtually superseding the Medical branch of the Poor Law, with its test of destitution. It has even been suggested that the Public Health Authorities should be restrained in their new activities.

On the other hand, it has been suggested that the new departures of the Public Health Authorities are indispensable, and that their action has no 'pauperizing' effect. The category

---

60 Other than her own diaries the best account of Beatrice Webb's activities on the Commission is McBriar, *Mixed Doubles,* 175–339.

61 Beatrice Webb, *Our Partnership,* ed. Barbara Drake and Margaret I Cole (New York, London, Toronto: Longmans, Green & Co., 1948), p. 348. The typescript diary on which this published work is based is in the British Library of Political and Economic Science, London School of Economics. Portions of this quotation are also published in *The Diary of Beatrice Webb,* vol. 3, *The Power to Alter Things,* ed. Norman and Jeanne MacKenzie (Cambridge, Mass.: Harvard Univ. Press, 1984), 45. Hereafter cited as Webb, *Diary,* 3.

62 Webb, *Our Partnership,* 348–9, 351, 356–7.

63 The responses were the ostensible basis for her address to the Society of Medical Officers of Health in November 1906. Beatrice Webb, "The Relation of Poor-Law Medical Relief to the Public Health Authorities," *Public Health,* 19 (1906–7): 129–38. Notice also the mixed reception her address received, ibid., 139–44.

of infectious diseases is being constantly widened, so that almost every case of illness may come, as a source of contamination, to be regarded as a public health nuisance. Moreover, it has been urged that the Public Health view leads to a method of treatment of the individual which is superior to that of the Poor Law Medical Officer substituting, in fact, a training in better habits of life for the grudgingly doled out 'bottle of physic.'[64]

Given the Webbs' bald appeal to M.O.H. fears and ambitions, it is not surprising that many of her respondents answered in the affirmative her one specific question, Would it be practical to bring the Poor Law Medical Officer under the Public Health Department? What is surprising as well as indicative of the range of opinion within the public health field was that some M.O.H. disagreed strongly with her assumptions and assertions. H. E. Armitage, M.O.H. of Newcastle, for example, denied that there was friction or overlapping between the Poor Law and the public health authorities, and H. Renney, M.O.H. of Sunderland, replied that he regarded the reference to the "grudgingly doled out bottles of physic" a "gratuitous libel" and claimed that saying that "almost every case of illness may come to be regarded as a 'public nuisance' is really too absurd."[65]

Replies like the last one were probably the kind she secretly removed in late October 1907, before she agreed to share her responses with other members, when opponents on the Commission protested her private investigations and demanded to see her information.[66] It was only one of many instances of her highhandedness and intrigue which infuriated Commission members and provoked strong pangs of conscience in Beatrice Webb which she rationalized away in her diary.[67]

It was during her study of the activities of local health authorities and her search for allies among Medical Officers of Health that Beatrice Webb learned of Arthur Newsholme. McCleary and Newman may first have suggested him. They were very familiar with his work in Brighton and would have recognized his influence in the public health world. His response to her circular letter was encouraging. He wrote that if the treatment of phthisis in workhouse infirmaries could be divested of all "parochial taint," and if the diet could be improved and the institution were managed more sympathetically, "we should be doing more towards the annihilation of Tuberculosis than by any other single measure."[68] Newsholme's interview with Webb's assistant on December 22, 1906, reinforced their impression that he was an energetic and bold public official who could be very

64 Undated draft letter to Medical Officers of Health in Webb, Local Government Collection, vol. 286a [no item number].

65 "Letters from Medical Officers of Health in Reply to a Letter from Mrs. Webb" [a summary], Webb, Local Government Collection, vol. 286c [no item number].

66 Webb, *Our Partnership*, 392–3; and J. Jeffrey [Assistant Secretary to the Royal Commission] to Beatrice Webb, 4 Dec. 1907, Webb, Local Government Collection, vol. 286. See also McBriar, *Mixed Doubles*, 231–5.

67 Webb, *Our Partnership*, 392, 395, 424. See also Webb, *Diary*, 3: 80, 105–6.

68 Transcribed excerpt of Newsholme's letter of 13 Aug. 1906 in Webb, Local Government Collection, vol. 335.

useful.[69] The assistant brought back a copy of his Annual Report for 1905 describing the municipal treatment of tuberculosis in Brighton and notes of the interview which stressed the comprehensive nature of his tuberculosis program and its successful operation. They also noted the high priority Newsholme attached to finding adequate institutional treatment of tuberculosis free from the deterrent policy of the Poor Law and the need for unifying under one authority all local health functions.

By the spring of the following year Newsholme had joined Newman, McCleary, and Robert Morant, the dynamic Permanent Secretary of the Board of Education, in her circle of advisers. This group pooled information, some of it privileged information from civil service offices, and it shared a conviction that a strong administrative remedy could be proposed, one that concentrated all health activity in one local administration.[70] The record shows that Newsholme supplied Beatrice Webb with technical information, on accommodation in isolation hospitals, for example, and made estimates for her: of the costs of providing a universal public system of medical care, of infant mortality in Poor Law institutions, and of the relative contribution of various diseases in causing destitution.[71] He seems to have brought to her attention certain anomalies in local health administration which she used to illustrate the harm done to the public health by the overlapping of public authorities and by the deterrent policy of the Poor Law authorities.[72] He also read and criticized memoranda she wrote for the Royal Commission.[73]

She and her circle in turn had a hand in molding Newsholme's opinions. She arranged social events calculated to impress her medical advisers with her political influence, such as the March 1907 dinner for her two most important M.O.H. and two Poor Law doctors with Arthur J. Balfour, leader of the Conservative Party. She believed the doctors had been duly impressed, but she was frustrated that the philosopher-statesman seemed more interested in discussing pathology than social policy.[74] Correspondence with the Webbs and the conversations at

---

69 Minutes of interview with Newsholme, 22 Dec. 1906, Webb, Local Government Collection, vol. 335.

70 For discussions of the working of this group, see Gilbert, *Evolution of National Insurance,* 144–7.

71 Arthur Newsholme to Beatrice Webb, 1 May 1907, Webb, Local Government Collection, vol. 297, B12; Arthur Newsholme to Beatrice Webb, 8 May 1907, ibid., B15; and Arthur Newsholme to Beatrice Webb, 6 June 1907, ibid., B23. See also Webb, *Our Partnership,* 416.

72 See, for example, the use she made of the failure of the Midwives' Act, 1902 to provide funds to pay the doctor's fees in difficult cases, Sidney and Beatrice Webb, *The State and the Doctor* (London, New York: Longmans, Green & Co., 1910), 243–4. Newsholme had earlier used the same illustration in Arthur Newsholme, testimony, *Report of the Royal Commission on the Poor Laws and Relief of Distress,* Appendix Vol 9, B.P.P. 1910, XLIX, [Cd. 5068], pp. 157 & 167 #92609–16, hereafter cited as Newsholme, Poor Law Commission, 9.

73 Arthur Newsholme to Beatrice Webb, 6 June 1907, Webb, Local Government Collection, vol. 297, B23; and Arthur Newsholme to Beatrice Webb, 17 Sept. 1907, ibid., B33. For evidence that Newsholme influenced other members of this group, see Robert Laurie Morant to Beatrice Webb, 12 May 1907, ibid., 297, B16.

74 Webb, *Our Partnership,* 374; or Webb, *Diary,* 3: 68–9.

their luncheon and dinner parties encouraged Newsholme to recast his dissatisfaction with local health services in more definite administrative terms. The changes soon began to appear in his public statements. He was President of the British Medical Association's Section on State Medicine in 1907, and he planned to use his opening remarks during the discussion of the coordination of public medical services during the B.M.A.'s 1907 annual meeting as a manifesto and as a trial balloon for the testimony he would give before the Royal Commission.[75] He showed his draft to Beatrice Webb, made some revisions following conversations he had at her home with Gerald Balfour, and told her afterward how the discussion at the annual meeting had gone.[76]

Historians who have studied the Poor Law Commission have recognized that Newsholme, Newman, and Morant had an important hand in shaping what would become the Minority Report of the Commission.[77] "The medical question is developing splendidly," Beatrice Webb wrote to Edward Pease in April. "Dr. Newsholme has sent in a ripping memo. in favour of free medical assistance organized by the Town and County Council. Newman, McCleary and ½ dozen others are following suit."[78] The testimony of M.O.H. before the Royal Commission was critical in discrediting the Poor Law and in moving most Commission members to accept the need to transfer at least some wards of the Guardians to other social agencies. At the annual dinner of the Society of Medical Officers of Health in October 1909, Sidney Webb paid tribute to the testimony of the M.O.H. and attempted, rather transparently, to promote the Minority Report by playing to both professional pride and fear:

> Up to that point it had been a question of how to deter people from applying. The medical officers of health brought in the ideas of searching out cases, of insisting on treatment at the incipient stage, of regarding even one 'missed case' as an evil and a public danger; and the Commission came to see what was wanted was not the relief of destitution but its prevention. It was this new principle learnt from the medical officers of health that the Minority Report worked out into a complete scheme. . . .
>
> Those who clung to the old notion of relieving destitution rather than preventing it, were already talking of what they called the encroachments of the Health Authority and the Education Authority. It was a significant thing that the Majority Report actually decided to retain the phthisis patient in the Poor Law, and thus exclude this disease in England from the sphere of Public Health, and to reclaim for the Poor Law the medical treatment of children at school. It had even been suggested by high official authority, that the medical officer of health should be stripped of his isolation hospitals and of his

75 The address was published as Arthur Newsholme "A Discussion on the Co-ordination of the Public Medical Services," *Br. Med. J.* (1907), no. 2: 656–60.
76 Arthur Newsholme to Beatrice Webb, 6 June 1907, Webb, Local Government Collection, vol. 297, B23; and Arthur Newsholme to Beatrice Webb, 5 Aug. 1907, Webb, Local Government Collection, vol. 297, B32.
77 Gilbert, *Evolution of National Insurance*, 145.
78 Beatrice Webb to Edward Pease, 18 April [1907], Fabian Papers, Nuffield College Library, Oxford in *The Letters of Sidney and Beatrice Webb*, ed. Norman MacKenzie (Cambridge: Cambridge Univ. Press, 1978) 3: 252. Hereafter cited as Webb, *Letters*, 3.

bacteriological laboratory, and relegated to what these people seemed to think was his proper position as a sort of superior sanitary inspector.[79]

Both Newman and Newsholme appeared before the Poor Law Commission in February 1908.[80] It is hardly surprising that there were strong parallels between their prepared memoranda and their answers to questions.[81] They both drew attention to the recent expansion of free medical services offered by local authorities, and Newman in particular explicitly pointed out that the emphasis in public medicine was moving from environmental to personal services. They both decried the failure of the medical services offered by the Guardians. Not only did those services not encourage prevention, but the deterrent tradition of Poor Law administration frustrated preventive work by the local health authorities. Finally both witnesses called for the creation of a unified public medical service to be initiated by transferring the medical services of the Poor Law to the local Public Health Authority.

Newsholme was the Webbs' prize witness, the "most emphatic and impressive of all."[82] From his experience in Brighton he effectively illustrated the forces (financial, institutional, and legal) that discouraged working-class patients from seeking medical attention early and the failure of medical practitioners to correctly diagnose infectious cases, to properly notify such cases to the M.O.H., to correctly certify the causes of death, or to inform the M.O.H. of conditions they discovered in their practices which were hazardous to the public health.[83] Newsholme pointed out anomalies in health legislation that undermined preventive work such as the failure of the Midwives Act, 1902, to provide funds to pay the physicians whom midwives were required to recommend be called in difficult births. As a result physicians were seldom called. The example worked well at the Commission; the Webbs used it effectively in later writings.[84] More important, Newsholme argued for a much broader, more comprehensive vision of public health. He had already voiced the complaints of the M.O.H. about recent innovations that created divided authority for health, such as the Factories and Workshops Act, 1895, which required notification of several industrial diseases not to the M.O.H. but to the Chief Inspector of Factories in the Home Office, or the appointment of school doctors and nurses by local educational authorities, who in too many instances worked independently of the local health department.[85] Before the Commission and in his manifesto to the

79 Sidney Webb as reported in "The Annual Dinner," *Public Health*, 23 (1909–10), 65, 66.
80 Newman's memorandum and testimony are found in *Report of the Royal Commission on the Poor Laws and Relief of Distress*, Appendix Vol. 9, B.P.P. 1910, XLIX, [Cd. 5068], pp. 262–88; Newsholme's memorandum and testimony are found in ibid., 155–82.
81 For the following discussion, see Newman, Poor Law Commission, 9: 267, 273, 274, 286–7; and Newsholme, Poor Law Commission, 9: 163–4, 174–5 #92806–25.
82 Webb, *State and the Doctor*, 221.
83 Newsholme, Poor Law Commission, 9: 160–1, 176–7 #92845–50, 178 #92888–900, 179 #92934–45.
84 Newsholme, Poor Law Commission, 9: 157 & 167 #92609–16.
85 Arthur Newsholme, "A National System of Notification of Sickness," *Br. Med. J.* (1895), no. 2: 530; Arthur Newsholme, "A National System of Notification and Registration of Sickness," *J. Roy.*

B.M.A.'s Section on State Medicine, he not only argued that the scope of public health work must extend far beyond the acute infectious diseases to include all preventable diseases but that such work must include the treatment of disease.[86] The division between curative medicine and preventive medicine was entirely arbitrary. "Medical aid," he told the Commission in a statement he would echo for the next thirty years, "will continue to be defective so long as medicine is regarded as chiefly curative rather than chiefly preventive."[87]

It is clear, therefore, that preventive medicine embraces in its true scope not only all the acute and chronic infective diseases, and the many noninfective diseases which can be prevented by personal hygiene, but also the early and systematic treatment of many diseases the early treatment of which prevents more serious and obstinate after-conditions.[88]

In fact, by this time he was building the case that local health authorities must not only be authorized to provide treatment but that they should organize and supervise such treatment.

Social inefficiency is caused by every form of disease in proportion to its duration and severity. The prompt and early treatment of disease in its widest definition being one of the chief means for securing social efficiency, the better communal organization of the treatment of the sick from whatever disease must be regarded as a chief object of the preventive medicine of the future.[89]

This was an idea with radical implications, indeed. It was probably the success of the tuberculosis program Newsholme started in Brighton, more than any other factor, which led him to think boldly about the future. Here was a scheme in which private practitioners cooperated with the local health authority without apparent friction in voluntarily notifying an important disease. Here was a scheme provided by the local authority which offered comprehensive services: diagnostic and educational, preventive and therapeutic, domiciliary and institutional. Here was a system of public medicine which aimed not only at treating illness among the poor as the Poor Law authorities did, but also at preventing illness in the first place by modifying both the environment and human behavior. Here was a scheme whose functioning parts were supervised and coordinated by one person, the Medical Officer of Health. In discussions during the first decade of the twentieth century of what should be done with the medical services for the poor, it was Newsholme's favorite example, his benchmark of success.[90]

Statist. Soc., 59 (1896): 26–7; Arthur Newsholme, "Address on Possible Medical Extensions of Public Health Work," *J. State Medicine,* 9 (1901): 550–1; and Newsholme, "Discussion on the Co-ordination," 659.
86 Newsholme, Poor Law Commission, 9: 158–9; and Newsholme, "Discussion of the Co-ordination," 656. See also Newsholme, "National System of Notification," *Br. Med. J.,* 530.
87 Newsholme, Poor Law Commission, 9: 158.
88 Newsholme, "Discussion on the Co-ordination," 656.
89 Newsholme, "Conditions of Social Efficiency," 407.
90 Newsholme, "Discussion on the Co-ordination," 659; and Newsholme, Poor Law Commission, 9: 158, 165–7 #92540–605.

In his memorandum and testimony for the Poor Law Commission, Newsholme championed locally administered, publicly financed, comprehensive medical services. "Every man should have the right to call for gratuitous diagnosis, treatment, and provision of medicine."[91] This system would be supported by the rates and supervised by the Medical Officer of Health. It would include the preventive and curative services then offered by the local health department, the medical treatment of the destitute presently undertaken by the Guardians, and publicly subsidized services to be offered to working-class families by private practitioners, by friendly society and dispensary doctors, and by hospital outpatient departments.[92] In short, he advocated turning over all preventive and therapeutic services for the working classes, other than inpatient services provided by voluntary hospitals, to the local health authority. Newsholme was not at all dogmatic about how this transition could be carried out or specific about details. He did recognize that the sudden appearance of a free medical system would create a demand for consultations which would exceed the capacity of local authorities. He trusted that the gradual evolution of the system would allow time for adjustment and that earlier detection and treatment would mean greater efficiency. He did not believe that private medicine would disappear,[93] but he recognized that some people would pay twice, once in rates for a service they did not use and a second time in fees for private service. This circumstance, Newsholme argued, was not a valid objection to his suggested system, because a similar situation had developed and was generally accepted in education.[94] It is not clear if medical practitioners working for the local authority health scheme would be full-time or part-time or precisely how they would be paid. Newsholme was clear, however, in his expectation that if a practitioner accepted public money for treating a patient, he would be subject to supervision by the local health department.[95] This supervision would be a great advantage, he predicted, in ending the careless or incompetent care the poor too often received and in ensuring an efficient coordination of services. A practitioner who treated a consumptive patient for chronic bronchitis without bothering to examine the chest or the sputum "would certainly get his knuckles rapped."[96]

His proposal was a bold attempt to stake a claim on behalf of local health authorities to all publicly funded health services and to gain a great measure of supervision over ordinary private practitioners as well. It was also an effort by strong administrators and their Fabian allies to centralize social services and to turn their administration over to experts. The scheme may be understood in part as an attempt to do for health what the controversial 1902 Education Act, an act which Robert Morant and the Webbs had energetically supported, had done for education: abolish ad hoc boards and administrative authorities and turn responsibility for running the schools over to education committees of town or county

91 Newsholme, Poor Law Commission, 9: 164.
92 Ibid., 164, 168 #92639–44, 172 #92727, 173 #92778, 175–6 #92826–9.
93 Ibid., 168 #92639–4.   94 Ibid., 181 #92988–90.
95 Ibid., 176–7 #92846–53.   96 Ibid., 179 #92934.

councils, where expert opinion was of greater moment and democratic forces less influential.[97] During the deliberations of the Poor Law Commission, for example, Robert Morant imagined that the public health and education committees of the local authorities would divide responsibility for children then under the supervision of the Guardians.[98] Under questioning at the Commission Newsholme revealed his dislike of divided administrative responsibility.[99] It is significant that he used the beneficial effects of the 1902 Education Act to explain his position. Before the Act school attendance officers in Brighton seldom reported cases of infectious disease, although the school board had agreed to cooperate with the health department in this matter. But after education was transferred to a committee of the Town Council, such reporting had become routine. Significantly, however, Newsholme did not agree that a similar coordination between the public health department and medical treatment of the destitute could be accomplished by simply transferring Poor Law authority from the Guardians to a statutory committee of the town or county council. He believed that a single health administration was necessary.

One aspect of Newsholme's tuberculosis program in Brighton that attracted the Webbs was the emphasis he placed on patient training during the stay in the Sanatorium. Newsholme drew attention to this feature of the program in his prepared memorandum to the Poor Law Commission, and Beatrice Webb noted it during her cross-examination and encouraged him to generalize.[100] Wasn't it true, she asked, that medical treatment which simply gave bottles of medicine to diabetics did little good? Was it not necessary to teach the patient to avoid sugar? Newsholme agreed and went on.

I think the same argument would apply generally. Take bronchitis, for instance; a person who has a dusty occupation must take certain precautions; he must wear a respirator or adopt certain means of getting rid of the dust. That is a great nuisance, and the workpeople do not like it, and they would almost rather have the bronchitis. Under a system of preventive medicine, pressure will be brought to bear upon them to use the respirators or other means that were needed.[101]

How much encouragement, how much compulsion, was necessary or tolerable? What should be done with those who did not want the new social services? The Minority Report of the Royal Commission shows that the Webbs were willing to use autocratic measures.[102] It proposed that the recipients of aid be classified

97 For the opinion of Morant and the Webbs on the Education Act, see Searle, *National Efficiency,* 207–10.

98 Webb, *Our Partnership,* 378–9.

99 For Newsholme's answers to questions on administrative centralization, see Newsholme, Poor Law Commission, 9: 174 #92789–99.

100 Ibid., 156, 173–4 #92781–8.

101 Ibid., 174 #92786.

102 For a discussion of the authoritarian elements in the Minority Report, see Searle, *National Efficiency,* 241–3. See also Cormack, *Welfare State,* 16–17. It is ironic that while the Webbs wanted to dismantle the Poor Law, they wished to retain for medical officials the disciplinary functions

without regard to their wishes and turned over to the appropriate authority for the type of assistance they were judged to need. No aid was to be unconditional. All was to depend on appropriate behavior. The recalcitrant, able-bodied unemployed were fated for a particularly unhappy lot: transportation to a training establishment for compulsory testing, exercise, and training. Idlers and the uncooperative would be treated to the sort of discipline and detention usually reserved for criminals. This contempt for liberal principles – she once noted in her diary that she expected that the Tories rather than the Liberals would enact her plans and that that would be preferable in many ways as "there would be no nonsense about democracy!"[103] – more than her persistent and sometimes transparent intrigue repelled members of both parties. "The observation of [C.F.G.] Masterman [Liberal M.P. for West Ham and Parliamentary Secretary of the L.G.B. 1908–9], that he hoped he would never fall into Mrs Webb's hands as a member of the unemployed, represents what must have been a very common reaction – particularly on the Liberal side of the House."[104]

Because neither the Minority Report nor Newsholme's more modest plan for a unified public medical system was enacted, it is impossible to say how he would have carried his principles into operation. He did tell the Royal Commission he believed that medical assistance was different from other gratuitous aid in not demoralizing the recipient. This was because cooperation and even personal sacrifices were required of the patient.[105] When asked whether he thought medical aid would be abused by people who did not need it, he replied. "I do not think so. Castor oil is not a favorite beverage; if it were whisky it would be a different matter. I think the medical attendance would be so disciplinary that it would be prohibitive of abuse."[106] How he planned to deter frivolous calls for medical attention without deterring necessary ones was not ascertained. His testimony, however, leaves little doubt that in planning a unified public medical system he did not have in mind the sort of compulsion implied in the minority report, especially in its recommendations for dealing with the able-bodied unemployed. He was questioned at the Royal Commission by members representing Guardians, the Charity Organization Society, and the Poor Law Medical Service on just this point.[107] He replied repeatedly that compulsion should be used only in very rare instances. Not only would public opinion at present not tolerate it, even in cases where the sick were a danger to members of their household, but in most instances the use of compulsion with the sick was unnecessary. "My own experience at Brighton is that compulsion is very rarely needed. If you take time to get into sympathetic touch with the patients and spend time over it, you can exercise discipline without compulsion."[108]

that Poor Law medical officers had assumed. This idea is developed in M. A. Crowther, "Paupers or Patients? Obstacles to Professionalization in the Poor Law Medical Service before 1914," *J. Hist. Med.*, 39 (1984): 47–50.

103 Webb, *Our Partnership*, 418; or Webb, *Diary*, 3: 103.
104 Searle, *National Efficiency*, 242.   105 Newsholme, Poor Law Commission, 9: 164–5.
106 Ibid., 172 #92731.   107 Ibid., 177 #92854–6, 179 #92944–6.   108 Ibid., 177 #92854.

Newsholme believed himself in full agreement with the Webbs' medical recommendations. "I do not see," he wrote to Beatrice Webb in September 1907, "how anyone can withstand the logical consequences of the 'principles of 1907,' " their working consensus.[109] He supported and publicized the medical recommendations of the Minority Report and was mute about its recommendations for the unemployed.[110] He does not seem to have noticed or at least to have worried unduly about the possibility that local authorities might abuse the broad powers the Minority Report would give them. As we will see, this was a problem he would have to confront directly during his visit to the Soviet Union in 1932.[111] As a highminded health administrator he can, perhaps, be expected to assume that other officials would invariably have his benign intent and would exercise his restraint. In his planning he had in mind the well-run British municipal borough.[112] The fact that the Town Councillors were responsible to the electorate guaranteed representation of democratic interests. Since those Councillors were amateurs who were advised by officials with specialized expertise whom they had grown to trust, expert administration was possible at the same time. It seemed to him an ideal combination of efficiency and democracy. But more was at work in conditioning his response than Newsholme's own administrative experience. His belief in the necessity for character transformation, a belief founded in his Evangelical background, made him responsive to the Webbs' insistence on behavior modification as a condition for public assistance. In Newsholme's vision the public doctor would have an elevating moral influence.

The form in which medical aid would be given would be such as constantly to enforce on the minds of the patients their duty to the community and to themselves in matters of health. Though they would pay nothing, they would not be merely passive recipients of advice and attention. The influence of the doctor would demand from them habits of life and even sacrifices of personal taste in the interest of the health of the community, their families and themselves, which would leave them conscious of a sensible discharge of duty in return for the attention which they received. The discipline of responsibility into which the system would educate them should, in my judgment, suffice to avoid the loss of self-respect liable to arise from the merely passive receipt of gifts; and it would introduce into the national life an attitude towards matters of personal health that would have an indirect influence upon conduct, while directly restricting disease.[113]

To bring about this transformation Newsholme preferred education, sympathetic persuasion, and incentives for right conduct, but, as we have seen, when these

---

109 Arthur Newsholme to Beatrice Webb, 17 Sept. 1907, Webb, Local Government Collection, vol. 297, B33.
110 For an example of his popularizing among his colleagues, see Newsholme, "Conditions of Social Efficiency," 403–14. The Webbs popularized the Minority Report's application to medicine in Webb, *The State and the Doctor.*
111 The literary product of this visit was Arthur Newsholme and John Adams Kingsbury, *Red Medicine: Socialized Health in Soviet Russia* (Garden City, N.Y.: Doubleday, Doran & Co., 1933).
112 Newsholme, "Conditions of Social Efficiency," 413. He continued to argue this position in later decades. See, for example, Newsholme, *Public Health and Insurance,* 47–8.
113 Newsholme, Poor Law Commission, 9: 164–5.

measures failed, he was prepared to recommend compulsory measures for those who did not, in his terms, evolve with the rising tide of public morality.

In these years the Webbs' plans called not only for taking control of the Royal Commission on the Poor Laws but also for placing allies in high administrative positions. Beatrice Webb had even considered trying to arrange the appointment of her M.O.H. allies to the Commission itself. In April 1907, when testimony from M.O.H. was beginning to influence the deliberations of the Commission, and when its Secretary was considering adding a medical member to represent the interests of private practitioners, Webb wrote to John Burns, President of the Local Government Board, to suggest the appointment of Newsholme, Newman, or McCleary – hardly physicians to represent the private practitioner but perfect appointees to further her plans.[114] She apparently did help secure George Newman's appointment as Chief Medical Officer of the Board of Education by introducing him to Robert Morant.[115] She also claimed credit for convincing John Burns to appoint Newsholme Medical Officer of the Local Government Board. In November 1907 at one of her luncheons which included H. G. Wells and John Burns, she learned that Burns was about to appoint a replacement for William H. Power, the current L.G.B. Medical Officer. After the other guests had left, she pressed Newsholme's candidacy. Burns, she reported, considered Newsholme a publicist and a better candidate for Registrar-General. She disagreed. "He is an administrative genius, with an entirely new outlook on the whole question of public health." Appealing to Burns's vanity, which she considered his great weakness, she continued, "If you appoint him, you will make your reputation as a public health reformer."[116] She followed up this conversation with a long letter and with visits to Morant and Newman to suggest they also urge Newsholme's appointment on Burns. Beatrice Webb probably flattered herself with the extent of her influence over Burns, and historians have been too willing to accept her assessment.[117] Burns was already beginning to distrust her and was unlikely to undertake the struggle to overcome the departmental resistance to the appointment of an outsider just to please her, and as his biographer points out, Burns had already met Newsholme and liked what he saw.[118] Newsholme's own account of his appointment strengthens the impression that Burns was not simply moving at Beatrice Webb's prodding.[119] Newsholme had noticed how closely Burns had read the reports of M.O.H. and was pleased to see his own annual

114 Webb, *Our Partnership*, 376.
115 At least Newman credited her with making the appointment possible. George Newman to Beatrice Webb, 19 Sept. 1907, Passfield Papers, II, 4, C 99, f. 277. See also Searle, *National Efficiency*, 243–4.
116 Webb, *Our Partnership*, 394.
117 See, for example, Searle, *National Efficiency*, 244.
118 Kenneth D. Brown, *John Burns* (London: Royal Historical Society, 1977), p. 133.
119 For Newsholme's account, see Arthur Newsholme, *The Last Thirty Years in Public Health: Recollections and Reflections on My Official and Post-Official Life* (London: George Allen and Unwin, 1936), pp. 28–9.

reports quoted in some of Burns's speeches. When Burns visited Brighton in 1907, apparently before his luncheon with Beatrice Webb and H. G. Wells, he took Newsholme aside to inquire whether Newsholme would like to join the L.G.B. as an Inspector. Newsholme declined his offer, and volunteered that the only government post he coveted was the job of medical statistician for the General Register Office, Farr's old post and a position for which Newsholme had been one of three candidates in 1893. This conversation in Brighton apparently prompted Burns's remark to Webb that Newsholme would make a better Registrar-General than a Medical Officer for the L.G.B.

Regardless of whether she was as responsible for Newsholme's appointment as she liked to believe, Beatrice Webb could well take pleasure in that appointment.[120] It gave her allies in important places: Morant and Newman at the Board of Education and Newsholme at the L.G.B. She also counted Leslie MacKenzie, Medical Officer of the Scottish L.G.B., among these allies.[121] Early in 1908 anything looked possible, but soon her hopes of reform from within would be ruined and within a few years the congenial working relations between her allies in upper ranks of the civil service would turn into bitter competition.

120 She was very pleased when she learned of the appointment; Beatrice Webb, diary entry 13 Jan. 1908, Webb Diary, 26: 2526. She took a pleasure in noticing "a certain sullenness" among her opponents on the Royal Commission at this news. Webb, *Our Partnership*, 399.
121 Ibid., 383–4.

8

The Local Government Board and the nation's health policy

John Burns offered Arthur Newsholme the position of Medical Officer of the Local Government Board on January 11, 1908, and Newsholme arranged to take up his duties in Whitehall on February 4, one day after testifying before the Royal Commission on the Poor Laws.[1] He became the Board's sixth Medical Officer in a line stretching back to Sir John Simon. In making this move, Newsholme went to the nation's central health and social welfare authority, to a bureau with important responsibilities in areas where major social reforms were presently under political consideration. The appointment was a great opportunity for a reform-minded Medical Officer. However, its organization, tradition, and leadership made the L.G.B. a very unlikely engine of reform.

Writing in 1936, R.C.K. Ensor sounded the tone which historians have followed for two generations in describing the L.G.B.

Set up to guard against extravagance in the granting of poor relief, it had imbued its officials with the idea that Whitehall's sole duty towards local authorities was to prevent them from doing what they ought not. But at this time what the local authorities . . . really needed from the centre was positive stimulus, enlightened guidance, and constructive advice based on research. . . . It is difficult to over-estimate what the country lost through having its local authorities down to 1914 placed under a central department constantly on the alert to hinder them and rarely, if ever, to help.[2]

While recent scholarship has begun to reevaluate this view of the L.G.B. as obstructionist and hopelessly reactionary and to portray more sensitively the Board's mission in terms that Victorians would have understood, as a guardian of

---

1 John Burns, Diary, 11 Jan. 1908, British Library, Add. Mss. 46326, hereafter cited as Burns, Diary, Add. Mss. 46326. See also "Sir Arthur Newsholme, K.C.B., M.D., F.R.C.P.," *Br. Med. J.* (1943) no. 1: 680.

2 R.C.K. Ensor, *England 1870–1914* (Oxford: Clarendon Press, 1936), 126. Also quoted in part in Roy M. MacLeod, *Treasure Control and Social Administration,* Occasional Papers on Social Administration No. 23 (London: G. Bell & Sons, 1968), 8.

local interests and of the public purse,[3] the fact remains that by the time News-holme went to Whitehall, the Board had an administrative culture that technical experts deplored. In announcing Newsholme's appointment, *The Lancet* labeled the post "the highest and the most onerous" in the public health service. While the editor conceded that the L.G.B. and its medical department could take credit for some health progress in recent years, he added "it would be interesting to know how many schemes of constructive sanitary policy in matters both large and small which have entailed endless inquiry and work by Simon's successors, could be unearthed from the Board's pigeon-holes."[4]

The L.G.B. was staffed by an ingrown bureaucracy. Although its Medical Department had attracted the services of some able officers, like the rest of the Board, it normally made its upper appointments from within. A number of its staff had served as M.O.H. to a local authority, but only two of the five previous Medical Officers had done so, and only the first of these, Simon, had been brought in from the outside to fill the position.[5] In the ordinary course of events the retiring Medical Officer, William Power, would have been succeeded by the staff member with the greatest seniority. In this case the successor would have been either H. Franklin Parsons, the Assistant Medical Officer, or perhaps R. Bruce Low, the Second Assistant Medical Officer. The appointment of an outsider was both unprecedented and, to the permanent staff at least, most unwelcome. Burns faced strong opposition from his senior civil servants and from the Medical Department, but he swept aside objections and told his staff, as he recorded in his diary, "The interests of the public must override Departmentalism and everyone must adapt themselves w. this or go."[6] Burns was pleased to see that his decision had wide support outside of the department.[7] George Newman wrote Burns a flattering letter about the appointment, claiming "I am & always have been of one opinion as to his [Newsholme's] unique qualifications for the post" and closed by claiming that he was "delighted to have the privilege of working w. a great friend."[8] The press welcomed the appointment of an able M.O.H. and took it as a sign of "Mr. Burns' determination to bring his department into the closest possible touch with local public health needs and enterprise."[9] In Fabian circles the appointment raised high expectations. Beatrice Webb heard of Newsholme's

3 For a very helpful recent analysis of the L.G.B. which is sensitive to the Board's political context, see Christine Bellamy, *Administering Central–Local Relations, 1871–1919: The Local Government Board in Its Fiscal and Cultural Context* (Manchester: Manchester Univ. Press, 1988).
4 "The Medical Officer of the Local Government Board: a New Appointment," *Lancet* (1908), no. 1: 242.
5 For brief sketches of the careers of these officers, see Arthur S. MacNalty, "The History of State Medicine in England. Lecture No. 3. – The Medical Department of the Local Government Board," *J. Roy. Inst. Pub. Health,* 11 (1948): 9–11; Newsholme, *Last 30 Years,* 32–9.
6 Burns, Diary, 13 Jan. 1908, Add. Mss. 46326.
7 Ibid., 16 Jan. 1908, Add. Mss. 46326.
8 Newman to Burns, 18 Jan. 1908, Burns Papers, British Library, Add. Mss. 46300, ff. 5–6.
9 See, for example, "Dr. Newsholme's Appointment and What It Means," *London Daily News,* 20 Jan. 1908, 6.

appointment within two days and noted in her diary, "I am awaiting curiously the result."[10] She hoped that "the gifted Arthur Newsholme" could move "that home of reaction, the Local Government Board," and make it an ally in the restructuring of social services that would follow the adoption of the minority Report of the Royal Commission on the Poor Laws.[11]

But much at the L.G.B. belied such expectations. A technical expert like Newsholme who had gained his administrative experience in a county borough in which he was able to exert a direct influence on local policy decisions and to oversee all administrative activity related to health was bound to be frustrated at the L.G.B. The Board had been created to supervise the activities of local authorities over a wide field, and it had an administrative tradition and an organization which limited administrative initiative by its technical experts. John Simon, the Board's first Medical Officer, found arrangements at the L.G.B. intolerable and resigned to censure them in his *English Sanitary Institutions.*[12] Edwardian social reformers, like the Webbs, who favored bold initiatives led by strong administrators, found the Board nearly hopeless. Coached by Newsholme in details, they soon used the L.G.B. to demonstrate the illogic, inefficiency, and watertight departmentalism of contemporary central welfare administration.[13] At the L.G.B. responsibility for sanitation and disease prevention was divided by the middle 1890s among five of its divisions or departments.[14] Each worked independently and reported to a different Assistant Secretary, who reported in turn to the Permanent Secretary, the civil servant head of the Board, and to the President, the political head and Cabinet member. This division of public health responsibilities within the L.G.B. did little to promote coordination or uniformity. Poor Law infirmaries and the isolation hospitals of the Metropolitan Asylums Board, for example, came under the Poor Law Division, but isolation hospitals outside the Metropolis came under the Public Health, Local Finance, and Local Acts Division. The latter division also supervised the vaccination services offered by the Guardians, and water supply, rivers pollution, and the food and drug acts. The administration of the other public health acts as well as drainage were under yet another division, the Sanitary Administration and Local Areas Division, and a fourth, the Legal and Order Division, oversaw bylaws local authorities made under the public health acts and regulations dealing with the water supply and milk. None of these four divisions devoted its attention exclusively to public health matters. The Public

---

10 Webb, Diary, 13 Jan. 1908, 13: 2526, British Library of Political and Economic Science. London School of Economics.

11 Webb, *Our Partnership,* 442.

12 John Simon, *English Sanitary Institutions, Reviewed in their Course of Development, and in Some of Their Political and Social Relations* (London: Cassell & Co., 1890), 354–8, 390–1, 398–400.

13 Sidney and Beatrice Webb, *The State and the Doctor* (London, New York: Longmans, Green & Co., 1910), 222–3.

14 For the following example, see ibid., 222–3. See also the organizational charts in MacLeod, *Treasury Control,* 59–62; and M. Heseltine, "The Functions of a Ministry of Health in Relation to the Present Local Government Board" [Memorandum for Christopher Addison, Minister of Reconstruction], 17 Nov. 1917, P.R.O. MH78/80.

Health, Local Finance, and Local Acts Division also was responsible not only for a host of problems dealing with local authority finance but also for public libraries and canal boats. The Sanitary Administration and Local Areas Division oversaw housing and roads, as well as gas and water facilities. The Legal and Order Division had responsibilities for automobiles and for overseeing the administration of the Unemployed Workman Act, 1905 and the Old Age Pension Act, 1908.

The Medical Department was the fifth administrative unit of the L.G.B. with public health functions. While the other four divisions we have mentioned were administrative units, the Medical Department was a technical department and functioned like the Architect's and the Engineering Departments. Each of these departments was directed by a technical expert: the Medical Officer, the Architect, or a Chief Inspector, each of whom reported to one of the Assistant Secretaries who administered the administrative departments. What galled Medical Officers like Simon and Newsholme was that in this position they had no direct access to the Permanent Secretary or to the President of the Board. Newsholme found that he could have an interview with the President or with the Permanent Secretary, if he requested it, but he had no assurance that he would be consulted on important decisions.[15] In conferences of the President, Permanent Secretary, and certain Assistant Secretaries where such decisions were often made, his written advice might simply be summarized by an Assistant Secretary who had read his minutes or reports.[16] In reaching a decision the assembled group might overrule the Medical Officer's advice without further consultation with him.

Newsholme was particularly annoyed to find that the Board's legal and secretarial staff took it upon themselves to oppose before Parliamentary Committees bills presented by local authorities which would authorize innovation or experimentation in local public health work.[17] In several instances he learned of the opposition L.G.B. officials had raised in these hearings to bills which he favored only when colleagues working for local authorities accosted him wanting to know why he had advised against their requests. He was dumbfounded and angry. In these matters he usually sympathized with local officials. His memories of Brighton Corporation's thwarted attempts to gain legal authority to ban the sale of sewage-contaminated shellfish were still keen. Throughout his career he remained unusually sympathetic to the viewpoint of local health officials.

As Newsholme later explained, arrangements at the L.G.B. reflected the late Victorian view that while scientific or technical advice should be available to administrators and ministers, it should be kept in a clearly subordinate position – as one minister put it, "on tap but not on top," a sentiment Newsholme labeled "profoundly foolish."[18] Newsholme resented his subordination to general administrators who lacked specialized training and local administrative experience. These administrators, he later complained, considered themselves competent to judge

15 Newsholme, *Last 30 Years*, 49.　　16 Newsholme, *Ministry of Health*, 91–2.
17 Newsholme, *Last 30 Years*, 46.
18 The unnamed minister is quoted with Newsholme's assessment in ibid., 50.

when technical or scientific advice was needed and able to decide whether that advice might be used in the future as a precedent in reaching other decisions.[19] He was thought of, in other words, as a dictionary or encyclopedia, which could be consulted at will and then shelved.[20] The more one knew, so it seemed, the less influence one had on policy formation. Newsholme quoted with approval Lord Sydenham's caricature of the administrative chain of responsibility in the civil service, where "one had to fight for a necessary improvement through an ascending series of officials, each knowing less than the last, until one reached the deciding authority, who knew nothing at all."[21]

The secretariat of the L.G.B. expected that the Medical Officer would be available to give advice, to answer technical questions, and to consult with local officials. Otherwise he was to occupy himself with the routine administration of his Department. There was certainly much routine work to do. The Medical Officer supervised and reported on the work of a large professional staff which conducted local inspections, special field investigations, and laboratory work. At the outbreak of the War, for example, at the end of a period of modest expansion, his Department comprised a First Assistant Medical Officer, three Second Assistant Medical Officers, seventeen Medical Inspectors, one Assistant Medical Inspector, four Inspectors of Foods, and the Bacteriologist at the Government Lymph Establishment, which maintained the supply of lymph for vaccinations.[22] All of these were medically qualified. In addition there were a few scientifically or technically trained staff members who were not medically qualified – an Assistant Inspector, an Inspector and an Assistant Inspector of Foods, and an Assistant Bacteriologist at the Lymph Establishment – as well as several clerks and laboratory technicians. Much of his time was taken up with reviewing reports and proposals and writing minutes to the secretarial staff. He reported that during his first year at the L.G.B. he and his two assistants dealt with some 13,000 such papers.[23] In addition he had a fairly heavy schedule of conferences with Medical Officers of Health and with representatives of local authorities. He took seriously his responsibility for advising local sanitary authorities on scientific and medical questions.

From the Fabian point of view the biggest obstacle at the L.G.B. was its President, John Burns. Burns was an anomaly in the Cabinet. He was England's first working-class Minister, a Liberal who had begun his political life as an inflammatory orator for the Social Democratic Federation (S.D.F.) and who twice had been tried for inciting riots.[24] By the late 1880s his radicalism had begun to cool, and in its place there emerged a more pragmatic socialism which emphasized working-class self-help and trade unionism. He began to find it easier to work with the radical members of the Liberal Party than with his former colleagues in

19 Ibid., 62.   20 This is Newsholme's analogy. Newsholme, *Ministry of Health*, 21.
21 Cited in Newsholme, *Ministry of Health*, 91, and also in Newsholme, *Last 30 Years*, 58.
22 *The Imperial Calendar*, 1915, 401–2.   23 Newsholme, *Last 30 Years*, 50–1.
24 For a study of Burns, see Kenneth D. Brown, *John Burns* (London: Royal Historical Society, 1977). Older Sources include G.D.H. Cole, "John Elliot Burns," *D.N.B.*, 1941–50: 121–4; and William Kent, *John Burns: Labour's Lost Leader* (London: Williams and Norgate, 1950).

the S.D.F. and in the Independent Labour Party. He was elected to the London County Council for Battersea in 1889 and continued on the L.C.C. until 1907. Amid great controversy he became the Liberal Party candidate for Battersea in 1892 and won a seat in Parliament. He remained a popular figure and was considered an asset to the Liberal Party, one who could be counted on to bring in working-class votes. Following the Liberal landslide victory in the 1906 election Campbell-Bannerman gave him the presidency of the L.G.B.

Although Burns had joined the Fabian Society in 1893, and although he had served on the L.C.C. with Sidney Webb following Webb's election in 1892, he had never been close to the Webbs. Beatrice had twice hoped that he might prove useful to them, once in Parliament and again in the Cabinet, but he resisted being drawn into her orbit.[25] The two came to distrust each other during the deliberations of the Royal Commission on the Poor Law. She had shown him a draft of her proposals, and he strongly disapproved of her scheme. He disliked the Webbs' intellectualized approach and their propensity for social engineering.[26] He came to hate them and to oppose anything that smacked of their influence, when he learned of their attempt to force their ally Robert Morant on him as Permanent Secretary.[27] For as long as he remained in office Burns continued to distrust Morant and to resent his intrigue. He reported in his diary at the end of July 1913: "A long conference with Morant as elusive as ever, as evasive as C. M. [Charles Masterman] and as determined to go in by every other way than the front door."[28] His feelings toward the Webbs and their allies in the civil service were returned in kind. "John Burns," Beatrice Webb concluded

has become a monstrosity . . . blinded by vanity and malice . . . overgrown by a sort of fatty complacency with the world as it is: an enormous personal vanity, feeding on the deference and flattery yielded to patronage and power. He talks incessantly, and never listens to anyone except the officials to whom he *must* listen, in order to accomplish the routine work of his office. Hence, he is completely in their hands and is becoming the most hidebound of departmental chiefs. . . .[29]

Her anger aside, there is some truth here. Burns genuinely wanted a better life for the working classes, but he lacked legislative vision and became an "unimaginative administrative plodder, obsessed with economy and detail."[30] He thus began to identify with the views of his permanent administrators and to share their suspicions of reform proposals. In fact Burns disliked both reports of the Poor Law

25 Brown, *John Burns*, 77, 118.
26 Burns, Diary, 23 March 1900, Add. Mss 46318; ibid. 12 Dec. 1913, Add. Mss. 46335; John Burns, Memorandum, 14 Dec. 1917, Burns Papers, British Library, Add. Mss. 46308, f. 173. All three citations in Brown, *John Burns*, 194.
27 A. M. McBriar, *An Edwardian Mixed Doubles: The Bosanquets versus the Webbs, A Study of British Social Policy 1890–1929* (Oxford: Clarendon Press, 1987), 308–11. See also George Newman, Diary, 1 (25 May 1908), P.R.O., MH 139/1. Hereafter cited as Newman, Diary.
28 Burns, Diary, 29 July 1913, Add. Mss. 46335.
29 Webb, *Our Partnership*, 393; or Webb, *Diary*, 3: 79–80.
30 Brown, *John Burns*, 167, 200–1.

Commission, and he distrusted his colleagues, David Lloyd George and Winston Churchill, who would formulate the new social policies of the Liberal Party. To resist fundamental change, Burns did not need to exercise any extraordinary political skill; his Department gave him ample means of obstruction. When Asquith replaced Campbell-Bannerman as Prime Minister in 1908, he considered replacing Burns with Churchill, but Churchill considered the post a political liability and declined.[31] Burns was kept in place. The Prime Minister, in fact, found him a convenient way of thwarting the Webbs.[32] The Webbs' last hopes for the Department were lost when Burns was allowed to reshuffle the Department when Samuel Provis retired as Permanent Secretary in December 1909. Burns insisted on promoting the Department's old guard. Horace Monro, a former Assistant Secretary, became the new Permanent Secretary, and Burns's former Private Secretary, W. T. Jerred, took over Monro's former post. Beatrice Webb now realized that their plans of sweeping reform from within might fail. If Burns had made these changes with Asquith's approval, she recognized in January 1910, it meant that the Liberals did not intend to reform the Poor Law.[33] In this she was right, as events were soon to prove.

In view of Burns's suspicion and his opposition to fundamental change, it is a credit to Newsholme's tact and persuasiveness that the Medical Officer was able to win and retain the President's trust and his support for important initiatives in public health, particularly in tuberculosis prevention and infant welfare.[34] These were areas where Burns's sentimental reform sympathies could be given concrete form by a technical adviser who had vision. Important initiatives did come from within the L.G.B. even during Burns's presidency. But under his presidency great opportunities were lost as major initiatives in social policy were diverted elsewhere. By the time Burns retired in 1914, the momentum for reform had passed the L.G.B. by. With the outbreak of the War, the Board and the local authorities it supervised soon found themselves overtaxed, understaffed, and scarcely able to cope with their routine responsibilities. In addition the repeated shuffling of the Cabinet after 1914 gave the Board six Presidents in as many years and robbed the Department of continuity and informed political leadership.[35] Even if its officials had had the will to lead, they were now unable to do so.

---

31 For Churchill's famous quips on refusing the appointment, see Gilbert, *National Insurance*, 248–9, fn. 32; McBriar, *Mixed Doubles*, 310n.

32 Brown, *John Burns*, 136–7.

33 Webb, *Our Partnership*, 443. There are, of course, many reasons why the campaign to break up the Poor Law failed. For a discussion of the failure of the campaigns of both the Majority and Minority Reports, see McBriar, *Mixed Doubles*, 313–39. At least one historian has seen the administrative reshuffling of 1910 as an effort, admittedly a belated one, to breathe new life into the L.G.B. and to bring it into touch with new political realities, MacLeod, *Treasury Control*, 49–51.

34 For the pride Burns took in Newsholme's work while Medical Officer at the Board, see Burns, Diary, 27 July 1910, Add. Mss. 46332; ibid., 26 Feb. 1911, Add. Mss. 46333; and ibid., 21 Oct. 1911. See also Burns to McCleary, [c. Nov. 1918], Burns Papers, Add. Mss. 46303.

35 Newsholme makes this complaint in Newsholme, *Last 30 Years*, 47, 48.

THE L.G.B. AND THE COMING OF NATIONAL INSURANCE

Nothing demonstrates more clearly how isolated from Liberal social planning and political strategy making the L.G.B. and its President had become than the fact that the Board and its chief officials had almost nothing to do with the creation of National Insurance. Lloyd George, Chancellor of the Exchequer, had begun considering a scheme as early as the fall of 1908, visiting Germany, holding conferences with officials of the friendly societies, many of which already offered their members insurance against sickness and incapacity, and obtaining estimates from actuaries.[36] The pace of planning quickened during 1910, and by the end of the year the Chancellor had chosen William Braithwaite, an able young Treasury official, to work out the details of the scheme. By February 1911 Braithwaite had finished the first of many drafts. During all this time the L.G.B., which Braithwaite acknowledged should have been the department to undertake social insurance, was kept in the dark. It was only in March 1911, after news of the scheme had already appeared in medical and public health journals and just before the scheme was presented to the Cabinet, that Lloyd George consulted Burns. The two had a heated interview in the Chancellor's office on March 31 which both Burns and Braithwaithe have described.[37] Burns was angry about being shut out of the planning. Lloyd George, quite clearly, considered Burns no more than a nuisance. Braithwaite's account portrays Burns as the fool.

A most amusing interview. Chancellor very anxious to conciliate him, but almost unable to sit still under the mass of irrelevancy poured forth. I wondered when it *would* end. There was always one thing more!

Finally there *was* one thing more, as J. B. got close up to the Chancellor and shaking hands with him said, 'You know, this is a bigger thing than either the Majority or Minority Report, and renders them both unnecessary.' When he went out I know we both nearly exploded. . . .'[38]

The insurance scheme did in fact help ruin the campaign for the Minority Report, and its passage symbolized the failure of the Fabian strategy of permeation. National insurance provided state-subsidized and -supervised benefits against two of the major causes of destitution: unemployment (Part II of the act) and sickness or injury (Part I). Not only did it offer an alternative to the recommendations of the Minority Report, but it operated on principles which were anathema to the Webbs and their allies in the civil service. Part I, the portion

---

36 For the planning and passage of National Health Insurance, see Gilbert, *National Insurance*, 289–399; E. P. Hennock, *British Social Reform and German Precedents: The Case of Social Insurance 1880–1914* (Oxford: Clarendon Press, 1987), esp. 143–51, 168–215; E. P. Hennock "The Origins of British National Insurance and the German Precedent 1880–1914," in *The Emergence of the Welfare State in Britain and Germany 1850–1950*, ed. W. J. Mommsen (London: Croom Helm, 1981), 84–106; and William J. Braithwaite, *Lloyd George's Ambulance Wagon: Being the Memoirs of William J. Braithwaite 1911–1912*, ed. Henry N. Bunbury (London: Methuen & Co., 1957), 71–7.

37 Braithwaite, *Ambulance Wagon*, 140.   38 Ibid.

of the act of greatest interest to us here, was directed, the Webbs alleged, toward the treatment of disease not toward its prevention, and, worse, it offered unconditional assistance, giving, the Webbs alleged, the providers of the benefits little chance to control the behavior of recipients and encouraging malingering by permitting free choice of doctors.[39]

The Webbs had raised objections to social insurance as a remedy for poverty and dependency at a meeting with Lloyd George, Winston Churchill, and Richard Haldane in the autumn of 1908, when the Chancellor was just beginning to consider state insurance.[40] By February 1911 they were alarmed to learn that a national insurance scheme had been formulated and would soon come before the Cabinet. Their feelings ran so high that when the Chancellor belatedly consulted them at a breakfast at 11 Downing Street on February 28, they were so aggressive that they "burnt their boats with the Liberal ministers."[41]

Although Sidney Webb wrote to acknowledge his "unpardonable truculence" and to offer further advice,[42] the Webbs had no significant influence on the scheme. They did try to find a way to salvage key elements of their plan. In a memorandum Sidney sent the Chancellor under his own name and in another he prepared for a delegation of Medical Officers of Health who called on Lloyd George, he argued that the contributions of the insured who were not members of approved friendly societies along with those of their employers should be turned over to the local authorities on condition that these authorities provide a comprehensive set of preventive and therapeutic services.[43] Lloyd George was not tempted, and the New Liberals continued to revise their plan. Beatrice Webb watched in dismay as the Chancellor's scheme won support, unable to understand the political success of a scheme she believed flawed in principle. "It is clear that public opinion has got firmly into its silly head that insurance has some mystical moral quality, which even covers the heinous sin of expenditure from public funds. It is an amazingly foolish delusion."[44] All that the Webbs secured at their famous breakfast with Lloyd George was a promise from the Chancellor to consult the Medical Department of the Local Government Board. They apparently hoped that Newsholme would offer irrefutable evidence that the scheme would not work.

39 See, for example, Webb, *The State and the Doctor*, 229, 230–1; and Webb, *Our Partnership*, 468, or Webb, *Diary*, 3: 151–2.
40 Webb, *Our Partnership*, 416–17; or Webb, *Diary*, 3: 100–1.
41 McBriar, *Mixed Doubles*, 314. See the account of the meeting in Braithwaite, *Ambulance Wagon*, 115–16.
42 Braithwaite, *Ambulance Wagon*, 117.
43 "Memorandum by Mr. Sidney Webb to the Chancellor of the Exchequer," in ibid, 307–10. Robert A. Lyster, M.O.H. of Hampshire, was the spokesman for the delegation of M.O.H. See Robert A. Lyster, "Sickness Insurance and Public Health," *Br. Med. J.* (1911), no. 1: 507–8 or *Public Health*, 29 (1910–11), 239–40. On the meeting with the delegation of M.O.H., see Braithwaite, *Ambulance Wagon*, 122–3. For the opposition of the Society of Medical Officers of Health to the insurance scheme, see Porter [Watkins], "English Revolution," 235–9.
44 Webb, *Our Partnership*, 470; or Webb, *Diary*, 3: 153. See also Webb, *Our Partnership*, 473–4; or Webb, *Diary*, 3: 158–9.

By the end of March Newsholme and other L.G.B. officials had seen Braith-waite's draft and were in regular consultation with him about its provisions. But by this time there was little prospect of change. The drafting of the insurance scheme is best understood as a grand exercise in interest-group politics, a masterful balancing and neutralizing of special interests.[45] In preparing his scheme Lloyd George worked to placate and to win support of primarily three groups: first, the friendly societies, who had a large working-class membership and experience in administering sickness and disability benefits; second, commercial insurance companies, who had a huge financial stake in small life insurance policies sold to working-class families by weekly premiums and hence a potentially great political force in their army of collecting agents; and third, the British Medical Association, whose members were necessary to implement Part I of the scheme. By compari-son the views of local authorities, their Medical Officers of Health, and the L.G.B. counted for little in the Chancellor's political equations.

By this time it had already been decided that the insurance plan would apply to all manual workers, and that weekly contributions would come compulsorily from the employee – by deductions from the pay envelope – and the employer in equal amounts with the Treasury adding a smaller additional sum.[46] In return for these contributions the insured would be entitled to the unlimited services of a general practitioner, including drugs and appliances, to special medical services in the event of tuberculosis – the Sanatorium Benefit – and to certain cash benefits: sick pay for the first twenty-six weeks of illness, and disability benefit thereafter. Lloyd George added a cash maternity benefit in early April, soon after negotiations began between the L.G.B. and the Treasury. The insured were to be enrolled in approved societies, which would receive the weekly contributions made on behalf of the insured and administer the benefits. While any group meeting minimum standards of democratic governance and nonprofit status might qualify under the scheme as an approved society, most approved societies were friendly societies, divisions of commercial insurance companies, or trade unions. The Chancellor had at first intended that the approved societies would administer all benefits, just as friendly societies then provided both cash and service benefits, but in the face of strong opposition from the B.M.A., whose members had long chafed under the terms of club practice, he turned the administration of the medical and the sanatorium benefit over to local insurance committees (during the planning known variously as joint health committees or local health committees). He also added representatives of local practitioners to these proposed committees whose other members represented the insured and local authorities. At the center, the government scheme was to be administered by the National Health Insurance Joint Committee operating under the Treasury.

The scheme had certain guarantees of fiscal soundness, and as an additional

45 This interpretation is persuasively made in Gilbert, *National Insurance*, 289–416. ⸱
46 For detailed accounts of this stage of the planning, see Braithwaite, *Ambulance Wagon*, 91–143; and Gilbert, *National Insurance*, 339–52.

protection of approved society funds, at Braithwaite's suggestion, the plan included an Excessive Sickness Clause.[47] This clause provided that if the sickness among the insured in a region was for three consecutive years 10 percent or more in excess of the ordinary rate, the local health committee could collect compensation for the added burden on the insurance fund from employers who permitted hazardous industrial conditions, from homeowners who were responsible for unhealthy housing, and from local authorities who tolerated unsanitary conditions.

The insurance plan caused alarm among the staff of the L.G.B. that was nearly as intense as that in Fabian circles. By creating a new local and central administrative apparatus independent of the L.G.B., the Chancellor's bill signaled the intention of the New Liberals to bypass the L.G.B. in social welfare initiatives. The L.G.B. sent strong representations to Braithwaite and to the Chancellor, defending its territory and opposing the plan.[48] Braithwaite reported that the Board's officials treated him like an interloper during their negotiations.[49] The Board's officials claimed that in creating a new unit of local government, the joint health committee, the plan would cause administrative confusion and upset the orderly development of local government which had been going on successfully for some fifty years. The plan would also cause unnecessary duplication of services, inefficiency, and friction with local authorities. The excessive sickness clause was especially objectionable and would provoke strong political opposition from local authorities who, the Board's officials predicted, would embarrass the government in the House of Commons. Furthermore, by providing a Sanatorium Benefit, the bill would discourage voluntary contribution to charitable institutions and would duplicate the services offered by local authority hospitals.

We know indirectly that Newsholme had strong reservations about the national insurance bill. In the twenties and thirties, after he had left the civil service, he wrote about these at length in a number of his publications that we will consider in Part III of this book. But at the time, he made no public statements about the plan, and we must try to reconstruct his views from surviving L.G.B. memoranda and from Braithwaite's memoirs. Newsholme prepared memoranda on the public health and medical aspects of the plan for Braithwaite's eyes[50] and on the administrative implications of the scheme for the secretarial staff of the Board.[51] Surviving

47 The clause became Clause 63 of the National Insurance Act, 1 & 2 Geo. 5, C. 55. Braithwaite claimed authorship of this clause in Braithwaite, *Ambulance Wagon*, 128, 136–7. For a copy of the clause at this stage, see Clause 34 of draft bill dated 4 April 1911 in P.R.O., Pin 3/3, 74.

48 See, for example, the following L.G.B. memoranda: "Insurance Scheme," 3 April 1911, P.R.O., Pin 3/3; and "National Insurance Bill," 26 June 1911, P.R.O. Pin 3/4.

49 Braithwaite, *Ambulance Wagon*, 70.

50 Arthur Newsholme, "Critical Notes on Insurance Scheme, made from the standpoint of Preventive Medicine," 28 March 1911, P.R.O., Pin 3/3. This paper was sent directly to Braithwaite. See Newsholme to Braithwaite, 28 March 1911, ibid.

51 Arthur Newsholme, "Skeleton of Administrative Arrangements under Sickness Insurance Scheme," 31 March 1911, P.R.O., Pin 3/3; Arthur Newsholme, "Memorandum on Clause 41 of National Health Insurance Bill (Draft of 7th April, 1911)," 8 April 1911, ibid.; and Arthur Newsholme, "Memorandum on the Present Position of the National Insurance Bill, in relation to Public Health Administration," 15 June 1911, P.R.O., Pin 3/4.

evidence suggests that he provided much of the substance of the L.G.B. opposition to the Chancellor's bill. It was Newsholme, for example, who provided the examples and arguments that the Excessive Sickness Clause would prove unworkable.[52] Not only would enforcement prove counterproductive, provoking hostility between the joint health committee and the local authority and its officials, but the resulting high legal fees would erode the insurance fund and lower benefits. The entire proposal to assess financial damages for illness was misguided. Only in exceptional circumstances, examples of which he provided, was it possible to demonstrate conclusively that a particular amount of sickness was caused by specific negligence. It is quite likely that Newsholme had in mind the trouble he had experienced in Brighton trying to demonstrate that illness was caused by diseased meat or by contaminated shellfish.

As time would demonstrate amply, there were major defects in the Chancellor's plan. The medical benefits were a comparatively late addition to the scheme and were never intended as a comprehensive national system of health care but merely as part of a plan for income protection for working-class families.[53] These facts coupled with the effect of crafting the proposal during private conferences of interested parties help account for some of the proposal's structural defects. Newsholme, like many medical spokesmen, was troubled that the medical provisions of the plan would expand and provide government subsidy for club practice.[54] Friendly society medical services, he asserted, were notoriously inadequate. Care was offered by general practitioners who worked without the benefit of consultations with specialists or access to hospital facilities. Furthermore, the Chancellor proposed to continue the system of paying these doctors by capitation. In the hands of the clubs, this system resulted in levels of remuneration so low that most doctors devoted too little time to each patient for proper examination. In the government plan, because physicians' incomes depended upon the number of patients they could attract to their panel, and because patients would be able to choose the doctor whose panel they joined, Newsholme worried that undue pressure would be placed on panel doctors to certify sickness or disability. This had been the result, he alleged, in the friendly societies where members annually elected their club doctor. Such an arrangement, he predicted, would encourage malingering and deplete insurance funds. This concern to prevent malingering and to protect the fund probably reflects Fabian mistrust of the friendly societies as well as Newsholme's realization that such cautionary points were most likely to gain attention in the Treasury.

Newsholme demanded changes in the medical benefits that reflect both medical distrust of club practice and a preference for administration by experts: access to

52 Newsholme, "Memorandum on Clause 41."   53 Gilbert, *National Insurance*, 289, 314, 315–16.
54 For the following comments, see Newsholme, "Critical Notes on Insurance Scheme," 1 & 2–3; and Newsholme, "Skeleton of Administrative Arrangements," 2–3, 9. In this context Newsholme also referred to his testimony before the Royal Commission on the Poor Laws, Newsholme, Poor Law Commission, 9: 160 #20.

specialist consultations, the use of medical referees in cases where certifications of sickness or disability were in dispute, and the transfer of the medical benefit from approved societies to the local health committees.[55] He was much more worried, however, about the effect of the national insurance proposal on the nation's public health apparatus and on the system of municipal health services which local authorities were constructing. The Chancellor's plan threatened the unified system of municipal health services Newsholme had championed before the Poor Law Commission. Like the other chief officials at the L.G.B., Newsholme argued that the adoption of the government's insurance scheme would produce duplication and competition with the medical services local authorities were offering and would, in effect, create a third system of publicly administered medical services alongside those of the local sanitary authorities under the L.G.B. and of the local education authorities under the Board of Education.[56] He was especially concerned with the Sanatorium Benefit and argued that the treatment of tuberculosis ought to be left to local authorities.[57] In fact, as we will see in the next chapter, the implementation of the Sanatorium Benefit caused great administrative difficulty, and the benefit was removed from the Insurance Commissioners soon after the Armistice. Newsholme did not accept Lloyd George's decision to make a special case of tuberculosis. Newsholme would have the treatment of tuberculosis left to local sanitary authorities who would bear the cost of treatment jointly with the Treasury. He hoped that the national insurance bill would provide the occasion for Parliament to require local authorities to make adequate provision for the treatment not only of tuberculosis but of all the major acute infectious diseases.

In this respect, as in others, Newsholme intended to make National Insurance promote the system of preventive medicine local authorities were evolving. This could be done within the proposed scheme, he reasoned, if the planned local or joint health committees (the future local insurance committees) were to become statutory committees of the County or the County Borough Council in the same way that the local education authority was a statutory committee of the County or County Borough Council. This was his most fundamental suggestion, the one he made consistently during the negotiations with Treasury officials.[58] Newsholme had in mind filling the new committee not only with representatives of the insured and of local practitioners but with a significant number of members from the local sanitary committee. This arrangement would assure proper communication between insurance and public health authorities. It would also permit the

55 Newsholme, "Critical Notes on Insurance Scheme," 3.
56 Newsholme, "Skeleton of Administrative Arrangements," 11.
57 He made this suggestion early in the negotiations with the Treasury: Newsholme, "Skeleton of Administrative Arrangements," 10. In June after Lloyd George had promised the medical profession higher capitation fees and it seemed that the scheme would prove more costly, Newsholme made this suggestion again even more directly, Newsholme, "Memorandum on Present Position," 2–4.
58 For the following discussion, see Newsholme, "Critical Notes on Insurance Scheme," 7–8; Newsholme, "Skeleton of Administrative Arrangements under Sickness Insurance Scheme," 1, 4–8; and Newsholme, "Memorandum on the Present Position," 2.

insurance committee to use local officials – M.O.H., Town Clerk, Accountant – in conducting its work. Efficiency and economies of scale would result, and administrative friction would be reduced, as would overlap between the work of the insurance committee and the substantial medical services some local authorities already offered, including sanatoriums, diagnostic laboratories, medical services to schoolchildren, and supervision of midwives.

If the insurance scheme were coordinated with the work of sanitary authorities through this sort of administrative consolidation, health insurance would not only palliate and provide treatment, but it would also help raise the level of public health. To this end Newsholme wanted to be assured that the boundaries of the districts overseen by the insurance committees would coincide with those of sanitary authorities, that the insurance committees would be required to keep good records of sickness among the insured, and that Medical Officers of Health would be given access to these records and would be required to include a section on them in their annual report.[59] This information on sickness in his district would materially assist the M.O.H. in locating the causes of preventable illness, and in so doing, it would render the Excess Sickness Clause unnecessary.

In trying to protect the preventive programs local authorities had initiated, Newsholme was doing what might be reasonably expected of the Medical Officer of the Local Government Board. But his memoranda suggest that he had other intentions as well. During the negotiations over the Chancellor's proposal, Newsholme hoped that properly constituted insurance committees of the local council would "swallow up" club practice.[60] In his proposal that the Sanatorium Benefit be dropped from the insurance scheme, he concluded, "I hope that these proposals would lead to the Councils of the County Councils and County Boroughs taking over the control of clinics for all diseases and the arrangements for institutional and expert treatment of disease: but I have preferred to confine the proposals to Tuberculosis."[61] Further indication of his intent is suggested in his memorandum of March 28. "Although the system of medical attendance under the 'Public Health Board' [i.e., insurance committee] will at present in most instances remain independent of the other branches of medical work of the Sanitary Authorities and their Education Committees, it is important that the arrangements should be such as will lend themselves to future amalgamations."[62] He still held to the hope that a way might be found through national health insurance to create a unified system of medical services under local authority control.

During these negotiations Newsholme's efforts won the respect of Treasury officials. In his memoirs Braithwaite portrayed no other L.G.B. official in favorable light, but he remembered Newsholme with appreciation. He considered Newsholme a "whole hearted L.G.B. man," but he acknowledged that Newsholme gave

59 Newsholme, "Memorandum on Clause 41," 5.
60 Newsholme, "Skeleton of Administrative Arrangements," 1.
61 Newsholme, "Memorandum on the Present Position," 5.
62 Newsholme, "Critical Notes on Insurance Scheme," 8.

"very good advice and much help."[63] He recognized the cogency of Newsholme's arguments, which he credited with causing certain changes in the insurance plan. Newsholme's memoranda guaranteed, for example, that the local insurance committee would not have the administration of the Sanatorium Benefit. But while Newsholme and other L.G.B. officials were able to win concessions on details, they failed to win their major objectives. The local insurance committee was not made a statutory committee of the County or the County Borough Council. This Lloyd George adamantly refused to allow. In order to gain the support of the friendly societies, he had promised that this would not happen, and he proved very happy to honor this promise.[64] He might also have anticipated strong opposition from organized medicine, if he gave control of the scheme to local authorities.[65] The architects of national insurance also refused to let local authorities have a majority on the local insurance committee. Braithwaite reported that Lloyd George would have given the ratepayers a majority on the committee, only if they would agree to share financial liability for the insurance scheme, but that there was no political support for that alternative.[66] The Chancellor also would not agree to remove the Sanatorium Benefit from the plan as Newsholme recommended. Lloyd George, from nearly the beginning, had insisted on special arrangements for tuberculosis within the insurance plan. Although there are several probable reasons that the Sanatorium Benefit was included in the insurance scheme, Lloyd George seems to have had a singular interest in tuberculosis. Braithwaite believed it sprang from the Chancellor's personal fear of the disease.[67]

Finally, there was the matter of the Excessive Sickness Clause. So certain was Newsholme that the clause was impossible, that he bet Braithwaite £1 that it would not make it into the Act, a bet he settled in the Gallery of the House of Commons when the clause was adopted without opposition.[68] Once again, Lloyd George's personal interest in the clause seems to explain its legislative success. The Chancellor turned a deaf ear to the predictions of local authorities and the L.G.B. that it would be unworkable and counterproductive, and he refused to "take the ginger out of the bill" by removing the clause.[69] In the House of Commons, he answered objections to it by reading juicy selections from M.O.H. and L.G.B. reports describing the sanitary shortcomings in his opponents' districts.[70]

The political triumph represented in the passage of national health insurance

63 Braithwaite, *Ambulance Wagon*, 138, 139.
64 Gilbert, *National Insurance*, 419.
65 Newsholme gives this as the reason for Lloyd George's refusal. Newsholme, *Last 30 Years*, 114. The British Medical Association did mount strong opposition to the implementation of the scheme. See Gilbert, *National Insurance*, 362–8, 401–16.
66 Braithwaite, *Ambulance Wagon*, 134.   67 Ibid., 71.
68 Newsholme, *Last 30 Years*, 114; and Braithwaite, *Ambulance Wagon*, 138–9, 221.
69 Braithwaite, *Ambulance Wagon*, 142.   70 Ibid., 221.

should not obscure the very real deficiencies of the 1911 Act.[71] Only a portion of the population was covered – one-third in 1911 rising to about one-half by the Second World War. Not only were nonmanual laborers earning more than the allowable maximum income excluded, but so were the self-employed, the unemployed, and dependents of the insured. Those who were covered were guaranteed only a minimum of medical services and modest cash benefits. Although they might be provided as additional benefits out of approved society surpluses, dental, optical, or nursing services were not assured. Nor was the attention of specialists or hospital treatment guaranteed except in the event of tuberculosis. While the Act guaranteed a cash maternity benefit for insured women and for the wives of insured men, the Act also provided no prenatal services or medical or midwifery attention at the time of delivery.

Most seriously of all, the system of administering the Act, pieced together so carefully with a practical political eye, proved to be a great liability. The price Lloyd George believed he had to pay to secure the Act's passage was to turn over the administration of much of the Act to private organizations – friendly societies, trade unions, and even divisions of commercial insurance companies – each of whom stood to benefit from administering the Act.[72] The requirement that approved societies be run democratically proved to be a fiction, so that complying proved to be no great burden for commercial insurance companies. These companies in fact found it very advantageous to operate approved societies to help finance the cost of their large staff of agents and as a means to sell commercial insurance policies to those enrolled in their approved societies.

Approved societies were free to compete for members throughout the kingdom. This meant that these societies differed greatly in size, in the geographical distribution of their members, and in their financial soundness. There would eventually be some 8,000 approved societies and their branches, whose membership varied between a mere 50 to over 2 million insured.[73] Persons working in the same workshop or factory might belong to many different approved societies, and the membership of any society might be scattered throughout the kingdom. At one time during the middle twenties, for example, ninety-eight approved societies had only one member in Glasgow.[74] The result was very great inefficiency in administration. The British national insurance scheme in fact had the highest

---

71 1 & 2 Geo 5, Ch. 55 became law 16 Dec. 1911. Contributions to the scheme began 15 July 1912, and benefits were awarded beginning on 15 Jan. 1913. For a discussion of the deficiencies of the National Insurance Act, see Harry Eckstein, *The English Health Service: Its Origins, Structure, and Achievements* (Cambridge, Mass.: Harvard Univ. Press, 1958), 19–29; *Health Insurance in Great Britain, 1911–1948: Social Security Series, Memorandum No. 11* (Ottawa: Department of National Health and Welfare, 1952), 111–33; and Charles Webster, *The Health Services Since the War*, I: Problems of Health Care, The National Health Service before 1957 (London: HMSO, 1988), 11, 14.
72 Eckstein, *English Health Service*, 23–6.   73 *Health Insurance in Great Britain*, 9.
74 Ibid., 126.

administrative cost, despite its comparatively low benefits, of any of the early twentieth-century European schemes.[75]

This inefficiency reduced the amount of money available for benefits. The system also distributed these benefits very unequally. Since an insured member's access to additional benefits depended on the surplus in his or her approved society, those insured who had the misfortune to have enrolled with a society which drew its members largely from hazardous industries or from less healthy areas were more likely to receive only the guaranteed benefits. Those with chronic health problems who were unable to find any approved society willing to enroll them fared even worse. Their only alternative might be to become Deposit Contributors. As such they were treated as a special category for which the insurance scheme assumed only minimal responsibility. Not only were Deposit Contributors ineligible for any supplemental benefits, but unlike the rest of the insured population they faced a strict limit in cash benefits, the amount that had actually been contributed in their behalf. The collective effect of features such as these was that some people who needed benefits the most were the least likely to receive them. The fact that benefits might vary so greatly, although each insured worker contributed the same amount weekly to the fund, has led some critics of the scheme to label its financial arrangements "a regressive head tax," and to suggest that the insured would have done much better for the same contributions if the Act had been administered differently.[76] Others have made much harsher judgments: "These arrangements constitute one of the more absurd chapters in the history of public health administration and the way they were worked out one of the more shoddy episodes in the evolution of British social legislation."[77]

Judgments such as these are made with the benefit of hindsight and from the perspective of an age when the National Health Service had become a reality and the novelty of the 1911 legislation was long forgotten. Those who debated the terms of the insurance bill in those anxious months in the spring and summer of 1911 could not anticipate exactly how the insurance system would unfold. It is remarkable, all the same, to notice how accurately Newsholme anticipated some the scheme's consequences and faults. The Excessive Sickness Clause did prove unworkable and was never used. Even Braithwaite admitted that it soon became "another rusty, musty weapon in the armoury of law."[78] Similarly the Sanatorium Benefit was retained in the insurance scheme only through the War and then eliminated in 1921 and the treatment of tuberculosis turned over to local authorities as Newsholme had suggested a decade earlier.[79] Newsholme had also foreseen that the appearance of a state insurance system would have serious implications for voluntary hospitals, and he predicted that they would eventually become state

75 Eckstein, *English Health Service*, 26.   76 *Health Insurance in Great Britain*, 122.
77 Eckstein, *English Health Service*, 21.
78 Braithwaite, *Ambulance Wagon*, 221. See also Newsholme, *Last 30 Years*, 114.
79 *Health Insurance in Great Britain*, 19; and F. B. Smith, *The Retreat of Tuberculosis 1850–1950* (London, New York, Sydney: Croom Helm, 1988), 108.

institutions.[80] In this, of course, he was proven wrong in the short run but correct in the long, when the National Health Service Act nationalized most of the nation's private hospitals.[81]

Most important of all, experience demonstrated that it had been a mistake to separate national health insurance from the nation's other health services and to insulate the administration of the medical benefits from the public health and welfare services local authorities provided. Upon the creation of the Ministry of Health, National Insurance was for the first time in the same ministry as the public health service, but that consolidation did not remedy the more fundamental administrative problems. By the time the Royal Commission on National Health Insurance met in 1926, informed opinion was nearly unanimous that the benefits offered under the insurance scheme were too limited in nature, too limited in distribution, and that the medical benefit must be brought into closer coordination with the work of local health authorities.[82] The Majority Report of this Commission recommended that the local Insurance Committee be abolished and its responsibilities be turned over to local authorities. The Minority Report agreed and suggested that the Approved Societies suffer the same fate, and local authorities take over all local administration of national insurance. The majority report concluded that in the long term the deficiencies in medical services under national health insurance would best be met by "divorcing the medical service entirely from the insurance system and recognizing it along with all the other public health activities as a service to be supported from the general public funds."[83] What such a recommendation would have meant in detail cannot now be ascertained, but the spirit of the recommendation is certainly like that Newsholme had suggested before the Royal Commission on the Poor Laws and in negotiations with Treasury officials over Lloyd George's insurance scheme.

Although history has vindicated many of Newsholme's assessments of the National Insurance scheme, and although he fought doggedly to secure changes in the scheme, his efforts were at best rear-guard actions. The campaign to secure National Insurance was nearly won before the L.G.B. joined the fight. Some of his critics blamed him for his failure to effect more successfully policy changes from within the civil service,[84] but such judgments are hardly fair. Any fair assessment of Newsholme's performance at the L.G.B. must recognize the restraints of his office and the circumstances under which he served. It must also be based on criteria more closely related to his official responsibilities rather than on

80 Newsholme, "Critical Notes on Insurance Scheme," 6.
81 See Brian Able-Smith, *The Hospitals 1800–1948: A Study in Social Administration in England and Wales* (Cambridge, Mass., Harvard Univ. Press, 1964), 488–502; and Eckstein, *English Health Service,* 178–92.
82 For a summary of the recommendations of the Majority and the Minority Reports, see *Report of the Royal Commission on National Health Insurance,* B.P.P., 1926, XVI, Cmd. 2596, 274–91, 327–9. For a discussion of these recommendations, see *Health Insurance in Great Britain,* 111–12, 127–31.
83 *Royal Commission of National Health Insurance,* 65–6.
84 See, for example, George Newman's report of his conversation with the Webbs, Newman, *Diary,* 2 (18 Dec. 1913).

the outcome of complex political decisions such as whether the Minority Report of the Poor Law Commission was implemented, National Insurance created, or a Ministry of Health established. Much more directly related to Newsholme's office were major initiatives in disease prevention made during his years in Whitehall. It is fair to ask what Newsholme thought of these initiatives and what influence he had on the shape the new programs took. In this context we will emphasize the evolution of measures to prevent tuberculosis, syphilis, and infant mortality. These proved to be very important new ventures, not only extending the role of the state in protecting the health of its citizens but changing the character of public health work. Besides these policy innovations Newsholme can also be judged on how well he carried out the Medical Officer's responsibility to monitor the health of the nation and to investigate outbreaks of disease. It was here that Newsholme's experience as an epidemiologist was particularly important. Some of his most ambitious epidemiological studies were undertaken at the L.G.B., where he had greater opportunity for national and international studies than he had had at Brighton. We will consider in particular the five major studies he and his staff prepared on infant, child, and maternal mortality, which appeared as supplements to his Annual Reports.[85]

85 Arthur Newsholme, *Infant and Child Mortality, Suppl. Ann. Rep. Med. Off. L.G.B.* 39 (1909–10); Arthur Newsholme, *Second Report on Infant and Child Mortality, Suppl. Ann. Rep. Med. Off. L.G.B.,* 42 (1912–13); Arthur Newsholme et al., *Third Report on Infant Mortality Dealing with Infant Mortality in Lancashire, Suppl. Ann. Rep. Med. Off. L.G.B.,* 43 (1913–14); and Arthur Newsholme, *Report on Child Mortality at Ages 0–5 in England and Wales, Suppl. Ann. Rep. Med. Off. L.G.B.,* 45 (1915–16).

9

Launching a national tuberculosis program

NOTIFICATION AND ITS USES

At the top of Newsholme's agenda when he joined the Local Government Board was the launching of a national tuberculosis program. His experience in Brighton led him to envision a comprehensive strategy operating on national guidelines but organized and administered by local health authorities. Notification of cases to the Medical Officer of Health would be the starting point. He never thought of notification as a mere statistical or administrative exercise. It must be the beginning of constructive action by local authorities. While M.O.H. in Brighton, he held that towns should not initiate notification of tuberculosis until they were prepared to offer the patient whose case was notified "all possible help" in return.[1] Once in Whitehall and after notification was compulsory, he continued to insist that the justification for notification was what followed.

It is only when the medical officer of health, the tuberculosis officer and the medical practitioner co-operate in securing the patient's welfare, by improving the conditions under which he lives and works, by measures of cleansing and disinfection, by safeguarding the health of the patient's family, and by a course of institutional treatment when this is indicated, that the possible utility of notification is realised.[2]

We have seen in Chapter 6 that there had been some professional opposition to notification of tuberculosis and a widely held apprehension that compulsory notification would be followed by social and economic discrimination against the disease's victims. While in Brighton, Newsholme stayed well clear of trouble by relying on voluntary notification. But by the time he joined the L.G.B., he was convinced that opinion in local government and in the medical profession had changed. Notification, both voluntary and compulsory, had been in force in a

---

1 Arthur Newsholme, "The Voluntary Notification of Phthisis in Brighton," *J. Roy. Sanitary Inst.*, 28 (1907): 34. Near the end of his career in Whitehall he repeated the claim that the utility of notification was to be measured by the benefit to the patient in Arthur Newsholme, "The Relations of Tuberculosis to War Conditions. With Remarks on Some Aspects of the Administrative Control of Tuberculosis," *Lancet* (1917), no. 2: 593.
2 Newsholme, *Ann. Rep. Med. Off. L.G.B.*, 46 (1916–17): xxiv.

number of towns for several years, and local authorities now were petitioning the
L.G.B. with increasing frequency in favor of compulsory notification and requesting permission to add tuberculosis to the list of infectious diseases already
notifiable in their jurisdictions.[3] Furthermore, resolutions favoring notification
were issued by prominent organizations: the International Congress on Tuberculosis in 1908, the Council of the British Medical Association in 1909, and the
Association of Municipal Corporations in 1910.

Newsholme concluded that the nation would accept the compulsory notification of all cases of the disease if such notification were implemented gradually and
did not result in added hardship for patients or their families. Accordingly, in April
1908 he proposed that compulsory notification be introduced in stages beginning,
as he had in Brighton, with those in receipt of poor relief, that is, the socially
most dependent and those whose privacy was least precious to public opinion.[4]
Gradually the scheme could be broadened. As he explained to his superiors, this
"step by step" approach would permit the Board to "educate public opinion &
prepare san[itar]y authorities for the further administrative control of this disease."[5]

This plan was eventually carried out in four stages, each initiated by an order from
the L.G.B. The Board first ordered Poor Law doctors to notify cases they discovered
in paupers beginning on the first of January 1909.[6] The order was limited to cases of
pulmonary tuberculosis and required that notification be made within forty-eight
hours to the M.O.H. of the district in which the patient lived and, when a patient
was about to be discharged from a Poor Law institution, to the M.O.H. of the district to which the patient was bound. The next stage extended notification to the
working poor. Beginning May 1, 1911, notification was required of pulmonary
cases discovered in hospital and dispensary practice.[7] The third order applied to pulmonary cases discovered in the entire population and went into effect January 1,
1912.[8] Finally the previous orders were consolidated, and tuberculosis in all its forms
was made universally notifiable on February 1, 1913.[9]

This orderly progression of regulations, each extending the scope of people and
pathologies coming under the scrutiny of public officials, disguises the strong
conflicts involved in issuing these orders. It is worth considering the way in which

3 For these petitions and the following resolutions, see Arthur Newsholme, "Proposal for the Compulsory Notification of Cases of Pulmonary Tuberculosis Coming under the Care of the Physicians of
Public Hospitals and Dispensaries," 23 April 1910, 3–5, P.R.O., MH55/525
4 Newsholme to Sir S. Provis (Permanent Secretary) and President (John Burns), 14 April 1908,
P.R.O. MH55/523. He repeated his plan in Newsholme to Provis and President, 7 Aug. 1908, ibid.
5 Newsholme to F. J. Willis, 17 Oct. 1911, P.R.O., MH55/526.
6 Public Health (Tuberculosis) Regulations, 1908. The order and accompanying circular letter can be
found in *Ann. Rep. Med. Off. L.G.B.*, 38 (1908–9): 221–32.
7 Public Health (Tuberculosis in Hospitals) Regulations, 1911. For the order and accompanying
circulars, see ibid., 40 (1910–11): 253–8.
8 Public Health (Tuberculosis) Regulations, 1911. For copies of the order and circulars, see ibid., 41
(1911–12): 188–95.
9 Public Health (Tuberculosis) Regulations, 1912. See ibid., 42 (1912–13): 312–24 for the order and
circulars.

these regulations appeared, because the process is indicative both of how the
L.G.B. conducted its business and of the unsettling effect the National Insurance
Act had on the Board's plans. Surviving evidence suggests that Newsholme was
the moving force in the L.G.B. behind these orders, although it is also clear that
at critical times he had the backing of John Burns, the President, and of F. J.
Willis, the newly appointed Assistant Secretary to whom Newsholme reported.[10]

The first order, the one requiring notification of pauper cases, brought protests
from the Board's Poor Law Medical Officers, who were under the Poor Law
Department, not the Medical Department. This intra-agency contest of authority
was couched in terms of economy and efficiency and worries that notification
would deter patients from seeking medical attention.[11] Newsholme answered
these objections with cost estimates of his own which were much lower than
what the Poor Law Department projected.[12] Of greater moment was the serious
objection the Legal Department raised to the authority the Board proposed to use
to issue these orders. The L.G.B.'s senior officials preferred not to seek new
legislation for tuberculosis notification.[13] Short of obtaining a new law they might,
of course, have permitted local authorities to add tuberculosis to the list of diseases
compulsorily notifiable under the Infectious Disease (Notification) Act, 1889, or
the Infectious Disease (Notification) Extension Act, 1899. As we have seen, the
Board had steadfastly refused to let local authorities act in this way, fearing such
action would create additional hardship and greater economic dependency among
tuberculosis victims.[14] A third approach open to the Board was to require notification using the authority it possessed under more omnibus legislation. After some
hesitancy in 1908, during which time it considered issuing the first order using its
authority under the Poor Law, it issued all four orders under the broad powers
granted to it in Section 130 of the Public Health Act, 1875, as amended in 1891
and 1896. This section authorized the Board to issue regulations for the treatment
or the prevention of cholera or other epidemic, endemic, or infectious disease.

10 The most important sources of information on the struggle within the L.G.B. over these orders are
   the following Ministry of Health files in the Public Record Office: MH55/523, MH55/525,
   MH55/526, and MH55/521. For suggestions of Burns's support of Newsholme's position, see
   Newsholme to Willis, 28 July 1910, P.R.O., MH55/525; Alfred Adrian, "Notification of Pulmonary Tuberculosis," 1 Oct. 1908, P.R.O., MH55/523; and Burns, minute, 8 Dec. 1908, P.R.O.,
   MH55/523. When he signed the draft of the 1908 regulations, Burns noted in his diary with
   characteristic brevity, "Thus begins a new stage of warfare against this social disease"; Burns
   Appointment Diary, 20 Aug. 1908, Add. Mss. 46330. The diary shows that he followed the process
   of drafting these orders and that he noted his pleasure in signing each successive order. See, for
   example, Burns, Diary, 9 March 1911 and 15 Nov. 1911, Add. Mss. 46333. For Willis's support of
   compulsory notification, see Willis to Monro, 25 May 1910, P.R.O., MH55/525.
11 Arthur Downes (Medical Inspector for Poor Law Purposes), minute of 6 Oct. 1908, P.R.O.
   MH55/523.
12 Arthur Newsholme "Notification of Pulmonary Tuberculosis," memorandum of 21 Oct. 1908,
   ibid.
13 S.B.P. (Provis) to President, 22 Aug. 1908, ibid.
14 Under Newsholme the Medical Department continued to oppose proposals to make pulmonary
   tuberculosis notifiable under these acts. H. F. Parsons, minute of 25 Sept. 1908, ibid.

The Legal Department favored a narrower reading of Section 130 than the Medical Department proposed. Two successive legal advisers questioned whether tuberculosis was a contagious, epidemic, or endemic disease under the meaning of Section 130. In 1910 the new Legal Adviser, John Lithiby, a former Assistant Secretary, even questioned whether the Board had acted properly in issuing the 1908 Regulations under authority of Section 130.[15] That section, he claimed, was clearly intended to apply to sea-borne epidemics such as Asiatic cholera and could not have been intended for use against a disease such as pulmonary tuberculosis, which was not even recognized as contagious in 1875. He vigorously objected to Newsholme's suggestion that the Board use Section 130 again and predicted that hospitals would challenge the Board's legal authority to require notification of pulmonary tuberculosis among their patients. In repeated conferences and in memoranda and minutes Newsholme argued that tuberculosis was in fact an infectious disease and that it was not unreasonable to consider it both contagious and endemic under the terms of Section 130.[16] This dispute was resolved to Newsholme's satisfaction only on appeal to the Law Officers of the Crown.[17] This was an important administrative victory, because it allowed the Board to escape some of the limitations of the Infectious Diseases (Notification) Act, 1889, and Infectious Diseases (Notification) Extension Act, 1899. By invoking Section 130, not only could the Board make a disease notifiable in all administrative areas at once, but it could require additional information about patients, place conditions on the use of that information, and suggest action that should follow notification. Following Newsholme's advice, the Board acted in this way to require notification of acute poliomyelitis and cerebrospinal fever (cerebrospinal meningitis) in 1912, ophthalmia neonatorium in 1914, and measles and German measles in 1915.[18]

Other objections to the notification orders for tuberculosis came from outside the Board. During the first year that pauper cases were notified, M.O.H. and sanitary authorities wrote to complain about incomplete forms or wrong addresses and to object that doctors were being overcompensated by being allowed to file

15 J. Lithiby to H. C. Monro (now Permanent Secretary), 1 July 1910, P.R.O., MH55/525.
16 For the following arguments by Newsholme, see Newsholme to Sir S. Provis, 19 Aug. 1908, P.R.O., MH55/523; and H. C. Parsons (Assistant Medical Officer), minute of 25 Sept. 1908, ibid. Parsons was writing at Newsholme's instruction.
17 This appeal is referred to in several L.G.B. minutes. See J. Lithiby to H. C. Monro, 1 July 1910, Arthur Newsholme minutes to H. C. Monro, 9 July 1910, 28 July 1910, 17 Nov. 1910, P.R.O., MH55/525.
18 The orders in question are Public Health (Cere-spinal Fever and Acute Poliomyelitis) Regulations, 1912; Public Health (Ophthalmia Neonatorum) Regulations, 1914; and Public Health (Measles and German Measles) Regulations), 1915. A copy of the order of cero-spinal fever and poliomyelitis may be found in *Ann. Rep. Med. Off. L.G.B.*, 42 (1912–13): 326–8. The year before the Board had issued a circular and memoranda by Newsholme on these diseases and advised local authorities to take action to prevent them, including requiring notification of them under the Infectious Diseases (Notification) Acts. See ibid., 41 (1911–12): 198–202. For Newsholme's comments on the advantages of using the newer strategy for requiring notification, see Newsholme, testimony, Royal Commission on Venereal Diseases, *Appendix to Final Report*, B.P.P., 1916, XVI, 217.

frequent notifications for the same patient.[19] Some Poor Law doctors objected however, to the added work and to the small size of the remuneration. A year or so later came the reaction of hospital managers and medical staff to the proposal to extend notification to hospital and dispensary cases. Although many hospitals acknowledged that notification might be desirable from a public health standpoint, and while some welcomed a compulsory scheme because it would free their staff from having to decide which cases to notify voluntarily, friction with local sanitary authorities over the working of some voluntary schemes had soured a few hospitals on notification in any form.[20] Other hospital managers feared that notification would deter patients with tuberculosis from seeking help early, especially if hospitals were singled out and made responsible for notifying while private practitioners were exempt.

The struggle to issue the second order, the one requiring notification in hospital and dispensary practice, proved to be the most contentious. It was at this point that Newsholme found an important ally in F. J. Willis. The Assistant Secretary, in fact, urged bolder action than Newsholme was recommending. In May 1910 Willis wanted to know why the Board should not move at once to make pulmonary tuberculosis compulsorily notifiable in all patients.[21] He correctly foresaw the objections voluntary hospitals would raise, and he warned that by acting in piecemeal fashion the Board would leave itself open to charges of creating one law for the rich and another for the poor. Perhaps with a mind to strengthening Newsholme's hand in the intra-agency conflict, Willis suggested that the Board investigate how well compulsory notification of pauper cases had worked, specifically what local authorities had done with the information they obtained. The Medical Department was in fact already at work collecting this information, and in late June and early July Newsholme presented John Burns with collections of extracts from M.O.H. reports and responses to questions addressed to M.O.H. and hospital managers which, he insisted, demonstrated that notification had wide support and that the notification of pauper cases had been implemented smoothly with benefit to the public health.[22] Again he was able to carry the day.

Newsholme was well aware that the success of notification depended on the cooperation of medical practitioners and of hospitals, and he worked to see that the Board's policy did not weaken the support that existed in those quarters. He pressured the secretariat of the Board to resist its normal impulse to put economy and efficiency first and instead to use the payment of small fees to foster goodwill

19 See in particular Charles Porter (Honorary Secretary of the Metropolitan Branch of the Incorporated Society of Medical Officers of Health) to Secretary, L.G.B., 3 Feb. 1910, P.R.O., MH55/524; and E. Claude Taylor (Medical Officer, Workhouse, Parish of St. John, Hamstead) 24 May 1910, ibid.
20 See the comments by the M.O.H. of Hamstead and the Secretary of the Mount Vernon Hospital in the collection of extracts presented by Newsholme to John Burns, 23 June 1910, P.R.O. MH55/525; and Newsholme, "Proposal for the Compulsory Notification of Cases," 6–7.
21 F. J. Willis to H. C. Monro, 25 May 1910, P.R.O., MH55/525.
22 Newsholme to President, 23 June 1910, ibid.; and Newsholme to Monro, 9 July 1910, ibid.

and cooperation. The Board should instruct local authorities to pay the prescribed fees even for forms that were not completely filled out and to pay the fees for renotification, even if a second notification came so soon after the first that it seemed superfluous.[23] Newsholme also joined with hospital authorities in unsuccessfully urging that hospital staff be paid at a higher rate than the Board's secretariat proposed, at the same rate (2s6d) that private practitioners were paid under the Infectious Disease (Notification) Acts and not at the rate (1s) at which Poor Law doctors were paid for the compulsory notification of pulmonary tuberculosis.[24]

While the issuing of the first two tuberculosis notification orders was a lengthy, contentious process, the final two orders appeared very quickly and without either conflict within the Board or consultation with health care providers. The order extending compulsory notification of pulmonary tuberculosis to the entire population was drafted, reviewed, approved, and issued in a mere five weeks.[25] The final order, the one extending compulsory notification to nonpulmonary cases, was not issued in such haste, but it was produced within seven months and appeared thirteen months after the third order.[26] The reason for the Board's great hurry is not hard to find. As we saw in the preceding chapter, the Board's officials learned of David Lloyd George's national insurance bill only in late March 1911. They had been successfully outflanked and spent the following few months catching up with the Chancellor and his advisors. During the spring and summer they tried unsuccessfully to secure fundamental changes in the bill. When it became clear that the Chancellor would resist their demands and that the Sanatorium Benefit along with other objectionable clauses would be retained, the officials at the Local Government Board recognized that they had no choice but to move quickly, if they were to salvage any influence on the nation's future health policy. The Sanatorium Benefit promised medical treatment to the insured who suffered from tuberculosis and would thus bring within the realm of the public medical service a much wider segment of the population than that presently covered by the notification orders. Newsholme's and Willis's minutes of mid-October 1911 show that they sensed the need for immediate action and worried that implementation of the Sanatorium Benefit would jeopardize local authority public health schemes.[27] Newsholme more specifically predicted that the local insurance committees, which were to be set up to administer the medical benefits

---

23 Newsholme minutes to John Lithiby (Assistant Secretary), 9 March 1909, and 7 April 1909, P.R.O., MH55/524.

24 Newsholme to Willis, 10 Feb. 1911, P.R.O., MH55/525; and Willis to Monro, 6 March 1911, ibid.

25 For background to the issuing of Public Health (Tuberculosis) Regulations, 1911, see the minutes and drafts in P.R.O., MH55/526 from mid-October to mid-November 1911.

26 For background to the issuing of Public Health (Tuberculosis) Regulations, 1912, see Newsholme, to Willis, Monro, and President, 3 May 1912, and the correspondence between L.G.B. officials and the officials of the Home Office and the National Insurance Commission in September, November, and December 1912 in P.R.O., MH55/521.

27 Willis to Newsholme 12 Oct. 1911, and Newsholme to Willis, 17 Oct. 1911, P.R.O. MH55/526.

under the national insurance scheme, would establish their own systems of notification independent of local health authorities. In view of the importance he placed on unified local authority health administration, that would be a most undesirable outcome.

Throughout the deliberations on the notification orders, Newsholme and the other officials at the L.G.B. were eager to demonstrate that patients would not suffer disadvantages from notification. While the order of 1908, the regulations requiring the notification of Poor Law cases, urged sanitary authorities to use the information obtained from notification to initiate preventive work, it explicitly forbade action which

renders the poor person, or a person in charge of the poor person, or any other person, liable to a penalty, or subjects the poor person to any restriction, prohibition, or disability affecting himself, or his employment, occupation, means of livelihood, or residence, on the ground of his suffering from Pulmonary Tuberculosis.[28]

The later orders carried similar language to protect other sets of patients. Newsholme had supported the inclusion of this section, and early in 1910 he advised that each form for notification of hospital and dispensary cases carry a warning that the information on the form was to be held in strict confidence.[29]

He relied on his experience with notification in Brighton to counter dire predictions. During the deliberations over the first order he observed, "My experience on a large scale of voluntary notification of phthisis, which has included notification of all poor law cases, shows that no disability or inconvenience, but on the contrary increased help to the patient attaches to such notifications."[30] When L.G.B. officials were hearing the concerns of hospital managers about the effects of the proposed hospital notification order, Newsholme argued more emphatically,

I have had ten years experience in active local administration of the notification of Phthisis, the vast majority of the cases notified having been hospital, workhouse and dispensary cases. In no single instance has any occupational disability to patients been incurred *through notification*. The same experience has been testified to in Sheffield under a system of universal compulsory notification. It could not happen under a reasonable system of administration; (of course, persons are, apart from notification, nervous about intimate contact with consumptives; and the absence of notification will not prevent this occasional nervousness being manifested). Compulsory notification is now in force for about half the population of Scotland, and in several towns in England, and there is throughout no evidence of any injury to patients *by notification*.[31]

Experience, however, was to prove this view dubiously sanguine. By 1914 Newsholme acknowledged that some employees whose cases had been notified

28 Public Health (Tuberculosis) Regulations, 1908, Art. IX in *Ann. Rep. Med. Off. L.G.B.*, 38 (1908–9): 228.
29 Newsholme to Willis, 28 July 1910, P.R.O., MH55/525.
30 Newsholme, minute of 15 Oct. 1908, P.R.O., MH55/523.
31 Newsholme to Willis, 10 Feb. 1911, 2, P.R.O., MH55/525.

subsequently had been dismissed by their employers, although he insisted that it was not certain that this dismissal was because of notification.[32] It also became clear that the interests of the individual patient sometimes conflicted with the public interest. Newsholme acknowledged that this might be the case with particular classes of workers: domestic servants, nursemaids in charge of small children, and milk handlers.[33] He insisted that the confidentiality of even these patients was to be protected; the M.O.H. was not justified in notifying the employer in such cases, and he was to ensure that the utmost tact be exercised in contacting these patients. A representative of the health department was not, for example, to try to visit such patients at their place of employment. In most instances a patient could be instructed to act in a way that did not endanger others and could safely remain at his or her present job. But in some instances the health officer should advise the patient to change occupations. There was no hint, however, that compulsion was contemplated to enforce this suggestion. But Newsholme came to believe that there were some circumstances in which the protection of the public might justify the breach of confidentiality. The example he used was a schoolteacher with a case of "open" tuberculosis. In a case like this one the school medical officer might find it necessary to notify the education authority of the teacher's condition and to recommend that the teacher be dismissed and pensioned.[34] It is quite clear that Newsholme thought that such instances would be exceptional. By the outbreak of the First World War the L.G.B. believed that in general notification procedures had successfully protected patients' interests. It continued to encourage local authorities to keep notifications confidential by directing local authorities to allow no one other than a member of the health department or persons specifically authorized by the council to have access to the register of notified cases kept by the M.O.H. It specifically applied this ban to local insurance committees.[35]

Newsholme was even more concerned to see that local authorities did not try to isolate compulsorily patients whose cases were notified. When the Board heard from an alarmed rural district council whose M.O.H. had advised them that tuberculosis was "one of the most contagious diseases," that no infectious disease needed isolation more than tuberculosis, and that under existing regulations local authorities were quite powerless to protect themselves, Newsholme urged his administrative superiors to remind the council of the constructive actions it could take, short of compulsory isolation, and to warn the M.O.H. against making exaggerated and alarmist statements.[36] When another rural district council wrote of a tubercular child whose guardians would not permit her removal to the sanatorium for isolation, Willis, the Assistant Secretary, proposed suggesting stat-

---

32 For this and the following comments, see Newsholme, *Ann. Rep. Med. Off. L.G.B.*, 43 (1913–14): lviii.

33 For the following discussion, see ibid., 41 (1911–12): xliv; and ibid., 42 (1912–13): xxxviii.

34 Ibid., 43 (1913–14): lviii.   35 *Ann. Rep. L.G.B.*, 43 (1913–14), III: xlvi.

36 A. L. Lewis [Assistant Clerk, Kiveton Park Rural District Council] to Secretary, Local Government Board, 15 June 1913, P.R.O., MH55/520; and Arthur Newsholme, minute, 26 June 1913, ibid.

utes and case law the local authority could use as precedents to try to isolate the child compulsorily. However, Newsholme counseled otherwise, suggesting that Willis's advice would encourage the local authority to place the child in the workhouse. He also pointed out that the Board could hardly agree that isolation was necessary, since it did not know what type of tuberculosis the child had or anything about the domestic accommodation of the family. He advised the M.O.H. and the County Tuberculosis Officer to confer about the case and to report to the Board afterward.[37] When the County M.O.H. from Worcestershire wrote about two cases he regarded as dangerous but which he had been unable to isolate – a child with tuberculosis bacilli in her sputum who slept in the same room with her siblings, and a man with advanced pulmonary tuberculosis who served in a confectioner's shop – Newsholme repeated that the Council could do nothing that would interfere with the man's livelihood, but that this did not prohibit the M.O.H. from giving the man advice on limiting his infectiousness or urging him to find another job. In this instance as well Newsholme preferred informal solutions. He kept the Board from issuing an official reply and urged the M.O.H. to stop for a conversation the next time he was in London.[38] As we will see in the next chapter, the War severely tested Newsholme's resolve that compulsory isolation not be used for tuberculosis cases.

Notwithstanding his insistence that notification be followed by meaningful prevention action, Newsholme highly valued the notification returns for statistical purposes and used them together with data supplied to him by special agreement with the General Register Office to undertake extensive analyses of the morbidity and mortality patterns of tuberculosis.[39] But he realized that the returns contained serious inaccuracies. The number of notifications did climb steeply in the early years. During 1911, the second full year of Poor Law notification and the first nine months of notifications from hospital and dispensary practice, Medical Officers of Health in England and Wales received 35,107 notifications: 13,464 from poor law practice, 11,804 from hospital and dispensary practice, and 9,839 notifications made under local acts and voluntary notification schemes.[40] Voluntary notification continued to be important for several years. The Board's officials claimed that the order to notify Poor Law cases had produced an indirect benefit; it stimulated local authorities to initiate voluntary notification for their entire populations.[41] The next year, 1912, was the first year that all pulmonary cases were compulsorily notifiable, and tuberculosis notifications jumped

37 Ernest Crundwell [Clerk, Farnham Rural District Council] to Secretary, Local Government Board, 2 Dec. 1913, ibid.; F. J. W[illis], minutes of 8 and 9 Dec. 1913, ibid.; and Arthur Newsholme, minute, 10 Dec. 1913, ibid.
38 G. H. Fosbroke [M.O.H., Worcestershire County Council] to Secretary, Local Government Board, 12 Dec. 1913, ibid.; Newsholme, minute, 18 Dec. 1913, ibid.; Newsholme to Fosbroke, 14 Jan. 1913, ibid.; and Newsholme to Barnes, 29 Jan. 1914, ibid.
39 See his sections "Statistics of Tuberculosis," in Newsholme, *Ann. Rep. Med. Off. L.G.B.*, 42 (1912–13), xxvii–xxxv, 234–43; ibid., 43 (1913–14), xci–ci, 143–50.
40 Ibid., 41 (1911–12): xxxvi.   41 *Ann. Rep. L.G.B.*, 40 (1910–11), II: xxxiii.

from 35,000 to over 110,000.[42] The following year the figure reached 134,743, including the 38,190 nonpulmonary cases notified during the last eleven months of the year.[43]

Error and confusion undoubtedly inflated these figures through duplicate notification. The figures stated are for "primary notifications," notifications made by medical officers or practitioners who did not have reason to believe that the case they diagnosed had previously been notified. Previously notified cases might also be reported, but they were to be reported separately as supplemental notifications. Under such an arrangement it was likely that some cases were notified more than once as new cases. Based on a 1914 survey of the notification records kept by Medical Officers of Health, the L.G.B. concluded that about 10 percent of primary notifications were duplicates.[44]

A greater and less easily corrected source of error was the failure of practitioners to notify cases at all. Newsholme recognized that this problem was greatest among the upper classes, but it was not confined to the nation's more fashionable practitioners.[45] As early as 1913 and frequently thereafter he attempted to demonstrate that noncompliance was rampant by calculating for various administrative areas the ratio of notified cases to registered deaths from pulmonary tuberculosis.[46] He found a wide variation in this ratio. In small areas there might be as many as 400 or as few as 100 notifications to every 100 deaths. If one compared whole administrative counties, the notifications ran as high as 250 per 100 deaths in Cumberland and as low as 140 in Nottingham. At first rather tentatively and then more forcefully, Newsholme suggested that M.O.H. who found that the notifications for pulmonary tuberculosis in their jurisdiction were less than twice the registered deaths from the disease should suspect that cases were escaping notification, and that they should seek defects in their tuberculosis program and put pressure on local practitioners to comply with the law. Noncompliance with the notification orders remained a problem throughout his tenure in Whitehall. In his last official report, Newsholme presented the results of a study by the County M.O.H. of Derbyshire of 412 deaths from tuberculosis that had been registered in his county in 1917.[47] Thirty-nine percent had never been notified and another 31 percent were notified only within the last twelve weeks of the patient's life. Notification practiced this way served no public health purpose, and it probably did nothing to help the patient.

42 There is a slight discrepancy in the reported figures. Newsholme, *Ann. Rep. Med. Off. L.G.B.*, 42 (1912–13), xxix, and *Ann. Rep. L.G.B.*, 42 (1912–13), III: xxvii both give 110,706. *Ann. Rep. L.G.B.*, 43 (1913–14), III: xlvii gives the correct figure as 110,551.
43 *Ann. Rep. L.G.B.*, 43 (1913–14), III: xlvii.   44 Ibid., xlix.
45 Arthur Newsholme, testimony, Royal Commission on Venereal Diseases, *Appendix to the Final Report*, B.P.P. 1916, [Cd. 8190]. XVI, 220.
46 Newsholme, *Ann. Rep. Med. Off. L.G.B.*, 42 (1912–13), xxix; ibid., 43 (1913–14), c; and ibid., 44 (1914–15), xix–xx.
47 See, for example, ibid., 47 (1917–18), lxiv–lxv.

Recent historical studies have suggested that the tuberculosis campaign was all too often identified with the sanatorium.[48] In view of Newsholme's sustained efforts to prove that institutional confinement was the most important single factor in the past decline of tuberculosis and the fact that he was in place at the L.G.B. when the national tuberculosis program was begun, it is tempting to see the prominent place the sanatorium came to occupy as a product of Newsholme's influence. But to view the history of the new state tuberculosis program in this way is to misunderstand what Newsholme intended, to overestimate his influence on national policy, and incorrectly to see the formation of that policy as an orderly, rational exercise. Here again the passage of National Insurance interrupted his scheme and forced the L.G.B. and local authorities to improvise a set of services that no administrator or theorist would have designed. Newsholme's performance as M.O.H. in Brighton, an extended section of his 1908 monograph on tuberculosis,[49] and a memorandum he composed at the L.G.B. for distribution to local health authorities in February 1909[50] show us what sort of local programs he had in mind, before the passage of the National Insurance Act made gradualism impossible and directed available public resources into a narrower channel. This 1909 memorandum was issued just three months after the first tuberculosis order, but it looked forward to the day when notification would be universal and it outlined for Medical Officers of Health and members of local health authorities the essential features of a complete tuberculosis scheme for a community. It is our best evidence of Newsholme's original intentions in tuberculosis policy at the L.G.B., and it deserves some attention here.

His brief exposition of the nature of tuberculosis emphasized both its specific bacterial cause and the importance of environmental conditions in facilitating transmission of the bacillus. The transmission of human tuberculosis occurred most frequently through human sputum. While persons suffering from pulmonary tuberculosis might expel tuberculosis bacilli in coughing or spitting, bacteriological studies had shown that the bacilli were present in the sputum only intermittently during the course of the disease. This fact should go some way to allaying

---

48 See, for example, the prominent place residential institutions play in F. B. Smith, *The Retreat of Tuberculosis 1850–1950* (London, New York, Sydney: Croom Helm, 1988); and Linda Bryder, *Below the Magic Mountain: A Social History of Tuberculosis in Twentieth-Century Britain* (Oxford: Clarendon Press, 1988). Smith, for example, believes the tuberculosis dispensary was often regarded as simply a recruiting station for the sanatorium; Smith, *Retreat of Tuberculosis*, 66–7. See also Neil McFarlane, "Hospitals, Housing, and Tuberculosis in Glasgow," *Social Hist. Med.*, 2 (1989): 59–85.

49 Newsholme, *Prevention of Tuberculosis*, 301–414.

50 For the following discussion, see Arthur Newsholme, "Memorandum by the Medical Officer of the Local Government Board on Administrative Measures against Tuberculosis," *Ann. Rep. Med. Off. L.G.B.*, 38 (1908–9), 232–9.

public fear of tubercular patients. But of greater importance was the fact that the disease did not spread with the ease of many acute infectious diseases such as smallpox. Exposure to large amounts of contagium or prolonged exposure to smaller doses was usually necessary for tuberculosis infection to occur.

The fundamental strategy for preventing tuberculosis was to ensure that no one suffered such exposure. The fact that substantial exposure was needed for transmission, coupled with the knowledge that some cases completely recovered and that many more went into remission, suggested that it should be possible to so arrange things that those diagnosed with tuberculosis could safely live in their community and remain self-sufficient for prolonged periods, possibly for the remainder of their normal lifetimes. In early 1909 Newsholme was, in fact, very optimistic. "Tuberculosis is not only a preventable disease, but it can also be arrested, especially in its earlier stages; and indeed the vast majority of those attacked by it recover."[51]

Such a happy outcome, in fact the success of all other measures against tuberculosis, depended on what was then unattainable, early diagnosis. Many cases were undetected until the disease was well advanced, until after there was cavitation or consolidation of lung tissue, after the patient had become too weak to continue working, and after the infected person had spread bacilli for prolonged periods. While it would be best, Newsholme observed, if the disease could be diagnosed before the bacilli appeared in the sputum, the public provision for free bacteriological diagnosis of sputum samples was an essential first step toward dealing effectively with the disease.[52]

Early diagnosis should be followed by a vigorous educational campaign beginning with the patient. The patient should be told candidly of his condition, so that he could protect his health and the health of those around him. Ever optimistic about human nature, Newsholme placed great faith in the power of instruction. In this 1909 memorandum he explained that tuberculosis was a disease of both misery and ignorance. "Many of the measures for its treatment and relief . . . have among their most valuable results the hygienic training of the patient."[53] It was particularly important that family members and others who nursed tuberculosis patients be informed of the nature of the disease, the risks of indiscriminate spitting, and simple strategies for containing and disinfecting infected sputum. Such knowledge could reduce the risk of infection at home, the place where he was convinced most infection took place. He also recommended special educational campaigns in industries where the incidence of tuberculosis was high as well as more general public tuberculosis education and the enactment of local antispitting ordinances.

Printed material was of some use in promoting this education, but Newsholme insisted that personal contact among patients and their families and health authority officials was much more effective. These conferences could most easily take

51 Newsholme, "Administrative Measures against Tuberculosis," 233.   52 Ibid., 234.
53 Ibid., 234, 236.

place during the home visits which should follow notification. Newsholme counseled tact and discretion as well as candor in these interviews. Neither patients, their families, nor their doctors should be alienated. During these visits the health department could provide information. It could inspect the condition of the home and seek to remedy such defects as insanitary conditions and overcrowding, and it could provide appliances and materials whose use would help prevent the spread of infection. It should also, perhaps more tactfully on a second visit, seek to obtain information on the health of other family members with an eye to identifying unrecognized cases. Regular home visits would serve to encourage patients to follow hygienic precautions, and such visits in conjunction with renotification when patients changed lodgings would permit the health authority to clean and to disinfect patients' dwellings before they were occupied by other tenants.

Tuberculosis dispensaries, provided either by the local health authority or by voluntary efforts, should be central to any local tuberculosis program.[54] The dispensary would be the hub of public tuberculosis work. It would serve as the center for diagnosis of cases and for treatment of ambulatory patients. It would also help link the more strictly medical services to the social services tuberculosis patients often need.

The object of this institution is to secure early diagnosis for patients suspected to be suffering from pulmonary tuberculosis, and to direct their treatment in the light of knowledge not only of their medical, but also of their domestic and industrial needs. The idea of the dispensary implies therefore, a careful system of domiciliary visitation and investigation.[55]

Newsholme recognized that patients might need help in finding suitable work or financial subsidies to improve their diet or to secure better housing. His later descriptions of tuberculosis schemes recommend the formation of care committees, voluntary agencies which would work in close connection with the local tuberculosis scheme and which would offer social services such as these which public authorities were not authorized to provide.[56]

The final element in the tuberculosis scheme was the sanatorium. Newsholme's early plans for the nation's tuberculosis policy reflected his experience in Brighton. His preferred use of the sanatorium was to provide beds for short periods of confinement. This strategy was dictated partly by cold calculation, by the need to stretch scarce resources. Cases were seldom diagnosed in the early stage, when hope of cure was greatest, and at present, Newsholme reasoned, even those patients still able to work would require lengthy sanatorium treatment to offer much hope of recovery. The nation simply could not afford to provide institutional accommodation of such length for all ambulatory working-class tuberculosis patients. But it might offer patients shorter stays. Even one month's treatment had decided advantages for the patient, his family, and the community.

54 Ibid., 237–8.   55 Ibid., 237.
56 See, for example, Newsholme, *Ann. Rep. Med. Off. L.G.B.,* 42 (1912–13), li.

The patient usually does not lose his place by the short absence from work contemplated; he is willing to come into a sanatorium for such a short stay, when he would not accept more protracted treatment; and the improvement experienced during such a short stay in a sanatorium is often most remarkable. This, however, is not the only gain. When the patient enters the sanatorium his dwelling is disinfected; his relatives are relieved temporarily from a source of anxiety; and the patient while in the sanatorium is trained in the methods of disposal of sputum, and in general hygienic regulation of his life in a practical manner that is scarcely possible at home. On his return home he is therefore no longer likely to be a source of infection, and the general hygiene of his home is almost certain to reflect the good influence of his stay in the sanatorium.[57]

But the problem remained of what to do with the thousands of late and terminal cases, cases which Newsholme believed were likely to pose the greatest risks of infection to others, especially in the crowded homes of the poor. These patients often required care and an environment that could not be provided at home. He was convinced that patients would willingly seek institutional care. This had been the case in Brighton. "So far from the patients objecting to notification, a not infrequent difficulty has been that they persist in applying for sanatorium treatment, apart from the advice and certificate of a private doctor, upon which we always insist."[58] At the L.G.B. he continued to hope that institutional care of late cases could be made as attractive to the patient as he believed it would be beneficial to his family and community. "The hospital treatment of the bedridden consumptive in the ideal state will be made so popular that domestic infection will become much less frequent than at present."[59] While residential institutions were necessary and likely to be used, it seemed impossible to contemplate the construction of new institutions for the nation's bedridden cases, although in his 1909 memorandum Newsholme held out the hope that the peak need for institutions for such cases would be brief and that the number of advanced cases needing institutional care would fall as diagnosis and prevention improved.[60] It seemed that the best hope for these cases lay in the Poor Law institutions.[61] But this option could be entertained only if the Poor Law Infirmary were cleansed of its unhappy associations with the indignities and deterrent principles of the Poor Law.[62]

While infirmary treatment involves the stigma of pauperism, far more patients will struggle against the disease till they are past recovery, in the hope of avoiding the workhouse, than will apply for infirmary treatment at a stage at which it can have a fair chance of producing recovery, and before they have sown widespread infection in their environment. . . . The Boards of

57 Newsholme, "Administrative Measures against Tuberculosis," 238.
58 Arthur Newsholme and H. C. Lecky, "An Account of the System of Voluntary Notification of Phthisis in Brighton, and of the Treatment and Training of Patients in its Isolation Hospital," *Tuberculosis*, 4 (1906–7): 237.
59 Newsholme, "Administrative Measures against Tuberculosis," 239.   60 Ibid.
61 See, for example, his first report to the Brighton Sanitary Committee on the prevention of tuberculosis: Newsholme, *Ann. Rep.* (Brighton), 1901, 48, 51–2.
62 Ibid., 51–2, and minutes of interview with Newsholme, 22 Dec. 1906, Webb, Local Government Collection, vol. 335.

Guardians have, in fact, the accommodation and arrangements for treatment without being able to secure the patients at the most favourable time; the Sanitary Authority can secure the patients, but seldom or never has the accommodation and arrangements for treating them. This inefficient state of things points to the need for finding a way of combining the resources and functions of the two Authorities in respect to the treatment of the sick.[63]

So committed was Newsholme to rehabilitating and using Poor Law facilities in the nation's tuberculosis program that he continued to recommend this policy even while the National Insurance Bill was being drafted.[64]

It is impossible to predict what form the tuberculosis campaign in Britain would have taken had it not been for the Sanatorium Benefit of the National Insurance Act. This enactment not only greatly accelerated the pace but also changed the course of that campaign. Among various service and cash benefits the Act promised the insured "treatment in sanatoria or other institutions or otherwise when suffering from tuberculosis, or such other diseases as the Local Government Board with the approval of the Treasury may appoint."[65] This section was unique in the Insurance Act in making special provision for a specific illness and in promising more than general practitioner services as a basic medical benefit. But in making this provision the Act promised much more than the nation could then deliver. In order to provide the Sanatorium Benefit local Insurance Committees were empowered to make arrangements with either private parties or with local authorities which maintained sanatoriums.[66] The only important restrictions on these agreements were that such institutions must be approved by the L.G.B. and that they could not be Poor Law institutions. Newsholme estimated soon after the L.G.B. learned the terms of the insurance bill that there would be constantly about 45,000 cases of pulmonary tuberculosis among the insured in England and Wales, and that the absolute minimum number of beds needed to provide sanatorium treatment during part of the duration of each insured case would be 7,500.[67] At the time there were 3,700 beds in private tuberculosis institutions, of which he thought, for unspecified reasons, as many as 1,400 might prove to be available for the insured. In addition local authorities collectively had provided about 600 beds for pulmonary tuberculosis. Even on the basis of this rather optimistic estimate, the nation had only about 27 percent of the beds it would need, leaving a deficit of about 5,500 beds. The Finance Act, 1911, went some way toward addressing this problem by making available from the Treasury £1.5 million for grants in aid of sanatoriums.[68] This fund for capital improvement was to be divided among the

63 Newsholme, *Prevention of Tuberculosis,* 369.
64 Arthur Newsholme, to H. C. Monro, 29 June 1911, P.R.O., Pin3/4; and Arthur Newsholme, "On the Policy in Administering the Sanatorium Benefit, with Special References to the Authorities Concerned," 23 Aug. 1911, pp. 7–10, P.R.O., Pin3/5.
65 1 & 2 Geo. 5, C. 55, sect. 8.   66 Ibid., sect. 16, 64.
67 Arthur Newsholme, "Estimate as to Number of Beds Required for Pulmonary Tuberculosis in England and Wales," 5 April 1911, P.R.O., Pin3/3.
68 1 & 2 Geo. 5, C. 48, Sect. 16. The estimated distribution of the fund is from the *Interim Report of the Departmental Committee on Tuberculosis,* B.P.P. 1912–13, [Cd. 6164], XLVIII, 8.

nations of the United Kingdom on the basis of their population, leaving an estimated £1.1 million for England and £81,000 for Wales to be distributed by the L.G.B. with the consent of the Treasury and after consultation with the Insurance Commissioners.

But money for construction was not the only problem. Who would provide the benefit and under what terms? Action was urgently needed. The Act received Royal assent on December 16, 1911, and was scheduled to go into effect on July 15, 1912. Clearly the additional beds that were needed could not be provided by new construction in that time. Furthermore, the Insurance Committees had to be organized before any thoughts of locating institutional beds could be entertained. The Insurance Committees were themselves not authorized to build and operate sanatoriums but were obliged to locate space in existing or new institutions. The best hope, in fact probably the only hope, of implementing the Sanatorium Benefit on time was to induce local authorities to cooperate, in the short term by converting empty beds in their isolation and smallpox hospitals for the use of tuberculosis patients and in the longer term by undertaking to build additional facilities for this purpose with the help of capital grants from the Treasury.

But would local authorities cooperate? There was much in the act to make them wary, even resentful, just as officials of the L.G.B. had predicted while the insurance bill was being drafted. As we saw in Chapter 8, not only had Lloyd George insisted on an ad hoc administration for the sanatorium and medical benefits, refusing to turn local administration over to a committee of the local authority as Newsholme had suggested or even to give the local authority a majority of places on the local Insurance Committee, but he drafted a bill which threatened the ratepayers with great financial liabilities. In addition to the Excess Sickness Clause, which made local authorities financially liable for excessive demands on the insurance fund caused by high local sickness rates which were deemed due to negligence on the part of local authorities, the Act established conditions in which local authorities would be liable jointly with the Treasury for any deficit in the funds earmarked for the Sanatorium Benefit.[69] To pay for the Sanatorium Benefit each Insurance Committee was to receive annually a fund equal to 1s 3d per insured person in its jurisdiction. The Act had provided an additional 1d from a Parliamentary grant, but that sum was soon earmarked for research. The Insurance Committee could extend the Sanatorium Benefit to the dependents of the insured and pay the cost of their care out of this same fund, but if the fund ran short, the County Council or the County Borough Council was expected to help guarantee the financial soundness of the fund. The only way a council could avoid this liability was to refuse to permit treatment to continue when a deficit was projected, and such refusal would be difficult. Even more important than the specific features of the Act were the longstanding problems in the relationship of the central government and local authorities which the Insur-

69 1 & 2 Geo. 5, C. 55, sect. 63, 17.

ance Act helped bring into the open. By the turn of the century there was a strong feeling in local government that the central government was thrusting upon local authorities obligations for performing national services and expecting the local ratepayers to shoulder the burden of these services without compensation from the national Treasury.[70] This feeling was manifest on a number of initiatives in the late nineteenth and early twentieth centuries, but the prospects of building costly institutions for tuberculosis, which the Insurance Committees were not even obliged to use, and the fear of being financially liable for the deficits in sanatorium funds made local officials particularly resentful. Why should the ratepayers agree to make the Sanatorium Benefit work, especially since only part of the population within the jurisdiction of the local authority stood to benefit?

The reluctance of local authorities strengthened the hand of L.G.B. officials in their intense negotiations with the Treasury and the Insurance Commission that, as we saw in Chapter 8, had begun while the bill was being drafted and continued into 1913, while the Act was being implemented. In a series of memoranda and conferences the Board reminded the Chancellor and Treasury officials that local authorities were not obliged to provide institutions for treating tuberculosis, that they were unlikely to do so unless they received a better deal, and that since very few private sanatoriums at this early stage had expressed an interest in participating, there was nowhere else for the Government to turn.[71] The L.G.B. and Newsholme in particular also continued to insist that it made little sense to treat only the insured. To be effective, action against tuberculosis must apply to the entire population and must include prevention as well as treatment.[72]

Even before the insurance bill became law, the L.G.B. had proposed the appointment of a Departmental Committee to consider the administrative problems that would be involved in beginning the Sanatorium Benefit, and it drew up a list of members it wanted to see appointed.[73] Lloyd George resisted appointing

70 For a very informative discussion of this issue, see Christine Bellamy, *Administering Central–Local Relations, 1871–1919: The Local Government Board in Its Fiscal and Cultural Context* (Manchester: Manchester Univ. Press, 1988), esp. chap. 2–3.

71 These points were made repeatedly. See for instance the L.G.B. memorandum "National Insurance Bill," 21 June 1911, pp. 3–4, a copy of which was sent to Braithwaite in P.R.O., Pin3/4; John Burns to David Lloyd George, 19 June 1912, P.R.O., MH55/522; "Deputation from the County Councils Association. The Position of County Councils with Regard to the Administration of Sanatorium Benefit," 29 July 1912, ibid.; "Government Grant in Aid of Sanatorium Schemes. Institutional Treatment," 15 Nov. 1912, pp. 1–2, ibid.; and untitled L.G.B. memorandum in preparation for a conference of local authority representatives with Lloyd George, 6 Feb. 1913, ibid.

72 Arthur Newsholme, "On the Policy in Administering the Sanatorium Benefit, with Special Reference to the Authorities Concerned," 23 Aug. 1911, p. 3, P.R.O., Pin3/5; Arthur Newsholme, "The Administration of the Sanatorium Benefit," 14 Oct. 1911, pp. 26, 29–30, P.R.O., Pin3/5; and John Burns to David Lloyd George, 19 June 1912, P.R.O., MH55/522.

73 There are two recitations of this history. See F. J. Willis to H. C. Monro, 22 July 1912, pp. 2–4; this is obviously an L.G.B. minute, but I have been unable to find it at the P.R.O. A copy is preserved in Newsholme Papers. See also untitled L.G.B. minute, 6 Feb. 1913, P.R.O., MH55/522.

such a Committee until the bill had passed, and in the meantime planning continued within the L.G.B. After passage of the National Insurance Act, the L.G.B. proposed to issue at once a circular to County and County Councils, urging them to formulate tuberculosis schemes and establishing guidelines. However, the Treasury and the Insurance Commission opposed this plan as well, insisting now that a Department Committee first consider the matter, and the Chancellor appointed such a committee in February 1912 with Waldorf Astor as chair. The Astor Committee was dominated by members with medical training. Among them were prominent civil servants: Newsholme, George Newman, and, from the L.G.B. for Scotland, Leslie MacKenzie, as well as M.O.H.: James Niven, Harold Richards, and John McVail. Also included were practitioners who were closely associated with sanatoriums and tuberculosis dispensaries such as Noel Dean Bardswell, Marcus Paterson, Arthur Lathan, and Robert Philip. Christopher Addison, the anatomist turned Liberal M.P., who had been instrumental in securing the passage of the Insurance Act and who would eventually hold a number of Cabinet posts, including Minister of Health, was an important force on the Committee.

Newsholme joined the Committee with well-formulated ideas on how the Sanatorium Benefit should be implemented. These had taken shape in the course of drafting numerous planning documents for his administrative superiors.[74] His views were informed and practical, and the more fundamental of them were confirmed by the Interim and Final Reports of the Committee.[75] The Committee agreed that the Sanatorium Benefit should be used to deal with tuberculosis in the entire population, not just in the insured, and that the provision of the benefit should form part of a comprehensive tuberculosis program having both preventive and therapeutic goals. The Committee also agreed that these schemes should apply to large areas and be in the hands of the County Councils or County Borough Councils or, in more sparsely settled areas, in the hands of joint boards representing several of these authorities. Care under the Sanatorium Benefit did not necessarily mean institutional treatment. Newsholme and the Committee both believed that the Sanatorium Benefit should be extended to the treatment of patients in their own homes. The Committee also stressed the need for economy in providing sanatoriums. Each should hold at least 100 beds to be efficient, and they should be plain and inexpensive. It established cost guidelines and recom-

74 See in particular Arthur Newsholme, "The Importance of Sanatoria as a Means for Diminishing Tuberculosis," 12 May 1911, P.R.O., Pin3/4; Arthur Newsholme, "Memorandum on the Present Position of the National Insurance Bill, in Relation to Public Health Administration," 15 June 1911, ibid.; Arthur Newsholme, "On the Policy in Administering the Sanatorium Benefit, with Special Reference to the Authorities Concerned," 23 Aug. 1911, P.R.O., Pin3/5; Arthur Newsholme, "The Administration of the Sanatorium Benefit," 14 Oct. 1911, ibid. See also Arthur Newsholme, "The Relative Functions of the Local Sanitary Authority and of the Local Insurance Committee in the Treatment of Tuberculosis," 1 March 1912, Newsholme Papers.
75 Interim Report of the Departmental Committee on Tuberculosis, B.P.P. 1912–13, [Cd. 6164], XLVIII; and Final Report of the Departmental Committee on Tuberculosis, 2 vols., B.P.P. 1912–13, [Cd. 6641 & 6654], XLVIII.

mended capital grants from the Exchequer to help defray the cost of building sanatoriums and establishing dispensaries.[76] The Committee's reports differed somewhat from Newsholme's previous statements in recommending that this tuberculosis work be carried out primarily through two units: a dispensary unit and a sanatorium unit.[77] The tuberculosis dispensary would be the center for observation, diagnosis, consultation, and referral. This unit should be managed by the Tuberculosis Officer, a salaried, full-time tuberculosis expert, who was expected to advise the Insurance Committee, to work closely with the M.O.H., and to serve as a consultant for local medical practitioners. The creation of sanatoriums should be planned so that there was a minimum of one bed per 5,000 population in the area served. The Committee laid great stress on the importance of finding properly qualified and experienced medical practitioners to serve as Tuberculosis Officers and Medical Superintendents of sanatoriums and stressed the need of offering high salaries, but it conceded that qualified candidates would be scarce and that initially it would be necessary to make appointments on the condition that the appointee agree to acquire the necessary clinical training.[78]

With this confirmation of some of its contentions about administering the Act, the L.G.B. issued its first circular to local authorities on the Sanatorium Benefit on May 14, 1912, just two months before the Act was to come into effect.[79] The circular explained the terms of the legislation of 1911, enclosed copies of the Interim Report of the Departmental Committee and sections from the Insurance Act, and made recommendations for action by local authorities that were in keeping with the Interim Report. To spur local authorities into immediate action, it also asked for a report on what had been accomplished in each county and county borough by June 8. What it learned from local authorities was not at all encouraging.[80] Only four local authorities had special sanatoriums for tuberculosis, and these contained a mere 170 beds. Fifty-seven local authorities had contracted to use a total of 200 beds in private sanatoriums, and another 970 beds in local authority infectious disease hospitals were currently used by tuberculosis patients. The Board's circular of July 6, issued just a week before the insurance scheme began, acknowledged that institutional treatment could not begin in many areas for some time.[81] While it urged local authorities and insurance committees to begin planning permanent schemes that conformed to the recommendations of the Astor Committee, it called on them to submit provisional schemes at once.

76 *Interim Report of the Departmental Committee*, 27.
77 For a discussion of these two units, see ibid., 11–16.   78 Ibid., 13, 15–16.
79 H. C. Monro, "Parliamentary Grant for Sanatorium Purposes. Finance Act, 1911, and National Insurance Act, 1911. Circular Letter to County, Town, and Urban and Rural District Councils (England)," 14 May 1912, in *Ann. Rep. L.G.B.*, 41 (1911–12), II: 46–9.
80 For the following, see the L.G.B. memorandum "Sanatorium Benefit," 11 July 1912, pp. 1–2, P.R.O., MH55/522.
81 "Treatment of Tuberculosis: Provisional and Permanent Arrangements. Finance Act, 1911, and National Insurance Act, 1911. Circular Letter to County and County Borough Councils (England)," 6 July 1912 in *Ann. Rep. L.G.B.*, 42 (1912–13), III: 2–15.

Where a Tuberculosis Officer had not been found, the M.O.H. might temporarily take on these duties. Treatment in homes or at a dispensary might be all that could be offered under these provisional schemes.

By mid-July only twenty-four of forty-seven county councils and twenty of the seventy borough councils had submitted schemes for L.G.B. approval.[82] Local authorities were worried about the cost of operating the new facilities, especially when they had received no guarantee that the Insurance Committee would use the facilities they provided. The problem was magnified by the prospect of providing the Sanatorium Benefit to the entire population. The Insurance Act seemed to commit the Treasury to sharing equally with local authorities any deficit caused by providing the benefit to the insured and their dependents in approved schemes, but to that unknown financial liability must be added the cost of offering the benefit to the uninsured, a cost which was apparently to be met entirely from the rates. These anxieties culminated in meetings in late July between a delegation from the County Councils Association, first with the chief officials of the L.G.B. and then with the Chancellor.[83] The delegation asked that the responsibility for treating tuberculosis be taken away from the insurance scheme and turned over to local authorities and that the government make direct grants to cover 75 percent of the cost of this work. The L.G.B. realized that Lloyd George would not permit a change in the Insurance Act; it had tried repeatedly to secure such a change, but it urged that something be done to appease local authorities. On July 31, 1912, in a letter to Henry Hobhouse, the President of the County Councils Association, the Chancellor announced that the Treasury would promise annual grants through the L.G.B., for 50 percent of the cost of providing the Sanatorium Benefit for the uninsured and dependents of the insured.[84]

While the L.G.B. did not formally announce the Hobhouse Award until December 6, 1912, the Treasury offer was widely known, and it was apparent well before December that local authorities were still not satisfied and continued to demand that their liability be limited to 25 percent of costs.[85] Their apprehensions were renewed when, to satisfy the demands of medical practitioners for more money under the insurance scheme, it was decided that 6d of the 1s 3d per insured individual from the insurance fund that had been earmarked for the Sanatorium Benefit would be diverted to pay private practitioners for home treatment of insured patients with tuberculosis.

In negotiations with the Insurance Commissioners and the Treasury in the following months L.G.B. officials proposed some radical restructuring of the

---

82 "Sanatorium Benefit," 11 July 1912, pp. 3–4, P.R.O., MH55/522.
83 See the L.G.B. memorandum "Deputation from the County Councils Association. The Position of County Councils with Regard to the Administration of Sanatorium Benefit," 29 July 1912, ibid.; and untitled memorandum, 31 July 1912, ibid.
84 A copy of his letter may be found in *Ann. Rep. L.G.B.*, 42 (1912–13), III: 35.
85 "Schemes for Institutional Treatment of Tuberculosis. Circular Letter to Councils of Counties and County Boroughs (England), 6 Dec. 1912 in ibid., 30–4.

scheme.[86] Since the Chancellor insisted that it was unfair to give the uninsured services free of charge for which the insured paid, the Board suggested that institutional treatment of tuberculosis offered by local authorities be free to all, that two-thirds, or in some proposals three-fourths, of the costs of this treatment be covered by government grants, and the entire sanatorium fund be used to pay private practitioners for home treatment of insured tuberculosis cases. The Permanent Secretary sought to strengthen the case for this course of action by arguing that the uninsured as taxpayers and ratepayers were in fact contributing to the building and maintenance of tuberculosis institutions and hence had a claim on them. He also briefly considered the feasibility of charging the uninsured fees to cover part of the cost of their treatment for tuberculosis. He dropped the idea quickly, however, when he was reminded that fees for institutional treatment of other infectious diseases had deterred the use of isolation facilities and that some local authorities were already treating cases of tuberculosis gratis. By January nerves were raw in Whitehall. The L.G.B. responded sharply and defensively to the suggestion that it was to blame for the delays in getting the Sanatorium Benefit launched.[87] It blamed the Treasury and the Insurance Commission for refusing local authorities the 75 percent grant they wanted. The struggle to remake the Sanatorium Benefit under the National Insurance Act into a comprehensive national tuberculosis program came to a head on February 6, 1913, when a combined delegation from the County Councils Association, the Borough Councils, and the Association of Municipal Corporations met with David Lloyd George and officials from the Treasury, Insurance Commission, and Local Government Board.[88] After hearing their demands, the Chancellor refused to up the ante. If local authorities were unwilling to act under these terms, the nation would have to get along by treating only the insured for tuberculosis. Local officials and medical officers had pushed as far as they could. Local authorities might use the Sanatorium Benefit to initiate local tuberculosis programs, but they could not expect more help from the Treasury. Insurance committees and local authorities would hereafter have to manage as best they could.

The decision to extend treatment to the uninsured under the auspices of local authorities made the shortage of beds for tuberculosis even more critical. The Astor Committee had estimated that initially for the United Kingdom 18,000 beds would be needed to provide sanatorium and hospital care for tuberculosis in the whole population.[89] A year and a half later Newsholme calculated that England and Wales alone would need 14,000 beds, assuming that 9,000 paupers with

86 For the following information, see the documents from Sept. 1912 to Feb. 1913 in P.R.O., MH55/ 522 in particular "Sanatorium Schemes," Sept. 1912; "Treatment of Tuberculosis," 11 Oct. 1912; "Government Grant in Aid of Sanatorium Schemes. Institutional Treatment," 15 Nov. 1912; and H. C. Monro, "Maintenance Grant for Institutional Treatment of Tuberculosis," 22 Nov. 1912.
87 L.G.B. Memorandum forwarded with John Burns to David Lloyd George, 24 Jan. 1913, ibid.
88 For an account of the meeting, see a summary, 6 Feb. 1913 in ibid.
89 *Interim Report of the Departmental Committee*, 26.

tuberculosis continued to occupy beds in Poor Law institutions.[90] We have seen that in June 1912, a month before the Sanatorium Benefit was to begin, the L.G.B. could learn of only 1,340 local authority beds for tuberculosis.[91] Over the next two years the number of beds available for state-aided treatment of tuberculosis grew rapidly but fell far short of the projected need. By the end of August 1913 the L.G.B. had approved the use of 7,764 beds in 219 institutions.[92] Voluntary bodies provided 4,367 of these beds and local authorities the remaining 3,397. There were still serious shortages, particularly in some regions. Insured patients were given top priority for treatment, but in 1913 the Insurance Commission reported to the L.G.B. that insurance committees were having difficulty finding beds for insured patients they had approved for the Sanatorium Benefit.[93] There were 300 such patients without beds in London. In the counties things were often even worse. Using the Astor Committee's standards, the Insurance Commission concluded that Kent should have had 136 beds, but it had only 45; Durham needed 124 but had only 27, and only 12 of these were in approved institutions; Derbyshire should have had 75 but possessed a mere 12, none of which were in approved institutions; and Cambridgeshire needed 17 and had none. By July 1914 beds in approved institutions reached 8,846.[94] Most of the addition since 1912 had been through the reassignments of local authority beds in isolation and smallpox hospitals and from the approval of private institutions for insurance or state-aided treatment. The National Insurance Act, 1913, had helped ease the shortage in London by permitting the use of beds operated by the Metropolitan Asylums Board.[95] These institutions would not hereafter be considered Poor Law institutions as far as the Sanatorium Benefit was concerned. But there was little new construction. By June 1914 the L.G.B. had received plans for institutions to house 5,000 new tuberculosis beds.[96] It had approved plans for 3,668 of these, but of the £1.116 million fund for capital grants, the Board had promised only £232,054 and had actually paid out only £62,026.[97]

The L.G.B. realized that it would be much easier to establish dispensaries than to arrange for the residential treatment of tuberculosis. At first it encouraged local authorities to establish a dispensary and appoint a Tuberculosis Officer as a first installment toward a complete and permanent scheme, and in these first years it gave a higher percentage of its capital grants toward the founding of dispensaries than toward residential institutions.[98] By June 1914 the Board had approved in

90 Newsholme, *Ann. Rep. Med. Off. L.G.B.*, 43 (1913–14): lxxx.
91 "Sanatorium Benefit," 11 July 1912, pp. 1–2, P.R.O., MH55/522.
92 *Ann. Rep. L.G.B.*, 42 (1912–13), III: xiv–xv.
93 For the following estimates of shortages, see two lists compiled for the L.G.B. by the Insurance Commission in 1913 in P.R.O., MH55/522.
94 Newsholme, *Ann. Rep. Med. Off. L.G.B.*, 44 (1914–15), xxiii.
95 3 & 4 Geo. 5, C. 37, sect. 39.
96 *Ann. Rep. L.G.B.*, 43 (1913–14), III: xxxvii.   97 Ibid., xxviii–xxix.
98 For this and the following figures on dispensaries and Tuberculosis Officers, see *Ann. Rep. L.G.B.*, 43 (1913–14), III: xxii–xxvi.

England 255 dispensaries, of which 216 were new, and the appointment of 177 Tuberculosis Officers. The approval of dispensaries or of residential institutions required that, among other things, the institution be part of a local authority tuberculosis scheme. By September 1914 the schemes submitted to the L.G.B. covered 95 percent of the population of England.[99] However, not all of these schemes had been approved and even fewer of them were complete schemes. The Board sometimes approved just the dispensary in order to encourage the local authority to begin. It was also true that some institutions did not meet L.G.B. standards and were only given provisional approval for temporary use. Nonetheless, the treatment program was running. On March 31, 1914, 4,555 insured and 1,231 uninsured were receiving treatment for tuberculosis provided by the insurance fund or by grant-aided local authority programs in residential institutions, and 7,898 insured and 14,201 uninsured were being treated at tuberculosis dispensaries.[100]

We have considered in some detail the administrative problems of implementing the Sanatorium Benefit in order to make two points. First, the Sanatorium Benefit did prove to be very difficult to administer, just as the civil servants at the L.G.B. had predicted. Once the wisdom of the Astor Committee's recommendations had been conceded, it made no sense administratively to continue to treat the insured with tuberculosis as a separate category and to unnecessarily multiply the number of public authorities and special funds in administering this benefit. It was with good reason that the treatment of tuberculosis was taken from the national insurance scheme in 1920 and given to local authorities to administer, just as the L.G.B. and the local authorities had requested between 1911 and 1913.[101] Second, we have tried to demonstrate how this issue could dominate the attention of Newsholme and the Board's Medical Department, as it did for three and a half or four years. During 1913 and most of 1914 Newsholme assigned six of his sixteen medical inspectors to work full-time on the review of tuberculosis schemes and the inspection of institutions.[102] He devoted much of his own time to the same work. Negotiations with local authorities were sometimes difficult and protracted. It took some three years of negotiations, for example, to work out a satisfactory arrangement in Berkshire.[103]

During these difficult years Newsholme did not change his ideals for community tuberculosis work. He and the L.G.B. continued to insist that dispensaries and sanatoriums supported by public money function as part of the public health work of local authorities. This advice applied particularly to the dispensary and its

99 Ibid., xv–xvi, li–cxii; Newsholme, *Ann. Rep. Med. Off. L.G.B.,* 43 (1913–14), lxiv, lxvi.
100 Ibid., xviii–xix.
101 This change was made by the National Health Insurance Act, 1920, 10 & 11 Geo. 5, C. 10, sect. 4. For its implementation see *Ann. Rep. Ministry of Health,* 2 (1920–1): 8–10.
102 Newsholme, *Ann. Rep. Med. Off. L.G.B.,* 43 (1913–14), lvii.
103 See the correspondence between the Berkshire County Council, the L.G.B., the National Insurance Commission, and the Board of Education between Feb. 1914 and Aug. 1917 in P.R.O., MH48/6.

staff. While the Departmental Committee on Tuberculosis had recommended that Tuberculosis Officers have clinical autonomy, the L.G.B. wanted them to be administratively subordinate to the Medical Officer of Health, who should have access to dispensary records.[104] Newsholme made a point of calling the M.O.H. the Administrative Tuberculosis Officer and the head of the tuberculosis dispensary the Clinical Tuberculosis Officer.[105] He recommended that the latter be part of the M.O.H.'s staff, but this arrangement could not always be made, especially when dispensaries were provided by voluntary organizations or by joint boards. The work of examining and treating patients at the dispensary, Newsholme insisted, must be carefully coordinated with the notifying of cases, the tracing of contacts, and the home visiting of known cases. It was very undesirable to have two unrelated medical staffs visiting the same patient in his home.

In his annual reports Newsholme continued to urge local authorities to provide the comprehensive preventive services he had outlined in his 1909 memorandum, but in their allotment of space to treatment and to prevention these same reports amply demonstrate how the struggle to provide treatment for recognized cases consumed the attention of the L.G.B. as well as the resources of the nation.[106] Newsholme was aware that certain crucial services whose establishment he believed should have preceded large schemes of institutional treatment were not getting the attention they deserved. Facilities for the bacteriological examination of sputum were initially in very short supply. Newsholme had prepared for the Astor Committee a special report on the pathological services available to local authorities, and he found that some county and county borough councils had made no provision to provide laboratory diagnosis. In 1911 the rate at which samples of sputum were examined for the tuberculosis bacillus in all the county boroughs collectively was only 1.27 examinations per 1,000 population, while in the counties the figure was a mere 0.38 per 1,000.[107] Even where facilities were available, they were often underutilized. The following year, after reading the reports of M.O.H. he noted

In one county borough with a population of about 100,000, 281 cases of pulmonary tuberculosis were notified, and 75 died during 1912; but only 47 specimens of sputum were sent by practitioners for examination. In this borough there are 60 registered practitioners, only 15 of whom sent specimens. Although it is possible that some practitioners examined specimens in their own laboratory, there is little doubt that many patients continue to be

104 *Interim Report of the Departmental Committee*, 17; and *Ann. Rep. L.G.B.*, 42 (1912–13), III: xx, xxvi.
105 Newsholme, *Ann. Rep. Med. Off. L.G.B.*, 43 (1913–14), lxiv–lxv, lxviii–lxix.
106 Notice, for example, the proportions of space devoted to treatment and schemes for providing treatment in his sections on the administrative control of tuberculosis in ibid., 42 (1912–13), xxxv–lv; and ibid. 43 (1913–14), lvii–xci.
107 Arthur Newsholme, "Memorandum submitted by the Medical Officer of the Local Government Board on the Pathological Work Undertaken by or on Behalf of Public Health Authorities and by Voluntary Hospitals, and on the Need for Great Extension and for Co-ordination of This Work," *Final Report of the Departmental Committee*, II: 128. The report was also reprinted, giving slightly different figures in Newsholme, *Ann. Rep. Med. Off. L.G.B.*, 42 (1912–13), 217.

treated for bronchitis, &c., long after they might have been recognized as tuberculous if sputum had been repeatedly examined.[108]

This deficiency was remedied sooner than most. By the end of 1913 most counties and county borough councils had provided free sputum examinations, although the willingness of practitioners to use such services still varied greatly from place to place.[109] Other problems were not easily solved. Newsholme warned repeatedly that M.O.H. and Tuberculosis Officers were not doing an adequate job in investigating home conditions and in examining contacts following notifications of tuberculosis. This deficiency was especially serious with notifications for non-pulmonary cases.[110] Such cases, Newsholme predicted, if properly investigated, would lead to the discovery of undetected cases of pulmonary tuberculosis.

Perhaps the gravest oversight during the fight to remake the Sanatorium Benefit and the rush to provide institutional treatment was the failure to take effective action against bovine tuberculosis. During 1911, the year that was so eventful for tuberculosis policy, the final report of the Third Royal Commission on Tuberculosis appeared. This Commission had been established to investigate the relationship between animal and human tuberculosis and the risk to humans from tuberculosis in animals, especially cattle. The Commission had been at work for a decade collecting clinical and experimental data, and it concluded unequivocally that infected meat and milk posed a very real danger to humans and were the frequent cause of tuberculosis, especially in children. The L.G.B. arranged to continue this research by transferring two of the Royal Commission's scientists to its own laboratory, where they devoted their attention to some of the unanswered questions concerning the etiology of tuberculosis and to demonstrating the frequency with which tuberculosis bacilli could be found in food brought to market.[111] Newsholme summarized the findings of the Royal Commission for the Astor Committee and for the readers of his Annual Reports.[112] While not all the scientific questions had been settled, he concluded that the policy implications of this important work were clear: A concerted attack on tubercular milk must be made.

The Board of Agriculture and Fisheries did issue an order in 1913 requiring notification of bovine tuberculosis (with emaciation; with tuberculosis of the udder; or with other chronic disease of the udder) and making provision for the slaughter of such animals.[113] Arthur Eastwood, the former scientific consultant for

108 Ibid., lii.
109 *Ann. Rep. L.G.B.,* 43 (1913–14), III: xix; and Newsholme, *Ann. Rep. Med. Off. L.G.B.,* 43 (1913–14), lx–lxi.
110 Ibid., lix; ibid., 44 (1914–15), xx, xxii–xxiii.
111 Newsholme, "Memorandum . . . on Medical Research," 122–5; and Newsholme, *Ann. Rep. Med. Off. L.G.B.,* 41 (1911–12), xlii–xliv.
112 Arthur Newsholme, "Memorandum submitted by the Medical Officer of the Local Government Board on Medical Research, with Special Reference to Tuberculosis," *Final Report of the Departmental Committee,* II: 122; Newsholme, *Ann. Rep. Med. Off. L.G.B.,* 41 (1911–12), xxxvii–xlii.
113 For a summary of the provisions of the order, see *Ann. Rep. L.G.B.,* 42 (1912–13), III: lx.

the Royal Commission who became the director of the L.G.B.'s small laboratory, proposed a pilot scheme which involved providing a bonus to farmers for maintaining herds of tuberculin-negative cattle.[114] But no concerted effort was made to insist on the tuberculin testing of herds or the pasteurization of milk. There were undoubtedly several reasons why more effective action was not taken, including resistance from the dairy industry, fears that the market would not repay the increased costs of producing tuberculosis-free milk, and a deep-seated medical suspicion that the boiling or pasteurizing of milk would rob it of its nutritive value for infants. It seems quite likely, however, that the pressure of implementing the Sanatorium Benefit did divert the attention of the L.G.B. from the implications of the Royal Commission's findings and delay effective action against bovine tuberculosis. The outbreak of World War I further frustrated the implementation of the tuberculosis program and imposed additional burdens on the L.G.B. while robbing it of resources.

114 "A Scheme for Inscreasing the Supply of Milk from Non-Tuberculous Dairy Stock," in News-holme, "Memorandum . . . on Medical Research," 125–6.

10

The Great War and the public health enterprise

CONTRACTION: PUBLIC HEALTH ON THE HOME FRONT

Almost five of Newsholme's eleven years at the Local Government Board were occupied by the demands of the First World War. He recalled two decades later that these demands had produced contradictory effects on the Board's activities. They "impeded much valuable work" and "stifled some progressive schemes at their birth," but they also prompted some important initiatives.[1] We begin by looking at the way in which the war tested the public health service and made the continuance of even routine activities extremely difficult and most innovation impossible. We will then turn to two areas in which the war prompted bold initiatives and major expansions of public health services: the prevention of venereal disease and the promotion of infant welfare.

"In Britain the time-honoured association between war and disease was broken during the Great War."[2] J. M. Winter reminds us of the great loss of human life to infectious disease during the war in Central and Eastern Europe and suggests that in Britain the "vagaries of disease," improvements of nutrition, and a system of recruiting of medical practitioners that preserved a skeleton of general practitioner services at home may have been responsible for a happier fate. It may be impossible to determine in retrospect why anticipated events, a series of epidemics for example, did not occur, but it is historically useful to observe whether contemporaries foresaw danger and what they did to try to forestall it. In Britain the wartime public health service was mobilized early to use all available means to prevent the spread of infectious disease.

Once war had been declared, the L.G.B. (like other civil service departments) put itself on a special footing to promote the war effort and to see that local authorities did the same. In the first month of the conflict the Board and the War Office worked out a set of agreements intended to protect both the civil popula-

---

1 Newsholme, *Last 30 Years*, 18.
2 J. M. Winter, *The Great War and the British People* (Cambridge, Mass.: Harvard Univ. Press, 1986), 154.

tion and the military forces.[3] Newsholme's commission as a Lieutenant Colonel in the Territorial Sanitary Corps and his membership on the Army Sanitary Committee allowed him to work directly with military medical authorities. In these early months of the war the Board instructed Medical Officers of Health to see that there was no deterioration of public health work among civilians and to provide information and assistance to military authorities in their areas. Newsholme's memoranda to M.O.H. dwelt on the establishment of camps and the billeting of troops, on water supply and drainage, on sanitation and the disposal of waste, and on the provision of isolation facilities for cases of infectious disease among the troops. The War Office ordered commanding officers to seek this advice from M.O.H. and to work cooperatively with local sanitary authorities. A system of mutual notification of infectious diseases was soon established so that civilian and military authorities would be aware of cases of infectious diseases that occurred in each other's population. In addition the L.G.B.'s Inspectors of Foods agreed to supervise the work of contractors who supplied food to the troops. The Board asked the assistance of M.O.H. farther up the supply chain by informing them of army suppliers in their jurisdiction and asking them to inspect these operations. During the first year of the war much of the effort of the L.G.B.'s Medical Department was given over to making this system of cooperative sanitation work. Newsholme assigned twelve of his medical inspectors to the task.

The wartime movement of people, especially the return home of sick troops and the arrival of infected immigrants, posed special risks of disease outbreaks. During the first year of the war Newsholme sought to relieve overburdened local officials and to stimulate vigilance by sending medical inspectors to help local M.O.H. conduct examinations of arriving immigrants.[4] He also worried about domestic cases of smallpox and about typhoid fever. Within two weeks of the declaration of war he sent to M.O.H. a memorandum on special measures that should be taken to guard against smallpox in the conditions of war. He urged special efforts in locating and properly isolating cases, in tracing contacts, and in seeing that contacts were vaccinated or revaccinated. An order of the L.G.B. in 1916 sought to facilitate the latter step by empowering M.O.H. to vaccinate rather than having to rely on public vaccinators.[5] The Board also stepped up the Government Lymph Establishment's production of vaccine to meet both the needs of the armed forces and an anticipated larger civilian demand.

To control typhoid fever in army camps, Newsholme warned against the use of the pail system for the disposal of human wastes in camps, and he recommended the use of the new typhoid vaccine.[6] But he worried especially about the move-

3 For the following discussion of these early agreements, see Arthur Newsholme and F. J. Willis, "Public Health Work of the Local Government Board in Relation to the War," in *Report of the Special Work of the Local Government Board Arising out of the War*, B.P.P., 1914–16, XXV, 30–2; Newsholme, *Ann. Rep. Med. Off. L.G.B.*, 44 (1914–15): iii–ix; and ibid., 45 (1915–16): iv–vi.
4 Newsholme and Willis, "Public Health Work," 32.
5 Public Health (Smallpox Prevention) Regulations, 1917 were issued on 12 Feb. 1916.
6 Newsholme, *Ann. Rep. Med. Off. L.G.B.*, 44 (1914–15): iv, viii–ix.

ment of the sick and convalescent troops. He saw to it that military authorities were instructed to notify M.O.H. when soldiers or sailors convalescing from typhoid fever were moved to a new location. He also instructed M.O.H. to investigate carefully all sporadic cases of enteric fever and to see that precautions were taken to prevent further transmission of the infection.

Dysentery was much feared and called for special precautions. As the war progressed, soldiers from the front suffering from dysentery were constantly being brought to hospitals in England. With each returning sick soldier came the potential for an outbreak in Britain. Civilian and military sanitary authorities agreed that military dysentery cases would be admitted to only a few hospitals, that strict isolation and disinfection procedures would be followed during the railway transport of these patients, that the discharge of convalescents would be delayed until the microscopic examination of their dejecta indicated that they were no longer infectious, and that the M.O.H. of the district to which convalescents were bound would be notified when these patients were discharged.[7]

As the war continued and tuberculosis was recognized as a major medical problem for the military, the L.G.B. encouraged local sanitary authorities to help the military screen recruits for tuberculosis. In May 1916 the Board issued two circulars and an order.[8] It first asked local authorities to allow their Tuberculosis Officers to assist in the medical examination of recruits. It then required M.O.H. to review their lists of notified cases of tuberculosis and to send to the Army Council a list of all men of military age whose names appeared on that list and to send thereafter a weekly list of newly notified cases.

After several years of war Newsholme could report that these special wartime measures had helped break the link between war and pestilence. Although there had been a few small civilian outbreaks of dysentery during the war, Britain had escaped the extensive epidemics that had taken place on the Continent. He recognized that Britain's more fortunate experience was due in part to its less disturbed food supply and to its higher level of nutrition, but he also believed that preventive action by civil and military authorities deserved much of the credit.[9] Similarly typhus and trench fever had occurred among British troops in the war zone, but these diseases had not spread to civilians in Britain, even though by some accounts part of the British population was now more louse infested.[10] Cases of bubonic plague had appeared at British ports and a few human cases had occurred in East Suffolk, apparently as a result of contact with infected local rodents, but prompt action by port sanitary officers and M.O.H. had kept the disease from spreading further.[11] When an outbreak of smallpox occurred in south

7 Ibid., 45 (1915–16): xvii–xviii.
8 For a brief discussion, see ibid., 46 (1916–17): xx. The order in question is Public Health (Tuberculosis) Regulations, 1916.
9 Ibid., 47 (1917–18), xlvi–xlviii.
10 Ibid., 45 (1915–16), xviii–xix; and ibid., 47 (1917–18), li–lii.
11 Ibid., 46 (1916–17), viii; and ibid., 47 (1917–18), xlix–li.

Lancashire and south Wales in the spring of 1916 and when in 1917 cases of malaria began to appear in troops who had never been outside of the United Kingdom but who were stationed in the areas famous for endemic ague in the nineteenth century, the Board conducted special field investigations and assisted local officials.[12] Finally, typhoid fever – in Newsholme's opinion the best indicator of the sanitary condition of the community – had continued its forty-year decline right through the war.[13]

The L.G.B.'s medical department felt itself helpless to respond effectively to two epidemic diseases during the war, however. The first was cerebrospinal fever (meningitis), which was very prevalent in 1915–17. Medicine simply did not know enough about this disease for Newsholme to recommend effective action. This disease seemed to be infectious, although not highly infectious. The meningococcus seemed to be associated with it, but the epidemiology of the disease was complicated, because meningococci had been found not only in the sick and in healthy contacts but also in those who had no known contact with a case. Newsholme probably did all that could be done.[14] As we have seen, he urged that the Board make cerebrospinal fever notifiable; he drew the attention of M.O.H. to the disease and summarized current knowledge for them, and he saw that the Board's pathologists conducted research on the disease.

The second disease with which the Board was unprepared to deal was influenza. The pandemic of 1918–19 was an exceptional experience by any standard and a mortality disaster against which no Western nation was able to defend itself. George Newman, who, as we will see, was unlikely to miss any opportunity for faulting Newsholme's administration, explained in 1919 that the pandemic of influenza of 1918–19 could not have occurred at a worse time for the civilian and military health authorities, and that these authorities did all that could be done under the circumstances.[15] Before the Royal Society of Medicine in November 1918, Newsholme discussed how poorly the disease was understood and how nothing that any health authorities had tried seemed to prevent the spread of the disease. He also suggested that the government had concluded that during the war it simply could not attempt the sort of rigid isolation and quarantine that might have helped prevent the disease. He had prepared, he explained, a memorandum on the disease in July 1918 which the Board never issued. "There are national circumstances in which the major duty is to 'carry on' even when risk to health and life is involved." Soldiers, sailors, and munitions and transport workers had to remain at their posts.

In each of the cases cited some lives might have been saved, spread of infection diminished, great suffering avoided, if the known sick could have been isolated from the healthy; if rigid exclusion of known sick and drastic increase of floor-space for each person could have

12 Ibid., 45 (1915–16), x–xiv; ibid., 46 (1916–17), viii–xi; ibid., 47 (1917–18), liii–liv; *Ann. Rep. L.G.B.*, 45 (1915–16), III: 10; and ibid., 46 (1916–17), 35–6.
13 Newsholme, *Ann. Rep. Med. Off. L.G.B.*, 45 (1915–16): xix–xx.
14 Ibid., xxi–xxv; and ibid., 47 (1917–18), liv–lvi.
15 George Newman, *Ann. Rep. Med. Off. L.G.B.*, 48 (1918–19), 11–13.

been enforced in factories, workplaces, barracks, and ships; if overcrowding could have been regardlessly prohibited. But it was necessary to 'carry on,' and the relentless needs of warfare justified incurring this risk of spreading infection and the associated creation of a more virulent type of disease or of mixed diseases.[16]

These are grim words from the leader of a nation's public health service. The lack of a more active policy from the Board and from local authorities which looked to it for leadership provoked criticism from contemporaries which recent historians have echoed, and it has been argued that the only effective action taken in the face of the epidemic was initiated by laypersons acting at the local level.[17]

The difficulty health authorities had in responding to the influenza pandemic becomes more intelligible, and their success in continuing normal public health services during the conflict and in taking on additional war-related work seems more remarkable, when we recognize how the war depleted their ranks. Eventually half of the nation's medical practitioners would join the armed forces. The British government delegated the task of recruiting medical practitioners and much of the responsibility for weighing the social costs of inducting particular practitioners to the medical profession acting through the Central Medical War Committee (C.M.W.C.), which was made up of officials and elected members of the British Medical Association.[18] The C.M.W.C. relied on local medical committees to determine which practitioners were willing to serve, to put pressure on the reluctant to enlist, and eventually to find ways of sharing responsibilities so that still more might be taken. In the early phases of the war, private practitioner suspicion of public or contract practice raised its head, and the C.M.W.C. established a ranking of eligibility for recruitment that placed physicians in public service and those with national insurance practices before those in private practice. It quickly backed down, however, in the face of fierce opposition from both the Local Government Board and the National Health Insurance Commission.[19]

Hereafter more consultative procedures were followed, with the L.G.B. sending two representatives to each meeting of the C.M.W.C.[20] By agreement with the War Office and the C.M.W.C., before a local authority medical officer could be commissioned, the L.G.B. had to give its approval.[21] In the early phases of the war

16 Arthur Newsholme, "Discussion on Influenza," *Proc. Roy. Soc. Med.*, 12 (1918–19) part 1: 13. Newsholme's remarks were reprinted in Arthur Newsholme, "Introductory Remarks on Epidemic Catarrhs and Influenza," *Lancet* (1918), no. 2: 692.
17 Sandra M. Tomkins, "The Failure of Expertise: Public Health Policy in Britain during the 1918–19 Influenza Epidemic," *Social Hist. Med.*, 3 (1992), 437, 444, 452–3.
18 Winter, *Great War*, 154–73.
19 Central Medical War Committee, minutes of Executive Subcommittee, 24 Nov. 1915 (Document 100); minutes of committee meeting 24 Nov. 1915; "Memorandum as to Question of Certain Classes of Medical Practitioners Being Urged to Join the Services in Preference to Others . . ." (Document 108); and "Report on Interview with L.G.B. on December 1st, 1915" (Document 115), British Medical Association Archives, Central Medical War Committee. Hereafter cited as B.M.A., C.M.W.C.
20 Newsholme, *Ann. Rep. Med. Off. L.G.B.*, 45 (1915–16): xxxi–xxxii.
21 Ibid., xxxi–xxxii; ibid., 46 (1916–17): vii; and ibid., 47 (1917–18): lxxvii.

it gave its approval to most inductions proposed, and it tried to determine which medical officers were willing to serve. It was concerned, however, to determine that the local authority for whom the medical officer worked could make other arrangements to see that statutory health services continued to be provided, that the public health would not be seriously jeopardized, and that the local authority agreed to the induction.[22]

At the beginning of the war there were 1880 sanitary districts in England and Wales employing 1,618 M.O.H.[23] The arrangements under which these officers served were Byzantine, with many officers holding more than one public appointment and some rural districts being served by more than one officer. Three hundred eighteen of these M.O.H. served full-time. The remainder were part-time appointees. In addition to these M.O.H., sanitary authorities by that time also employed 237 Tuberculosis Officers, in addition to Assistant Medical Officers, Assistant Tuberculosis Officers, and Medical Officers of isolation hospitals. The staffs of local health departments also included at the beginning of the war in excess of 2,300 sanitary inspectors who were not medically qualified but whose services and experience would be missed as the needs of the army and navy drew off public health workers.

The number of M.O.H. receiving commissions grew rapidly. By March 1915, seven months into the conflict, it had reached 155 and by the end of the year 248.[24] Tuberculosis Officers, typically young and newly appointed, were particularly liable to be taken. Eighty-four had been commissioned by the end of December 1915, and by the following April that number reached 110, or 46 percent of the number of such positions at the beginning of the war.[25] Local authorities filled in the gaps by combining appointments and districts in ways the L.G.B. ordinarily would not have permitted. They also sought the services of older practitioners, and, for the first time, hired medically qualified women as medical officers. Women served during the war as Tuberculosis Officers, Assistant Medical Officers, and M.O.H., a few as M.O.H. for counties. The L.G.B. asked that posts be held for incumbents who had to serve in the military. Substitutes should be appointed only temporarily and should be over military age or otherwise ineligible for military service.[26]

Local authorities found it more difficult to manage by the spring of 1916. By April over 500 medical officers – M.O.H., Assistant M.O.H., Tuberculosis Officers, Assistant Tuberculosis Officers, and Medical Officers to infectious disease

22 "Memorandum by Mr. Stutchbury [Principal Secretary, L.G.B.] on Medical Men Holding Offices under the Control of the L.G.B., and Giving Their Whole Time to These Offices," (Document 331), B.M.A., C.M.W.C.
23 For the following figures, see *Ann. Rep. L.G.B.,* 43 (1913–14), III: cxxxix–cxlii; and "Report of Interview with L.G.B. on December 1st, 1915, Document 115, B.M.A., C.M.W.C.
24 *Ann. Rep. L.G.B.,* 44 (1914–15), III: 26; and Willis's comments in "Report of Interview with L.G.B. on December 1st, 1915," Document 115 (1915–16), B.M.A., C.M.W.C.
25 Willis's comments in "Report of Interview with L.G.B. on December 1st, 1915," Document 115 (1915–16), B.M.A., C.M.W.C.; and *Ann. Rep. L.G.B.,* 45 (1915–16), III: 5.
26 Newsholme, *Ann. Rep. Med. Off. L.G.B.,* 45 (1915–16), xxxii.

hospitals or sanatoriums were in the armed forces.[27] The ranks of sanitary inspectors had also been seriously depleted, and Newsholme observed that many untrained men and women were carrying on as best they could in these posts. "Unless considerable readjustments are made," he reported, "more officers cannot be spared consistently with the public safety."[28] But the worst was yet to come.[29] During the next year the age for compulsory service by doctors was raised to fifty-five and their recruitment passed to the Ministry of National Service. The Central Medical War Committee hereafter served as a tribunal for appeals. By stricter scrutiny of civilian needs and the induction of men recently hired to replace those already taken, the authorities raised the number of medical officers supplied to the military by another 10 percent. In early August 1917 the C.M.W.C. informed the Government that the well was dry. No more medical men could be safely withdrawn from the public health service.[30]

The L.G.B. also felt the pressure of military manpower needs. By war's end 421 of its 510 male staff members of military age had served in the military, and 51 had been killed in combat.[31] When the war began, the Medical Department employed 26 medically qualified officers and inspectors in addition to Newsholme.[32] Eleven of these would serve in the armed forces. In addition Newsholme lost two other male officers, one to retirement and another to death unrelated to the war and the Department's only woman employee, Janet Lane-Claypon, then an Assistant Medical Inspector, who resigned to become Dean of the Household and Social Science Department, King's College for Women. Newsholme was authorized to appoint temporary replacements more slowly than the departures occurred. During the war five older men, two of them retired officers from the Indian Medical Service, and three women doctors joined the staff, the men as Temporary Medical Inspectors and the women as Temporary Assistant Medical Inspectors. The net result was that the Department was chronically understaffed, at the worst of times by 25 percent of its former size.

Such reduction in staff both at the center and at the periphery could not be made without curtailing the work of public health authorities. Before the war, the L.G.B. had regarded local inspections as an important device to maintain a high standard of services. In normal years this work occupied a large share of its efforts.[33] As the war dragged on, such inquiries became rare, except when out-

27 Ibid., 46 (1916–17), vii–viii.   28 Ibid., vii.

29 For the following discussion, see ibid., 47 (1917–18), lxxvii.

30 Executive Subcommittee, Central Medical War Committee, to Lord Derby, Sir A. Keoh, the Local Government Board, and National Health Insurance Commission, 3 Aug. 1917, Document 9 (1917–18), B.M.A., C.M.W.C.

31 *Ann. Rep. L.G.B.,* 48 (1918–19), 150, 151.

32 For the following information, see *British Imperial Calendar* (1915): 399–400; Newsholme, *Ann. Rep. Med. Off. L.G.B.,* 44 (1914–15), v; *Ann. Rep. L.G.B.,* 44 (1914–15), III: 65–66; Newsholme, *Ann. Rep. Med. Off. L.G.B.,* 45 (1915–16), xxxii–xxxiii; ibid, 46 (1916–17), xxxix–xl; and ibid., 47 (1917–18), lxxiv–lxxv.

33 See, for example, the list of inspections the Medical Department conducted in the administrative year 1913–14 in ibid., 43 (1913–14), 76–80.

breaks of dangerous disease were reported. Such inquiries following an epidemic were aggressively undertaken at the beginning of the war, but that standard was harder to maintain as the war effort drained the resources of civilian health authorities. Newsholme reported with regret in 1917 that recently prompt action had not been taken in some outbreaks of disease because of the inexperience of local officials, and he worried that the nation stood at risk should more cases of smallpox appear.[34] The L.G.B. also had to allow several new prevention programs to languish. In February 1915 it had issued an order aimed at preventing the spread of typhoid fever through contaminated shellfish, but it soon found that neither it nor local medical officers had the time or energy to enforce the new regulations.[35]

Although the war curtailed many public health programs, its cost fell most heavily on the tuberculosis work. It was a bitter disappointment to Newsholme to have to preside over the stunting of the program in which he had such high hopes. When the war began, no local authority scheme had been in operation very long, and some of the largest were only getting started. London County Council's scheme, for example, began only one month before war was declared.[36] Furthermore, most of the schemes then in operation were incomplete, frequently consisting of little more than a dispensary. During the war some planning continued. A few local authorities submitted tuberculosis schemes, and the L.G.B. continued to pay capital grants for construction that had begun before the war. But capital grants for new construction were no longer considered after July 1915, and shortages of money, labor, and materials meant that several institutions begun before the war remained unfinished throughout the conflict.[37] The number of beds in residential institutions approved for the treatment of tuberculosis under the state scheme increased somewhat during the war, from 8,846 in July 1914 to 12,441 by the spring of 1918.[38] But this increase was brought about mainly by the reassignment of existing beds, usually those in local authority isolation hospitals, and the effects were neutralized first by the transferring of pauper tuberculosis patients into local authority sanatoriums as Poor Law institutions were converted into military hospitals, and then by the loss of entire sanatoriums for use as war hospitals.[39]

The war meant not only that there was little expansion, but in most areas the tuberculosis work deteriorated. With the beginning of the war, Newsholme felt obliged to end routine inspection of local authority tuberculosis programs and to

34 Ibid., 46 (1916–17), vii.
35 Public Health (Shell-fish) Regulations, 1915. See also Newsholme, *Ann. Rep. Med. Off. L.G.B.*, 45 (1915–16), xxi.
36 For a description of its first year, see *Ann. Rep. L.G.B.*, 44 (1914–15), III: 17–21.
37 *Ann. Rep. L.G.B.*, 45 (1915–16), III: 6; Newsholme, *Ann. Rep. Med. Off. L.G.B.*, 47 (1917–18), lxi.
38 Ibid., 44 (1914–15), xxiii; and ibid., 47 (1917–18), lxi.
39 *Ann. Rep. L.G.B.*, 44 (1914–15), III: 9, ibid., 45 (1915–16), III, 6; ibid., 46 (1916–17), 30; and ibid., 47 (1917–18), 9.

reduce the number of full-time inspectors he assigned to tuberculosis work from six to two.[40] To lighten the administrative load on local authorities, the L.G.B. eased its accounting requirements, and it postponed indefinitely the required reports from sanatoriums and dispensaries.[41] It also ceased requiring M.O.H. to submit an annual summary of notifications. Notification of cases, never satisfactory before the war, now decayed to a state which by 1918 Newsholme labeled "deplorable."[42] The Board was also forced to tolerate a deterioration in standards of services. As local authorities found it increasingly difficult to find medical officers, the Board first relaxed and then withdrew entirely its requirement that those appointed as Tuberculosis Officers have or agree to acquire special training. It also was forced to continue to approve inadequate dispensaries and sanatoriums it had originally approved on a temporary basis to launch a local authority scheme.[43] The results of this stagnation were particularly unfortunate for children with tuberculosis who, Newsholme believed, were especially poorly served by the nation's sanatoriums.[44]

As resources dwindled, the L.G.B. decided that effort must be focused on providing treatment to tuberculosis patients.[45] This decision was dictated by the statutory obligations the Sanatorium Benefit imposed on local Insurance Committees and on those local authorities which had entered into agreements with these committees. In this retrenchment some of the work Newsholme thought was most important, such as the tracing of home contacts and the formation of after-care committees, had to be abandoned. "This is regrettable," he lamented, "as the reduction of tuberculosis can best be secured by this and other preventive and social work, which should go hand in hand with the actual treatment of patients."[46]

Newsholme's frustration can be clearly seen in a section on tuberculosis and the war in his annual report for the administrative year 1916–17, which he republished in *The Lancet.*[47] He noted the increase in tuberculosis mortality – up 12 percent in 1916–17 from the level of 1913, and he recognized as contributing factors certain wartime conditions – overcrowding in camps and factories and the movement of infected peoples, including the induction or employment of unrecognized cases of tuberculosis, plus fatigue and dust in industrial employment – as well as the prevalence in 1915 and 1916 of influenza, a serious complication for those

40 Newsholme, *Ann. Rep. Med. Off. L.G.B.,* 44 (1914–15), xviii.
41 *Ann. Rep. L.G.B.,* 45 (1915–16), III: 6; Newsholme, *Ann. Rep. Med. Off. L.G.B.,* 45 (1915–16), xv.
42 Ibid., 47 (1917–18), lxiv. 43 Ibid., 44 (1914–15), xxi.
44 Ibid., xxv–xxvi; ibid., 47 (1917–18), lxi–lxii; and *Ann. Rep. L.G.B.,* 44 (1914–15), III: 12–13.
45 *Ann. Rep. L.G.B.,* 44 (1914–15), III: 10.
46 Newsholme, *Ann. Rep. Med. Off. L.G.B.,* 45 (1915–16), xiv, xv–xvi.
47 For the following discussion, see ibid., 46 (1916–17), xviii–xxx; and Arthur Newsholme, "The Relations of Tuberculosis to War Conditions with Remarks on Some Aspects of the Administrative Control of Tuberculosis," *Lancet* (1917), no. 2: 591–5. In the following discussion, citations will be to the latter publication.

with pulmonary tuberculosis.[48] He rejected the claim that nutritional deficiencies were responsible for this mortality increase as well as the argument that housing reform was the best strategy for controlling tuberculosis.[49]

The war, he also claimed, altered human behavior in ways which hampered preventive work.[50] In normal times patients were often reluctant to consult a physician or to undergo treatment. The uninsured feared the expense, and even the insured often delayed using the Sanatorium Benefit, preferring to wait until their twenty-six weeks of sick pay were about to end and their insurance benefits to drop by half when their disability pay began. The war had provided additional incentives for delay and concealment: a patriotic sense of duty to contribute to the war effort in some, and a reluctance to miss out of high wages in war industries in others. Even when patients sought medical attention, there were troubles. General practitioners were even more overworked than usual, and many failed to diagnose accurately or to notify cases as they were required to do. They also frequently failed to consult the local Tuberculosis Officer. There had been trouble, Newsholme conceded, between local practitioners and Tuberculosis Officers in some places and even difficulties between M.O.H. and Tuberculosis Officers. Some Tuberculosis Officers were too young and inexperienced to win the confidence of more experienced local doctors. Local doctors were sometimes suspicious of the new initiatives in municipal medicine.

Newsholme was most frustrated by what had happened to sanatoriums.[51] While in his planning he had intended these institutions for patients in the early stages of the disease, for whom the prospects of recovery or a permanent arrest of the disease were believed good, he found that most were filled with advanced cases who stayed for long periods. Because many of these patients were insured, they were hard to refuse. Every person suffering from tuberculosis, including those for whom there was no hope of recovery, deserved treatment, but that treatment must be suited to the nature of his or her case. The filling of sanatoriums with advanced or chronic cases resulted in inadequate treatment of these cases and the denial of those peculiar features of the sanatorium to those most likely to benefit from receiving them. Many of those found in sanatoriums, Newsholme claimed, should be nursed at home following a period of training in an institution, or in a hospital, if they needed surgery or when their condition deteriorated to the point that they could no longer safely remain at home. While Newsholme did not explicitly frame the issue in this way, his frustration shows the conflict between two views of the purpose of the public sanatoriums. Put crudely, he believed that the nation was sending the wrong patients to the sanatorium and defeating their preventive

48 Newsholme, "Relations of Tuberculosis to War," 591.
49 Newsholme to C.-E. A. Winslow, 7 Nov. 1919, Yale University Library, Winslow Papers; Winslow to Newsholme, 19 Nov. 1929; Arthur Newsholme, "Housing and Tuberculosis" [lecture notes, audience unspecified], 22 Oct. 1937, Newsholme Papers, uncatalogued materials; and Newsholme, "Relations of Tuberculosis to War," 594–5.
50 Newsholme, "Relations of Tuberculosis to War," 592–5.   51 Ibid., 593–4.

purpose. Some of these advanced cases were the ones who had declined to enter the institution at an earlier time, when their treatment would have done both them and their community the most good. Newsholme did not consider framing the situation in other terms. Perhaps the nation had provided the wrong type of institution for its tuberculosis victims. Perhaps Lloyd George had a better sense of what the people wanted: a medical benefit they could choose when they wanted it and not an institution-based public health program.

Newsholme continued to believe that it was possible to balance the rights and wishes of patients with the needs of the community. Institutional treatment of advanced cases, he claimed cannot

be considered solely from the standpoint of the patient's own interest. Nothing should be done, and nothing need be done, contrary to these interests; but public and personal interests alike point to the desirability of treating the consumptive under conditions which will minimise the possibilities of acquirement of infection by contacts.[52]

Wartime conditions made health authorities even less tolerant of difficult tuberculosis patients than they had been before the war and put greater pressure on Newsholme and the L.G.B. to permit the use of compulsion against these patients. Beginning in 1911 when St. Helens successfully sponsored a private bill giving it powers of compulsory isolation for tuberculosis, nine local authorities had acquired this power by private legislation before the end of 1914.[53] During the war, councils, citizens' groups, and insurance committees demanded that powers of compulsory isolation be granted as a matter of general policy.[54] In April 1916 the President of the L.G.B., Walter Long, faced a question in the House of Commons on the issue.[55] By early 1917 the campaign became more organized as insurance committees endorsed the model resolution drafted by the Insurance Committee of the East Riding of Yorkshire, which demanded the repeal of Article XVI of the L.G.B.'s Public Health (Tuberculosis) Regulations, 1912. That article was the most recent version of the Board's guarantee that patients would not suffer civil or economic disabilities from local authority action following notification. By July 1917, fifty committees and local authorities had supported the petition.[56]

Local authorities were worried about both public danger and public expense. The Huddersfield Citizens' Guild of Help, for example, was indignant when patients in the public sanatorium demanded to return home for the Christmas holidays in 1914 "with all the attendant risks" and the waste of "costly sanatoria."[57] To buttress their demand, local officials sent accounts of cases they believed

52 Ibid., 594.   53 *Ann. Rep. L.G.B.*, 44 (1914–15), III: 15–16.
54 See, for example, the correspondence between these local groups and the L.G.B. during 1915, 1916, and 1917 in P.R.O., MH55/520.
55 Great Britain, *Parliamentary Debates*, House of Commons, 5th series, 81 (12 April 1916), 1775–6, question 121.
56 A manuscript list of those supporting the resolution of the East Riding of Yorkshire Insurance Committee may be found in P.R.O., MH55/520.
57 George T. Lowe [Honorable Secretary, Huddersfield Citizens' Guild of Help] to Home Secretary [sic.], Local Government Board Offices, 20 March 1915, ibid.

proved that powers of compulsory confinement were necessary. The East Riding Insurance Committee provided an extended history of an insured seventeen-year-old who lived with his parents and four siblings in an overcrowded four-room cottage. In September 1916 he had been admitted to a sanatorium but had left four days later complaining of the food and of the treatment he had received from the nurses. The sanatorium staff denied the complaints and claimed that the patient had been "badly behaved" and had left because he found that he was not free to go out to town at night. The young man refused to reenter the institution, although he was urged to do so by the County Medical Officer of Health, an assistant to this M.O.H., and by his panel doctor. He finally promised to return at some indefinite time in the future. During the interview with a member of the Insurance Committee where that promise was made he is reported to have had a fit of coughing where he brought up a mass of sputum which he promptly spat on the floor. "It is no exaggeration to say," the Insurance Committee concluded, "that this youth is in his present condition a serious menace to the health of the community," and if he is "left free to spread the infection" as he is doing, the large sums, £2,500 per year, being spent on this work in East Yorkshire will be wasted.[58]

The behavior of soldiers and sailors who had been discharged with tuberculosis alarmed and angered some local authorities. With the encouragement of the L.G.B. and with funds for the uninsured provided by the Ministry of Pensions, local authorities had given discharged servicemen priority in their sanatoriums.[59] However, many of these men refused institutional treatment, and some had left the institution soon after entering. James Niven, M.O.H. of Manchester, wrote to Newsholme in February 1916 demanding that something be done to stop the "wasteful, irritating, and dangerous coming and going" from sanatoriums.[60] The medical superintendents of these institutions also complained of discipline problems with patients recently discharged from military service. Some superintendents suggested that such patients be treated only in military hospitals or that sanatorium officers be given military rank.[61]

In the face of this demand for greater authority over patients, Newsholme continued to hold that compulsory powers were unnecessary and that patient rights must be respected. He reminded those who wanted tuberculosis patients returning from the armed forces subjected to strong discipline that "unrest and insubordination" had occurred in civilian sanatoriums before the war and were best seen as a reflection of poor institutional management, in particular of instances where the superintendent "is not possessed of a strong personality and is not imbued with a high sense of the importance and value of his work."[62] He

58 John Bickersteth [East Riding of Yorkshire Insurance Committee] to Secretary, Local Government Board, 19 Oct. 1916, ibid.
59 *Ann. Rep. L.G.B.*, 45 (1915–16), III: 4–5; ibid., 46 (1916–17), 29; and ibid., 47 (1917–18), 7–8.
60 James Niven to Newsholme, 4 Feb. 1916, P.R.O., MH55/520.
61 Newsholme, *Ann. Rep. Med. Off. L.G.B.*, 45 (1915–16), xv; and ibid., 47 (1917–18), lxiii.
62 Ibid., 47 (1917–18), lxiii.

emphasized the importance of "straight talk" with soldiers and of the need to keep body and mind occupied while in the institution. In answer to Niven he provided a legal answer, the provisions under which the local authority might try to enforce institutional isolation, but he then strongly advised against trying this approach and recommended instead the continued use of persuasion.[63] He did not, however, oppose the renewal of compulsory powers in St. Helens when their initial five-year period was about to lapse, and he reported that the limited use St. Helens had made of its powers had not "infringed the spirit" of Article XVI of Public Health (Tuberculosis) Regulations, 1912, or caused "appreciable local friction or hardship."[64] However, he continued to oppose the removal of Section XVI from the Board's regulations, although he recognized that in the future the Board might have to consider "modified powers of compulsory segregation of advanced cases." For the present he thought it best to observe how these powers were used in those few local authorities that had them. Until the way was clearer, Newsholme urged his administrative superiors to deprecate the sweeping views of local authorities who demanded broad powers to isolate tuberculosis patients and to explain that tuberculosis cases need not be a "serious source of danger to others," if patients have learned the "elementary rules of life suited to their condition."[65]

There is thus plenty of support for Newsholme's retrospective claim that the war stifled important public health work. It did try the resources and patience of public health authorities. The deterioration of tuberculosis work and the increase in tuberculosis mortality were especially bitter for Newsholme. We turn next to the two examples of bold new initiatives during the war. In the remainder of this chapter we consider the venereal disease clinics; in the next, local authority child-welfare work.

EXPANSION: THE STATE VENEREAL DISEASE SERVICE

There is little doubt that the war hastened public action against syphilis. The prospect of thousands of infected troops returning home became horrible for public authorities to contemplate. As an emergency wartime measure the venereal disease service had an unusual birth.[66] Seldom had the central health authority acted so swiftly on so major a program. Seldom had the recommendations of a Royal Commission been enacted with so little change. Seldom had the L.G.B. acted more boldly and with less consultation or consideration of objections. With strong incentives to act, with support from highly placed individuals in government, social reform, and the professions and without competition from within the

---

63 Newsholme to Niven, 25 Feb. 1916, P.R.O., MH55/520.
64 Newsholme, *Ann. Rep. Med. Off. L.G.B.*, 45 (1915–16), xvi.
65 Newsholme, minute, 26 May 1915, P.R.O., MH55/520.
66 For an informative account of the establishment of the new service, see David Evans, "Tackling the 'Hideous Scourge': The Creation of the Venereal Disease Treatment Centres in Early Twentieth-Century Britain," *Social Hist. Med.* 3 (1992): 413–33.

civil service, it was free to follow the blueprints set out by its technical experts. Never was Newsholme so much of an insider in the creation of a new medical service. What emerged was closer than any other of the new state medical services to his ideal of a unified, local authority medical service.

While the war may have hastened public action, it did not determine the basic preventive strategy. That strategy had already been articulated before the war opened. For several years advocates of a new approach to venereal disease both warned of the dangers of these diseases and insisted that they could be controlled if cases were diagnosed early and treated effectively. Newsholme made this point in February 1908 in his memorandum for the Poor Law Commission.[67] The context for his remarks was his call for a local authority medical service which would diagnose and treat all diseases, including venereal diseases. His first official pronouncement on venereal disease came in his *Annual Report* for 1913–14 and reflected a greater sense of urgency and opportunity. "For several years past it has been evident that the social convention of silence respecting these diseases and the absence of direct measures for their prevention was accompanied by very serious injury to the public health."[68] Like other medical advocates of a public venereal disease policy, he pointed to recent scientific discoveries to demonstrate that the continuance of the conspiracy of silence was a public menace. Within less than a decade there had been a revolution in the knowledge of syphilis. First came the successful production of experimental cases in laboratory animals (1903); then the discovery of the causal organism, the *Treponema pallidum* – then known as *Spirochaeta pallida* – (1905); next the development of a reliable serological test for syphilis – the Wassermann test (1906); and finally the introduction of an effective chemotherapeutic agent – Salvarsan (1910).[69] The remarkable claims for Salvarsan attracted intense medical interest and were soon verified in Britain by clinical trials, some of the most important of which took place in military hospitals. Very successful results were reported in a series of papers at the British Medical Association's annual meeting in 1911, and in a leading article in the issue of the *British Medical Journal*. These and other articles on the new treatment of syphilis sounded an optimistic chord.[70] The implications for public health work were very clear. It was now possible to diagnose cases with much greater certainty and with proper treatment to render them noninfectious to others. The prospects of dealing with gonorrhea were not nearly so good, but the medical optimism about syphilis affected professional attitudes toward that disease as well.

67 Newsholme, *Poor Law Commission*, 9: 160.
68 Newsholme, *Ann. Rep. Med. Off. L.G.B.*, 43 (1913–14), ci.
69 For a short contemporary historical discussion of the pathology and therapeutics of syphilis and gonorrhea, see Harry F. Dowling, *Fighting Infection: Conquests of the Twentieth Century* (Cambridge, Mass.: Harvard Univ. Press, 1977): 86–94; and Allan Brandt, *No Magic Bullet: A Social History of Venereal Disease in the United States Since 1880* (New York: Oxford Univ. Press, 1985), 40–1.
70 For the articles presented at the Section on Therapeutics of the B.M.A. annual meeting at Birmingham, see *Br. Med. J.* (1911) no. 2: 673–87. See also the lead article "Recent Developments in the Diagnosis and Treatment of Syphilis," ibid., 692–3; and Carl H. Browning and Ivy McKenzie, "The Treatment of Syphilis by Salvarsan," ibid., 654–5.

This improvement in medicine's capacity to deal with syphilis came at a very opportune time, for the disease now loomed larger in Western consciousness. Pathologists in the second half of the nineteenth century had demonstrated that the damage syphilis caused was not limited to the primary and secondary stages of the disease. Years after infection, long after the victim considered himself cured, the horrible wastage of tertiary infection – aneurysms and other damage to the heart and great vessels, paralysis, or insanity – might appear.[71] Similarly gonorrhea was shown not only to have immediate and previously recognized effects but to cause chronic suffering and to produce sterility. Were this catalogue of horrors not enough, pathology also elucidated gonorrheal ophthalmia of the newborn, a major cause of blindness, and congenital syphilis. Following these discoveries the consequences of these venereal diseases could no longer be regarded as rewards reserved for those who had placed themselves at risk of contracting them. They included among their victims the next generation as well. To a nation already uneasy about the declining birth rate of its upper and middle classes and suspicious that the urban working classes were degenerating, these revelations from the death house were chilling.

In March 1912 the Local Government Board decided to conduct an investigation of the prevalence and treatment of venereal diseases in England. To undertake this study Newsholme chose one of his senior medical inspectors, Ralph W. Johnstone. Johnstone's report, which was based on a review of the scientific literature, on an analysis of available statistics, and on visits to select hospitals and Poor Law institutions, appeared as a Parliamentary Paper in August of the next year.[72] It was a short but influential report. In fact, it accurately pointed in the direction which both the Royal Commission on Venereal Diseases and subsequent state policy would follow.[73] Johnstone first tried to determine how prevalent venereal diseases were.[74] No one who had considered the matter seriously believed that the reported mortality rates for syphilis were accurate. Not only had there been unavoidable difficulties in correctly diagnosing venereal infections of long standing, but since the death registers were not confidential, there were strong incentives for private practitioners to obscure or even to falsify the reported cause of death when syphilis was involved. The Registrar-General's reports did show a decline of syphilis mortality since 1875, and Johnstone tried to determine whether these figures reflected a real decline or merely the transference of a larger number of deaths to other categories such as general paralysis of the insane, aneurysm, or locomotor ataxy. He also sought proxies in military records: rejections for syphilis or other diseases of the genital organs at recruitment examinations, and admissions to military hospitals for venereal disease. Such weighing of the admittedly unsatis-

---

71 For a short summary of this pathological research, see Brandt, *No Magic Bullet,* 9–13.

72 R. W. Johnstone, *Report on Venereal Diseases,* B.P.P. 1913, [Cd. 7029], XXXII.

73 For Newsholme's assessment of the importance of this study, see his announcement of Johnstone's death in Newsholme, *Ann. Rep. Med. Off. L.G.B.,* 45 (1915–16): xxxiii.

74 For the following comments, see Johnstone, *Report on Venereal Diseases,* 4–10, 19.

factory evidence led Johnstone to conclude that it was impossible to know not only how many people were infected with syphilis but even whether the infection rate were really falling. It did seem certain, however, that syphilis was very common and that the number infected with gonorrhea was probably even higher.

The most important finding of Johnstone's report was that most of this un-known multitude of venereal disease sufferers were not receiving proper treatment and hence posed a serious public health hazard. He found the nation's hospitals "wholly inadequate for the needs of the country" as far as the treatment of venereal diseases was concerned.[75] None of the general hospitals he visited had set aside beds for syphilis in its infective stages, and some categorically refused admission to such cases. Ironically and tragically, all treated in their wards patients suffering from the late complications of venereal diseases. Syphilis patients were free, he was told, to attend the outpatient department, but it was apparent to Johnstone that in many hospitals there was much to discourage such attendance. Hospital governors and staff often found dealing with such patients repugnant. "Not long ago the committee of one of the London general hospitals seriously debated the advisability of continuing to treat certain prostitutes in their district on the grounds that they were thereby helping to support the brothels to which these women belonged."[76] To discourage prostitutes from attending, a number of hospitals refused outpatient treatment of syphilis to unmarried women, although they treated unmarried men. The discouraging thing about these policies was that the general hospitals were capable of providing excellent medical services for these diseases. All of the general hospitals in London had facilities to diagnose syphilis and gonorrhea, and most of them had admitted a few patients for treatment with Salvarsan. In the provinces one-third of the general hospitals Johnstone visited had the facilities for performing the Wassermann test, and two-thirds of them had used Salvarsan on a small scale.

Poor Law institutions more frequently treated venereal disease. Johnstone visited thirty-five of these institutions, and found that all had venereal disease wards.[77] Those in separate infirmaries were usually modern in construction and satisfacto-rily run, but the "lock wards" in many general workhouses were the worst in the house – worn, cheerless, ill-ventilated, and inadequately lit. In some the managers offered the inmates neither occupation nor reading material. It is no wonder that medical officers complained that they had a hard time convincing paupers with syphilis to remain in the institution long enough to complete treatment. The treatment offered was usually only a course of mercury. Salvarsan had been employed in only a couple of institutions. Few Poor Law institutions employed Wassermann tests.

Johnstone demanded a new policy toward venereal diseases, a policy based on medical rather than legal or moral priorities.[78] The failure of the Contagious

75 Ibid., 21. For the discussion of the general hospitals that follows, see ibid., 19–21.
76 Ibid., 20.   77 For a discussion of the Poor Law institutions, see ibid., 21–3.
78 For the following discussion of control measures, see ibid., 25–9.

Diseases Acts (1864–86) had proved the futility of trying to control venereal disease by police regulation of prostitution and the injustice of applying punitive measures to one sex while leaving the other free from prosecution. It was also growing abundantly clear that public attitudes which regarded venereal disease as the just punishment for sin frustrated efforts to prevent these diseases.

Even if venereal diseases were spread by sexual inter-course alone, which is not the case, a retribution which falls upon innocent women and children, and with equal force upon the raw youth or girl, as upon the vicious and abandoned, is not remarkable for its justice. This attitude of mind . . . prevents the charitable from subscribing towards the proper cure and treatment of venereal diseases, it influences our general hospitals through their lay committees against the provision of accommodation for these diseases, and it emphasises the stigma and disgrace attached to the inmates of lock hospitals and the lock wards of our Poor Law institutions. While it operates as a deterrent to the provision of proper treatment, it operates still more seriously by leading to concealment of the disease, and by preventing sufferers from seeking the aid and advice which is [sic] essential for their cure and for the prevention of the spread of the disease.[79]

The nation's health policy, he maintained, should encourage all infected to obtain treatment early in the disease and to continue such treatment long enough to obtain a cure. In order for this to happen, all barriers between the infected and qualified medical attention must be removed. "In short the essence of the problem is how to get a willing patient at the earliest time to the doctor from whom, or to the institution from which such advice and treatment is to be had."[80] Johnstone recommended that free laboratory diagnosis be made available to all, that venereal diseases not be made notifiable at the present, and that free, anonymous treatment be provided for all those found to be infected.

Here in outline was the strategy the nation would soon adopt – one that emphasized medical not moral initiative, one relying on voluntary compliance not compulsion. In introducing this report Newsholme praised its analysis, endorsed its recommendations, and pointed out that venereal diseases proved even more clearly than tuberculosis that in modern public health work prevention could not be divorced from treatment.[81] Effective treatment was essential to prevention. He would carry this argument along with the evidence Johnstone had collected to the Royal Commission on Venereal Diseases, of which he was one of twelve members. The Commission was appointed in November 1913 and issued its final report in February 1916.[82] It was charged with framing a venereal disease policy. The only restriction on its work was that it might not recommend a return to the principles embodied in the Contagious Diseases Acts. The work of the Commission was dominated by its medical members, among whom Newsholme was a major influence.[83] News-

79 Ibid., 26–7.   80 Ibid., 27.
81 Arthur Newsholme, "Introduction by the Medical Officer," in ibid., i–iv.
82 Royal Commission of Venereal Diseases, *First Report*, B.P.P. 1914, XLIX; *Appendix to the First Report*, ibid.; *Final Report*, B.P.P. 1916, XVI; and *Appendix to the Final Report*, ibid.
83 Evans, "Tackling the Hideous Scourge," 416–20.

holme prepared an extensive memorandum for his fellow Commissioners dealing with the activities of local authorities in disease notification and prevention and with the special problems posed by venereal diseases, and he was one of eighty-five witnesses examined.[84] Johnstone's report of 1913 was frequently referred to by the Commission, and Johnstone was asked to prepare additional evidence for the Commission on hospital facilities.[85]

The Royal Commission collected much evidence which confirmed Johnstone's initial findings, and it considered several topics which he had either ignored or dealt with only superficially. Among the latter were the diagnosis and treatment of venereal diseases in private or insurance practice, the role of quackery or self-medication in discouraging or delaying adequate treatment, and the need for medical students to receive thorough training in venereal diseases. It also went well beyond Johnstone's report in proposing specific legal and administrative measures. The Commission discounted the recommendations of the British Medical Association, which wanted treatment in the hands of private practitioners whose work could be subsidized with government funds, and it accepted Newsholme's conclusions that only a state service would do.[86] Private practitioners might play a role in controlling venereal disease. The Commission recommended that the L.G.B. make Salvarsan or its wartime equivalent available to properly trained practitioners, foresaw that infected persons who could afford to pay for treatment might be advised to see their own doctors, but it agreed with Newsholme that most practitioners were neither equipped nor trained to diagnose or to treat venereal diseases by modern methods. Furthermore only public authorities could manage a treatment scheme.

No adequate system of treatment would be organized unless responsibility for the measures to be adopted were undertaken by the State. . . . The diseases are so widespread and their consequences are . . . so serious not only to the individual but also to the race, that concerted action by a public authority is in our view essential.[87]

The Commission recommended that county and county borough councils be asked to draw up venereal disease schemes as they had done for tuberculosis.[88] For diagnostic services they should enter into agreements with medical schools or with the larger hospitals which had the required laboratory facilities and trained staff. For the Wassermann tests the Commission had in mind collecting specimens locally and having these sent to regional diagnostic laboratories. Treatment for most of the population would be best provided by agreements between local

---

84 Arthur Newsholme, "Memorandum," Roy. Comm. V.D., *Final Report*, Appendix 98–118; and Arthur Newsholme, testimony, Roy. Comm V.D., *Appendix to Final Report*, 217–26.

85 "Note on Visits made by Dr. Johnstone on behalf of the Royal Commission to Towns Having No Hospitals with Laboratories near Them in Which the Modern Diagnosis and Treatment of Venereal Diseases Could Be Carried Out." Roy. Comm. V.D., *Final Report*, Appendix XXV, 175–6.

86 Evans, "Tackling the Hideous Scourge," 420; and Roy. Comm. V.D., *Final Report*, 46. See also ibid., 36, 42, 43.

87 Ibid., 46.

88 For the Commission's recommendations on diagnosis and treatment, see ibid., 45–8. For a summary of the Commission's general conclusions, see ibid., 62–6.

health authorities and general hospitals. Such hospitals, it felt sure, would be willing to establish venereal disease wards and outpatient departments. Physical examination, some microscopic examination of smears, and the taking of specimens for laboratory diagnosis could take place in the outpatient department. Salvarsan could be administered there too, although beds must be provided for at least an overnight stay following the intravenous injection of Salvarsan, as well as for complicated cases. The Commission clearly considered this to be a national service, most of whose costs should be met by the Exchequer. It recommended Treasury grants for 75 percent of approved expenditures.

The Commission agreed that all barriers between the infected and proper treatment must be removed. Both diagnosis and treatment in the state scheme, it asserted, must be free, regardless of the income or insurance status of the patient. If a patient able to pay for his own treatment were reluctant to consult his own physician, he should be entitled to free treatment at the public treatment center. These clinics should be accessible to the working class and should, for example, be open in the evening. The treatment they provide should protect the confidentiality of patients and avoid stigmatizing them. For this reason the Commission advised against the creation of additional separate venereal disease institutions. It also recommended that although clinics would be provided by local authorities, infected persons should be free to use any facility, not merely the one provided by their own local authority. This desire to remove fear of exposure and the penalties that even National Insurance permitted for venereal infection led the Royal Commission to rule out, at least for the immediate future, three control measures which had strong advocates: the compulsory notification of venereal disease, the requirement of a medical certificate of freedom from venereal infection for marriage, and, with a couple of exceptions, the compulsory detention of patients until treatment was completed.[89]

The Commission was led by witnesses appearing before it to believe that unqualified practice was a major threat to their planned scheme. Quacks and herbalists, it believed, spread false information, and their practice deterred the infected from seeking proper treatment in a timely manner.[90] It recommended that the advertisement of cures for venereal disease be made illegal. It also wanted to recommend the banning of the treatment of these infections by the medically unqualified, but it felt that under the present circumstances such a ban could not be made. It also recommended expanded educational work both in the training of medical practitioners and among the public.[91]

In closing, the Royal Commission stressed that immediate action was needed

89 Ibid., 48–50, 51–3, 55–6. For the provisions of National Insurance practice which deterred patients with venereal disease from applying for the treatment to which they were entitled, see ibid., 43.
90 Ibid., 53–4. Medical Officers of Health had for some years argued that the treatment of venereal disease by unqualified persons was a public health menace. See, for example, *Report as to the Practice of Medicine and Surgery by Unqualified Persons in the United Kingdom*, B.P.P., 1910, [Cd. 5422]. XLIII, 15–16.
91 Roy. Comm. V.D., *Final Report*, 59–62.

even though the nation was at war. That war in fact made action even more pressing.

The diminution of the best manhood of the nation, due to the losses of the war, must tell heavily upon the birth-rate – already declining – and upon the numbers of efficient workers. . . . Now and in the years to come the question of public health must be a matter of paramount national importance, and no short-sighted parsimony should be permitted to stand in the way of all means that science can suggest and organization can supply for guarding the present and future generations upon which the restoration of national prosperity must depend.[92]

Here was a bold plan for national action. The National Council for Combating Venereal Diseases had been lobbying L.G.B. officials for several years and had been influential in the choice of Royal Commissioners.[93] Once the Commission's Final Report had appeared, the National Council stepped up its pressure, demanding that the major recommendations of the Royal Commission be carried out at once. They found Newsholme to be an effective ally within the L.G.B. He urged his superiors to receive a delegation from the National Council and to invite the Chancellor to attend, and he prepared a briefing paper for the President of the L.G.B., Walter Long, on the findings of the Royal Commission.[94] Within the Board Newsholme argued that public action was urgently needed, and that Treasury grants of at least 75 percent of cost should be sought, estimating the cost for the first year between £75,000 and £100,000. He tried to anticipate Treasury objections and to answer them. To demonstrate that such public expenditures would be more than adequately repaid, he offered dramatic estimates, some of them from the Royal Commission's evidence, of the social and military costs of venereal diseases.[95]

Long agreed to meet a delegation of distinguished civic leaders and medical authorities representing the National Council on April 14, and at that meeting he promised the full cooperation of the L.G.B. and announced that the Treasury had agreed earlier that day to authorize and fund L.G.B. grants for 75 percent of approved costs.[96] Actually the Board had tried to secure even more. It attempted unsuccessfully to convince the Treasury to pay the entire cost of the venereal disease program as a special war measure.[97]

92 Ibid., 66.
93 See, for example, John Burns's diary entries for 19 Jan. 1911, B. L. Add. Mss. 46333; 2 Feb. 1912, ibid. 46334; 8 Aug. 1913, 11 Aug. 1913, 14 Aug. 1913, 24 Oct. 1913, and 25 Oct. 1913, ibid. 46335.
94 See Newsholme to Willis, 24 March 1916, P.R.O., MH55/531; and Newsholme, untitled memorandum for The President, 6 April 1916, ibid. See also Willis to President, 28 March 1916, ibid.; and Walter Long, minute, 28 March 1916, ibid.
95 Newsholme, memorandum, 6 April 1916, Appendix A, 8–9.
96 An account of this meeting dated 14 April 1916 may be found in P.R.O., MH55/531. The formal Treasury announcement of these grants did not come for another two weeks. See T. L. Heath [Joint Secretary, Treasury] to Secretary, Local Government Board, 3 May 1916, ibid.
97 Willis to Secretary, Treasury, 13 April 1916, ibid.; and H. P. Hamilton [Second Class Clerk, Treasury] to F. L. Turner [Private Secretary to President, L.G.B.], 14 April 1916, ibid.

Newsholme would later claim to be the author of the specific regulations that would govern the state venereal disease service.[98] Surviving documents from the L.G.B. substantiate this claim. Newsholme attached great importance to seeing that the new scheme was universal. For this to happen, the Board must depart from the precedent of most disease control measures and claim the authority to compel local authorities to act. When the Board's secretariat objected that such power could be claimed only if there were an emergency, Newsholme countered that the nation in fact did face an emergency with venereal disease.[99] Making this case was one of the most influential things he did. He was able to gain the support of F. J. Willis, the Assistant Secretary, and with Willis's backing convinced the reluctant Permanent Secretary, H. C. Monro, to agree.[100] Within a week Newsholme was circulating a draft of his memorandum outlining the steps local authorities should take to combat venereal disease, a document he hoped would be printed and sent to local authorities with the forthcoming regulations.[101]

During May 1916 the L.G.B. prepared that set of regulations and a circular letter for county and county borough councils. By the end of May the drafts were ready, and the Board invited comments from public authorities and other interested parties. Copies of the draft regulations, circular letters, and Newsholme's memorandum on medical measures were sent to the Treasury, the National Health Insurance Commission, the County Council Association, the Association of Municipal Corporations, the British Medical Association, the Royal College of Physicians, the Royal College of Surgeons, and the National Council for Combatting Venereal Diseases.[102] Curiously enough, the Board does not seem to have sought the reaction of hospitals. The Board's response to the resulting objections and suggestions shows its sense of urgency, its impatience with the usual process of formal negotiations, and Newsholme's determination to defend the principles outlined in the Royal Commission report and to enforce its recommendations with as little modification as possible. It was not that he refused all advice. He readily agreed to a small list of changes in his memorandum, mainly on technical points, suggested by a committee of the Royal College of Surgeons, when the committee's chairman, D'Arcy Power, showed them to him privately.[103] Several respondents also worried about the recommendation that local practitioners and medical students be admitted to the venereal disease clinics as

98 Arthur Newsholme, *Health Problems in Organized Society: Studies in the Social Aspects of Public Health* (London: P. S. King, 1927), 167.
99 A. B. M[aclachlan] to Willis, 26 April 1916, P.R.O., MH55/531; and Newsholme to Willis, 26 April 1916, ibid.
100 F. J. W[illis] to Monro, 17 April 1916, ibid.; and Monro, minute of 28 April 1916, ibid.
101 Newsholme to A. B. Maclachlan, 5 May 1916, ibid.; and Arthur Newsholme, "Memorandum on the Organisation of Medical Measures against Venereal Diseases," undated, ibid. The latter source will hereafter be referred to as Newsholme, "Memorandum," May 1916.
102 See the correspondence for June and July 1916 in ibid.
103 Newsholme to A. B. Maclachlan, 22 June 1916, ibid.; and "Report of a Subcommittee of the Council of the Royal College of Surgeons of England upon the Local Government Board's Organisation of Medical Measures against Venereal Disease," 21 June 1916, ibid.

observers in order to learn the new methods. To allay the anxiety that such arrangements would endanger the confidentiality of patients, he agreed to add a clause to his memorandum emphasizing the obligation of observers to strict professional secrecy.[104]

But when faced with two sets of objections, Newsholme was adamant. The first was the localist claim that in some districts the proposed regulations would prove unworkable. Typically these critics argued that there were no facilities in the area to do the work and that in any event such regulations should be permissive not compulsory. Newsholme insisted that for the venereal disease service to be a success the regulations must be universal and hence local authorities must be required to adopt schemes.[105] Those who offered such criticism, he suggested, had usually misunderstood the regulations. There was no necessity for there to be either a diagnostic laboratory or a general hospital in the immediate vicinity. The Royal Commission expected and the L.G.B. regulations assumed that both diagnostic and treatment facilities would be regional and thus frequently shared. Both economy and efficiency had led the Royal Commission to urge that Wassermann tests be performed at only a few sites. There should, it was true, be more clinics than laboratories, but most regions had a hospital within reasonable distance. In some cases it might be necessary for local schemes to underwrite the cost of transporting patients to a more distant clinic. Where no hospital was accessible, the Board could approve new, independent establishments or set up a few ad hoc clinics at isolation hospitals or Poor Law institutions. Newsholme accused some of the proposal's critics, the Medical Officer of Health for Somerset County, for example, not only of failing to grasp the intended policy but of "making a ringed fence around the County."[106] He even suggested that some councils would be grateful to have the new service be made an obligation.

As to compulsion, there is strong reason to believe, in the light of our experience as to Tuberculosis and Maternity & Child Welfare Schemes that Local Authorities will welcome *shall* instead of *may* throughout the Order, as obviating difficulties with ratepayers.[107]

The second set of objections that Newsholme strongly resisted included claims made on behalf of private practitioners. The draft versions of his memorandum had specified that private practitioners might attend the practice of the clinic to

---

104 The change can be seen in comparing Newsholme, "Memorandum," May 1916, paragraph 24 with the published version, Arthur Newsholme, "Memorandum by the Medical Officer of the Local Government Board on the Organisation of Medical Measures against Venereal Diseases," July 1916, paragraph 19. The latter was not published in either *Ann. Rep. L.G.B.* or in News-holme, *Ann. Rep. Med. Off. L.G.B.* A copy may be found in P.R.O., MH55/533. The published version will hereafter be cited as Newsholme, *Memorandum,* July 1916.

105 For the following argument, see Newsholme to Willis, 16 May 1916 and 14 June 1916, P.R.O., MH55/531. For an example of these objections, see M. S. Johnson [Assistant Secretary, County Councils Association] to Willis, 8 June 1916 and the accompanying observations of W. G. Savage [M.O.H., Somerset County] in a letter of Henry Hobhouse, 6 June 1916, ibid.

106 Newsholme to Willis, 14 June 1916, ibid.

107 Ibid.

observe and that they were encouraged to consult with the medical officer of the clinic and the pathologist of the laboratory. Practitioners were to be supplied with apparatus for collecting specimens for diagnosis and with instructions for doing so, and, when necessary, they were to be assisted in taking a specimen. The diagnostic laboratory would make a diagnosis free of charge for any practitioner and would supply the practitioner with a confidential report of the results. Private practitioners might refer any of their patients to the clinic for treatment with Salvarsan, and the Medical Officer of the clinic might supply Salvarsan free of charge to any practitioner he recognized as being trained and sufficiently experienced to use the new drug safely and effectively.[108] The new service did, in fact, promise some important benefits to the average general practitioner. But organized medicine was already growing uneasy with the expansion of public health clinics for tuberculosis and for infant welfare.[109] The appearance of another state service offering free treatment by salaried medical officers seemed not only a threat to the practice of private practitioners but another step toward an entirely salaried medical service. The Board, with Newsholme's concurrence, added a paragraph to its circular letter, drawing attention to the role which private practitioners could play in treatment. A person attending a clinic might be asked whether he or she had a personal or panel physician and were willing to be treated by that doctor. "If the patient has no doctor or, being an insured person, has not yet chosen a panel doctor, but is willing to be referred to a private practitioner for treatment in association with the treatment provided at the institution, he should be advised to choose a doctor who would co-operate in his treatment."[110] Newsholme added to his memorandum a short section somewhat less flattering to private practice: "Some parts of the treatment required can in many cases be given by the patient's own doctor, and, in cases where this is arranged, the Medical Officer should furnish the practitioner with a report on the patient's treatment at the clinic, with suggestions as to continued treatment."[111] Newsholme hastened to repeat the Royal Commission's warning that patients found to be suffering from venereal disease must not be referred to their own doctors against their will, and, should the patients desire, they should be treated at the clinic. It is clear that Newsholme, like the majority of the Royal Commission, regarded most private practitioners as incompetent to deal with venereal disease, and he feared that most patients would forgo treatment if there were no alternative to seeing a panel doctor or a private practitioner.

While he agreed to such minor changes to placate medical anxieties, he refused

---

108 See Newsholme, "Memorandum," May 1916, paragraphs 3, 23–4, 30–3.
109 See for example Winter, *The Great War*, 173–7. Lord Dawson of Penn also reflected this suspicion of local authority clinics and their employment of full-time specialists. See his "Medicine and the State," *Br. Med. J.* (1920), no. 1: 744.
110 "Prevention and Treatment of Venereal Diseases," [Circular Letter of the Local Government Board], 13 July 1916, 10 in P.R.O., MH55/533. For Newsholme's agreement to the addition of this paragraph, see Newsholme to Maclachlan, 20 June 1916, P.R.O., MH55/531.
111 Newsholme, *Memorandum*, July 1916, paragraph 24.

to accede to the demand that organized medicine have a voice in the planning and managing of local venereal disease schemes. Both the National Health Insurance Commission, which was indignant that it had not been consulted earlier about the regulations, and the British Medical Association demanded that in drawing up their schemes county councils and county borough councils be required to consult with local doctors.[112] The National Health Insurance Commission specified that such consultation should be with the Local Medical Committee, the body that the National Insurance Act had created to represent the interests of medical practitioners in the insurance scheme. "The proposal," Newsholme responded, "is merely one for Trades Union representation of doctors in private practice. Why not have this also for patients, as distinguished from the general public?"[113] The proposed regulations, he pointed out, were closely patterned on the recommendations of the Royal Commission, which carefully gathered the advice of private practitioners. Newsholme could speak with some authority on this point. Early in the Commission's deliberations he had consulted privately with the B.M.A.'s Medico-Political Committee, urging it to represent the views of general practitioners before the Commission, and it was he who delivered the invitation to the B.M.A. to send witnesses to the Commission.[114]

Once a scheme was established, Newsholme insisted, local practitioners could make their views known to the M.O.H. or to the medical staff of the hospital which sponsored the venereal disease clinic.[115] Medical practitioners could also seek representation on the county council or county borough council just as patients could. The local authority already had plenty of expert medical advice from its M.O.H., from the scheme's pathologist, and from the medical staffs of the clinic and the sponsoring hospital. Although a local authority was free to seek the advice of the Local Medical Committee in planning or managing its scheme, requiring it to do so would in Newsholme's opinion have "a mischievous effect"; it would "merely imply delay & embarrassment."[116] His superiors at the Board initially agreed and refused to comply with this demand although pressured to do

---

112 For this demand and Newsholme's response, see Vivian to Secretary, 16 June 1916; Newsholme to Willis, 14 June 1916; and Newsholme to Maclachlan, 20 June 1916, P.R.O., MH55/531. The British Medical Association supported the recommendations of the Royal Commission on Venereal Diseases, but it insisted that local medical practitioners must have a voice in the planning and management of local schemes and a hand in running the clinics. See the lead article, "State Provision for the Treatment of Venereal Disease," *Br. Med. J.* (1916), no. 2: 115–16. See also British Medical Association Archives, Medico-Political Committee, minutes of Parliamentary Sub-Committee meeting, 24 May 1916; Document 62 (1915–16) draft report of the Joint Sub-Committee of Medico-Political, Public Health, and Hospitals Committees, 8 June 1916. This series of minutes and documents will hereafter be cited as B.M.A., Med. Pol. Comm.

113 Newsholme to Willis, 14 June 1916, P.R.O., MH55/531.

114 B.M.A., Med. Pol. Comm., minutes of meeting 25 Nov. 1914, and Document 46 (1914–15) Alfred Cox to Committee Members, 12 Dec. 1914, B.M.A. Archives.

115 For Newsholme's position on the issue, see Newsholme to Willis, 14 June 1916, P.R.O., MH55/531; and Newsholme to Maclachlan, 20 June 1916, ibid.

116 Newsholme to Maclachlan, 20 June 1916, ibid.

so right down until the time it issued its regulations.[117] However, the B.M.A. continued to put pressure on the Board, passing a series of resolutions at its annual representative meeting at the end of July that supported the general provisions of the Board's venereal disease order but decried the absence of local consultation with organized medicine, and in August it sent first a memorandum and then a delegation to the President of the L.G.B..[118] The secretariat of the Board relented and in a circular of August 29, 1916, formally recommended but did not require that local authorities invite two medical representatives to attend the meeting of their local venereal disease advisory committee.[119]

The L.G.B. issued its Public Health (Venereal Diseases) Regulations, 1916, on July 12 and the circular letters to county and county borough councils, to hospitals, and to the Clerks of Guardians on the following day. These documents with Newsholme's memorandum on medical measures were sent out to interested parties immediately.[120] In requiring local authorities to adopt the measures it described, the Board claimed authority under the Public Health (Prevention & Treatment of Disease) Act, 1913, which permitted the Board to issue compulsory orders to county councils in the face of an emergency.[121] The schemes it called for followed very closely the recommendation of the Royal Commission and the Board's Medical Officer. County councils and council borough councils were to arrange schemes which would provide free, confidential diagnosis and treatment to all sufferers of syphilis, gonorrhea, and soft chancre regardless of income or place of residency. The councils were encouraged to enter into agreement with larger hospitals or medical schools to provide such services rather than to establish new facilities. They were to keep records for statistical and financial purposes, but they were admonished to see that the names or addresses of patients were never divulged. They were also given authority to begin programs of public education about venereal diseases. The L.G.B. promised reimbursement for 75 percent of all approved expenses. These documents also made a place for the Poor Law medical service in the state venereal disease program. Poor Law doctors and their patients, like other practitioners and patients, were entitled to free diagnostic, consultive, and therapeutic services, and the L.G.B. extended its grants to approved venereal disease work undertaken by Guardians.

117 For later exchanges on this point, see S. Vivian to Secretary, Local Government Board, 3 July 1916, ibid.; and A. B. Maclachlan to Secretary, National Health Insurance Commission, 13 July 1916, ibid.

118 For the resolutions at the annual meeting, see *Br. Med. J.* (1916), no. 2, Suppl.: 47–52. For the B.M.A.'s Memorandum and an account of its deputation to the L.G.B., see "Diagnosis and Treatment of Venereal Diseases," *Br. Med. J.* (1916), no. 2, Suppl.: 69–70. See also B.M.A., Med. Pol. Comm., Document 2a (1916–17) minutes of Joint Meeting of Medico-Political, Public Health and Hospitals Committees, 4 Oct. 1916, and unnumbered document at beginning of document collection for 1916–17 stating the B.M.A. position for President, L.G.B., Aug. 1916.

119 L.G.B., "Venereal Diseases. Circular to County and County Borough Councils," 29 Aug. 1916. A copy may be conveniently found in "Diagnosis and Treatment of Venereal Diseases," *Br. Med. J.* (1916) no. 2, Suppl.: 77.

120 A printed copy of this collection may be found in P.R.O., MH55/533.

121 3 & 4 Geo. 4, C. 23.

Since the new service was to use existing facilities rather than to build new ones, it was hoped that county councils and county borough councils could be prodded into beginning their schemes quickly in spite of the dislocations and shortages of the war. Medical inspectors from the L.G.B. were sent out at once to hold conferences with councils and with hospital boards. They also inspected laboratories where the diagnostic work might take place. In December the Board issued a set of printed forms which it hoped would help local authorities begin: public announcements of services, leaflets of instruction for patients undergoing treatment, and forms for submitting specimens to laboratories and for reporting the pathologist's conclusions. Accompanying these forms was a memorandum, which Newsholme had helped draw up, specifying the records which were to be submitted periodically to the Medical Officer of Health and to L.G.B. on the services rendered and expenses incurred.[122]

Within nine months a start had been made. By the end of March 1917, 86 of the 145 local authorities charged with the duty of providing these services had submitted schemes, and the Board had approved 45 of these.[123] The Board also reported that between 130 and 140 hospitals had expressed a willingness to participate, but only 30 had begun work. A year later the service was nearly complete. The schemes of 124 local authorities had received approval by then, and within the jurisdiction of those authorities lived nearly 92 percent of the population of England and Wales.[124] Work had begun at 121 clinics, and 49 laboratories had been approved to undertake this work.[125]

Newsholme was gratified to have the system in place so quickly, but he acknowledged that there were problems. The service worked least well in sparsely settled areas.[126] In his planning Newsholme had underestimated the difficulty of getting patients to a hospital from districts having none. Patients in Westmoreland, for example, would have to travel to the Royal Infirmary in Manchester. Even though local authorities were authorized to pay the traveling expenses of such patients, Newsholme recognized that such traveling involved inconvenience and loss of wages for venereal disease patients. If additional clinics were not established in more remote areas, patients would be encouraged to forgo treatment or to stop attending the clinic prematurely. On the other hand he also recognized that in

122 "Prevention and Treatment of Venereal Diseases," [Circular to Councils of Counties and County Boroughs, Common Council of the City of London], 22 Dec. 1916; P.R.O., MH55/534; and "Memorandum as to the Records to be Kept and the Returns to Be Made by Institutions Approved by the Local Government Board for the Diagnosis or Treatment of Venereal Disease," n.d., ibid. There was pressure on the Board to issue these forms. See in the same folder A. C. Gotto [Joint Honorable Secretary, National Council for Combatting Venereal Diseases] to Newsholme, 30 Oct. 1916; Edmund M. Smith [M.O.H., City of York] to Newsholme, 9 Nov. 1916; and Newsholme to Willis, 6 Dec. 1916.

123 Newsholme, *Ann. Rep. Med. Off. L.G.B.*, 46 (1916–17): xxxi.

124 Ibid., 47 (1917–18): lxv.   125 Ibid.; and *Ann. Rep. L.G.B.*, 47 (1917–18): 10.

126 For the following discussion, see Newsholme, *Ann. Rep. Med. Off. L.G.B.*, 46 (1916–17): xxxii; and ibid., 47 (1917–18): lxv.

sparsely settled areas, especially in the ad hoc clinics that were established where no hospital was within convenient distance, it had sometimes proved difficult to ensure patient confidentiality.

He was also disappointed with the response of some hospitals. A number had been reluctant to deal with venereal disease patients, fearing a loss of subscriptions.[127] A more common problem was staffing the clinic.[128] Newsholme had wanted a single medical officer with special training in venereal diseases to be in charge of the clinic. To overcome the shortage of qualified practitioners during the war, the L.G.B. had arranged with the Royal Army Medical Corps for the part-time release of army doctors experienced with venereal disease to help staff local authority clinics. Very few hospitals availed themselves of this offer or sought a specialist they could add to their medical staff. Some tried to give the task of running the clinic to a hospital resident. This the Board refused to approve. More common was the practice of dividing the work of the clinic among several members of the medical staff or among the entire staff. The L.G.B. discouraged this arrangement and tried to insist that a single practitioner be responsible for the clinic. Record keeping was sometimes lax, and clinics frequently had little success getting patients to complete a course of treatment. One M.O.H. reported that in the clinic in his area 55 percent of men and 75 percent of women stopped attending the clinic before the treatment was finished. Patients must be told, the L.G.B. insisted, how important it was to complete the treatment.

The gender difference just noted points out how poorly the service reached infected women.[129] Newsholme's recommendations that separate clinics be established for women and that women be included on local advisory committees and on clinic medical staffs were ignored. Women attended in small numbers and discontinued treatment early. Newsholme also reported that in a few clinics the quality of medical attention had been poor for both men and women. The clinic staff had not exercised sufficient care in preparation and administration of Salvarsan or its substitutes, or it had not properly observed patients who had received the drug for side effects. Information Newsholme received about such shortcomings in the clinics was troublesome, but there was a limit to what he or other L.G.B. officials could do about it. The Board had promised that it would not interfere in the internal administration of hospitals, and its officials were aware that they needed to retain the cooperation of hospitals, which, unlike local authorities, were not legally bound to participate in the venereal disease service. Short of disapproving a local authority scheme for using a particular institution, the Board had to

127 Ibid., 46 (1916–17): xxxi.
128 For the following discussion, see ibid., xxxii; ibid., 47 (1917–18): lxvii–lxviii. For the arrangements with the Royal Army Medical Corps, see Newsholme, memorandum to President, 6 April 1916, P.R.O., MH55/531; and "Prevention and Treatment of Venereal Diseases" [Circular Letter Addressed by the Local Government Board to the Governing Bodies of General and Special Hospitals], 13 July 1916, 1 in P.R.O., MH55/533.
129 Evans, "Tackling the Hideous Scourge," 427.

deal with hospitals by making the best use it could of persuasion and appeals to professional pride and a sense of public service.

Once patients were given an opportunity to have free, confidential diagnosis and treatment, the question arose whether the state should do more to see that all cases were promptly and adequately treated. The L.G.B. had pressed on it the demands that venereal diseases be made compulsorily notifiable, that the medically unqualified should be banned from treating these diseases, and that advertisement of cures should be made illegal. The first proposal stood no chance of passage. Too much informed opinion was against it. Organized medicine opposed it; Newsholme and the Royal Commission on Venereal Diseases considered that at least for the immediate future requiring notification would defeat the purposes of the new state service, and the new President of the Local Government Board, Lord Rhondda, advised the Prime Minister against pursuing the idea.[130] The Royal Commission, however, had thought that it was desirable, although probably then impractical, to ban unqualified practice, and it had recommended that the advertising of cures be made illegal. Newsholme's position was that both should be made illegal in areas where the state scheme was in operation and patients had qualified treatment available to them. By the fall of 1916 he was urging the Board to sponsor legislation that would do just that.[131] He circulated clippings from the *Daily Mail* to demonstrate how common and misleading such advertisements were, and he suggested terms for a bill. However, while Walter Long remained President, the leadership of the Board remained skeptical, especially of the idea of making unqualified practice illegal. Horace Monro, the Permanent Secretary, in fact regarded it as just another attempt by the medical profession to eliminate competition.[132] But there was strong support in local government, in the medical profession, and from the National Council for Combatting Venereal Diseases.[133]

130 We have considered the views of Newsholme and the Royal Commission on this point already. See Rhondda to Prime Minister [David Lloyd George], 10 Jan. 1917, H.L.R.O., Lloyd George Papers F/43/5/4. For the opposition of the British Medical Association, see "Compulsory Notification," *Daily Telegraph*, 11 Nov. 1916, 5.

131 Newsholme to Willis, 30 Sept. 1916, P.R.O., MH55/530; Newsholme to Willis, 19 Oct. 1916, ibid.; Newsholme to Willis, 1 Nov. 1916, ibid.; Newsholme to President, 7 Nov. 1916, ibid.; Newsholme to Willis, 14 Nov. 1916, ibid.; and Newsholme to Willis, 17 Nov. 1916, ibid.

132 H. C. M[onro] to President [Walter Long], 8 Nov. 1916, P.R.O., MH55/530. See also W. H. L[ong] to Solicitor General [Sir George Cave], 13 Nov. 1916, and accompanying memorandum, ibid.

133 See, for example, J. W. Johnson [Assistant Secretary, County Councils Association] to Secretary, Local Government Board, 5 Dec. 1916; and W. Watson Cheyne [President, Royal College of Surgeons] to Lord Rhondda [President, Local Government Board], 11 Jan. 1917. Resolutions in favor of such legislation also came from the Association of Municipal Corporations, the Public Health Committee of the County Councils Association, and from the Royal College of Physicians. These resolutions are described in "Venereal Diseases: Deputation from the Association of Municipal Corporations, the County Councils Association, the Royal College of Physicians, the British Medical Association, the National Council for Combating Venereal Diseases, and the London County Council to the Right Hon. Lord Rhondda, President of the Local Government Board, 24 Jan. 1917, P.R.O., MH55/530.

Soon after becoming President of the Board, Lord Rhondda agreed to receive a prominent delegation from the bodies most active in pressing for legislation: the National Council, the County Councils Association, the Association of Municipal Corporations, the Royal College of Physicians, and the British Medical Association.[134] Their representatives argued that venereal disease was a special case and required a policy that departed from that used to deal with other infectious diseases. The chronic nature of these infections, the damage they inflicted on the unborn, the shame they caused in their victims, and the vulnerability of those victims to exploitation by the unscrupulous set these diseases apart. Rhondda received the delegation sympathetically and promised that he would urge the government to bring forward legislation. The L.G.B. did sponsor a bill, which became the Venereal Disease Act, 1917.[135] The Act adopted the approach Newsholme had been advocating. Section Two banned the advertisement of cures for venereal diseases throughout the Kingdom, and in districts where an adequate public venereal disease scheme was in operation it permitted the L.G.B. to apply Section One, which banned the treatment of venereal disease by the medically unqualified. The policy of the L.G.B. consistently limited compulsion to the providers, qualified or unqualified, public or private, of medical services for venereal disease patients. Its strategy stood in stark contrast to the action of the War Cabinet in dealing with venereal disease in the armed forces through the use of Regulations 13A and 40D under the Defence of the Realm Act, whose punitive measures are reminiscent of the Contagious Diseases Acts.[136]

In just a little more than a year the nation had launched an important new medical service. The venereal disease clinics were in full operation well before the war ended. Just to be sure that all was in readiness for demobilization, on December 10, 1918, Newsholme presided over a conference for clinicians on the treatment of venereal disease.[137] Newsholme was proud of the new service, and he had done much to give it form. It embodied what he believed was the rational, scientific response to a national health crisis, although, as we will see, he continued to believe that venereal diseases would not be conquered by medical means alone. Special circumstances, the anxieties of the war, and public and medical attitudes toward venereal disease, permitted Newsholme and the L.G.B. to act with unprecedented speed and directness. What had emerged was a public service unusual in its universality, in its reliance on treatment as the primary means of disease prevention, and in its aim of restricting treatment to qualified medical practitioners and of concentrating it in the hands of salaried medical officers. The creation reflected Newsholme's belief that the future of public health lay in the provision of comprehensive medical services by local authorities. It demonstrated that when there existed a strong mandate for public action and no competition from within

---

134 "Venereal Diseases: Deputation . . . Lord Rhondda."   135 7 & 8 Geo. 5, C. 21.
136 Evans, "Tackling the Hideous Scourge," 429.
137 *Minutes of Discussion at a Conference of the Treatment and Cure of Venereal Diseases* (London: Local Government Board, 1918).

the civil service, the L.G.B. was capable of acting quickly and decisively, and that under these circumstances its Medical Officer could exercise a great deal of influence. We turn next to another critical wartime issue where there was wide support for public action, but where the Board found itself in a vastly different administrative and political circumstance.

11

Infant and maternal mortality, interdepartmental conflict, and Newsholme supplanted

In the years between 1910 and 1916 Newsholme published five book-length official reports on infant, childhood, and maternal mortality.[1] Collectively these reports represented the most intensive empirical studies of these subjects to date in English. They should be understood historically as part of an ongoing debate about the meaning of death among the very young that took new form with the investigations of national efficiency and physical fitness following the Boer War. As such, these reports had immediate policy intentions. Newsholme was intent not only on demonstrating that recent national initiatives, undertaken in the wake of the Boer War, to promote the health of schoolchildren through school meals, medical examination, and medical treatment should be extended to children of preschool ages, but also on answering eugenists who warned that such ameliorative efforts merely hastened the pace of the nation's physical and mental degeneration.[2]

Newsholme's investigations may have been the most extensive, but they were not the first. Studies of infant mortality had become more common in M.O.H. reports and in medical journals, and several other monographs on infant mortality had appeared in the decade preceding 1916.[3] The General Register Office had

---

1 Arthur Newsholme, *Infant and Child Mortality: Suppl. 39th Ann. Rep. Med. Off. L.G.B.* (London: HMSO, 1910); Arthur Newsholme, *Second Report on Infant and Child Mortality: Suppl. 42nd Ann. Rep. Med. Off. L.G.B.* (London: HMSO, 1913); Arthur Newsholme, *Third Report on Infant Mortality dealing with Infant Mortality in Lancashire: Suppl. 43rd Ann. Rep. Med. Off. L.G.B.* (London: HMSO, 1914); Arthur Newsholme, *Maternal Mortality in Connection with Childbearing and Its Relation to Infant Mortality: Suppl. 44th Ann. Rep. Med. Off. L.G.B.* (London: HMSO, 1915); Arthur Newsholme, *Report on Child Mortality at Ages 0–5, in England and Wales: Suppl. 45th Ann. Rep. Med. Off. L.G.B.* (London: HMSO, 1916).

2 Simon Szreter has quite properly described these studies as part of a political and professional dispute between Newsholme and his allies at the G.R.O. such as Stevenson and Karl Pearson and his associates. See Simon R. S. Szreter, "The Genesis of the Registrar-General's Social Classification of Occupations," *Br. J. Sociol.*, 35 (1984): 525–30.

3 Dwork, 22–51. Among the monographs are George Newman, *Infant Mortality: A Social Problem* (London: Methuen, 1906); and Hugh T. Ashby, *Infant Mortality* (Cambridge: Cambridge Univ. Press, 1915). Ashby had obviously studied Newsholme's reports.

taken the lead by drawing attention to the problem long before the Boer War, providing the basic data and a tradition of analysis for these investigations. John Tatham, successor to William Farr and William Ogle at the G.R.O., took a special interest in infant mortality and applied to the problem the sorts of statistical and demographic analyses Farr had pioneered. In his report on the registration year 1891 Tatham produced a limited but very suggestive analysis.[4] In order to determine how mortality varied during the first year of life, he constructed a basic life table for a group of three industrial towns with high infant mortality and a group of three agricultural counties having low infant mortality. The table had monthly entries for the first year, weekly entries for the first month, and daily entries for the first week of life. He next produced tables showing the causes of death by week and month for these two life table populations. While this report was very brief – occupying fewer than seven printed pages including tables – and while it was based on very limited experience, it demonstrated the use that might be made of the registration returns in studying infant mortality, and it identified several of the most important mortality patterns that would be confirmed repeatedly over the next quarter century. As infant mortality gained greater policy significance, Tatham returned to the subject. He was a member of the Inter-Departmental Committee on Physical Deterioration, and he prepared for the Committee another analysis of infant mortality data.[5] He also wrote reports on infant mortality for the Registrar-General's annual reports for 1903 and 1905.[6] Tatham's attention to the subject was continued by his successor at the G.R.O., T. H. C. Stevenson, Newsholme's former Deputy at Brighton and coauthor with Newsholme of articles on life tables and fertility.[7]

Newsholme was one of several M.O.H. whose interest in infant mortality can be traced to the late 1880s.[8] In Chapters 2 and 3 we considered some of the best evidence of this interest: his studies of diarrheal diseases and his energetic efforts in Brighton to prevent these disorders. Before coming to the Local Government Board, Newsholme had also taken an interest in the health of school-age children. He wrote for teachers a textbook on school hygiene that went through many editions and several articles on the responsibility of sanitary authorities to maintain a healthy environment in schools.[9] He advocated the teaching of elementary

4 *Ann. Rep. Reg.-Gen.*, 54 (1891): x–xvi.
5 "English Mortality among Infants under One Year of Age," *Report of the Inter-Departmental Committee on Physical Deterioration*, Vol. I, Appendix Va, 130–7. B.P.P., 1904, XXXII.
6 *Ann. Rep. Reg.-Gen.*, 66 (1903): xxxvi–xxxvii; and ibid., 68 (1905): cxviii–cxxxiii.
7 See, for example, Stevenson's report on infant mortality in ibid., 71 (1908): cxxi–cxxvii. Newsholme and Stevenson jointly authored "Graphic Method of Constructing a Life Table Illustrated by the Brighton Life Table 1891–1900," *J. Hygiene*, 3 (1903): 297–324; "The Decline of Human Fertility in the United Kingdom and Other Countries as Shown by Corrected Birth-Rates," *J. Roy. Statist. Soc.*, 69 (1906): 34–87; "Improved Method of Calculating Birth-Rates," *J. Hygiene*, 5 (1905): 175–84, 304–10; and *The Second Brighton Life Table* (Brighton: King, Thorne and Stace, 1903).
8 Newsholme's recognition of the role of poor sanitation and artificial feeding in the causation of infant diarrhea was repeated by several M.O.H. Dwork, 38–41, 46–7.
9 Arthur Newsholme, *School Hygiene: The Laws of Health in Relation to School Life* (London, 1887); Arthur Newsholme, "The Health of Scholars: With Special Reference to the Education Code and

hygiene to schoolchildren.[10] And he argued for raising the age of entering school in the hope of sparing children at more vulnerable ages from the increased exposure to infectious diseases that occurred in schools.[11] We also have seen in Chapter 4 how he tried to control infectious diseases through a system of barring sick children and their siblings from school and occasionally by closing schools. The public alarm about child health in the wake of the Boer War encouraged Newsholme to think more boldly. He now discussed, using as an example what was then being done in Brighton, how school nurses and free school meals for needy children might be provided by voluntary agencies, and around 1906 he began to hold a weekly clinic for schoolchildren where he treated a limited number of common conditions such as impetigo, ringworm, and head lice.[12] He also began to discuss infant mortality as a national problem and to consider it statistically. However, his first statistical papers on infant mortality rather than infantile diarrhea were rather derivative, drawing heavily on the publications of Tatham.[13]

Once in Whitehall, however, Newsholme made infant mortality his number one epidemiological preoccupation. It is indicative of the significance that he and his administrative superiors attached to this issue, that in the war years, when the normally ponderous annual reports of the L.G.B. and of its Medical Officer were reduced to a few dozen pages, these studies of infant, childhood, and maternal mortality continued to appear as a series of substantial volumes. The series formed a logical whole, each study extending and refining the generalizations reached in the preceding ones. The first three reports focused in turn on infant mortality and on childhood mortality in the nation as a whole during 1908, in its most populous urban districts from 1907 to 1911, and then on infant mortality where it was highest, in Lancaster and its industrial towns.[14] The last two studies used data for

---

the Board of Education Act, 1899," *J. Sanitary Inst.*, 21 (1900): 269–79; and Arthur Newsholme, "Physical Inspection," *J. Roy. Sanitary Inst.*, 26 (1905): 64–8.

10 Arthur Newsholme, "On the Study of Hygiene in Elementary Schools," *Public Health*, 3 (1890–1): 134–6.

11 Arthur Newsholme, "The Lower Limit of Age for School Attendance: A Plea for the Exclusion of Children under Five Years of Age from Public Elementary Schools," ibid., 14 (1901–2): 570–83; and "The Lower Limit of Age for School Attendance," *Proc. 2nd International Congress on School Hygiene* [Aug. 1907] (London, 1908) II: 612–22. The latter paper was published under the same title in *Practitioner*, 79 (1907), 593–607.

12 Newsholme, "Physical Inspection," 66, 67–8. He describes his experiment in running this school clinic in Arthur Newsholme, *International Studies on the Relation between the Private and Official Practice of Medicine with Special Reference to the Prevention of Disease* (London: George Allen and Unwin, 1931), III, 367.

13 The chapter on infant mortality in Newsholme, *The Elements*, 120–35, for example, is heavily dependent on Tatham's analysis in the Registrar-General's *Annual Report* for 1891; and Arthur Newsholme, "Infantile Mortality. A Statistical Study from the Public Health Standpoint," *Practitioner*, 75 (1905): 489–500 likewise draw extensively on the published reports of the G.R.O. and on the statistical evidence Tatham prepared for the Inter-Departmental Committee on Physical Deterioration.

14 Newsholme, *Infant and Child Mortality;* Newsholme, *Second Report on Infant Mortality;* and Newsholme, *Third Report on Infant Mortality.*

1911 to 1914 to explore how the mortality of women in childbirth and how the death rates of preschool children were related to infant mortality.[15]

These studies were distinguished from the infant mortality reports coming from the G.R.O. not only by their scale but also by their use of observations by Medical Officers of Health to supplement the registration data. Beginning in 1905 the L.G.B. had required M.O.H. to include in their annual reports a tabulation for the infant deaths that had occurred in their jurisdiction, showing for each of the first four weeks and for each of the first twelve months of life the number of deaths due to each of twenty-seven specified causes.[16] Because these annual reports were forwarded to the L.G.B., Newsholme had information on early deaths and their causes independent of the special tabulations the G.R.O. occasionally undertook. He also made frequent use of the M.O.H. reports to explore local sanitary, social, and economic conditions, and he included excerpts from these annual reports in his discussion of the causes of excessive infant mortality.[17] In addition, for his report on infant mortality in Lancashire, Newsholme sent three of his Medical Inspectors to investigate conditions in seven towns. Their reports form a substantial portion of his third volume in this series.[18] He also sent Janet Lane-Claypon, then an Assistant Medical Inspector who was devoting much of her time to infant mortality, to report what was then being done in Lancashire to prevent this loss of life. She visited all the Lancashire boroughs and urban districts except the seven inspected by her three colleagues, and in most towns she not only interviewed the M.O.H. but also accompanied a health visitor to the homes of infants.[19]

Newsholme was at pains, especially in the first report, to demonstrate the importance of infant mortality to the nation and to suggest that it might be vastly reduced. If lives were to be saved, early life offered a great opportunity. During 1908, one-third of all deaths in England and Wales occurred under the age of five; one-fifth belonged to the first year of life; and one-ninth took place within three months of birth.[20] Similarly Illustration 11.1 shows graphically the distribution of deaths during 1911–14 according to age group. Recent mortality trends, especially the belated downturn in infant mortality, suggested that fatalism about high death rates among the very young was not warranted. (See Illustration 11.2.) Other proof that high infant death rates were not inevitable was to be found in the

---

15 Newsholme, *Maternal Mortality;* Newsholme, *Report on Child Mortality.*
16 W. H. Power, "Memorandum as to Annual Reports of Medical Officers of Health," *Ann. Rep. Med. Off. L.G.B.,* 35 (1905–6): 259–60, 261. Newsholme explains the significance of these tabulations to his studies of infant mortality in Newsholme, *Infant and Child Mortality,* 5; and Newsholme, *Ann. Rep. Med. Off. L.G.B.,* 43 (1913–14), xxii–xxiii.
17 He first made extensive use of this information in his second report. See, for example, the excerpts from M.O.H. on sanitation in Newsholme, *Second Report on Infant Mortality,* 60–3, 66–72.
18 S. Monckton Copeman reported on Burnley, Colne, and Nelson. R. A. Farrar reported on Wigan and Stretford, and E. P. Manby reported on Widness and Farnworth. Newsholme, *Third Report on Infant Mortality,* 31–136.
19 "Dr. Lane-Claypon's Report on Infant Welfare Work in Lancashire," in Newsholme, *Third Report on Infant Mortality,* 137–90.
20 Newsholme, *Infant and Child Mortality,* 74.

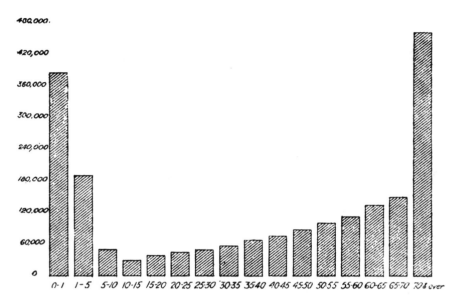

Illustration 11.1. Age-group distribution of deaths in England and Wales, 1911–14. From Newsholme, *Report on Child Mortality at Ages 0–5 in England and Wales*, Suppl. Ann. Rep. Med. Off. L.G.B., 45 (1915–16): 9.

experience of nations such as New South Wales, Norway, and New Zealand, which had infant mortality rates of 75, 69, and 62 per thousand births, respectively, while the rate for England and Wales, although beginning to fall, still exceeded 135 per thousand births in 1906.[21] Regional differences in England and Wales were as striking. In 1908, for example, the administrative counties of Hereford and Oxford had rates only half those of Durham and Glamorgan.[22] See Illustration 11.3. But most suggestive were local variations. In Wigan, Lancashire, whose average annual townwide infant mortality for 1911–13 was 165.4 per thousand, rates varied from 78 in All Saints Ward to 238 in St. Thomas Ward.[23] In fact, Newsholme's reports demonstrated fairly consistent patterns in the distribution of high infant death rates. Urban districts almost always had higher rates than rural districts. Textile-working, metal-working, and mining towns usually had much higher rates than other towns. Poor families and poorer neighborhoods generally had higher rates than their more prosperous neighbors.

The key to understanding why some infants were so much more likely to die than others lay, Newsholme believed, in a careful analysis of such differences. But first Newsholme felt obliged to answer those who insisted that high rates of infant mortality were eugenic and that society interfered at its peril with this weeding

21 See the table reproduced from the Registrar-General's reports in Newsholme, ibid., 41.
22 Newsholme, ibid., 8.   23 Newsholme, *Third Report on Infant Mortality*, 23, 93.

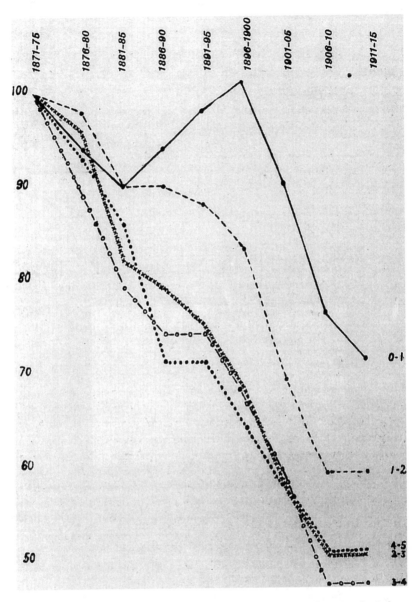

Illustration 11.2. Trends in relative age-specific mortality rates for infancy and childhood, 1875–1915. From Newsholme, *Report on Child Mortality at Ages 0–5 in England and Wales, Suppl. Ann. Rep. Med. Off. L.G.B.*, 45 (1915–16): 13.

out of inferior life. So important did Newsholme believe dealing with this objection to be, that he devoted the first section of his first report to demonstrating that extensive weeding out of infant lives did not produce a healthier population. Specifically he demonstrated that high death rates in the first year of life did not result in lower rates of mortality in succeeding years. He tried several different approaches. First he computed for a single year, 1908, the relative infant mortality (ages 0–1) and relative child mortality (ages 1–5) for four categories of large administrative areas.[24] He found that the rank order of these regions by their relative infant mortality was followed quite closely by the order of their relative childhood mortality. See Illustration 11.4. In this case the national rates for England and Wales were set equal to 100. Discrepancies in the relative order of these areas he thought could be accounted for by epidemics that year of whooping cough and measles. It seemed that the forces which produced high death rates in the first year of life continued to produce high rates in the next four years as well. Stated in other terms, infants who survived the greatest risks in the first year seemed to enjoy no advantages in the next four years. He next attempted to carry this sort of demonstration to later years by using published G.R.O. data for male mortality in the counties of England and Wales during 1908.[25] In this case he computed coefficients of correlation for the relationship of mortality in the first five years of life to those of each of the next three 5-year periods of life. The coefficients were + .74, + .57, and + .43. The third figure, for the correlation of mortality at ages zero to five to that for ages fifteen to twenty, was affected, he believed, by migration. Counties, it seemed, with high infant mortality generally continue to have high rates of mortality at least to the age of twenty, and counties with low infant mortality enjoy lower mortality until age twenty.

Two years later Karl Pearson responded in a paper to the Royal Society of London and more briefly in a lecture to a medical audience.[26] Pearson objected to Newsholme's method, because it compared children of different ages at the same time rather than following a cohort for a period of years. Pearson insisted that the difficulty would be overcome if age-specific mortality rates from the G.R.O.'s national life tables were used. He displayed male and female infant and childhood mortality rates drawn from the four latest national life tables: Farr's life table number 3 (1838–54), Ogle's table (1871–80), and two life tables by Tatham (1881–90 and 1891–1900). From this vast national experience Pearson observed

It is not generally realised that the infantile mortality in England and Wales has not been falling but steadily rising since the restriction in size of families. On the other hand, the child mortality has been steadily falling. . . . If we might suppose the environment of the country as a whole to have remained constant, we could only conclude that it is certain

24 Newsholme, *Infant and Child Mortality*, 9–13.   25 Ibid., 15–17.
26 Karl Pearson, "The Intensity of Natural Selection in Man," *Proc. Roy. Soc. Lond.*, Ser. B., 85 (1912): 469–76; and Karl Pearson, *Darwinism, Medical Progress, and Eugenics: The Cavendish Lecture, 1912, Eugenics Laboratory Lecture Series, IX* (London: Dulau, 1912), 12–16.

1908.—*Infant Mortality at different Ages and from various Causes, and Death-rates at Ages 1–5 in England and Wales, and in the Administrative Counties of Durham, Glamorgan, Hereford, and Oxford.*

Death-rate per 1,000 Births.	England & Wales.	Durham.	Glam-organ.	Hereford.	Oxford.
Under 1 week	24·3	33·8	24·8	18·2	20·9
Under 1 month*	40·3	52·1	46·1	31·2	30·6
Under 3 months†	64·4	77·9	76·7	43·4	44·6
3–6 months ...	23·6	30·9	34·5	16·6	13·1
6–12 months ...	32·4	42·2	43·1	15·8	15·3
Entire first year ...	120·4	151·0	154·3	75·8	73·0
Measles	1·9	1·8	3·6	—	—
Whooping cough	5·0	6·6	6·7	2·0	3·7
Diarrhœal diseases ...	19·9	26·9	27·1	5·7	8·1
Premature birth	19·9	23·6	15·5	15·8	17·5
Congenital defects ...	6·7	6·4	5·9	1·6	4·4
Injury at birth	1·0	1·3	·4	·4	·6
Want of breast milk, &c....	·8	·2	·3	1·2	—
Atrophy, marasmus, &c. ...	15·0	27·1	24·7	15·4	8·1
Tuberculous diseases ...	4·7	5·8	4·1	2·9	1·6
Convulsions	10·8	13·0	22·0	6·9	7·5
Bronchitis and pneumonia	20·4	25·3	24·7	14·2	10·9
Other causes	14·3	13·0	19·3	9·7	10·6
	120·4	151·0	154·3	75·8	73·0
Number of births ...	942,611	31,291	26,089	2,468	3,204
Deaths at ages 1–5 per 1,000 survivors to the age of 1 year.	61·8	75·4	77·5	43·0	26·3

* *i e.* from birth to 1 month.

† *i.e.* from birth to 3 months.

Illustration 11.3. Newsholme's table comparing the healthiest and the least healthy English counties according to infant mortality by age and cause. From Newsholme, *Infant and Child Mortality, Suppl. Ann. Rep. Med. Off. L.G.B.,* 39 (1909–10): 8.

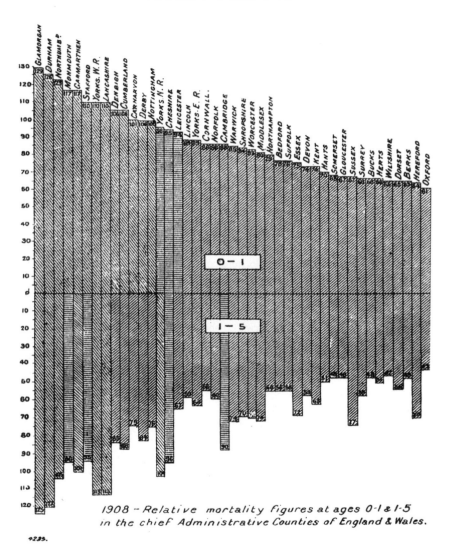

ADMINISTRATIVE COUNTIES.

RELATIVE MORTALITY FIGURES, 1908.

AT AGES 0–1 AND 1–5.

1908 – Relative mortality figures at ages 0-1 & 1-5 in the chief Administrative Counties of England & Wales.

Illustration 11.4. One of Newsholme's demonstrations that high infant mortality is not eugenic. From Newsholme, *Infant and Child Mortality*, *Suppl. Ann. Rep. Med. Off. L.G.B.*, 39 (1909–10): facing p. 10.

that a high infant death-rate in a given community implies in general a low death-rate in the next four years of life.[27]

It was probably with great delight that Newsholme pointed out Pearson's errors in his second report.[28] First, Pearson's demonstration ended in 1900, about the time when the death registers began to show a decline in infant mortality. While the life table for the decade 1900–10 had not yet been published, it was abundantly clear from the registration data that life table mortality figures for infancy would show a decline in this decade similar to the decline at later ages of childhood. Second, Pearson had ignored or failed to mention that the national life tables had been constructed using different methods in computing the entries for the most troublesome years, those under age five and those over age sixty-five. A paper to the Royal Statistical Society in 1901 had pointed out the differences in these methods and had demonstrated the errors that arose when values for the extremes of life from different life tables were used for comparative purposes.[29] It was for these reasons, Newsholme explained, that mortality for the first five years of life was best computed directly from the registers of births and deaths. When it was, the increase in infant mortality Pearson found between the decades 1871–80 and 1881–90 became a decrease.

Newsholme went on to answer some of Pearson's objections by comparing relative infant and childhood mortalities for a series of years, 1907–1910, this time for 241 urban districts.[30] The results here confirmed his earlier conclusions. In his first report he had also attempted a more ambitious demonstration that Pearson had not noticed.[31] Newsholme obtained from Stevenson an unpublished G.R.O. table showing annually the births and deaths for each of the first five years of life from 1855 onward. Newsholme tried to show in tables and in graphs that major annual fluctuations in the infant death rate were accompanied by fluctuations in the same direction in each of the four following years, although ages one to two followed the trend in infancy much more closely than any of the three succeeding years. Not content with these results, Newsholme asked the statistician George Udny Yule, Newmarch lecturer in statistics at University College, London, and former assistant of Pearson, to subject these data to more rigorous analysis.[32] Yule concluded that there might be a slight selective effect of high infant mortality on the mortality during the second year of life, but such effect did not extend beyond the third year, whereas the effects of a sickly infancy extended much longer. He

---

27 Pearson, "Intensity of Natural Selection," 470–1.
28 Newsholme, *Second Report on Infant Mortality*, 47–8. Newsholme quotes from Pearson's paper in this section.
29 T. E. Hayward, "A Series of Life-Tables for England and Wales for each successive Decennium from 1841–50 to 1881–90, calculated by an Abbreviated Method," *J. Roy. Statist. Soc.*, 64 (1901): 636–41. Newsholme cites this article in this discussion.
30 Newsholme, *Second Report on Infant Mortality*, 43–6.
31 Newsholme, *Infant and Child Mortality*, 14–15.
32 "On the Possible Selective Influence of Mortality in Infancy on Mortality in the Next Four Years of Life," Appendix I in ibid., 78–83. On Yule's career see *D.N.B.*, 1951–60: 1095–6.

cautioned that the data were too sparse and the problem was too complex to place much faith in this conclusion.

Newsholme concluded that the exact effect of high infant mortality on later life was a moot point. It could only be settled by a grand social experiment in which an equal number of infants who had survived the first year of life would be exchanged between a county with a very high infant mortality rate, like Durham, and a county with a low infant mortality rate like Oxford. Short of carrying out that experiment it was only fair to observe that

> If natural selection during infancy in the county of Durham has left a juvenile population less prone to disease, the effect of this selection is most effectively and completely concealed by the evil environment in that county, which causes the hypothetically stronger survivors to suffer from excessive mortality, so long as they can be traced through life.[33]
>
> There need therefore be no hesitation in making every practicable effort to reduce infant mortality. It is not only in accord with the highest feelings of humanity, but action which secures reduction of infantile mortality also secures reduction of mortality at higher ages.[34]

The medical community found Newsholme's demonstrations definitive and took comfort in his conclusions. The eugenic view of high infant mortality rates "has received a severe check, if not been actually destroyed, by the pains-taking and scientific investigation of Dr. Newsholme and his department."[35]

Having demonstrated that high infant mortality was not eugenic, Newsholme devoted the greater portion of these reports to testing contemporary explanations for such high rates.[36] It was easy to discredit simple climatic or geographic explanations. Infant mortality simply varied too widely within the wards of the same town to make these plausible. Newsholme referred to his earlier demonstrations of a relationship between high temperature or low rainfall and high mortality from diarrhea, but he reported that he could find no connection between temperature and rainfall records and recent trends in infant mortality as a whole.[37] Similarly, he found no relationship between a population's level of infant mortality and such other demographic indicators as its birth rate, fertility rate, its rate of illegitimacy, or its preponderance of male over female births.[38]

Infant mortality was commonly thought to be dependent on social class. G.R.O. figures for the census year, 1911, showed in fact that among upper- and middle-class families infants died at a rate of 77 per thousand births, but among the working class as a whole infant mortality rose to 133 per thousand, and among unskilled laborers it reached 152 per thousand.[39] Regional studies suggested that income was an important factor. The M.O.H. of Bradford, for example, had shown that in his town

33 Newsholme, *Infant and Child Mortality*, 18.   34 Ibid., 17.
35 Ashby, *Infant Mortality*, 11.
36 He gave a list of such explanations early in his first report, Newsholme *Infant and Child Mortality*, 40.
37 Ibid., 40–1, 43–4.
38 Ibid., 45–9; Newsholme, *Second Report on Infant Mortality*, 56–8; and Newsholme, *Report on Child Mortality*, 76–8.
39 See the table reproduced in Newsholme, *Second Report on Infant Mortality*, 73.

	0—1 year.		0—5 years.	
—	Deaths.	Percentage of Total Deaths.	Deaths.	Percentage of Total Deaths.
Measles	2,533	3·1 ⎫	11,812	9·3 ⎫
Scarlet fever	66	0·1	1,110	0·9
Whooping-cough	3,989	4·8 ⎬ 21·3	8,159	6·4 ⎬ 32·5
Diarrhœa and enteritis	6,734	8·1	8,493	6·7
Tuberculosis (all forms)	2,459	3·0	7,137	5·6
Venereal diseases	1,204	1·5	1,286	1·0
Other infective diseases	614	0·7 ⎭	3,266	2·6 ⎭
Bronchitis and pneumonia	15,623	18·9 ⎫	27,265	21·5 ⎫
Meningitis	1,120	1·4	2,462	1·9
Disease of eyes	5	0·0 ⎬ 20·7	12	0·0 ⎬ 23·9
„ ears	149	0·2	348	0·3
„ mouth	180	0·2 ⎭	238	0·2 ⎭
Heart diseases	37	0·0	195	0·2
Rickets	301	0·4	728	0·6
Cancer and other tumours	23	0·0	120	0·1
Scurvy	15	0·0	21	0·0
Other general diseases	166	0·2	345	0·3
Infantile convulsions	7,413	9·0	8,740	6·9
Premature birth, atelectasis, and injury at birth	19,521	23·6	19,521	15·4
Atrophy, debility, and marasmus ...	10,281	12·4	10,281	8·1
All other causes...	10,346	12·4	15,535	12·0
Total...	82,779	100·0	127,074	100·0

Illustration 11.5. Newsholme's table showing deaths and percentage of deaths by cause for infancy and childhood during 1912. From Newsholme, *Maternal Mortality in Connection with Childbearing and Its Relation to Infant Mortality, Suppl. Ann. Rep. Med. Off. L.G.B.*, 44 (1914–15): 18.

the infant mortality of families decreased as the rateable (assessed) value of their houses increased.[40] Newsholme agreed that infant mortality was highest in the poorest, most crowded districts of industrial cities, but he doubted that low income alone could explain this fact.[41] If infant mortality were determined primarily by low income, he reasoned, infant mortality should not have remained stationary in the late nineteenth century when the economic condition of the average English worker was improving. Newsholme's medical inspectors reported that there was little pauperism or dependency due to low wages in the Lancashire towns they visited, yet infants born in these industrial towns experienced the highest death rates in the

40 See the table of A. Evans reproduced in ibid., 75.
41 For the following comments, see Newsholme, *Infant and Child Mortality*, 54–6, 60, 61; Newsholme, *Second Report on Infant Mortality*, 73–8; and Newsholme, *Third Report on Infant Mortality*, 21; and Newsholme, *Report on Child Mortality*, 67–9.

nation. Foreign statistics suggested that in Ireland and Norway families were on average not only larger but also poorer than in England, yet the national infant mortality rates for these nations were lower than England's. In England some groups of workers, such as Durham miners, had high wages and very high infant mortality rates, while Jews living on very low incomes in some of the poorest quarters of industrial cities experienced low rates of infant mortality. Poverty, Newsholme insisted, was a complex social condition in which income was only one element. In order to understand why the offspring of the poor died at such frightful rates, one would have to analyze more carefully the conditions in which the urban working classes lived.

To investigate further, Newsholme considered the registered causes of infant deaths. As Illustrations 11.3 and 11.5 show, his search led him to finger five categories of causes: childhood infectious diseases, diarrheal diseases, bronchitis and pneumonia, convulsions, and a miscellaneous category of wasting and developmental diseases which he sometimes labeled the "Five Grouped Diseases" (premature birth; congenital defects; injury at birth; want of breast milk; atrophy, debility, and marasmus, or wasting).[42] The predominance of the first three were cause for optimism, Newsholme insisted, because these were diseases which could be controlled by known means. The meaning of the latter two categories was more problematic, although he suspected at first that improper feeding, syphilis, and inaccurate registrations of causes of infant deaths all helped elevate these numbers.[43] This analysis suggested what Newsholme sought to demonstrate: Infant mortality was both a sanitary and a social problem involving both individual and community responsibility. Newsholme deliberately chose to emphasize the sanitary aspects of the problem, because he believed that action here promised the most immediate results and because doing so placed responsibility where it belonged, on local authorities.[44]

The importance of communicable diseases and the fact that infant mortality was so high in the oldest and most densely populated sections of industrial towns suggested that overcrowded housing was an important contributor to infant mortality. Newsholme did find that in general counties or towns with high infant and child mortality rates had a higher percentage of their residents living in overcrowded houses than did counties or towns which had comparatively low infant death rates.[45] But as Illustration 11.6, compiled from registration and census data, and his department's field investigations of the seven Lancashire towns showed, there were important anomalies, most often high rates among uncrowded populations.[46] He concluded that overcrowded housing played an important part

---

42 For his introduction to the Five Grouped Diseases, see Newsholme, *Second Report on Infant Mortality*, 33.
43 Newsholme, *Infant and Child Mortality*, 26–8.
44 Newsholme, *Second Report on Infant Mortality*, 55.
45 Newsholme, *Infant and Child Mortality*, 68–9; and Newsholme, *Report on Child Mortality*, 68–71.
46 Newsholme, *Third Report on Infant Mortality*, 14.

PROPORTION PER CENT. OF POPULATION IN PRIVATE FAMILIES
WHO LIVE IN A CONDITION OF OVERCROWDING—I.E., IN
TENEMENTS WITH MORE THAN TWO OCCUPANTS PER ROOM.

Large Towns.

Large towns with the twenty highest death-rates, 0–5.			Large towns with the twenty lowest death-rates, 0–5.		
——	Per cent. of over-crowd-ing. (Census, 1911.)	Birth-rate, 1913.	——	Per cent. of over-crowd-ing. (Census, 1911.)	Birth-rate, 1913.
BURNLEY	9·5	22·8	Hornsey	3·2	16·2
WIGAN	12·9	28·1	Ilford	2·1	17·3
MIDDLESBROUGH	13·4	31·1	BOURNEMOUTH ...	1·6	15·6
ST. HELENS ...	17·0	32·2	Ealing	3·8	18·3
BARNSLEY ...	10·0	30·3	SOUTHEND-ON-SEA	3·6	18·5
STOKE-ON-TRENT	8·6	31·3	HASTINGS	5·5	14·5
LIVERPOOL	10·1	29·8	EASTBOURNE ...	4·3	16·0
PRESTON	5·6	23·9	BATH	4·8	15·7
OLDHAM	7·2	23·0	OXFORD	2·4	17·7
SALFORD	10·1	27·1	READING	3·1	20·9
WALSALL	7·2	30·0	Swindon	2·2	23·5
WEST BROMWICH	12·2	29·5	EAST HAM	6·4	25·5
MANCHESTER ...	7·2	25·7	Walthamstow ...	7·4	24·4
ROTHERHAM ...	8·2	30·2	Cambridge	2·3	19·5
BOOTLE	9·2	30·0	Wimbledon	4·0	19·2
GATESHEAD... ...	33·7	29·2	CROYDON	4·3	21·9
SHEFFIELD	8·4	28·2	SOUTHPORT ...	3·5	15·2
DUDLEY	15·0	28·6	Gillingham	2·3	22·5
SUNDERLAND ...	32·6	30·9	Leyton	5·5	22·3
Rhondda	5·6	33·1	WALLASEY	3·3	22·1
NOTTINGHAM ...	4·3	22·7	Willesden	13·0	24·8

Illustration 11.6. Newsholme's table showing overcrowding and infant mortality in large towns. From Newsholme, *Report on Child Mortality at Ages 0–5 in England and Wales, Suppl. Ann. Rep. Med. Off. L.G.B.,* 45 (1915–16): 70.

in the nation's excessive infant mortality and, for example, blamed Durham's "deplorably bad," colliery-owned housing for that county's excessive rate.[47] But, he concluded, housing could not be the most important cause.

As he had in Brighton when he studied diarrheal diseases, Newsholme blamed failures of community sanitation, particularly in the disposal of household waste and human excrement. Over wide stretches of the industrial North, he wrote dramatically, in regions where infant mortality was the highest, "a condition approaching sanitary barbarism" exists.[48] Conservancy methods, that is, privies or pail closets, were used for human excrement; covered, movable dustbins (garbage

47 Newsholme, *Infant and Child Mortality,* 68; and Newsholme, *Report on Child Mortality,* 69.
48 Newsholme, *Second Report on Infant Mortality,* 60.

cans) were rare, and household refuse was often stored in fixed pits in back yards from which it had to be carried through the house for removal; backyards were often unpaved; and the scavenging of streets was woefully inadequate.[49] It was in dealing with this subject that Newsholme made the greatest use of the reports of M.O.H. and of the reports of the Board's medical inspectors. Sections of these reports are reminiscent of Edwin Chadwick's classic report of 1842 in their graphic descriptions of revolting conditions. A County M.O.H. reported

In the County of Durham privies are almost universal. . . . Many of the midden privies are very large with uncovered receptacles sunk below the ground level, not watertight, and serving for two, four, or a much larger number of houses. In some districts many of these privies are greatly dilapidated and without proper doors, so that their contents escape on the surface of the streets. . . . The contents of midden privies have to be thrown out on the ground in many districts, from which they are shovelled into a cart or basket. In many instances the contents have to be conveyed through the dwellings in baskets, to be emptied into the cart in the street. Under these circumstances the ground of the streets and back streets and in many instances also the interiors of the dwellings become fouled with excremental filth.[50]

He postulated a similar mechanism to the one he had employed in his earlier studies of diarrheal diseases to link such environmental pollution to infant deaths.[51] Excrement and putrefying rubbish were brought from yard or street into the house on feet, hands, or clothing or by flies. Infants or young children ingested the filth in contaminated food or inhaled it as airborne dust. Infants who were artificially fed were especially vulnerable. In the poorest households there were often no places to prepare or store safely a baby's food. Such food was thus not only likely to spoil, but it was easily contaminated. The higher diarrheal death rate in the second six months of life, a time when many infants were weaned, strongly implicated the contamination of infant food.

"It is an accepted fact," Newsholme observed in his first report, "that defective scavenging and the retention of excremental matters in privies and pail closets are always accompanied by excessive infantile diarrhoea."[52] This was a conclusion that he confirmed with each subsequent study whether it was focused on whole counties, on towns, or on individual wards.[53] His preference for this environmental explanation for high infant mortality rates is easily seen in the way he handled unexpected results. Normally when comparisons of local statistics showed that the ranking of towns by infant mortality did not match their ranking by some

---

49 For discussions of these sanitary evils, see Newsholme, *Infant and Child Mortality*, 63–8; Newsholme, *Second Report on Child Mortality*, 58–72; and Newsholme, *Third Report on Infant Mortality*, 12–15.

50 From the report of the County Medical Officer of Health, Durham quoted in Newsholme, *Infant and Child Mortality*, 64.

51 For the following discussion, see ibid., 66–7; Newsholme, *Second Report on Infant Mortality*, 58–9; and Newsholme, *Report on Child Mortality*, 72.

52 Newsholme, *Infant and Child Mortality*, 66.

53 See, for example, Newsholme, *Second Report on Infant Mortality*, 60; and Newsholme, *Third Report on Infant Mortality*, 90–1.

proposed cause, Newsholme concluded that the factor in question was not of great importance. But this procedure was not used when the issue was waste disposal. When he found, for example, that some towns or parishes that had converted to water closets continued to have higher infant mortality rates than areas that had not, he went out of his way to find extenuating local circumstances. The town with water closets and a high infant death rate was more densely populated, or its water closets were of the inferior hand-flushed variety.[54]

His certainty that defects of community sanitation were responsible for the largest share of excessive infant mortality justified his claim that the primary responsibility for preventing infant deaths lay with local authorities. Throughout his extended investigation of infant mortality he was intent on collecting evidence that would shame local authorities into action. The recommendations of his first report on infant mortality listed the names of the twenty-five sanitary districts with the highest infant mortality rates and called for these authorities to meet their responsibilities.[55] In an address intended to publicize the results of that report, he described the high infant mortality rates in industrial towns as the result of "inexcusable municipal neglect and parsimony."[56] He had no doubt that local authorities must lead and bear much of the responsibility for the current state of infant health.

Among the other explanations of high infant mortality rates were two involving mothers: employment of married women outside the home, and maternal igno-rance and carelessness. Many of the recent historical studies of the infant welfare movement have emphasized the medical discussions of these causes. Carol Dy-house, for example, has described the Edwardian discussion of extradomestic maternal employment and has argued that public health authorities blamed work-ing mothers for preventable infant deaths and sought to keep married women out of the labor market.[57] She is certainly correct to insist that Newsholme believed that the industrial employment of women with infants was inadvisable, and potentially harmful to the babies themselves.[58] Employment in textile mills and other industries, he maintained, often involved physical strain and exhaustion, the early weaning of infants, and their care by baby minders (babysitters). It also erected one more barrier to domestic cleanliness.[59] He pointed out, that in poor families the extra income a working mother brought home might be more important to the health of her young children than the personal care she might

---

54 See, for example, his use of the M.O.H. reports in Newsholme, *Second Report on Infant Mortality*, 61, 62, 68–9.
55 Newsholme, *Infant and Child Mortality*, 77.
56 Arthur Newsholme, "The National Importance of Child Mortality," *J. Roy. Sanitary Inst.*, 31 (1910): 344.
57 Carol Dyhouse, "Working-Class Mothers and Infant Mortality in England, 1896–1914," in *Biology, Medicine and Society 1840–1940*, ed. Charles Webster (Cambridge: Cambridge Univ Press, 1981), 73–98.
58 Ibid., 93.
59 See Janet Lane-Claypon's report on infant welfare in Lancashire in Newsholme, *Third Report on Infant Mortality*, 138–40.

give them in greater poverty.[60] Nor was that all. Newsholme displayed for his readers statistics for counties and towns which demonstrated that both high and low rates of married women's industrial employment were associated with high infant mortality rates and that places where few women worked outside the home might still have very high infant mortality.[61] This evidence suggested to Newsholme that while in principle the employment of mothers outside of the home was a hazard to infant life, other dangers were then so much more important as to almost completely overshadow the influence of working women. Dyhouse's demonstration by linear regression that there was no correlation between infant mortality rates and rates of industrial employment of married women for county level data was not necessary to disprove Newsholme.[62] He had reached a similar conclusion using simpler methods. Wartime experience strengthened Newsholme's conviction on this point. He pointed out in 1918 that the infant death rate had continued to fall during the war, although an increasing number of mothers with young children had been working in industry.[63] Until public authorities did their duty of guaranteeing decent standards of housing and public hygiene, Newsholme held that it was misguided to expect that urging mothers to stay home and to keep a tidy house would have much effect on infant mortality.

In the final chapter of his first report on infant mortality, Newsholme included a section entitled "Ignorance and Fecklessness of Mothers."[64] He disposed of this topic very briefly – it occupied fewer than four pages of a thirty-three-page chapter in the first report, and it was not repeated in either his second or third report on infant mortality nor in the report on maternal mortality, although he did devote two and a half pages to the topics separately in the final report in this series.[65] As in the case of industrial employment of women, he minimized the importance of maternal ignorance and fecklessness. Nevertheless, the title Newsholme gave that section has proven irresistible to historians who have used it to characterize his position: "Newsholme continued to stress the many possible causes of diarrhoea and while he refused to reduce these to the one issue of maternal hygiene, he too came to regard 'the ignorance and fecklessness of mothers' as the most important factor causing infant mortality."[66] Even more misrepresentative of Newsholme's emphasis is this statement by Anna Davin:

Even as careful a statistician as Arthur Newsholme, in his report on infant mortality for the medical department of the Local Government Board in 1910, ended up ignoring the

60 Newsholme, *Infant and Child Mortality*, 57–8; Newsholme, *Second Report on Infant Mortality*, 56; and Newsholme, *Report on Child Mortality*, 75.
61 Newsholme, *Infant and Child Mortality*, 58; Newsholme, *Second Report on Infant Mortality*, 56; and Newsholme, *Report on Child Mortality*, 74–5; and Newsholme, *Third Report on Infant Mortality*, 17–18.
62 Dyhouse, "Working-Class Mothers," 97–8.
63 Newsholme, *Ann. Rep. Med. Off. L.G.B.*, 47 (1917–18): xxxv.
64 Newsholme, *Infant and Child Mortality*, 70–3.   65 Newsholme, *Report on Child Mortality*, 64–6.
66 Jane Lewis, *The Politics of Motherhood: Child and Maternal Welfare in England, 1900–1939* (London: Croom Helm, 1980), 65–6.

evidence of his own tables as to regional variation and the excessive incidence of infant mortality wherever particular features of working-class urban life were concentrated (most of all overcrowding and the failure of local authorities to introduce a waterborne sewage system in place of middens and ash pits), and sounding off interminably [sic] about the 'ignorance and fecklessness of mothers.'[67]

Newsholme acknowledged that poor mothers sometimes were careless or ignorant of their infants' needs, but he doubted that, taken as a group, they were more ignorant or feckless than mothers in other social classes. However, a poor mother's situation made her mistakes and ignorance more tragic.[68] She, after all, was unlikely to have domestic help or access to medical care when she or her infant fell sick. She was more likely to work outside the home and to be overworked and physically exhausted; her home was more likely to be crowded and insanitary. In short her economic vulnerability provided little margin for error or bad luck. Newsholme, in fact, was quite contemptuous of the maternal ignorance theory of infant mortality.

Maternal ignorance is sometimes regarded as a chief factor in the causation of excessive child mortality. It is a comfortable doctrine for the well-to-do person to adopt; and it goes far to relieve his conscience in the contemplation of excessive suffering and mortality among the poor.

This doctrine has found favour in occasional official reports and in miscellaneous addresses. It embodies an aspect of truth, but it is mischievous when it implies, as it sometimes does, that what is chiefly required is the distribution of leaflets of advice, or the giving of theoretical instruction as to matters of personal hygiene.[69]

Anna Davin has suggested that this is an enlightened view that Newsholme came to late in life. She cites a section of this passage from his autobiography which appeared in 1935 and claims that it shows that by the 1930s he was able to free himself from "the influence of maternalism."[70] In reality, when Newsholme wrote that section of his autobiography, he quoted from his *Report on Child Mortality* that appeared in 1916.[71] His was not a deathbed conversion.

Similarly, while Newsholme recognized that good domestic hygiene was critical in protecting the health of infants and young children, he was sympathetic to the plight of the families of unskilled workers, and he refused to place the major blame for infant mortality on individual homemakers. Writing of Clarendon Street, Paddington, where 784 one-roomed tenements were occupied by 1,889 people including 501 children and the infant mortality for 1909 was 220 per thousand births, Newsholme observed,

---

67 Anna Davin, "Imperialism and Motherhood," *Hist. Workshop,* 5 (1978): 14. This statement is even more surprising because later in this article she gives Newsholme's work a fairer reading, ibid., 31.

68 Newsholme, *Report of Child Mortality,* 65–6; and Newsholme, *Infant and Child Mortality,* 73.

69 Newsholme, *Report on Child Mortality,* 64.

70 Davin, "Imperialism and Motherhood," 31–2.

71 Compare Newsholme, *Report on Child Mortality,* 64, with Arthur Newsholme, *Fifty Years in Public Health: A Personal Narrative with Comments* (London: George Allen and Unwin, 1935), 372.

It may be justifiable to state that much of the excessive mortality in these tenements is caused by the shiftless, dirty, and drunken habits of many of the tenants; and to add that until the next generation which has learnt to appreciate a high standard of living takes the place of the present tenants, there is little hope of reform. But to say this, is to present only a portion of the truth. . . . When the mother has to fetch clean water up and to carry dirty water down several flights of stairs, domestic cleanliness becomes very difficult; and the fact that the water-closet is equally inaccessible, conduces to a condition of life most inimical to health, especially for children.[72]

It was quite unreasonable to expect that the insides of homes could be kept clean, when the immediate environment was filthy. In sections also reminiscent of sections of Chadwick's 1842 report, Newsholme described how an overworked mother's attempts to keep a clean house were "thwarted by the terrible condition of things outside the back door," and how she eventually became discouraged and wearied in her "house-pride."[73] Newsholme believed that there was little hope that domestic hygiene would improve until local authorities saw to it that the environment of every house was clean and established a higher minimum standard of housing.[74]

Newsholme did believe that parental behavior was an important factor. Parental drinking sapped family resources and put infant lives at risk. He even predicted that a great improvement would be brought about in towns such as Middlesborough if the pubs could be closed for six months.[75] He also believed that for real progress to be made in the fight against infant mortality better paid workers would have to give up some "ephemeral pleasures" to see that their families enjoyed greater "domestic comfort."[76] But he had great faith in the goodwill and good intentions of working-class parents, particularly mothers. "Happily it is beyond doubt that nearly every mother is profoundly wishful to secure the welfare of her offspring, and will welcome any aid which is judiciously offered in this direction."[77] Newsholme followed this axiom with the observation that working-class mothers offered their children the benefits of breast feeding more consistently than the higher classes. Given this great advantage, the harmful effects of the circumstances in which the urban working classes too often existed were brought into stark relief.

It was typical of him to assign responsibility both to the community and to the individual.

The responsibility of the Local Authorities consists in efforts to provide a decent environment for every home; in the training of scholars, especially of the elder girls, in domestic economy and hygiene; in arranging for visits, soon after the birth of infants and at

---

72 Newsholme, *Second Report on Infant Mortality,* 72.
73 Newsholme, *Infant and Child Mortality,* 63. See also Newsholme, *Second Report on Infant Mortality,* 59–60.
74 Newsholme, *Third Report on Infant Mortality,* 15, 21.
75 *Second Report on Infant Mortality,* 78–82; and Newsholme, *Report on Child Mortality,* 60, 66–7.
76 Newsholme, *Infant and Child Mortality,* 70.   77 Ibid.

intervals afterwards, of competent and tactful health visitors. The parents are responsible for abstinence from such indulgences as will lower the standard of domestic life by leaving insufficient margin for adequate housing, food and clothing. They are responsible also for the intelligent use of every available means for the improvement of personal health, including domestic cleanliness and their share in the sanitary control of the district in which they dwell.[78]

He insisted, however, that the reform process must be started by local authorities. Their action would have the most immediate effects, and it would facilitate better housekeeping and child care.[79]

Newsholme's report on maternal mortality is the most original, if least exhaustively pursued, of this series. It was one of the first on the subject in the English public health literature, and it remains an important source of data on maternal mortality in England in the early twentieth century.[80] It was methodologically sound, acknowledging, for example, that maternal deaths were too rare to be statistically studied except in large populations.[81] In it Newsholme reached conclusions, such as the cardinal importance of the nature of attendance at birth and the relatively minor importance of the direct effects of poverty on maternal mortality, which recent historical research has confirmed.[82] His attention was drawn to the subject by the high rates of infant mortality from the developmental or wasting diseases, sometimes labeled the Five Grouped Diseases: premature birth; congenital defects; injury at birth; want of breast milk; and atrophy, debility, and marasmus. Mortality from these conditions had declined less dramatically than the mortality from diseases which were more likely to kill later in the first year of life. As these disorders generally killed soon after birth, typically within the first month, Newsholme believed that they reflected conditions at or before birth.[83]

Newsholme dealt very briefly with this subject in his first report, merely showing that counties with high infant mortality also had high death rates in the first month of life and high mortality from developmental and wasting diseases.[84] Counties with low infant mortality likewise had low rates from these two other categories. Newsholme suspected that poor attendance during childbirth was a major contributing factor, and he promised further study. In their special investigation of Lancashire, Newsholme's staff paid attention to the Group of Five Diseases and to midwifery services, and they turned up some suggestive evidence. They reported that some of the stillbirths and part of the mortality from congenital

78 Ibid., 74.   79 Newsholme, *Second Report on Infant Mortality,* 55.
80 See, for example, the use made of it in the research of Irvine Loudon, "Maternal Mortality: 1880–1950. Some Regional and International Comparison," *Social Hist. Med.,* 1 (1988): 193, 206.
81 For Newsholme's comment on methodology, see Newsholme, *Maternal Mortality,* 23–25.
82 Compare Newsholme's major conclusions with those reached for England and other nations over a much larger time period in Loudon, "Maternal Mortality: 1880–1950," 208–9, 222–3; and Irvine Loudon, "Obstetric Care, Social Class, and Maternal Mortality," *Br. Med. J.* (1986), no. 2: 606–8. See also Irvine Loudon, *Death in Childbirth: An International Study of Maternal Care and Maternal Mortality 1800–1950* (Oxford: Clarendon Press, 1992), 45–8, 243–6, 371, 377–81, 492–6.
83 Newsholme, *Maternal Mortality,* 19–20.   84 Newsholme, *Infant and Child Mortality,* 50–2.

weakness or developmental disorders were probably caused by the taking of drugs, usually lead compounds, to produce abortion.[85] Lane-Claypon also reported that half of the midwives legally practicing in Lancashire in March 1914 were untrained.[86]

In his special report on maternal mortality Newsholme was unable to show a precise relationship between the quality of prenatal and maternity care and deaths of mothers or children during or soon after birth. The data for such a demonstration were either unavailable, unreliable, or incompatible with other data.[87] Much evidence, however, pointed in that direction. First was the toll of maternal lives due to preventable causes. Newsholme reproduced returns from the G.R.O. showing that, during 1913, 31 percent of maternal deaths associated with pregnancy or childbirth were due to puerperal fever, 17 percent to hemorrhage, and 10 percent to other accidents of childbirth.[88] All of these could be drastically reduced. Sepsis had almost disappeared from surgery. There was no excuse for its appearance at childbirth.[89] Newsholme also tried to show that other possible influences did not have much effect on maternal mortality. Using the sort of statistical comparisons and rankings of different administrative or geographic areas he had used in his previous studies, Newsholme showed that maternal mortality did not seem to depend to a large extent on birth rate, on the rate of illegitimacy, on the rate at which women worked outside the home, nor significantly on the state of community sanitation.[90] Various regional comparisons suggested, though, that the highest rates of maternal mortality occurred in places where attendance at childbirth was either remote or unskilled.[91] He expected that remoteness accounted for much of the high rates in Wales and in Westmoreland, Herefordshire, Cumberland, Devonshire, and Cornwall. The very high rates in the textile towns in Lancashire and the West Riding of Yorkshire contrasted dramatically with low rates for other industrial towns such as Manchester, Birmingham, Liverpool, and the Metropolis. Newsholme believed that in these textile towns women received poor care in pregnancy and childbirth. It is hardly surprising then that Newsholme spent the last third of this report discussing the state of midwifery services and recommending a set of prenatal and maternity services local authorities ought to establish.[92]

These five studies of infant, child, and maternal mortality were massive and ingenious. They are the more remarkable for having been completed during the Great War when the resources of the L.G.B. and local sanitary authorities were severely taxed. Newsholme clearly believed them to be of great public importance. He succeeded in documenting the needless loss of human life and the possibilities of its substantial reduction. He also effectively answered both the claim that this

85 See the reports of Copeman and Farrar in Newsholme, *Third Report on Infant Mortality,* 69–70, 86–7.
86 Lane-Claypon's report in ibid., 143.   87 Newsholme, *Maternal Mortality,* 23–5, 29–30, 47–8.
88 Ibid., 24.   89 Ibid., 22–3, 60.   90 Ibid., 54–9.
91 For the following discussion, see ibid., 32–45.   92 Ibid., 60–85.

loss was eugenic and hence ultimately desirable and the claim that its reduction must be left to the reformation of individual behavior. He did not deny that individual parental behavior was important; he simply believed that progress would come faster and be more certain if public authorities took the lead. While he certainly shared many of the beliefs of his age about home and family, his position on the influence of maternal ignorance and carelessness, on the role of housekeeping and the effect of maternal employment outside of the home demonstrates that Newsholme was more sympathetic to the plight of working-class women than many of his colleagues in the public health service and more than contemporary readers might infer from some otherwise useful recent histories.[93] Given the clear policy orientations of his discussions and his ordinary practice of preceding recommendations for public initiatives with epidemiological investigation, it is reasonable to assume that he would have recommended an orderly expansion of local authority sanitation, infant-welfare, and midwifery services. However, political forces, not Newsholme's methodical planning, determined the outcome of events.

INTERDEPARTMENTAL CONFLICT

By the time Newsholme finished these reports on infant, child, and maternal mortality not only was the new preventive work rapidly developing with encouragement from Whitehall but the Local Government Board found itself in bitter conflict with the Board of Education to control it. The episode demonstrates how poorly suited to the emerging welfare state existing administrative arrangements for health were. Not only was responsibility divided among several departments, making contested territory almost inevitable, but, as we have seen, the department with the most extensive public health responsibility, the L.G.B., was not well adapted to rapid, creative social planning. Its delay in acting on an issue of great public concern further tarnished its reputation with the Liberal leadership and exacted a very heavy political penalty.

There is also a personal side to this conflict, an intense personal rivalry between two former allies, Arthur Newsholme and George Newman, the Chief Medical Officer of the Board of Education. There is a great deal of irony in the roles played by the two Medical Officers. When Newman joined the Board of Education as its first Chief Medical Officer in 1907, he was a recognized expert on infant mortality, having published one of the early works on the subject the preceding year, but he had no claim to expertise in school medical services.[94] In 1907 the leading authority on school hygiene and the most likely candidate for the new medical post was Dr. James Kerr, School Medical Officer of the London County

93 See, for example, Dyhouse, "Working-Class Mothers, 93, 97–8; Jane Lewis, *The Politics of Motherhood: Child and Maternal Welfare in England, 1900–1939* (London: Croom Helm, 1980), 35, 62, 65–6, 67; and Anna Davin, "Imperialism and Motherhood," *Hist. Workshop*, 5 (1978): 14.
94 Newman, *Infant Mortality.*

Council. Kerr had been an effective and innovative administrator, and furthermore he claimed that in 1906 he had been promised the new post at the Board of Education.[95] Newman's appointment was greeted by protests from Kerr's supporters and from the enemies of the Webbs and of Robert Morant on the Education Committee of the London County Council and in the National Union of Teachers who correctly suspected that Newman was in league with the Webbs and Morant.[96] The protests spilled over into the *British Medical Journal*, where a lead article declared Kerr the better candidate and a letter from a subordinate of Kerr described Newman's appointment as an "absolute farce" since Newman "knew nothing" of school hygiene and had "been pitchforked into office" in place of the rightful candidate James Kerr.[97]

To secure and defend his appointment, Newman sought and obtained the warm support of Newsholme, who, with some difficulty, convinced Newman not to respond to the public attacks.[98] He relied on Newsholme to help him obtain support from the public health community. As he explained to Morant, Permanent Secretary of the Board of Education, two weeks later,

Newsholme wants to see me & I think I shall run down tomorrow (Thursday) to Brighton. He is editor of the M.O.H. monthly journal *Public Health* & we want to have this definitely on our side all along. The Soc. wanted me to be joint Ed. W. Newsholme. He & I are v. great friends – so I think this can be assured. It goes to every M.O.H. practically.[99]

Newman and Newsholme conferred on policy and appointments to the new medical department and saw quite a bit of each other in these first months after Newman's appointment.[100]

It was not only Newsholme's prominence among Medical Officers of Health that made him an important ally. He was also a recognized advocate of a school health service. He was, after all, the author of a standard text on school hygiene. Also in 1903, four years before the passage of the Education (Administrative Provisions) Act, 1907, he had written a lead article in the *British Medical Journal* that not only praised the efforts of public health authorities in the sanitary

95 J. D. Hirst, "A Failure 'Without Parallel': The School Medical Service and the London County Council 1907–12," *Medical Hist.*, 25 (1981): 281–4.
96 For a discussion of these relationships and events, see Gilbert, *Evolution of National Insurance*, 131–8.
97 "The Attitude of the Board of Education to School Hygiene," *Br. Med. J.* (1907), no. 2: 760–1, and A. H. Hogarth to Editor, ibid., 772–3. See also Hirst, "Failure," 284.
98 Newman describes his correspondence with Newsholme in Newman to Morant, 23 Sept. 1907, P.R.O., Ed 24/280. He agreed to heed Newsholme's advice but was clearly troubled by the criticism.
99 Newman to Morant, 9 Oct. 1907, P.R.O., Ed 24/280.
100 See, for example, Newman to Morant, 11 Oct. 1907, P.R.O., Ed 24/280; Newman to Mootie, 2 Nov. 1907, Wellcome Institute, Newman Letters; Newman to Mamma, n.d. [probably late 1907] ibid.; Newman to Mootie and Hattey, n.d. [probably early 1908], Wellcome Institute, Newman Letters; and Newman, Diary I, entries for 19 Dec. 1907, 7 Jan. 1908, 5 Feb. 1908, 13 Feb. 1908, 14 Feb. 1908, 18 Feb. 1908, 8 April 1908, 16 May 1908, 25 May 1908, 28 May 1908, 14 June 1908, 12 Dec. 1908; 3 Feb. 1909, P.R.O., MH 139/1. Hereafter cited as Newman Diary.

inspection of schools but also advocated the systematic medical inspection of pupils.[101]

While Newsholme respected the work of the early school medical officers and included in this lead article praise of James Kerr's efforts, he rejected Kerr's notion that school hygiene should be an independent public health activity and that the primary object of inspection was to find treatable defects.[102] Newsholme insisted both in print and in private dealings with those having political influence that school medical services must be considered public health functions to be directed by the M.O.H. and not ad hoc services of the education authorities.[103] In fact, in his opening paper in the discussion of the coordination of medical services at the 1907 meeting of the British Medical Association Newsholme used as his prize example of uncoordination the situation where school medical examinations were conducted without reference to the M.O.H.[104] In his last months in Brighton he resisted the attempt of the Town Council's Education Committee to hire its own Medical Officer and helped insure that the town's M.O.H. was also the Chief Medical Officer to the Education Committee.[105] Also early in 1907 he resigned in protest from a committee of prominent medical figures petitioning the Board of Education for the teaching of hygiene and temperance in all schools, when a clause was added calling for the establishment of a medical bureau in the Board of Education to function independently of the public health authorities.[106]

In the months surrounding Newman's appointment Newman and Morant espoused a view of the school medical service very much like Newsholme's. The claim that school medical work was public health work made Newman's prior experience as M.O.H. of the Metropolitan Borough of Finsbury and of Bedfordshire highly relevant to his appointment. This vision also clearly differentiated the Board of Education's new medical service from what Newman called the "thumping children's chests idea" of Kerr and associates, and he predicted it would reassure and win the confidence of local authorities.[107] Even before Newsholme joined the Local Government Board, Newman sought an alliance with the L.G.B. When he and Morant were planning the Board of Education's Circular 576 initiating the beginning of school medical examinations, Newman suggested the use of a sentence from the 1906 annual report of the then Medical Officer of the L.G.B., William Power. It will demonstrate, Newman explained, that this work is essentially public health work and will be "one more nail in Kerr's cof-

---

101 "The Organization of the Medical Inspection of Schools," *Br. Med. J.* (1903), no. 2: 1288. Newsholme claimed authorship of this article in Newsholme, *Fifty Years,* 391.

102 For Kerr's position, see Hirst, "Failure," 283–4, 287.

103 See, for example [Newsholme], "Organization of the Medical Inspection," 1288; and Newsholme to Arthur James Balfour, 15 May 1907, Webb, Local Government Collection, vol. 297, Item B18.

104 Arthur Newsholme, "A Discussion on the Co-ordination of the Public Medical Services," *Br. Med. J.* (1907), no. 2: 659.

105 Newsholme. *Fifty Years,* 394–5. See also Brighton, Proc. San. Comm. 24 (12 Dec. 1907): 159–63; ibid., (30 Jan.): 212–13; and Brighton, *Proc. Town Council,* 6 Feb., 69–70.

106 Newsholme describes this incident in Newsholme, *Fifty Years,* 393–4.

107 Newman to Morant, 6 Sept. 1907, P.R.O., Ed 24/280.

fin!"[108] He also suggested that Morant ask Power to include reference to their circular and emphasize the need to join together the school medical and public health work in each sanitary district. When Power agreed, Newman was delighted.

> It will show beyond all doubt that the L.G.B. and the Board are of one mind – & will stand no nonsense. It will frustrate their knavish tricks! because they[,] the Kerr folk[,] want to upset us by irritating the Sanitary Authorities – & setting them agst[.] us. If now the S.A. receive their usual orders from the L.G.B. and find the L.G.B. with us, the Enemy is *done*.[109]

Circular 576, which outlined the Board of Education's intentions for the new school medicine service, stated that school medical work "should rest upon a broad basis of public health" and that it should use "to the utmost extent the existing machinery of medical and sanitary administration, developing and supplementing it as required, rather than supplanting it by bringing into existence new agencies, partially redundant and possibly competing." The circular added that the Board of Education

> view the entire subject of school hygiene not as a speciality or as a group of specialities existing by and of themselves but as an integral factor in the health of the nation. The application of this principle requires that the work of medical inspection should be carried out in intimate conjunction with the public health authorities and under the direct supervision of the medical officer of health.[110]

Newsholme worked to win support in the M.O.H. world, reprinting the circular in the December 1907 issue of *Public Health* and writing an editorial which praised the document as a "landmark in the history of public health administration" which heralded the creation of a unified preventive service.[111] The latter prediction could not have been further off the mark.

This cooperation to secure Newman's appointment and to launch a school medical service was part of the strategy of the Webbs and their allies in the civil service, including Newsholme, Newman, and Morant. The Webbs and Morant had already agreed that, in breaking up the Poor Law, infants and probably also the infirm and the elderly should be transferred from the Guardians to the public health authorities and children should go to the education authorities but that school medical inspection should be in the hands of M.O.H.[112] When Sidney Webb and Morant appeared on the speaker's platform at the annual dinner of the Society of Medical Officers of Health in October 1909, they were predictably full of praise for the new service. Morant told the audience that 307 of the 328 local

108 Newman to Morant, 24 Oct. 1907, ibid. For Newman's effort to win the favor of the L.G.B., see also Newman to John Burns, 3 Nov. 1907, Burns Papers, British Library, Add. Mss. 46299.
109 Newman to Morant, 17 Nov. 1907, P.R.O., Ed 24/280.
110 Board of Education, Circular 576, 22 Nov. 1907, sect. 5, quoted in *Lancet* (1907), no. 2: 1557.
111 A[rthur] N[ewsholme], "The Children's Charter of Health," *Public Health*, 20 (1907–8): 161–63.
112 Webb, *Our Partnership*, 378–9; and Robert Morant to Sidney Webb, 22 March 1908, Webb, Local Government Collection, vol. 286.

education authorities had appointed school medical officers and that 224 of these appointees were also the local M.O.H. In other cases the education authorities and health authorities were cooperating. He reported that the L.G.B. and the Board of Education had "come into close touch" and spoke of "the happy cooperation which existed between Dr. Newsholme and Dr. Newman."[113]

This happy cooperation did not last very long. Some of the incentive for collaboration evaporated with the frustration of the Webbs' plans by the passage of the National Insurance Act, by further signs that the Liberal Party did not intend to reform the Poor Law, and then by Morant's forced departure from the Board of Education to administer, irony of ironies, the Liberal alternative to the Fabian scheme, as Chairman of the National Insurance Commission–England.[114] And then with each passing year Newman needed Newsholme and the L.G.B. less and his own political sense alerted him to much greater opportunity through an independent course.

That conflict soon arose is not surprising. Infant welfare had achieved high political priority, yet at the center there was a policy vacuum. The Board of Education had recently obtained special responsibility for the health of school-children; the Local Government Board continued to be responsible for supervising the work of local public health authorities; but no national programs for infant health existed, although a few local authorities had begun experimenting with milk depots and health visiting of infants, and voluntary agencies continued their work.[115] Legislation between 1902 and 1908 offered an opening. The Midwives Act, 1902, made county and county borough councils the local supervising authorities for the new system of certifying and regulating the practice of midwives under the new Central Midwives Board.[116] More significant in the present context was the Notification of Births Act, 1907, which provided that in districts where the act was in effect births had to be notified in writing to the M.O.H. within thirty-six hours of their occurrence.[117] This notification was in addition to the universal requirement of registration of births with the local registrar, a form of reporting which occurred at a much more leisurely pace and was not in the hands of the local health authority. The new legislation was intended to permit interested local authorities to initiate special health work among newborns, and like so many other general statutes touching local services, it was modeled on private legislation.[118]

113 "The Annual Dinner," *Public Health*, 23 (1909–10): 67.
114 See Gilbert, *Evolution of National Insurance*, 134.
115 For the roles of milk depots and health visiting in the infant welfare movement, see Dwork, 103–12; and G. F. McCleary, *The Early History of the Infant Welfare Movement* (London: H. K. Lewis & Co., 1933), 69–89.
116 2 Edw. 7, C. 17, sect. 8–9.
117 7 Edw. 7, C. 40.
118 See, for example, the experiment in infant welfare work at Huddersfield that was facilitated by the Huddersfield Corporation Act, 1906, Hilary Marland, "A Pioneer in Infant Welfare: The Huddersfield Scheme 1903–1920," *Social Hist. Med.*, 6 (1993), 25–50; & McCleary, *Early History,*

The L.G.B. might have used these acts, especially the Notification of Births Act, 1907, to aggressively promote a national infant welfare program. The legislation of 1907 required local authorities to obtain the approval of the L.G.B. before adopting the Act, and it authorized the Board to declare the Act in force in any district where it thought its adoption expedient. The Board did require local authorities wishing to adopt the Act to demonstrate that they were prepared to give advice on child care, preferably through a system of home visiting under the supervision of the M.O.H.[119] But the Board did not seize the opportunity to extend the Act to areas where the enthusiasm for this new work was tepid. Instead it recommended adoption and enforced conditions. Slowly local authorities complied. By the end of March 1915, 65 percent of the English and Welsh population lived in districts where the Act was in force.[120]

This failure between 1907 and 1914 to more actively address a public health problem that had excited such national interest only a few years before reflects the L.G.B.'s preoccupation with other problems, tuberculosis work and national insurance to name just two. It also reflects the presidency of John Burns.[121] In his own way Burns was an advocate of infant welfare.[122] In 1902 while still representative for Battersea to the London County Council, Burns had helped George McCleary, the borough M.O.H., establish what would become the best known British milk depot. He also helped found and served as President of the first National Conference on Infant Mortality in 1906. His diary shows that he retained his interest in infant mortality while President of the L.G.B.[123] However, Burns had reservations about active state involvement and favored efforts to promote infant health by reforming maternal behavior.[124] These reservations, coupled with his own lack of administrative vision, prevented him from seeing to it that the Board modified its procedures in dealing with local authorities when infant welfare work was an issue. The legal basis for local authority initiatives in this area was in fact dubious. Indicative of the crossed purposes at the L.G.B. is that fact that

90–4. Another local model was the London County Council (General Powers) Act, 1908, which encouraged health visiting in London by authorizing the appointment of female health visitors, 8 Edw. 7, C. 107, sect. 6.

119 "Legislation in 1907," [L.G.B. circular] 27 Sept. 1907, *Ann. Rep. Med. Off. L.G.B.*, 37 (1907–8): 184; and "Memorandum Submitted by the Local Government Board in regard to the Award made by Lord Haldane on the 4th July, 1914," P.R.O., Ed. 24/1378, pp. 2–3.

120 *Ann. Rep. L.G.B.*, 43 (1913–14), III: cli.

121 This was a view held by some Whitehall officials. See, for example, how L. A. Selby-Bigge, Permanent Secretary of the Board of Education, characterized the views of Horace Monro, Permanent Secretary of the Local Government Board, in Selby-Bigge to President [Joseph A. Pease], 27 July 1914, P.R.O., Ed 24/1377.

122 For the following discussion, see Dwork, 105–7, 113–15; McCleary, *Early History,* 73–4, 105–7; and Brown, *John Burns,* 152–3.

123 Burns, Diary, 2 May 1910, Add. Mss. 46332; ibid, 25 May 1910; ibid., 2 June 1910; ibid., 18 June 1910; ibid, 30 June 1910; ibid., 27 July 1910; 26 April 1913, Add. Mss. 46,335; ibid, 15 May 1913.

124 Dwork, 114.

in these years the Board's auditors routinely disallowed Battersea's expenditures on its milk depot, but the Board then permitted them on appeal.[125]

Newsholme's first studies of infant mortality, particularly his argument that public action more than maternal education was needed, were designed to influence opinion in his own Department as much as in local authorities. In retrospect he blamed his superiors at the L.G.B. for delay and lost opportunity. Writing two decades later with characteristic discretion, he recalled:

Writing as one whose steady endeavour was to stimulate the Local Government Board to proceed further and more quickly in the prevention of child mortality and the improvement of child health than appeared feasible in the complex conditions of official life, I can testify that the intrusive efforts of the Board of Education to occupy part of this field were a useful stimulus to increased effort in child welfare on the part of the Local Government Board.[126]

In the Board of Education there was none of the inertia that delayed the L.G.B. The Board of Education had a more flexible administrative apparatus, and its Medical Department was newer, smaller, and more narrowly focused than the department Newsholme headed. During its brief history the Board of Education's Medical Department had expanded its responsibilities dramatically, initiating medical inspection and then in rapid succession adding medical treatment of schoolchildren. Most important of all, the Board of Education had in Robert Morant and George Newman a pair of dynamic civil servants committed to reform through administrative means. The two formed a very close friendship which survived Morant's departure from the Board and which was an immense help to Newman on his rise in officialdom.[127]

Newman's post at the Board of Education gave him another advantage over Newsholme. Newman held administrative rank, Principal Assistant Secretary. He had as a result direct access to his own minister, insider status in the administration of his department, and a much clearer view of cabinet affairs than Newsholme. While he lacked Newsholme's scholarly disposition and was no match for Newsholme as an epidemiologist, Newman had links to academic medicine, and he had published important works on infant mortality and on the bacteriology of milk.[128] He was by nature a much more political animal than Newsholme. His diaries show that he followed political and cabinet affairs very closely. He recorded his meetings with important people carefully, occasionally even sketching seating diagrams for a dinner party or committee meeting.[129] While Newsholme was given to defending first principles and could be stubborn, Newman was flexible

125 McCleary, *Early History,* 80.   126 Newsholme, *Last 30 Years,* 196.
127 For evidence of this friendship and its help to Newman's career, see Morant to Newman, 17 Aug. 1913, in Newman, Diary I, 30; and Morant to Newman, 18 Oct. 1913, ibid.
128 He had lectured on bacteriology at King's College, London, and on public health at St. Bartholomew's Hospital and inspected medical schools in connection with Board of Education grants. See Newman, *Infant Mortality;* and Harold Swithinbank and George Newman, *The Bacteriology of Milk* (London: John Murray, 1903).
129 See, for example, Newman, Diary I (19 Jan. 1912 and 26–8 Feb. 1912).

and pragmatic, one might even say opportunistic. Unlike Newsholme, he was not affiliated with a department in disfavor with the leaders of the Liberal Party, nor had he gone on record opposing the Chancellor's scheme for National Insurance. He could be very charming even to those for whom he had no respect. It is remarkable, in view of Newman's low opinion of him, to find John Burns confiding in his diary about his delight in a rainy walk he shared with Newman and fellow Board of Education official L. A. Selby-Bigge.[130] It is testimony to Newman's political instincts and skill that he was able to win the confidence of Lloyd George while retaining, for a while at least, his contacts with the Webbs.

Newman quickly acquired in the highest political circles a reputation as a dynamic and promising administrator and soon became the favored medical administrator of the Chancellor of the Exchequer and his closest associates. He first met David Lloyd George during tea at the House of Commons in May of 1908.[131] But it was during the passage of the National Insurance Bill that Newman gained the ear of the Chancellor. On the night of Lloyd George's insurance speech, Newman dined at the House of Commons with a group of Liberal politicians, and by the end of the month he recorded his first extended conversation about national insurance with Christopher Addison, the anatomist turned Liberal M.P. who would prove invaluable to the Chancellor in securing passage and implementation of the Act.[132] During July and August he had frequent conversations with members of the Cabinet and those planning the insurance scheme, including an intimate conversation with Lloyd George and his advisers in the Chancellor's rooms at the House after which he wrote a memorandum for the Chancellor.[133] He had another lengthy conversation with Lloyd George on October 25. The Chancellor seems to have liked what he was hearing from this civil servant because on November 5 he tried to recruit Newman for the National Insurance Commission and promised him much greater reward in the future. Newman recorded in his diary

A wonderful day w. Mr. David Lloyd George. . . . Ll. Geo. & the Tuberc. children. He offered me the Vice Chairmanship of the Insurance Commission. We discussed the Bill – Sanatoria, Health Committees, Children. He wished me to start the Ins. Scheme & afterwards go to the L.G.B. as Chf. M. O. I declined provisionally. He pressed me a great deal & so I said I wd. think abt. it. But it filled me w. anxiety & trouble. I said I wd. only go to L.G.B. if I cd. take the chn. w. me.[134]

The interview fanned Newman's grand ambitions. He added on the same page, "Lloyd George's ideas! for me! L.G.B. & Ho. of Lords!"

130 Burns, Diary, 4 June 1910, Add. Mss. 46332.
131 Newman, Diary I (28 May 1908).
132 Ibid., 4 May 1911 and 30 May 1911. On Addison's involvement with the National Insurance Act, see Kenneth and Jane Morgan, *Portrait of a Progressive: The Political Career of Christopher, Viscount Addison* (Oxford: Clarendon Press, 1980), 10–21; and Frank Honigsbaum, "Christopher Addison: A Realist in Pursuit of Dreams," in *Doctors, Politics and Society: Historical Essays*, ed. Dorothy Porter and Roy Porter (Amsterdam and Atlanta: Rodopi, 1993), 230–2.
133 Newman, Diary I (3 Aug. 1911 and 7 Aug. 1911).
134 Ibid., 5 Nov. 1911.

Newman had regular contacts with Addison and Waldorf Astor during their service on the Departmental Committee on Tuberculosis, the Astor Committee, and during the spring of 1912 he saw them frequently to discuss the insurance scheme and the Medical Research Council. On the first Sunday of May Newman traveled by car with Addison to the latter's estate where he spent the day with Lloyd George, Astor, and Addison. On this outing Newman was pleased to discover that he was privy to gossip about other ministers and to discussion of housing, taxes on land and luxuries, and meals for children. He recorded that Lloyd George "thought J. Burns wholly obstructive & troublesome. L.G.B. reactionary."[135] Newman's star continued to climb. In August 1913 he was offered and declined the Chairmanship of the Board of Control for Lunacy and Mental Deficiency.[136] In December a more attractive offer came, the post of Secretary of the Medical Research Council. Again Newman declined in order to remain at the Board of Education, but in so doing demanded and obtained terms: a higher salary, and more money for pet projects.[137] His President, Joseph A. Pease, went to the Chancellor of the Exchequer and to the Prime Minister to get the extra money to keep Newman. In February 1914 Newman had lunch at the Grand Hotel with Lloyd George and Pease to discuss additional funding for the Board's health programs: school meals, medical treatment of schoolchildren, physical training, open air schools and institutions for tubercular children, and schools for mothers. The latter were recent creations, usually organized by voluntary bodies and offering formal classes in mothercraft, infant care, and sewing. The Board of Education had made its first grant to a school for mothers in 1907 under its authority to aid technical schools, and during the two years preceding the Board's efforts to dramatically expand its grants program, it had received applications from twenty-seven schools for mothers.[138] At this meeting the three also discussed the Board of Education and the Local Government Board. "A most satisfactory talk" Newman concluded in his diary.[139] In April Newman met the Chancellor of the Exchequer at the Treasury and was promised substantial increases in funding.[140]

It seems to have been during these negotiations with Lloyd George that Newman was given to understand that he might proceed to create an infant welfare program from the Board of Education.[141] Apart from a substantial increase in funds for schools for mothers, Newman did not record in his diary a specific understanding with Lloyd George. However, he did describe a conversation he had with Morant after a dinner at Lord Moulton's in which Morant predicted that

---

135 Ibid. 136 Ibid., II (4 Aug. 1913, 8 Aug. 1913, and 12 Aug. 1913).
137 Ibid., 12 Dec. 1913, 20 Dec. 1913, 6 Jan. 1914, 23 Jan. 1914, 12 Feb. 1914.
138 George Newman, *Ann. Rep. Chief Med. Off. Board of Education* (1912): 330–6; and ibid. (1913), 41.
139 Newman, Diary II (26 Feb. 1914). See also ibid., 12 & 13 Feb. 1916.
140 Ibid., 24 April 1914.
141 The circumstantial evidence is strengthened by the comment by the Permanent Secretary of the Board of Education that Lloyd George had cleared the way at the Treasury in February. See L. A. Selby-Bigge to the Viscount Haldane, 19 May 1914, Ed 24/1377.

the L.G.B. would be willing to cede all children's affairs to the Board of Education since "they were out after sanatoria & tubercle."[142]

In early April 1914 the Board of Education began to circulate a draft bill, one clause of which would have authorized it to supervise and provide grants to local authorities to provide schools for mothers, infant consultation centers, home visitors for mothers with young children, nursery schools, day nurseries, and crèches.[143] It conceded that local sanitary authorities should have responsibility for prenatal and neonatal work. The latter it considered to end four or six weeks after birth. In other words the Board of Education proposed to claim responsibility not only for the health of schoolchildren but of children and infants down to the age of four or six weeks. Although it realized that this bill had little chance of passage, the Board of Education proposed to begin by dramatically expanding its support of schools for mothers on the authority of the promise it had received from the Treasury.[144] The L.G.B. protested vigorously what it regarded as the invasion of its territory and the violation of the mutual understanding between the boards of seven years' standing. Years later Newsholme still held, "it is almost unbelievable that such preposterous proposals should have been advanced."[145]

Available sources place the historian at a disadvantage in studying this dispute. The surviving public records on this issue are much more complete from the Board of Education than from the L.G.B. Unlike George Newman, Arthur Newsholme left no diary of these years. The result is that we are forced to try to understand this episode mainly from the files of the Board of Education and from the perspective of one of its chief officials. Nonetheless, the interdepartmental rivalry produced a great quantity of paper, and the Board of Education files contain many of the L.G.B. memoranda, often aggressively annotated. It is still possible to gain a fairly good idea of what happened, if a sense of perspective is maintained.

In pressing its claims the Board of Education stressed the promise it had obtained from the Treasury and the fact that through its supervision of nursery schools it already had responsibility for the health of some 300,000 children between the ages of three and five years; it emphasized the size and experience of its staff of school doctors and nurses; and it argued that if it were to protect and promote the health of schoolchildren, it needed authority to work with preschool children.[146] It also attempted to cast infant welfare as a problem of ignorance and misinformation. The Board already gave grants in aid of nearly 3,000 classes in nursing, midwifery, and hygiene.

Supported by their new President, Herbert Samuel, who replaced John Burns

---

142 Newman, Diary II (19 March 1914).
143 For a copy of the clause, see Selby-Bigge to Haldane, 7 May 1914, P.R.O., Ed 24/1377.
144 Selby-Bigge to Haldane, 19 May 1914, P.R.O., Ed 24/1377.
145 Newsholme, *Last 30 Years*, 196.
146 For the position of the Board of Education in the early phases of this dispute, see Newman, minute [probably to Selby-Bigge], 23 April 1914, P.R.O., Ed 24/1377; Newman, to Secretary [Selby-Bigge], 5 May 1914, ibid.; and Newman, to President [Pease], 12 June 1914, ibid.

in 1914, the L.G.B. officials insisted on the position both boards had taken in 1907, that the health of children could not be effectively promoted in isolation from the other health and sanitary activities of local authorities.[147] For that reason the L.G.B. now insisted this work must remain in the hands of local health authorities and be under the supervision of the L.G.B. Its officials emphasized what opportunities the Midwives Act, 1902, the Notification of Births Act, 1907, and the London County Council (General Powers) Act, 1908, had given local authorities to initiate work with pregnant women and newborns as well as what some authorities had done. The health functions of the Board of Education were and should remain, the L.G.B. claimed, limited to those children enrolled in board-assisted elementary schools. The L.G.B. also demanded the right to give grants of its own in aid of maternal and infant welfare work.

At this early stage in the dispute the Medical Officers of the two boards played a prominent role in framing their departments' positions. Newman's notion of a school for mothers was a very expansionist one.[148] Such a school should include not only classes in mothercraft but also dinners for mothers, milk kitchens and depots, consultations, treatment centers, and home visiting.[149] The school for mothers should become, in other words, the center for all health work among infants and preschool children. For his part Newsholme drew a strong distinction between health and educational work.[150] The former, including antenatal programs, midwifery work and associated health work during pregnancy, home visiting following the notification of births, medical consultation associated with home visiting, and sanitary services in the environment of the mother and child, must be in the hands of the local health authorities and under the supervision of the L.G.B. Educational functions should be relegated primarily to formal classes in mothercraft. He conceded that there was a need for close cooperation between the local health and education authorities, but he now attempted to make the L.G.B.'s authority in early childhood clearer. He suggested that following the registration of a birth a file be started for each child and maintained by the health authority until the child entered school. At that time the file would be handed over to the education authority.

The Prime Minister and the Chancellor of the Exchequer delegated the responsibility of deciding between the rival claims of these two departments to the

---

147 The most complete statement of the L.G.B. position comes from the second phase of this conflict. It can be read profitably in the present context nonetheless. See "Memorandum Submitted by the Local Government Board in regard to the Award made by Lord Haldane on the 4th July, 1914," ibid. See also the L.G.B. memorandum "Ante Natal Hygiene and Infant Welfare Work," ibid.; Selby-Bigge to Haldane, 5 May 1914, ibid.; Newsholme to Lord Haldane, 13 May 1914, ibid.; and Selby-Bigge to Haldane, 19 May 1914, ibid.

148 See, for example, Newman, minute, 23 April 1914, ibid.; Newman, to Secretary, 5 May 1914, ibid.; and Newman, minute, 12 June 1914, ibid.

149 Newman to Secretary, 5 May 1914, ibid. Milk depots provided pure milk to working-class mothers at subsidized prices.

150 Newsholme to Haldane, 13 May 1914, ibid.

Lord Chancellor, Richard Burton Viscount Haldane.[151] Haldane first tried a compromise, suggesting that prenatal and neonatal work be supervised by the Local Government Board, the school health service by the Board of Education, and work with preschool ages by joint local committees and a joint central committee containing representatives and funding from both boards.[152] The Board of Education agreed to accept this arrangement provided it was interpreted broadly in its favor.[153] The L.G.B. refused, and the issue was thrown back into the lap of the Lord Chancellor.[154]

The dispute then went to formal arbitration. Haldane met with the Presidents and the Medical Officers of both boards and on July 4 made his determination, the first so-called Haldane Award, and in answer to a question in the House the Prime Minister announced Haldane's scheme as a settlement of the dispute.[155] Again Haldane tried to encourage compromise recognizing that some work would fall in disputed territory and that "interlacing, and even overlapping, must be provided for." Again he called for local and central joint committees to work out disputed claims. As a general principle medical services to children not enrolled in a school, including nursery school, day nursery, crèche, or school for mothers, should be supervised by the L.G.B. Medical services for children enrolled in any school, including a school for mothers, should be supervised by the Board of Education. He then came to the heart of the issue. What was a school for mothers, the legitimate recipient of Board of Education grants, and what was a baby clinic or infant dispensary, the legitimate recipient of L.G.B. grants? He defined a school for mothers as an educational institution that provided instruction in the care of infants by classes, home visiting, or infant consultations. Any medical or surgical treatment given in connection with a school for mothers must be "only incidental." A baby clinic, however, he defined as primarily an institution for providing "medical and surgical advice and treatment" for infants and young children. Any maternal instruction provided should be "only incidental."

Predictably the award, while entirely rational, did nothing to settle the dispute,

151 Early in the dispute Newman had dinner with Haldane and Elizabeth Sanderson Haldane, his sister and pioneer social worker, and tried to press his Department's position on the Lord Chancellor. George Newman, "Memorandum of Conversation with Lord Haldane," 30 April 1914, ibid.; and covering letter Newman to Secretary, 30 April 1914, ibid. See also Newman, Diary II (29 April 1914).

152 "Memorandum on L.G.B. v. Brd. of Ed. Dispute over Infant Welfare," c. 18 May 1914, P.R.O., Ed 24/1377. It seems that Addison may have helped Haldane conceive of this first proposal, Christopher Addison, *Four and a Half Years: A Personal Diary from June 1914 to January 1919* (London: Hutchinson & Co, 1934), I: 16–17.

153 Selby-Bigge, "Memorandum," 20 May 1914, P.R.O., Ed 24/1377; Selby-Bigge to President," 20 May 1914, Ibid.; and Pease to Lord Chancellor, 22 May 1914, ibid.

154 Herbert Samuel [President, L.G.B.] to Lord Chancellor, 19 May 1914, ibid. Samuel must have made a formal refusal on June 10 because several Board of Education documents refer to it. See, for example, Newman to President, 12 June 1914, ibid.

155 "The Relations of the Local Government Board and the Board of Education as regards the Care of Children's Health," ibid.; and Great Britain, *Parliamentary Debates,* House of Commons, 5th series, 65 (20 July 1914), 29, question 45.

and in fact relations between the two boards became decidedly more hostile. Not only were there mutual suspicions that the opposing board was trying to snare all voluntary agencies in its net, but ordinary standards of civil service courtesy and conduct broke down. Both boards began to draw up their regulations and circulars for their grants and, as was the custom, permitted the officials of the other board to offer suggestions. The L.G.B. requested that the Board of Education at least notice the fact in its circular that the L.G.B. was also offering grants for baby clinics, but on July 24 the Permanent Secretary of the Board of Education wrote to his counterpart at the L.G.B. saying that without his knowledge the Board of Education circular had been printed and sent out without the changes the L.G.B. had requested.[156] As a result the Board of Education circular went out nine days before the one from the L.G.B., although the L.G.B. had requested a simultaneous issue. About this time the L.G.B. also learned that the Board of Education was sponsoring a conference of schools for mothers and requested information on the meeting so that it could send a representative. The Permanent Secretary of the Board of Education wrote a sharp response reminding the L.G.B. officials of their refusal in May of joint administration and declining to accept an L.G.B. representative.[157] Privately George Newman insisted that under no circumstances should Newsholme or Janet Lane-Claypon be permitted to attend.[158] Without the knowledge of his officials Herbert Samuel wrote a confidential letter to Joseph Pease to protest several recent actions of the Board of Education and threatened to take the matter to the Cabinet.[159] By October both boards had written to the Treasury complaining about the behavior of the other. The Permanent Secretary of the L.G.B. stated his department's anger best in a letter to the Secretary of the Board of Education.

As for the controversy itself you know my views. Neither the Haldane award nor a long letter by the Bd of E really touch the question, which is, not what is or is not a school for mothers or baby clinic, but what are and are not the proper boundaries between the territories of the LGB and Bd of E.

I feel that in this matter we are in the position of a Belgium invaded by a hostile Power. The Bd of E's position seems curiously like that of Germany. They are impelled by the notion that the destiny of the Bd of E – or of its Medical Officer – demands that it shall be a Central Public Health Authority – This being a Divine decree it is obviously the duty of the Bd. of E to invade the territory of the LGB!

This doctrine strikes me as preposterous. – There really seems no more reason for the Bd of E to deal with the health of infants because they are concerned with the health of

156 Selby-Bigge to Monro, 24 July 1914, P.R.O., MH 55/540; and Board of Education, *Regulations under Which Grants to Schools for Mothers in England and Wales Will Be Made by the Board of Education During the Year Ending on the 31st March, 1915*, 21 July 1912 (London: HMSO, 1914).
157 Monro to Selby-Bigge, 24 July 1914, P.R.O., MH 55/540; and Selby-Bigge to Monro, 28 July 1914, ibid.
158 Newman to Selby-Bigge, n.d. [handwritten note on Board of Education Stationary], P.R.O., Ed 24/1377.
159 Samuel to Pease, 27 July 1914, ibid.

children in schools than for the Archbishop of Canterbury to claim to be Secretary of War because there are chaplains in the Army.[160]

The appearance of Treasury grants from both departments in July 1914 marked the beginning of a significant wartime increase in publicly funded infant welfare work. The L.G.B. circular of July 30, 1914, which announced the grants for baby clinics and urged local authorities to act, was accompanied by a short memorandum by Newsholme that outlined an ideal infant and maternal welfare scheme offering a comprehensive set of home, outpatient, and hospital services for pregnancy, birth, and infancy.[161] In November 1915 the Board issued a much longer Memorandum by Newsholme on maternal and child welfare schemes that offered specific advice on health visiting and on the staffing, equipment, and procedures of maternity and infant welfare centers.[162] Faced with strong competition from a rival, the L.G.B. now worked hard to encourage local authority initiatives. During the war Newsholme found that he spent more time on infant welfare than on any other subject other than war-related services, but he reported many difficulties.[163] The wartime shortages of medical practitioners often prohibited local authorities from recruiting medical officers for infant welfare programs.[164] This and other strains of war caused maternal and infant welfare programs to develop more slowly than local venereal disease schemes, whose creation was compulsory and for which Exchequer grants covered 75 percent rather than 50 percent of costs. But local authorities did act. By the end of 1917 all county boroughs except one, all Metropolitan boroughs except one, 51 county councils, and 360 smaller sanitary authorities had made a beginning.[165] Often the work was very incomplete. Ten county council schemes, for example, applied to only part of the county, and some centers had been unable to find even a part-time medical officer. By the end of 1917 there were 542 infant and maternal welfare centers provided by the local authorities and another 551 offered by voluntary societies. By July 1918 there were 1,278 centers, 700 local authority and 578 voluntary, which together received that administrative year £122,000 in grants from the L.G.B.[166] During the war, as these figures suggest, there was expansion in both the scale and scope of services, and there began a shift from voluntary to public initiative.[167] The Board of Education's grant program also grew. In the year ending March 31, 1915, the Board awarded grants totaling £6,100 to 157 schools for mothers and grants of

---

160 Monro to Selby-Bigge, 12 Oct. 1914, ibid.
161 For a copy see "Maternity and Child Welfare," Newsholme, *Ann. Rep. Med. Off. L.G.B.*, 44 (1914–15), 15–17.
162 Arthur Newsholme, "Memorandum on Health Visiting and on Maternity and Child Welfare Centres," ibid., 1–15.
163 Ibid., 45 (1915–16): xxxiv; and ibid. 46 (1916–17): xxxvi.
164 For suggestions of the difficulties local authorities were having finding qualified staff, see ibid., 45 (1915–16): xxxv; ibid., 46 (1916–17): xxxvi; and Ibid., 47 (1917–18): xx.
165 Ibid., 46 (1916–17): xxxvi.
166 Ibid., 47 (1917–18): 17, 20.   167 Dwork, 211.

another £5,100 to 80 day nurseries. Within four years the figures totaled £17,054 to 290 schools for mothers and £27,467 to 174 day nurseries.[168]

This expansion at the periphery did not make cooperation in Whitehall any easier. The two boards competed for applications, and the joint committee could not agree in whose bailiwick a number of applications fell. By the end of 1914 it was clear that further arbitration was needed. Lord Haldane met with a group of representatives from the two boards, including Newman and Newsholme, on January 29, 1915.[169] The fact that the L.G.B.'s regulations had been issued and the Board had begun to award grants to local authorities made its case more credible. Surviving accounts suggest that during this conference Newsholme and Newman each pressed examples on the Lord Chancellor which favored their positions. While Haldane refused to change any terms of his previous award, he now interpreted it more in the L.G.B.'s favor. Work with children up to nine months should be under the supervision of the L.G.B. Medical advice and baby weighing should be considered treatment and thus under the L.G.B.

This second award also failed to bring peace. The two ministers next agreed to leave the establishment of a working agreement to their respective Assistant Secretaries, Newman and Frederick Willis. Newsholme was thus removed from the front line of the battle. Newman and Willis decided to dissolve the joint committee and to personally decide disputed cases. They also agreed that their departments would issue a joint circular announcing the new arrangements.[170] But bickering continued during March and April over the precise meaning of this most recent agreement and over the wording of the joint circular. The Permanent Secretary of the Board of Education was especially worried that the L.G.B. could use this understanding to steal the whole show.[171] The joint circular finally appeared at the end of May.[172]

During late 1915 and for most of 1916 the tide in this rivalry ran in favor of the Local Government Board. The Notification of Births (Extension) Act, 1915 required the notification of births in all areas and thus provided an incentive for

168 For the following figures, see George Newman, *Annual Report of the Chief Medical Officer of the Board of Education* (1914), 37–41, 45–8; and ibid. (1918), 22.

169 For an account of the meeting, see E. H. Pelham [Assistant Secretary, Medical Department] to Newman, 2 Feb. 1915, P.R.O., Ed 24/1378; and F. J. Willis, minute, 30 Jan. 1915, ibid. For the cases of the two boards, see "Memorandum submitted by the Local Government Board in regard to the Award made by Lord Haldane on the 4th July, 1914," ibid.; and "Statement of the Position of the Board of Education in Regard to the Points in Controversy between Them and the Local Government Board upon the Interpretation of Lord Haldane's Award," ibid.

170 For the Newman-Willis agreement, see the untitled memorandum dated 23 March 1915, ibid., also in MH 55/544. For the Assistant Secretaries' accounts of the negotiations see Newman to Selby-Bigge, 23 March 1915, Ed 24/1378; and Willis to President, 24 March 1915, MH 55/544.

171 Selby-Bigge to President, 19 April 1915, P.R.O., Ed 24/1378. See also Willis to Selby-Bigge, 25 March 1915, ibid.; Selby-Bigge to Willis, 25 March 1915, ibid.; Selby-Bigge to Willis, 26 March 1915, ibid.; Selby-Bigge to Willis, 27 March 1915, ibid.; Selby-Bigge to Willis, 9 April 1915, ibid.; Selby-Bigge to Willis, 13 April 1915, Ibid.; Selby-Bigge to Willis, 16 April 1915, ibid.; and Selby-Bigge to Willis, 19 April 1915, ibid.

172 For a draft of the circular, see Local Government Board and Board of Education, "Grants in Aid of Maternity Centres and Schools for Mothers," May 1915, P.R.O., MH 55/544.

more local health authorities to begin infant welfare programs and swelled the number of applications for grants to the L.G.B.[173] Also the Retrenchment Committee noticed the waste and duplication of effort this rivalry caused, and it recommended that all infant welfare work be turned over to the L.G.B.[174] The medical press also seemed to favor consolidating the competing infant welfare work under the L.G.B. In reviewing George Newman's annual report for 1914, the *British Medical Journal* greeted the new initiatives sympathetically, but it expressed amusement with Newman's efforts to demonstrate that a school for mothers was fundamentally different from a baby clinic.[175] Using the Retrenchment Committee's recommendation as a lever during spring 1916, L.G.B. officials pressed their advantage with the Board of Education and the Treasury and in the Cabinet.[176] Board of Education officials recognized they were now at a great disadvantage. Their authority to issue grants had been given for one year only, and they hoped at best to maintain the status quo for another year.[177] In the end Reginald McKenna, then Chancellor of the Exchequer, agreed to extend existing arrangements.[178]

During most of this dispute the statutory power of local authorities to undertake infant and maternal health work had been in question. Robert Morant, Newsholme, and Newman all pointed out that the most likely source of such authority was a very dubious one, Section 133 of the Public Health Act, 1875, a section which permitted sanitary authorities to offer a temporary supply of medicine or of medical assistance to the poor.[179] The L.G.B. finally gained the upper hand, in the short term at least, by sponsoring new legislation giving local health authorities clear and unequivocal authority to provide health services to pregnant and nursing mothers and to preschool children subject to the supervision of the L.G.B. The legislation began life as the Notification of Births (Amendment) Bill which Walter Long, President of the L.G.B., brought before the Cabinet in December 1916.[180] Successive L.G.B. presidents pressed for this bill against opposition in the

173 "Notification of Births (Extension) Act, 1915," 5 & 6 Geo. 5, C. 64.
174 Committee on Retrenchment in the Public Expenditure, *Final Report,* B.P.P., 1916, XV, Cd. 8200, 15–16.
175 "The State and the Care of the Children," *Br. Med. J.* (1916), no. 1: 348–9. See also "Education and Infant Welfare," *Lancet* (1916), no. 1: 628–9.
176 Willis to Secretary of the Treasury, 18 March 1916, P.R.O., Ed 24/1379; Walter H. Long [President, LGB] to [Arthur] Henderson [President, Board of Education], 9 April 1916, ibid; Long to [Reginald] McKenna [Chancellor of the Exchequer], 26 May 1916, P.R.O., MH 55/544, and Walter Long, "Maternity and Infant Welfare Work," [a private Cabinet paper], Ed 24/1363.
177 Selby-Bigge to President, 10 April 1916, P.R.O., Ed 24/1379; and Newman, minute, 18 April 1916, ibid.
178 McKenna to Henderson, 27 July 1916, ibid.; and unsigned minute, 21 Sept. 1916, ibid.
179 38 & 39 Vict. C. 55, sect. 133. See also Morant to Willis, 14 Nov. 1914, P.R.O., MH 55/543; unsigned L.G.B. minute expressing Newsholme's views, [July 1914], ibid.; and Newman to Secretary, 9 July 1917, Ed 24/1363.
180 See several drafts of the bill in ibid. The version that Long took to the Cabinet on Dec. 5 was an emergency measure for the duration of the war plus six months.

Cabinet from the National Insurance Commission, and it eventually became the Maternity and Child Welfare Act, 1918.[181] During Cabinet deliberation of this bill the Board of Education struggled to retain any hold on health work with preschool children. Its President first offered to support the bill, if the L.G.B. would cede children above the age of two to the Board of Education, but the L.G.B. refused.[182] At the Board of Education George Newman spurred his superiors to put up a strong fight warning that the "prestige and usefulness" of the Board would suffer and that there would be public criticism if too much ground were given up, and he claimed that if not checked, the L.G.B. would try to gain control of the school medical service as well.[183] In February 1917 a truce seemed at hand when the newly appointed ministers of the boards came to an agreement which limited the Board of Education's health services to children enrolled in schools, including nursery schools, and granted to the L.G.B. health work among children not in schools as well as those attending crèches, infant-welfare centers, and schools for mothers.[184] These were concessions which Newman deplored.[185] In fact the agreement never came into effect. The Prime Minister failed to ratify it, and in July the Cabinet recommended that its implementation be delayed until a Ministry of Health could be created.

Schools for mothers and baby clinics were not the only areas where the two boards competed as health services were expanded in an ad hoc fashion under different departments. In 1912 the L.G.B. and the Board of Education had worked out an uneasy agreement for the inspection and financial support of institutions for children with tuberculosis.[186] The agreement was strained during 1913 and early 1914 when the Board of Education attempted to become the sole supervising authority for these institutions by claiming a portion of the Hobhouse Award, and the L.G.B. resisted.[187] For his part Newsholme saw that the Astor committee did

181 8 & 9 Geo. 5, C. 29. Section 1 is the provision in question. For an indication of the objections raised in the Cabinet see C[hristopher] A[ddison], "Maternity and Child Welfare Bill: Notes on Lord Rhondda's Memorandum (G.T. 1056)," P.R.O., Cab 24/18, G.T. 1268; Edwin Cornwall [Chairman, National Health Insurance Joint Committee], "Maternity and Child Welfare Bill," 2 Aug. 1917, Cab 24/21, G.T. 1594; and Edwin Cornwall, "Maternity and Infant Welfare," 31 Oct. 1917, Cab 24/30, G.T. 2460;

182 Lord Crewe [President, Board of Education] to Long, 14 Nov. 1916, P.R.O., Ed 24/1363; Selby-Bigge to Monro, 15 Nov. 1916, ibid.; Long to Crewe, Nov. 1916 [no day indicated], ibid.; and Monro to Selby-Bigge, 22 Nov. 1916, ibid.

183 Newman to Secretary, 15 Nov. 1916, P.R.O., Ed 24/1363; and Selby-Bigge's summary of Newman's views for H.A.L. Fisher, the new President of the Board of Education, in Selby-Bigge to President, 24 Jan. 1917, ibid.

184 Lord Rhondda and H.A.L. Fisher, "Health Work for Young Children: Agreement between the Board of Education and the Local Government Board," 12 Feb. 1917, P.R.O., Ed 24/1363.

185 See two minutes of Newman to the President, H.A.L. Fisher on the date of the Rhondda-Fisher agreement (21 June 1917), ibid.

186 G[eorge] N[ewman], "Memorandum of Interview at the Local Government Board, 17 Dec. 1912," P.R.O., MH 55/527; and "Institutional Treatment for Tuberculous Children," 17 Jan. 1913, ibid. See also Selby-Bigge to Monro, 2 Aug. 1912, P.R.O., Ed 24/1361; and Monro to Selby-Bigge, 16 Aug. 1912, ibid.

187 Selby-Bigge to Newman, 11 Oct. 1913, ibid.; Newman to Secretary [Selby-Bigge], 16 Oct. 1913, ibid.; and Selby-Bigge to Newman, 16 Oct. 1913, ibid.

not endorse the suggestion either.[188] The conflict over infant welfare brought an abrupt end to the shared supervision of tuberculosis institutions for children. The L.G.B. now insisted on its right to be the supervising authority of all such institutions, since it administered funds for tuberculosis provided by the Finance Act, 1911, and by the Hobhouse Award.[189] The Board's success delighted Newsholme. "This is a most satisfactory conclusion of recovery of raided territory. My congratulations!"[190]

Few administrative developments could have made ministers more conscious of the desirability of combining the state's major health functions in one ministry as this protracted competition over infant-welfare work. Although the competition probably hastened the development of infant welfare schemes at the local level, in Whitehall the stream of written arguments, complaints, and appeals to higher authority tried ministerial patience and absorbed energy and attention that might more profitably have been spent elsewhere. During the interdepartmental conflict the stakes changed from control of a new health program to control of the entire health service. Proposals for a new ministry of public health had been put forward before the war. In fact, Newsholme had been questioned repeatedly on the subject during his testimony before the Royal Commission on Venereal Diseases in July 1914.[191] By 1916 the minutes and memoranda between the chief officials of the Board of Education and the L.G.B. contain frequent reference to the likelihood of a new ministry, and Board of Education officials worried that the L.G.B. was trying to absorb the health services of the Board of Education and become that ministry.[192] The proposal for the new ministry was first formally brought before the Cabinet on April 6, 1917, by D. A. Thomas, Viscount Rhondda, the recently appointed President of the L.G.B., in a short and practical memorandum.[193]

188 See Newsholme's annotations, dated 5 Feb. 1913, to the draft of the Final Report of the Departmental Committee on Tuberculosis, 12 in Newsholme Papers, box of uncatalogued reprints. Newsholme crossed out the clause giving to the Board of Education the right to control the grant money to these institutions, and he called the attention of Willis to this section of the report. The clause in question did not appear in the Final Report.
189 See the letters and minutes from July 1914 to June 1915 in P.R.O., MH 55/527. See especially the new agreement, "Recognition of Institutions for Tuberculous Children."
190 Newsholme to A. B. Maclachlan, 22 June 1915, ibid.
191 Royal Commission on Venereal Diseases, *Appendix to Final Report*, B.P.P., 1916, XVI, Cd. 8190, 224–5, #19,110–16, 19,123–4, 19,140–1, 19,146–9.
192 Selby-Bigge to Monro, 15 Nov. 1916, P.R.O., Ed 24/1363; and Selby-Bigge to President, 24 Jan. 1917, ibid. See also Crewe to Long, 14 Nov. 1916, ibid.
193 Lord Rhondda, "The Urgent Need for a Ministry of Health," 27 March 1917, P.R.O., Cab 14/9, G.T. 361. For discussion of the creation of the Ministry of Health, see Bellamy, *Administering Central–Local Relations, 1871–1919*, 251–8; Bentley B. Gilbert, *British Social Policy, 1914–1939* (Ithaca, N.Y.: Cornell Univ. Press, 1970), 98–132; Frank Honigsbaum, *The Struggle for the Ministry of Health 1914–1919*, Occasional Papers on Social Administration, No. 37 (London: G. Bell & Sons, [1970]); John Turner, " 'Experts' and Interests: David Lloyd George and the Dilemmas of the Expanding State, 1906–1919," in *Government and Expertise: Specialists, Administrators and Professionals, 1860–1919*, ed. Roy MacLeod (Cambridge: Cambridge Univ. Press, 1988), 216–21. Honigsbaum discusses the competition between the Board of Education and the Local Government Board in this context. Bellamy and Gilbert do not. Turner alludes to it.

Rhondda recommended transferring the health and sanatorium benefits of the National Insurance scheme to a new Ministry of Health to be built upon the basis of the L.G.B. The consolidation of other official health work could follow.

Rhondda may have first raised the issue in the Cabinet, but it fell to Addison, Lloyd George's staunchest ministerial ally on matters of health, to see it through to completion. Addison was impatient with the interdepartmental rivalry, and his sympathies were decidedly with the Board of Education and its Chief Medical Officer.[194] In April 1914 when the Board of Education was first making its claims, Addison had written a letter of support to the *Times*.[195] He served at the Board of Education as Parliamentary Secretary from August 1914 to May 1915, leaving to follow Lloyd George to the Ministry of Munitions as Parliamentary Secretary. It was as Minister of Reconstruction, a post he assumed in July 1918, that Addison took the initiative in negotiating an agreement with interested parties that would permit passage of the Ministry of Health Bill, and he was promised the post of Minister of Health.[196]

Even before the proposal had been formally made, Newman was an insider in planning the new ministry, and he quite early staked his claim for its chief medical post. Two days after the first Haldane award in July 1914 he had lunch with Morant to consider the outcome, and they discussed how a ministry of health could be created by transferring National Insurance to the Local Government Board.[197] Newman called on Lloyd George at Number 11 Downing Street two days later and reported that the Chancellor of the Exchequer agreed with this idea and that he wanted Newman at the L.G.B.[198] By late 1916, when it looked as if a ministry of health would be created at the War's end, and especially after January 1917, when Lloyd George succeeded Asquith as Prime Minister, Newman began to lobby intensely among ministers and key civil servants: Robert Morant, Waldorf Astor, Christopher Addison, H. A. L. Fisher, the new President of the Board of Education, and Lord Rhondda.[199] Soon after Addison became Minister of Munitions, Newman met with him at the War Office. The two agreed that Newman

194 For his impatience and his suspicion that Newman exaggerated the importance of the issue, see Addison, *Four and a Half Years*, 18, 44.
195 Christopher Addison, "Mothers of the Race. The Opportunity of Education Authorities," *Times*, 10 April 1914, 10.
196 Gilbert, *British Social Policy*, 116–25, 130–2; Turner, " 'Experts' and Interests," 218–21, and Morgan, *Portrait*, 75–80. See also "Ministry of Health Bill: Memorandum by the Minister of Reconstruction," April 1918, P.R.O., Cab 24/49, G.T. 4399. For criticism of the bill and Addison's role in putting it forward by the present and former President of the L.G.B., see W. Hayes Fisher, "Observations by the President of the Local Government Board on the Draft Bill and Memorandum (G.T. 4399) Circulated by the Minister for Reconstruction," 13 May 1918, Cab 24/51, G.T. 4533; and W[alter] H. L[ong], "Memorandum for the War Cabinet," 28 May 1918, Cab 24/52, G.T. 4660.
197 Newman, Diary II (6 July 1914).
198 Ibid., 8 July 1914.
199 Discussions of the new ministry in Newman's diary are too numerous to mention separately. But see ibid., III, Dec. 1916 through Dec. 1918. See also Christopher Addison, diary entry for 9 Dec. 1916, Bodleian Library, Oxford, Diary Series 55.5, [p.] C. 514.

should stay at the Board of Education for the moment but eventually move to the L.G.B. They discussed how the health services should be divided between the L.G.B. and the Board of Education. Newman even drew an organizational chart. They also agreed to get rid of Newsholme and Willis.[200] Soon after Lloyd George formed his first Cabinet, Newman had lunch with Rhondda and Addison to discuss a ministry of health, and within two weeks Newman wrote to Addison claiming to have no personal ambitions in the matter, disclaiming any responsibility for the continuing conflict between his Board and the L.G.B., and asking what the Government planned for a new ministry.[201] On April 5, 1917, Newman recorded with satisfaction that at a lunch with Morant Rhondda had said he wanted Newman as his Chief Medical Officer at the new ministry, that Lloyd George approved this proposal, and that Rhondda had agreed that, if Newsholme and Willis decided to stay on, they would have to serve under Newman.[202] Newman secured the renewal of this promise in 1918, while the political struggle for the ministry was proceeding.[203] These private negotiations help explain Newman's and Addison's opposition to the L.G.B.'s Maternity and Infant Welfare Bill or to changes at the Board which would "queer the pitch" for the creation of the new ministry.[204]

By late November Newman learned from Addison what ultimately would transpire. Addison would be Minister of Health, Robert Morant would become Permanent Secretary, and Newman would be Principal Medical Officer with the right to continue advising the Board of Education.[205] Newman recorded that Addison was eager to get rid of Newsholme and Willis. It is clear that Newman was even more eager. After a conference at the L.G.B. in late October 1918 Newman described Newsholme as "weak, vacillating, incompetent, untrustworthy & vain."[206]

The promised changes were made in stages. Addison was named President of the L.G.B. on January 11, 1919. Within his first days as President he had angry conferences with his Medical Officer in which he must have told Newsholme that Newman, not he, would help lead the new ministry in the promised land, and Newsholme declared that he would not serve under Newman. On the seven-

---

200 Newman, Diary III (9 Dec. 1916). Addison's diary mentions the conversation and confirms his belief that Morant should be brought to the new ministry, but it does not mention either dismissing Newsholme or adding Newman. Addison, *Four and a Half Years,* I: 278.
201 Ibid., 317; Newman, Diary III (16 Jan. 1917); Newman to Addison, 28 Jan. 1917, Bodleian Library, Oxford, Addison Papers, Box 8.
202 Newman, Diary III (5 April 1917).
203 Ibid., 6 March 1918.
204 Newman to President, 21 June 1917, P.R.O., Ed 24/1363. See also Newman to Secretary, 22 Jan. 1918, ibid.; and C. A[ddison], "Maternity and Child Welfare Bill. Notes on Lord Rhondda's Memorandum (G.T. 1056)," [17 June 1917], Cab 24/18, G.T. 1268. Addison also privately campaigned against changes at the L.G.B. See Addison to Lloyd George, [22 Nov. 1918], H.L.R.O., Lloyd George Papers, F/1/4/30; Addison to Lloyd George, 25 Nov. 1918, ibid., F/1/4/31.
205 Newman, Diary III (30 Nov. 1918).
206 Ibid., 29 Oct. 1918.

teenth Addison demanded Newsholme's retirement pointing out that Newsholme had been eligible for retirement for two years and was within three years of mandatory retirement.[207] In the end Newsholme retired at the end of March 1919.[208] True to form, Newman campaigned for better terms, at first refusing the appointment, demanding a higher salary and criticizing the L.G.B. for giving its Medical Officer "no administrative functions and placing him in a subordinate position under an Assistant Secretary."[209] He got the higher salary and administrative rank. Addison completed his major appointments by choosing Waldorf Astor as his Parliamentary Secretary, thus bringing another close Lloyd George associate into the Board in preparation for its metamorphosis into the Ministry of Health. That event took place in June when the Ministry of Health Bill received the Royal signature and Addison was made Minister of Health.

While in retirement Newsholme's sense of decorum kept him from public criticism of Newman, his resentment can be detected nonetheless. In his copy of Hugh Cabot's The Doctor's Bill, a volume that went with his books and papers to the library of the London School of Hygiene and Tropical Medicine, someone, probably Newsholme, has placed exclamation marks in the margins in several places where the author attributed to Newman personally the achievements of the Ministry of Health.[210] But rather than quietly nursing his resentments, Newsholme continued writing prolifically and, when opportunity permitted, seeking a quiet retaliation. In his descriptions and historical accounts of the British public health and medicine that Newsholme wrote in retirement, mention of Newman is conspicuously absent. Instead Newsholme celebrated the achievements of Newman's major competitor for the post at the Board of Education, Sir James Kerr.[211] In retirement he ventured into new territory, the health care system of nations, offering in the process an alternative voice to the British government's current chief medical administrator. Most of these postretirement publications identify Newsholme not as former Medical Officer of the L.G.B., his actual title, but as former Chief or Principal Medical Officer, a title comparable to Newman's.

Newsholme's retirement works reflect his experience in Whitehall in another way as well. The work of establishing municipal clinics for tuberculosis, venereal

207 Addison to Newsholme, 17 Jan 1919, Bodleian Library, Oxford, Addison Papers, Box 43, Letter 31.
208 Monro to Meiklejohn [Assistant Secretary, Treasury], 8 March 1919, P.R.O., MH 78/92.
209 Newman to President [H.A.L. Fisher], 10 Feb. 1919, ibid. See also Newman to [probably Hatty, his sister], 1 Feb. 1919, Wellcome Institute, Newman Letters.
210 Hugh Cabot, The Doctor's Bill (New York: Columbia University Press, 1935), 171, 219. These marks were first pointed out by Honigsbaum, Struggle, 79, fn. 194, although the author has Cabot's name and one of the pages wrong.
211 See, for example, Newsholme, Fifty Years, 382–4, 388–9, 397–8, 409, where the author provides generous acknowledgment of Kerr's work, quoting from Kerr's reports. Compare these sections with the single reference to Newman which identified him merely as the Board of Education's "newly appointed chief medical officer," Ibid., 395. This neglect of Newman was pointed out by Bentley Gilbert in Gilbert, British Social Policy, 133.

disease, and especially for infants and young children had made him acutely sensitive to organized medicine's resistance to publicly funded schemes of treatment. He would find this resistance even more vociferous in America, and answering it with historical and international examples would become the focus of his final projects.

PART III

The old world and the new:
Newsholme as elder statesman

12

Newsholme's trans-Atlantic retirement

ANSWERS TO THE BIOMETRICIANS

Far from sinking into a quiet retirement when he left Whitehall, Newsholme continued to be professionally very active for a decade and a half. He held a number of those largely honorary appointments reserved for elder statesmen on advisory boards: the Executive Committee of the Imperial Cancer Research Fund, the Board of Governors of the London School of Economics, the Advisory Board of the Johns Hopkins School of Hygiene and Public Health as well as offices in the British Social Hygiene Council and the Society for the Study of Inebriety and Drug Addiction.[1] Most of his great energy, however, was channeled into public speaking and writing. His literary output in this period is remarkable. Between his retirement and his eightieth birth year, 1919 to 1937, he was the sole author of eight books totaling eleven volumes,[2] joint author of one volume,[3] and the author of some three dozen journal articles and chapters in books edited by others. He also brought out a new edition of his textbook on vital statistics and produced two volumes of collected public addresses.[4] His ever-active pen was now directed to new objects. He no longer undertook epidemiological investigation or composed

1 For Newsholme's appointment at the L.S.E., see William Beveridge [Director of L.S.E.] to Newsholme, 13 Feb. 1924, L.S.E., Beveridge Papers, IIb, 23.
2 Arthur Newsholme, *Prohibition in America and Its Relation to the Problem of Public Control of Personal Conduct* (London: P. S. King, 1921); Arthur Newsholme, *The Ministry of Health* (London and New York: G. P. Putnams, [1925]; Arthur Newsholme, *International Studies on the Relation between the Private and Official Practice of Medicine with Special Reference to the Prevention of Disease,* 3 vols. (London: George Allen and Unwin, 1931; Arthur Newsholme, *Medicine and the State: The Relation between the Private and Official Practice of Medicine with Special Reference to Public Health* (London: George Allen and Unwin, 1932); Arthur Newsholme, *Evolution of Preventive Medicine* (Baltimore: Williams and Wilkins, 1927); Arthur Newsholme, *The Story of Modern Preventive Medicine, Being a Continuation of the Evolution of Preventive Medicine* (Baltimore: Williams and Wilkins, 1929); Newsholme, *Fifty Years,* and Newsholme, *Last 30 Years.*
3 Arthur Newsholme and John Adams Kingsbury, *Red Medicine: Socialized Health in Soviet Russia* (Garden City, N.Y.: Doubleday, Doran, 1933).
4 Arthur Newsholme, *The Elements of Vital Statistics in Their Bearing on Social and Public Health Problems,* new ed. (New York: D. Appleton, 1924); Arthur Newsholme, *Public Health and Insurance: American Addresses* (Baltimore: Johns Hopkins Univ. Press, 1920); and Arthur Newsholme, *Health Problems in Organized Society: Studies in the Social Aspects of Public Health* (London: P. S. King, 1927).

detailed memoranda or official reports. Instead, a fair proportion of his writing and much of his public speaking was now health advocacy and commentary on current policy. The most important of Newsholme's productions in retirement are his comparative international studies of health care systems. To this work he devoted several years to travel, observation, and reading. These writings will be the focus of the last section of this chapter.

Newsholme's new life began at once. Immediately after his retirement he attended an international conference at Cannes on Red Cross work. At that conference the American delegation was led by William Henry Welch, who was then organizing the newly created Johns Hopkins School of Hygiene and Public Health. Welch evidently thought that Newsholme's reputation and experience would be useful in launching the new school, because he offered Newsholme a teaching post for the following academic year. The offer may not have been a complete surprise. The two men had first met in 1894 at the International Congress on Hygiene and Demography in Budapest, and they renewed their acquaintance in 1908 on Newsholme's first trip to America to attend the Sixth International Congress on Tuberculosis.[5] During the Great War Welch had discussed plans for the school with a group of British hygienists around Newsholme's dinner table in Westminster. Before the Cannes conference was over Newsholme had accepted Welch's offer, and he left for America within a month.[6]

Newsholme taught at the School of Hygiene for two academic years, 1919–20 and 1920–1 as Resident Lecturer on Public Health Administration. He was at first the only member of that department and one of only two senior faculty to hold the title of Resident Lecturer. At the time the other Resident Lecturer was Wade Hampton Frost in Epidemiology, then on loan to the School from the Public Health Service.[7] Newsholme's academic duties were quite light. In the first two trimesters he met his class two afternoons each week, and he participated in the school's public lecture series.[8] This schedule gave him ample opportunity to lecture off campus. Newsholme enjoyed the teaching and found the faculty company at Hopkins welcome and stimulating, but he was aware that his eclectic, highly autobiographical approach to his subject made his course an oddity in a highly specialized curriculum.[9]

5 Newsholme, *Last 30 Years*, 253. Newsholme described Welch's congress paper on the throat culture service the New York City Health Department had just initiated in Arthur Newsholme, "Report as to the Buda-Pesth International Congress on Hygiene and Demography," Newsholme, *Q. Rep.* (Brighton), 1894, no. 3: 7–11.

6 Newsholme, *Last 30 Years*, 237. Newsholme to Welch, 7 April 1919, Welch Papers.

7 *The Johns Hopkins University School of Hygiene and Public Health, Catalogue and Announcement for 1920–21;* and Elizabeth Fee, *Disease and Discovery: A History of the Johns Hopkins School of Hygiene and Public Health, 1916–1939* (Baltimore and London: Johns Hopkins Univ. Press, 1987), 67, 68, 70.

8 The syllabus for his course is preserved in Hopkins, Chesney Archives, School of Hygiene and Public Health, Office of Dean Correspondence, Box 5. See also *The Johns Hopkins University School of Hygiene and Public Health, Catalogue and Announcement for 1920–21,* 33–4, 54, 60, 63; and ibid., 1921–2, 35.

9 He included, for example, discussion of etiology and epidemiology in his course on public health administration, arguing that that administration needed to be firmly based in these two scientific

Newsholme was a tireless lecturer. On his arrival in the United States he set off on a six-week whistlestop, coast-to-coast tour in May and June 1919 for the Federal Children's Bureau, describing recent English child-welfare work, typically giving several lectures a day at each stop.[10] Thereafter he was a frequent speaker at American universities and professional meetings.[11] In addition to a trip to the West Indies in 1924 to attend a conference on tropical medicine the United Fruit Company sponsored in Jamaica, he returned to the States on four later occasions, lecturing, visiting friends, and spending the winters of 1927–8 and 1937–8 in southern California.[12] To American audiences he usually described what England was doing in public health. He was convinced that in social and medical services America was backward and dominated by special interests, and he was repelled by American machine politics and by the frequent corruption of city governments.[13] But in America he learned as well as instructed. New sources, studies by Louis Dublin, Frederick L. Hoffman, and other American statisticians, for example, began to appear among his citations.[14] American examples began to illustrate his addresses to British audiences as well.

His experience in America widened Newsholme's circle of professional friends. His acquaintance with prominent American public health officials had begun during his tenure at Brighton. Charles V. Chapin, the Commissioner of Health of Providence, Rhode Island, and influential American public health authority, visited Newsholme in Brighton in 1903 and again in 1906, and the two remained in touch for the remainder of their lives.[15] But most of Newsholme's American

subjects. Newsholme, *Last 30 Years,* 265–6. Welch's emphasis on a research basis for the school can be seen in the choice of the original faculty; see Fee, *Disease and Discovery,* 57–66.

10 Newsholme described this American tour in greater detail than any of his other ones. Newsholme, *Last 30 Years,* 241–4. A synthesis of these addresses was published in Newsholme, *Public Health and Insurance,* 240–67. For a contemporary description of his three talks in Minneapolis, see "Sir Arthur Newsholme, K.C.B., M.D., on Child-Welfare in London," *Journal-Lancet,* 39 (1919): 289–90.

11 Two of his books are collections of these addresses. Newsholme, *Public Health and Insurance;* and Newsholme, *Health Problems in Organized Society.* Others were published in medical and social work journals.

12 Newsholme delivered two papers at the Jamaica conference, "A Note on the Causes of the Historical Reduction of Leprosy," *Proceedings of the International Conference on Health Problems in Tropical America* (Boston: United Fruit Co., 1924), 791–5; and "Disease Records as an Indispensable Means of Disease Prevention," ibid., 940–50. His diary of this trip is preserved in the back of his Commonplace Book, Newsholme Papers, FA D1(4), and he published an account of the trip in Newsholme, *Last 30 Years,* 333–43. His itinerary in the States can be pieced together from his published speeches. He describes the travels before 1935 briefly in Newsholme, *Last 30 Years,* 250–2. For his final visit see Newsholme's letters to John Kingsbury, 12 Aug. 1937, 18 Nov. 1937, 18 Jan. [1938], 8 Feb. 1938, and 5 March 1938, Kingsbury Papers, B-16, Newsholme folder 3.

13 Newsholme, *Last 30 Years,* 279–90.

14 Arthur Newsholme, "National Changes in Health and Longevity," *Q. Pub. Am. Statist. Assn.,* 17 (1920–1): 697, 704, 711; Newsholme, "Causes of the Historical Reduction of Leprosy," 791–5; and Newsholme, *The Elements,* new ed., 74, 132, 153, 171–2, 323, 356–7, 490, 552–3.

15 James H. Cassedy, *Charles V. Chapin and the Public Health Movement* (Cambridge, Mass.: Harvard Univ. Press, 1962), 92, 119–20, 125. See also Newsholme to Chapin, 1 Jan. 1932, and 2 Nov. 1935, Chapin Papers, Brown University Library; and Newsholme's entry for Chapin in Newsholme, *Last 30 Years,* 261–3.

acquaintances were formed in the years after 1919. He became close to several of the Hopkins faculty, particularly William Howell and Wade Hampton Frost. In succeeding years he entertained them and dozens of other American friends in Britain.[16] Surviving letters attest to warm and active friendships between Newsholme and Welch, Charles-Edward Amory Winslow, Professor of Public Health at Yale University, and John Kingsbury, Secretary of the Milbank Memorial Fund.[17] His American experience also stimulated him to take up new projects and provided him with the means to do so, the most important of these being the studies he undertook with Milbank Fund sponsorship.

In his early retirement Newsholme also returned to a topic that had been smoldering for nearly a decade, his differences with the biometricians and eugenists over the efficacy of public health programs. Newsholme had not publicly argued with Karl Pearson and other biometricians since he published his second report on infant mortality in 1913. But his time at Johns Hopkins rekindled old animosities. Next to Wade Hampton Frost, with whom Newsholme remained on friendly terms, the senior faculty whose authority was most likely to be challenged by Newsholme's presence was Raymond Pearl, Professor of Biometry and Vital Statistics. Pearl in fact claimed to have strongly protested Newsholme's appointment and to have considered resigning over it.[18] Newsholme was not only a rival voice on vital statistics but a prominent representative of the old style of statistical investigations that Pearl detested. His simmering resentment of Newsholme and the special, and he believed undeserved, treatment Newsholme was receiving exploded after a dinner party in March 1920. Newsholme had dared criticize Pearl's ongoing study of tuberculosis statistics and to suggest that his results were likely to be biased. Pearl responded the next day with a short, venomous letter which ended with the statement that he held Newsholme and Newsholme's opinion on any subject in "unmeasured contempt."[19] Newsholme at once wrote a gracious note of apology expressing regret that he had unintentionally given offense and explaining that he had simply meant to caution against studies which failed to distinguish between familial infection and inheritance of a tuberculous proclivity.[20] The hot-headed Pearl would have no overtures of peace. Although William Stewart Halsted, the Professor of Surgery, urged him to let the matter quietly drop, Pearl responded with a haughty letter explaining his methodology to one he implied could not possibly understand it.[21]

Nor did this rivalry quickly lose its personal dimension. Pearl found in Major

16 Welch to Newsholme, 23 Sept. 1919, Welch Papers; and Newsholme to Welch, 13 Feb. 1932 and 25 Feb. 1932, Welch Papers. See the lists of American visitors in Newsholme to Winslow, 25 June 1923, Winslow Papers; Newsholme to Kingsbury, 11 Aug. 1931, Kingsbury Papers, B-79 folder 1; and Newsholme to Mabel Kingsbury, 5 Oct. 1938, Kingsbury Papers, B-16 Newsholme folder 3.
17 See the Welch Papers; Yale University Library, Charles-Edward Amory Winslow Papers; and Library of Congress, John Adams Kingsbury Papers.
18 Raymond Pearl to Major Greenwood, 12 May 1921, Pearl Papers.
19 Pearl to Newsholme, 11 March 1920, ibid.
20 Newsholme to Pearl, 12 March 1920, ibid.
21 Pearl to Newsholme, 13 March 1920, ibid. See also Pearl's diary entry for 11 March 1920, ibid.

Greenwood an ear very sympathetic to his pique at Newsholme. Greenwood, a former protégé of Karl Pearson, was then statistician at the Ministry of Health and a close associate of George Newman.[22] He thus had links to Newsholme's chief antagonists in Britain. Moreover, as Greenwood was angling for an academic appointment, in particular a post at the new School of Public Health at Harvard,[23] he regarded Newsholme as a potential obstacle. He and Pearl first feared that Newsholme would be appointed at Harvard and then that Newsholme might be made director of the London School of Hygiene and Tropical Medicine when it opened.[24] In their letters, interspersed with some reckless talk, Greenwood suggesting, for example, that it would be best for America to use its military and economic strength to dictate terms to Europe, and snide comments about other statisticians – John Brownlee, Frederick L. Hoffman, and the members of the American Statistical Association – and some vicious, anti-Semitic slurs about Louis Dublin, the two gossiped about Newsholme.[25] Pearl revealed that after the dinner party of March 1920 he had twice more threatened to resign because of Newsholme's presence in Baltimore, and he took credit for the fact that Newsholme was not returning for a third year. The two agreed that Newsholme was ignorant and incompetent, although because he was suave and a great talker, he was convincing to those who did not understand modern – that is, mathematical – statistics. Ironically in these same letters, Pearl asked Greenwood a series of basic questions about the English systems of administration and of collecting vital statistics, which, if he had read any of a number of Newsholme's works, he would have understood.[26]

The historic importance of this episode lies less in what it reveals about personal rivalries and more in its power to remind us how bitter was the conflict over the uses of vital statistics in the early twentieth century. It is tempting to describe this conflict as one between the older – arithmetical – and the newer, more highly mathematical approach to statistics. This is certainly how the biometricians would have characterized it, because it suggests that the struggle was between scientific progressives and reactionaries. The basic issue, however, was the autonomy of statistics as a science, its place in medicine and social administration, and attitudes of the biometricians toward public health programs.

22 For information on Greenwood, see the following obituaries: Lancelot Hogben, "Major Greenwood, 1880–1949," *Obituary Notices of Fellows of the Royal Society,* 7 (1950–1): 139–54; and "Major Greenwood, DSc., F.R.C.P., F.R.S.," *Br. Med. J.* (1949), no. 2: 877–9.

23 Major Greenwood to Pearl, 12 Feb. 1921, Pearl Papers; Pearl to Greenwood, 3 March 1921, ibid.; Pearl to Greenwood, 21 Dec. 1921, ibid.; Greenwood to Pearl, 13 Jan. 1922, ibid.; and Pearl to Greenwood, 4 Feb. 1922, ibid. For Greenwood's career, see Hogben, "Greenwood," 139–54.

24 Pearl to Greenwood, 11 April 1921, Pearl Papers; Greenwood to Pearl, 18 Dec. 1921, ibid.; Pearl to Greenwood, 5 April 1922, ibid; Greenwood to Pearl, 7 July 1923, ibid.; and Greenwood to Pearl, 5 Aug. 1923, ibid.

25 Greenwood to Pearl, 24 April 1921, ibid.; Pearl to Greenwood, 12 May 1921, ibid.; Greenwood to Pearl, 39 [sic] May 1921, ibid.; Pearl to Greenwood, 5 July 1921, ibid.; Greenwood to Pearl, 16 July 1921, ibid.; Greenwood to Pearl, 18 Dec. 1921, ibid.; Greenwood to Pearl, 13 Jan. 1922, ibid.; and Pearl to Greenwood, 4 Feb. 1922, ibid.

26 Pearl to Greenwood, 5 July 1921, ibid.

No letters comparable to those of Pearl and Greenwood survive from Newsholme. He had less personally at stake, and theirs were not his tactics in any case. But several times during his retirement Newsholme took up this subject in addresses and publications. The first occasion was on the eve of his departure from the States in April 1921, when he delivered a dinner address to the American Statistical Association in New York City.[27] In this speech Newsholme considered the role that modern statistics should play in public health work, arguing that mathematical statistics was merely one of several sources of guidance for public health officials. It had no special claim to authority. "In their present stage of development in most communities, vital statistics form an excellent servant but a very bad master for the health officer."[28] Quoting James Clerk Maxwell, he urged his audience to remember the uncertainty of statistical investigations. When the results of biometrical investigation called into question preventive work that was grounded in biology, pathology, chemistry, or other experimental sciences, the public health worker must trust the basic sciences.[29]

In short, in a large part of public health work we must content ourselves with the fact that our work is on the lines which our knowledge of physiology, pathology, and medicine – the institutes of medicine – shows to be important, and reserve to the future the possibility of securing non-fallacious measurements of complex social influences.[30]

He spoke even more bluntly at a Red Cross Conference on child health in Paris in February 1922.

As regards child welfare work and how to obtain major results, it is quite axiomatic that child welfare work has been a chief means of bringing about a reduction in infant mortality. Even in the absence of corroborative statistics, it is certain that such work decreases infant mortality. To think otherwise would be to assert that ignorance is as good as knowledge; that care of infants is no better than carelessness; and that educated skill, added to maternal instinct, is no better than maternal instinct alone.[31]

In his address to the American Statistical Society Newsholme took several pokes at the biometricians and conspicuously failed to mention Pearl among the American contributors to vital statistics. Pearl and Greenwood were enraged. The latter objected that Newsholme was trying to have it both ways. Statistics could be trusted, if they confirmed his views but not if they ran counter to them.[32] Newsholme was in fact backing away from the stance he had taken a quarter century earlier. In 1896 he had answered those who belittled the value of sickness

27 Arthur Newsholme, "The Better Use of Vital Statistics in Public Health Administration," *Q. Pub. Am. Statist. Assn.*, 17 (1921): 815–25; republished as "Vital Statistics: Their Better Use in Public Health Administration," *Lancet* (1921), no. 2: 833–6.
28 Newsholme, "Better Use of Vital Statistics," 815–16.
29 Ibid., 815–16.   30 Ibid., 817.
31 American Red Cross European Child Health Program 1921–22, *Medical Conference at Paris Headquarters February 2–3, 1922* (Paris: Medical Department of the American Red Cross, 1922), 75. I am indebted to John Hutchinson for bringing this source to my attention.
32 Greenwood to Pearl, 13 Jan. 1922, Pearl Papers; and Greenwood to Pearl, 31 May 1922, ibid.

registration because the reported diagnoses were often inaccurate by insisting that "erroneous and imperfect diagnosis could be made the basis of safe and certain calculations by means of the law of averages," and that "statistics founded on imperfect data might form the subject of valuable calculations."[33] Faced with challenges from the eugenists and the biometricians, he no longer suggested that statistics could produce results that were better than the data on which they were based. In his 1921 address, in another at the London School of Economics two years later, and at greater length in the new edition of his *Elements of Vital Statistics* he argued that the use of more sophisticated mathematics did not give a biometrical study special status. It must still conform to normal statistical standards.[34] Data must be appropriate, accurate, complete, unbiased, and compatible. Further, both investigator and reader must recognize that medical and social phenomena usually have multiple and interdependent causes. It was therefore difficult to isolate and to measure the influence of single factors. In fact in many social phenomena, including public health, the notion of cause had to be used in a restricted sense. "The phenomena are so complex that a specific cause is undeterminable; the real cause is a combination of forces, some inimical and some helpful to the result under investigation."[35]

Newsholme was careful to concede that sciences advanced by adopting quantitative methods, that quantitative methods would eventually replace qualitative methods in medicine, and that Karl Pearson and others of the biometrical school had made substantial contributions to mathematical statistics.[36] It was in the applications of these methods and in the inferences drawn from them that the biometricians often went wrong. In these papers and especially in his textbook he provided examples, many of them from the products of the Galton Eugenics Laboratory. He chose, for example, Pearson's claim to have demonstrated that heredity was more important than infection in pulmonary tuberculosis by showing that in a set of families the correlation between tuberculosis in parent and child was strong, while that for tuberculosis in both marriage partners was quite weak. This study, Newsholme objected, failed to test sensitively for conditions influencing infection between spouses: age of spouses, the length of their exposure to infection, and whether the infected spouse had taken simple precautions to prevent exposing others. More important, Pearson's study failed to recognize a biological fact that was becoming increasingly obvious: adult cases of pulmonary tuberculosis were often due to latent childhood infection activated by environmental stress or other disease.[37] Furthermore, in analyzing the nation's tuberculosis mortality curves in his critique of Newsholme's studies of tuberculosis, Pearson had commit-

33 Arthur Newsholme in discussion of his "National System of Notification," *J. Roy. Statist. Soc.*, 35.
34 Arthur Newsholme, "The Measurement of Progress in Public Health with Special Reference to the Life and Work of William Farr," *Economica*, 3 (1923): 196–201; and Newsholme, *The Elements*, new ed., 358–60, 365–6, 503–62, 586–8.
35 Newsholme, *The Elements*, new ed., 530.   36 Ibid., 542.
37 Ibid., 543–44. See also [Arthur Newsholme], "The Supposed Acquired Immunity of the Population against Tuberculosis," Newsholme Papers.

ted a basic statistical error, inferring changes in rates of change from arithmetical rather than from logarithmic curves, in effect confusing differences with rates of difference.[38] When logarithmic curves were used, Newsholme showed that tuberculosis mortality for males in England and Wales had declined at a steady rate since 1866 and not at a retarded rate as Pearson had asserted. He also pointed out that Pearson's contention in 1918 that not only had tuberculosis mortality stopped declining but was beginning to rise again had proven to be erroneous, a brief anomaly produced by the war.[39]

Similarly, he objected to a Galton Eugenics Laboratory study of parental alcoholism which purported to show that children did not suffer in health or height from their parents' alcoholism and that the children of one group of alcoholic parents were taller and slightly healthier than children of one group of nonalcoholic parents. This study had already been subjected to much criticism. No effort had been made to ensure that the two groups of families were alike except for the use of alcohol. Newsholme also pointed out that both sets of parents were in receipt of charity, and that it was possible that the alcoholic parents may have been initially the healthier and stronger of the two groups and may have been reduced to accepting charity by their alcoholism while the other group may have been dependent because of chronic ill health. Furthermore, it was not certain that the parents' alcoholism had begun before their children's conception.[40]

Newsholme did not deny the importance of heredity. In fact, he insisted that the capacity to reach old age that exists in some families apparently independently of environmental influences was a good example.[41] But he continued to defend preventive medicine from the charge that saving weak lives endangered the health of the future generations. In the twenties he was even more categorical than he had been at the turn of the century that natural selection's brutal reign had been suspended in modern society.

Under the circumstances of modern civilization the assumption that natural selection can act as under savage conditions is completely unwarranted. Civilized life, leading to progressive improvement of environment and of personal habits, submerges any possible influence of natural selection in removing those unfit for survival, substituting for it a process of steady uplifting in fitness of the general population.[42]

Newsholme's major worry about many of the biometrical studies of his day was that they demoralize health officials whose statistical limitations rendered them helpless to question the biometricians' assertions.[43] His new edition of *The Elements of Vital Statistics*, a quarter century after the last edition, was Newsholme's

---

38 Arthur Newsholme, *The Elements*, new ed., 586–8.
39 For Pearson's contention, see Karl Pearson, "The Check to the Fall in the Phthisis Death-rate since the Discovery of the Tubercle Bacillus and the Adoption of Modern Treatment," *Biometrica*, 12 (1918–19): 374–6.
40 Newsholme, *The Elements*, new ed., 547–9.
41 Newsholme, "National Changes in Health," 712.   42 Ibid., 717.
43 Newsholme, *Last 30 Years*, 208.

answer. This edition, like its predecessors, was intended as a practical textbook for public health workers. As he had done in previous editions, he showed how current vital statistics could be applied, using his own studies and administrative work as examples and now adding American illustrations as well. But he also wrote to prepare health officers to deal with the challenge posed by critics of public health initiatives who wielded sophisticated statistical methods. He explained some of the new statistical concepts and tools – normal distribution, standard deviation, probable error, coefficients of correlation, and partial or multiple correlation – and he provided his readers with references to more complete discussions of mathematical statistics.[44] He also offered more systematic criticism of biometrical studies than he had previously done. One finds him quoting, for example, the critique of the use of coefficients of correlation John Maynard Keynes offered in his *Treatise on Probability*.[45] Newsholme found allies in the American public health world, including C.-E. A. Winslow, with whom he discussed some of these quarrels.[46] "For personal reasons," he told Winslow, "I have not made use of Pearl's numerous fallacious statements as illustrations for my new book though the material was very tempting."[47] Winslow shared Newsholme's views, and as an answer to Pearl he sent Newsholme a copy of the statistical demonstrations of the value of public health programs produced by Isidore Falk, then in his department at Yale.[48]

SOCIAL HYGIENE AND MORAL EVOLUTION

During the first two decades of the twentieth century, individual behavior came to the forefront of public health discussion.[49] Many factors contributed to its new prominence, among them the campaigns for infant welfare and against venereal disease. Newsholme had played an early role in this change by his advocacy of incorporating the teaching of hygiene into the elementary school curriculum.[50] In the middle twenties he returned to the issue of personal behavior, pointing out that knowledge was not enough. It was not unusual to know the cause of a disease and the means by which it could be prevented and still fail to control the disease. The typhoid epidemic in the town with a parsimonious council was the classic

44 Newsholme, *The Elements,* new ed., 507–24.
45 Ibid., 525–6.
46 Newsholme to Winslow, 25 June 1923, Winslow Papers; Winslow to Newsholme, 10 March 1924, ibid.; and Newsholme to Winslow, 23 March 1924, ibid.
47 Newsholme to Winslow, 28 Aug. 1923, ibid.
48 Winslow to Newsholme, 11 Aug. 1923, Winslow Papers; and Winslow to Newsholme, 6 Sept. 1923, ibid. See also I. S. Falk, "A Differential Analysis of the Reduction in the Death-Rate," *Nation's Health,* 5 (1923): 435–6, 500.
49 Dorothy Porter, " 'Enemies of the Race': Biologism, Environmentalism, and Public Health in Edwardian England," *Victorian Studies,* 34 (1991): 171–2.
50 Arthur Newsholme, "On the Study of Hygiene in Elementary Schools," *Public Health,* 3 (1890–1): 134–6. See also Arthur Newsholme, *Lessons of Health: Containing the Elements of Physiology, and Their Application to Hygiene* (London, 1890).

instance.[51] More to the point were syphilis and alcoholism, two serious preventable conditions that were not being prevented. These two were "the greatest obstacle in our midst to health, happiness, and prosperity," and, he was convinced, they were linked together so closely that "the action required to reduce one will lessen the other."[52] The state could do some things to control them; in fact, Newsholme continued to point proudly to the venereal disease service Britain had established while he was at the Local Government Board, but he insisted that these diseases and some others of the most intractable health and social problems of his day would not be solved until human behavior was modified. To that end, he devoted some of his retirement energy to the work of the British Social Hygiene Council and to public lecturing on venereal disease, contraception, and alcoholism.[53]

What may seem surprising, given his role in establishing a state venereal disease service that offered confidential diagnosis and treatment to all, free of cost, free of means tests, and free of stigmatization, was how highly moralizing, one might even say morally apocalyptic, his public statements on social diseases were in the twenties.[54] We can understand this apparent change in part as a reflection of his retirement. No longer in public office, he was freer to speak his mind. In no other set of his writings are his own moral convictions and traces of his religious training so evident. It was also a reflection of his age. Now in his seventies, he found the changes in moral standards and sexual practices in the postwar era worrisome, and he increasingly found himself out of step with the times. His friend John Kingsbury, who fancied himself a modern man, considered Newsholme's responses to nude bathing and mixed-gendered sleeping cars on trains in the Soviet Union rather quaint.[55] He also recorded that Newsholme's attitudes toward Soviet laws on marriage and divorce startled the other Westerners en route to the Soviet Union in 1932. One of them commented to Kingsbury, "What a charming and intelligent old gentleman Sir Arthur is – but what an archaic mind!"[56]

By the middle twenties Newsholme's social and moral attitudes probably seemed archaic or prudish. It is worth noting about his writing on sexual behavior and on alcoholism, however, that he was able to revive the notion of moral evolution he had first used at the turn of the century in discussing poverty, physical degeneration, and social policy. I have argued in Chapter 7 and elsewhere that, following the example of Thomas Henry Huxley's Romanes Lectures,

51 Arthur Newsholme, "The Moral Aspects of Social Hygiene," *J. Social Hygiene,* 10 (1924): 514–15. Most of this article also appeared as Arthur Newsholme, "The Moral Aspects of Social Hygiene," *Hibbert J.,* 22 (1923–4): 279–293. Citations will be to the previous version.

52 Newsholme, "Moral Aspects of Social Hygiene," 515; and Newsholme, *Ministry of Health,* 228.

53 Newsholme served as chair of the Council's Social Hygiene Committee in 1926; see the list of committee members in *Foundations of Social Hygiene* (London: British Social Hygiene Council, 1926), 140.

54 See, for example, Arthur Newsholme, "The Community and Social Hygiene," in *Foundations of Social Hygiene* (London: British Social Hygiene Council, 1926), 126.

55 John Kingsbury, travel diary, 22 Aug. 1932, 29 Aug. 1932, Kingsbury Papers, B-67.

56 Kingsbury, travel diary, 2 Aug. 1932, ibid.

Newsholme used the notion of moral evolution to try to reconcile his politics with his science, to accept biological evolution without abandoning social welfare efforts or endangering personal liberty.[57] In the first decade of the century he had used the notion to defend public initiatives for human welfare. Now two decades later, he used it much more often to judge the behavior of individuals.

He continued to find in human history the gradual evolution of moral sensibility which witnessed the replacement of barbarism by civilization and selfishness by altruism.[58] Its effects could be detected socially in, for example, the string of reform and ameliorative efforts of the past century that protected the weak and vulnerable and promoted the welfare of society as a whole. This is the process he had emphasized twenty years before. Now he emphasized that it might also be seen in the recent fall in the per capita consumption of alcohol in Britain and in the evolution of monogamous family life, which he took to be the highest expression of social and moral progress, the pinnacle of moral evolution and human happiness.[59] Moral evolution also explained differences in values and individual behavior. "In our daily life we meet people representing all stages from the most rudimentary ethics to the highest Christian character."[60] He once considered drawing a parallel between stages of human history and McDougall's stages of individual development in which the child first responds only to instinct, then to fear, and finally is ruled by intellect and ideals.[61] The exemplary Christian, the person who exercised self-control and exhibited altruism, was morally the most highly developed. "The ideal of the ethical life is that of a man who is master of himself, the Christian holding that he obtains this mastery by Divine help, and that the goodness thus secured is the great object in life."[62] At the other end of the evolutionary scale were the drunkard and the sexually promiscuous, "the savage members of civilized communities, i.e. those who are unwilling or unable to exercise the self-control called for in communal life."[63] "The sexually immoral man," he claimed was "an enemy of society, who cannot be tolerated."[64]

Between the ethical supermen on the one hand and the moral barbarians on the other was a middle ground inhabited by moderate drinkers, by couples that

---

57 John M. Eyler, "Poverty, Disease, Responsibility: Arthur Newsholme and the Public Health Dilemmas of British Liberalism," *Milbank Quarterly*, 67, Suppl. 1 (1989): 109–26; John M. Eyler, "The Sick Poor and the State: Arthur Newsholme on Poverty, Disease, and Responsibility," in *Framing Disease: Studies in Cultural History*, ed. Charles E. Rosenberg and Janet Golden (New Brunswick, N.J.: Rutgers Univ. Press, 1992), 276–96. The latter was reprinted in *Doctors, Politics and Society: Historical Essays*, ed. Dorothy Porter and Roy Porter (Amsterdam and Atlanta: Rodopi, 1993), 188–211.

58 See, for example, Newsholme, *Health Problems*, 182–7.

59 Ibid., 175–6; Newsholme, "Moral Aspects of Social Hygiene," 520–1.

60 Newsholme, *Health Problems*, 119.

61 Newsholme, "Moral Aspects of Social Hygiene," 526–7.

62 Arthur Newsholme, "The Control of Conception," in *Sexual Problems of To-day*, ed. Mary Scharlieb (London: Williams and Norgate, [1924]), 167.

63 Newsholme, *Health Problems*, 215, 197. Also Arthur Newsholme, "The Story of Alcoholic Control in Great Britain," *Survey Graphic*.

64 Newsholme, *Health Problems*, 178.

used contraception for nonmedical reasons,[65] and by those who experienced occasional moral lapses – ordinary people we might say. It was here that the greatest challenge for social hygiene lay. Like others among its proponents, Newsholme preferred to rely on education and character building. He championed frank public discussion of sexually transmitted diseases. Educational authorities, employers, and local health authorities all could play a role.[66] The problem was partly one of information that could be given in adulthood, but more fundamentally it was one of self-control that had to be learned over a lifetime. The latter should begin in the home, and it would have to begin early. He even suggested that making an infant wait for meals on a regular schedule was the first step. "Thus in earliest infancy the judicious mother is giving her child the first lessons of postponement of pleasure, i.e., of self-control, on which character is based."[67] The training had to continue through childhood, so that social instincts and self-control were well-developed before puberty.

Like other social hygienists, he was occasionally led by his zeal to provide misinformation, as when he wrote that "the *sole source* [his italics] of infection by syphilis and gonorrhoea is through extra-marital sexual relations."[68] His writings also make it clear that the goals of the campaign were as much moral as medical. "Sexual vice is a serious enemy of family life, whether associated with venereal disease or not."[69]

The prevention of venereal disease, although an immediate, is not, indeed, the chief aim. Inasmuch as any relation between the sexes which implies the risk of venereal disease is either directly the result, or in an earlier relationship has been the result, of an infringement of chastity or marital fidelity, it is this breach of morality, this tampering with the ideas of love, that is the chief evil, needing to be attacked in the larger interests of public morality.[70]

Where persuasion and education failed, compulsion might be necessary. This was especially true where commercial interests were involved. Newsholme endorsed strong police action against prostitution and even supported the formation of vigilante groups, Law Enforcement Leagues, to help the police battle organized vice.[71] He also initially supported Prohibition in America. He was in the States when the Eighteenth Amendment passed, and he watched the experiment with great interest. He answered those who saw the American act as an unwarranted invasion of freedom by trying to demonstrate both that state restriction on access to alcohol was a well-established principle, in Britain dating to the sixteenth century, and by arguing that the prohibition of alcohol was but the "logical

---

65 Newsholme opposed the widespread use of contraception, arguing that it would have undesirable social and economic consequences and also that its use reflected selfishness and irresponsibility. See Newsholme, "The Control of Conception," 147–72; and Arthur Newsholme, "Some Public Health Aspects of 'Birth Control,' " in *Medical Views of Birth Control,* ed. James Marchant (London: Martin Hopkinson, 1926), 132–50.

66 Newsholme, "The Community and Social Hygiene," 124–5.

67 Newsholme, *Health Problems,* 193.   68 Ibid., 181.

69 Ibid., 176.   70 Ibid., 181.   71 Ibid., 177–8.

culmination" of the regulation of individual behavior by government in the interest of the welfare of all.[72] But Newsholme welcomed the use of compulsion only under certain conditions.[73] The end to be served must be of great social value and must be unattainable or unattainable in a reasonable time by education and voluntary initiatives alone. Compulsion must have the prospect of achieving the desired ends, and it must be supported by the majority of the people. At first Newsholme believed that the Eighteenth Amendment satisfied these conditions. He had no doubt that grave medical and social problems could be traced to the excessive consumption of alcohol.[74] The remarkable fall in alcoholic consumption and improved health that accompanied the wartime restrictions of alcohol in Britain proved that prohibition was practical.[75] Early statistical returns from America suggested that prohibition was having similar beneficial effects on health, welfare, and social order.[76]

In drawing attention to Newsholme's moral absolutism and his defense of compulsion, we risk distorting his position. While he never adopted a disease model for alcoholism, he also did not pursue the consequences of his moral evolutionary model. There were to be no draconian measures, no institutionalization or sterilization, for moral savages. As he had done throughout his career, he recalled that alcoholism was a consequence as well as a cause of social problems. Ignorance, the grinding lives of the urban poor, and well-established social customs all encouraged drinking.[77] Also he regarded Prohibition as an American experiment, a "short cut."[78] He never suggested that Britain follow the American example. Britain's wartime experience demonstrated that alcoholic excesses could be discouraged short of absolute prohibition.[79] He also changed his mind about Prohibition as the experiment proceeded. While he continued to defend the principle that a people might properly and with likelihood of great benefit to health, prosperity, and happiness enact an absolute ban on the use of alcohol as a

72 Newsholme, *Public Health and Insurance*, 197–205; Arthur Newsholme, "Some International Aspects of Alcoholism with Special Reference to Prohibition in America," The Ninth Norman Kerr Memorial Lecture, *Br. J. Inebriety*, 19 (1922), 107–10. This lecture appeared soon after in expanded form as Arthur Newsholme, *Prohibition in America and Its Relation to the Problem of Public Control of Personal Conduct* (London: P. S. King, [1922]), 49–56. See also Arthur Newsholme, "The Place of the Alcohol Question in Social Hygiene," *Br. J. Inebriety*, 26 (1928): 58–9.

73 For the following, see Newsholme, *Health Problems*, 102; or Arthur Newsholme, "Presidential Address on the Relative Roles of Compulsion and Education in Public Health Work," *J. Roy. Sanitary Inst.*, 43 (1922–3): 89.

74 Newsholme "Alcohol and Public Health," in *The Drink Problem in its Medico-Sociological Aspects*, ed. T. N. Kelynack (London: Methuen, [1907]), 123–4, 127–50; Newsholme, "Social Aspects of the Alcohol Problem," 217–18, 220–4; and Newsholme, "The Place of the Alcohol Question," 61–6, 67, 68–71; Newsholme, *Public Health and Insurance*, 124; and Newsholme, *Health Problems*, 101, 216.

75 Arthur Newsholme, "New Light on the Drink Problem," *Contemporary Review*, 125 (1924): 440–3; and Newsholme, *Health Problems*, 207–10.

76 Newsholme, *Prohibition in America*, 36–42; Newsholme, "International Aspects of Alcoholism," 103.

77 Newsholme, *Public Health and Insurance*, 149–50.   78 Ibid., 149.

79 Newsholme, "New Light on the Drink Problem," 438–43; and Newsholme, *Health Problems*, 207–10.

beverage, by the late twenties he conceded that the problems of enforcement were much greater than he or American advocates had anticipated, that national prohibition may have been premature, and that it might have been best to have left the matter a local option so that policy might reflect more closely the views of local citizens.[80] By the middle of the next decade he had become convinced that national prohibition had been a mistake, one that illustrated the power of dedicated minorities and special interests to distort the American political process and one that had proved corrupting to ordinarily law-abiding citizens and to public officials.[81] He remained convinced, however, that "rigid restrictions" on the sale of alcohol were called for, although he preferred the British system of indirect regulation through taxation and licensing.

We find a similar pragmatism in his recommendations for dealing with venereal disease. While he regarded syphilis as a consequence of moral failure, he insisted that it could not be dealt with exclusively as a moral problem. The first duty of government in regard to venereal disease was to remove all barriers to diagnosis and treatment.[82] Here Britain was far ahead of the United States. Newsholme was convinced that British policy had been effective in reducing new cases of syphilis and gonorrhea. While he believed that providing prophylactic disinfection kits to soldiers encouraged promiscuity, and while he found the kits personally repulsive – the provider became, he insisted, "a co-partner with the sensualist" – he recognized that, once a person exposed himself to infection, all means to keep that person from infecting others must be tried.[83] For that reason he recommended that medical practitioners give information on chemical prophylaxis to patients who had exposed themselves and requested such information. In preaching moral perfection he did not lose all sense of perspective. He counseled mercy for those who broke the strict ethical code he outlined, and he recognized that training in self-control had to be supplemented by healthy recreational outlets, financial encouragement of early marriage, reformed divorce laws, and social work among sex offenders.[84] There was a role for public authorities in even so private an area as character reform.

THE SOCIALIZATION OF MEDICINE: NEWSHOLME'S
INTERNATIONAL STUDIES OF HEALTH CARE SYSTEMS

Newsholme assumed that America would inevitably follow the road that Britain had taken in providing health care for its people. Many of his American addresses

---

80 Ibid., 221, 224–5.   81 Newsholme, *Last 30 Years*, 305–14.

82 For the following discussion, see Arthur Newsholme, "The Decline in the Registered Mortality from Syphilis in England. To What Is It Due?" *J. Social Hygiene*, 12 (1926): 513–23. This article was reprinted in Newsholme, *Health Problems*, 163–72. Future citations will be to the latter form.

83 Newsholme, *Public Health and Insurance*, 152; Newsholme, *Health Problems*, 108, 174; Newsholme, "Moral Aspects of Social Hygiene," 523; and Newsholme, "The Community and Social Hygiene," 109.

84 Newsholme, *Health Problems*, 180, 191–2; and Newsholme, "The Community and Social Hygiene," 121.

described the system of free public medical services that had evolved in Britain: the Poor Law medical service, the tuberculosis and venereal disease clinics, maternal and infant welfare centers, public health nursing under health visiting programs, the school medical service, local authority infectious disease hospitals, public asylums, and publicly provided laboratory diagnosis. Already the scale of this work was so great, he told an American audience in 1919, that it involved at least the part-time labor of a large segment of the British medical profession in the Poor Law, school medical, or public health services. In addition probably three-quarters of the nation's doctors had the panel practices under the tax-supported National Insurance system.[85] This expansion of public medical services reflected, Newsholme believed, both society's realization of its interests and the advancement of civilization, of moral evolution.

The real wealth of a nation does not consist in its money, in the volume of its trade, or in the extent of its dominion. These are only valuable insofar as they help to maintain a population – and not only a portion of it – of the right quality; men, women and children possessing bodily vigor, alert mind, firm character, courage and self-control. . . . Can we be satisfied while a large proportion of the population do not obtain medical and ancillary assistance to the extent of their needs? Does such a state of things conduce to the settlement of social unrest? Is it consistent with Christian principles?

If communal provision has been recognized as a duty for police protection, for sanitation, for elementary education, should it not likewise be admitted for the more subtle and maleficent enemies of health . . . ?[86]

The process had gone too far and its benefits were too obvious for there to be any fear that it would be reversed.[87] Before they, themselves, reached a ripe age, Newsholme rashly told an audience of medical students at Johns Hopkins, medical care would be provided to all in America who needed it and this care would be paid for by a graduated tax.[88]

But while Newsholme had every confidence that America would follow England in socializing its health care, he remained highly critical of many features of the English system, repeating publicly in the twenties criticisms he had made before the Poor Law Commission and in the negotiations over the National Insurance bill. The marvel of the British system, he told American audiences, was

85 He estimated that 5,000 of the 24,000 medical practitioners in England and Wales worked as Poor Law doctors. Another 4,000 to 5,000 held appointments in the public health service and some 500 in the lunacy service. The school authorities employed another 1,300. Newsholme, "The Increasing Socialization of Medicine" [The Wesley M. Carpenter Lecture, New York Academy of Medicine, 2 Oct. 1919] in Newsholme, *Public Health and Insurance*, 83–6. Future citations will be to *Public Health and Insurance*. He gave a more detailed breakdown with smaller totals than he had compiled in 1919 in Newsholme, *Ministry of Health*, 245–6.

86 Newsholme, *Public Health and Insurance*, 101.

87 Arthur Newsholme, "Insurance and Health" [Address to Quiz Medical Society, New York City, 14 Feb. 1920] in Newsholme, *Public Health and Insurance*, 115. Future citations will be to *Public Health and Insurance*.

88 Arthur Newsholme, "The Inter-Relation of Various Social Efforts" [Address to Alpha-Kappa-Kappa Club, Johns Hopkins University, 10 Dec. 1919] in Newsholme, *Public Health and Insurance*, 146. Future citations will be to *Public Health and Insurance*.

that it worked as well as it did in spite of politicians' mistakes.[89] The evolution of its medical and social services had been tarnished by the ad hoc vice, the creation of separate, inefficient, uncoordinated, and potentially competing authorities. The small, autonomous administrative units of the Poor Law, the deterrent policy in its medical service, and that service's emphasis on palliation of conditions rather than on prevention stood as a monument to the errors of the past.[90] The passage of the National Insurance Act might have been a "great stride in the socialization of medicine" but "it was done ill-advisedly; it continued a false and low level of isolated general medical practice; it has even been described as a fraud on the insured. . . ."[91] The system of approved societies, the limitations of benefits, payment by capitation, the mixture of cash and service benefits all conspired to produce a system which Newsholme, as well as some more recent critics, insisted was financially extravagant, actuarily unsound, and medically flawed.[92]

Health insurance might be a good complement to an adequate public system of preventive medicine, but it was no substitute for it. What would have been the effect, he asked his audiences, if Edwin Chadwick and John Simon had been content to ask Parliament to insure part of the population against smallpox and typhus?[93] The money and effort that had been "lavished" on the insurance scheme would have produced more beneficial results had it been turned over to local authorities in the form of conditional grants to expand and support their public health work.[94] Take, for example, the cash maternity benefit under National Insurance. The money thus granted unconditionally at the time of birth would have done much more good in advancing the health of mothers and infants if it had been used to provide medical and nursing services under local authority control. Turning again to analogy, he insisted that no one would pretend to argue that the education of the next generation would best be provided by small grants to families ostensibly to allow them to buy books for their children's education. We realize that the provision of skilled services, in the case of education state schools and public libraries, is both more efficient and productive of better results than unconditional cash payments.[95]

89 Newsholme, *Public Health and Insurance,* vi–vii.

90 Arthur Newsholme, "The Historical Development of Public Health Work in England" [Address to American Public Health Association, 27 Oct. 1919], *Am. J. Pub. Health,* 9 (1919): 909–10, 914; also in Newsholme, *Public Health and Insurance,* 48–9, 59–60. Subsequent citations will be to *Public Health and Insurance.*

91 Newsholme, *Public Health and Insurance,* 95.

92 Ibid., 33–6, 65–8, 88–96, 104–12. For a slightly later discussion, see also Newsholme, *Ministry of Health,* 186–95, 198–9, 203–4, 258–9. Later observers have pointed out similar deficiencies: Harry Eckstein, *The English Health Service: Its Origins, Structure, and Achievements* (Cambridge, Mass.: Harvard Univ. Press, 1958), 19–29; *Health Insurance in Great Britain, 1911–1948: Social Security Series, Memorandum No. 11* (Ottawa: Department of National Health and Welfare, 1952), 111–33; and Charles Webster, *The Health Services since the War,* I: Problems of Health Care, The National Health Service before 1957 (London: HMSO, 1988), 11, 14.

93 Newsholme, *Public Health and Insurance,* 35.   94 Ibid., 33–4.

95 Arthur Newsholme, "Some Problems of Preventive Medicine of the Immediate Future," *Canadian Practitioner and Review,* 44 (1919): 209; also in Newsholme, *Public Health and Insurance,* 134. Future citations will be to *Public Health and Insurance.*

Newsholme continued to champion a unified public medical system under local authority control as the best system of social medicine, and he lamented the political choices that had been made since he entered Whitehall. A common ground could have been found between the Majority and the Minority Reports of the Poor Law Commission which would have permitted the establishment of a truly national medical service.[96] Echoing his statements before the Commission, he argued in 1919 that had the Poor Law medical service been transferred to local health authorities, and had these authorities been empowered to absorb the school medical service, the nation would be well on the way to achieving this goal.[97]

Such a unified system would offer what was currently unavailable in England: hospital, consultation, pathological, and nursing services for the entire population. The basis of the system would be the work of the family doctor, but the organization of the system would make expert and institutional help available to that doctor and make possible medical teamwork. Doctors would be paid by salary and would have vacation time and opportunities for postgraduate education. They would be encouraged to take an interest in preventive medicine. Ideally each general practitioner should in effect become an M.O.H. in the sphere of his practice.[98]

Until every medical practitioner is trained to investigate each case of illness from a preventive as well as from what is often rather a pharmaceutical than a really curative standpoint, until a communal system of consultant and hospital services independent of any insurance system is made available for all needing it, and until every medical practitioner is related by financial and official ties to this communal system, full control over disease, – to the extent of our present available medical knowledge, – will not be secured.[99]

C.-E. A. Winslow has helped create the impression that Newsholme changed his mind about health insurance during his retirement.[100] There is substance to this statement, but it is a claim that can be easily misunderstood. For as long as he was able to write, Newsholme continued to point out the same major deficiencies of the National Insurance system, even quoting in the thirties from criticisms he had published in the early twenties.[101] Although he never became an enthusiastic

---

96 Arthur Newsholme, "Public Health Progress in England during the Last Fifty Years," *Commonhealth*, 6 (1919), 310–11; also in Newsholme, *Public Health and Insurance*, 29–31. Subsequent citations will be to *Public Health and Insurance*. This address was prepared for the celebration of the fiftieth anniversary of the Massachusetts State Board of Health, but it was never delivered because of expected disorder accompanying a police strike. Newsholme, *Last 30 Years*, 247. See also Newsholme, *Ministry of Health*, 186.

97 Newsholme, *Public Health and Insurance*, 32. Newsholme had made some of these same recommendations in his final report to the L.G.B., Newsholme, *Ann. Rep. Med. Off. L.G.B.*, 47 (1917–18): xiii–xx.

98 Ibid., 46 (1917–18): xi; Newsholme, *Public Health and Insurance*, 27, 99–100, 117–19.

99 Ibid., 68–69.

100 C.-E. A. Winslow, "Arthur Newsholme: 1857–1943," *Medical Care*, 3 (1943): 290.

101 See, for example, his characterization of health care under national insurance as a "false and low ideal of isolated general practice" in Newsholme, *Public Health and Insurance*, 95–6; and Newsholme, *Medicine and the State*, 241. In the latter case he omitted his earlier phrase that some considered the insurance scheme a fraud on the insured.

partisan of Lloyd George's creation, as his perspective changed, he began to make less of the insurance scheme's shortcomings. By the late twenties Newsholme was systematically studying Continental and American medicine. Seeing what was available abroad made him appreciate more fully the system that had evolved at home during his lifetime.

The changed perspective began with his trip to America in the spring of 1926. During this visit Newsholme was invited by the Milbank Memorial Fund to join the party of dignitaries observing the health demonstration projects the Fund was sponsoring in Syracuse and in Cattaraugus County, New York.[102] These projects, both in their third year, were two of the three demonstrations then underweigh with support from the Fund. The third was in the Bellevue-Yorkville area of New York City and was then in its second year.[103] The Cattaraugus County demonstration established the first full-time county health department in New York State and developed a program that few American health departments in rural areas could match. Newsholme was already familiar with some of the problems of providing health services in rural New York State. In 1920 he had written a memorandum in support of a proposal of Hermann Biggs, New York State Commissioner of Health, for the creation, under the auspices of the State board of health, of mobile speciality units which would bring consultation services to rural general practitioners.[104] When the State legislature refused to act, the Milbank Fund decided to attempt to show what could be done to improve the health of a select rural population. Newsholme spent a week observing the demonstrations in Syracuse and Cattaraugus County and giving several speeches at public meetings. He was impressed with what he found, especially with the comprehensiveness of the local schemes and with the intelligent coordination of official and voluntary work. He praised the demonstrations at a dinner meeting of the Milbank Trustees on the eve of his return to Britain, and he submitted

---

102 The tour of Cattaraugus County took place June 1–3 and was timed to correspond with the annual meeting of the State and Local Committees on Tuberculosis and Public Health of the New York State Charities Aid Association. A program and related material are preserved in Newsholme Papers, FA: D2(8). See also, "Health Leaders of State Conduct Observation Tour of Health Demonstration," *Olean Evening Times* (1 June 1926), 3; "Hundreds Throng State Park at Dedication of Milbank Pavilion Gift," *Olean Evening Times* (2 June 1926), 3; and "Olean Health Heads Explain Demonstration," *Olean Evening News* (2 June 1926), 9.

103 For information on these projects, see the trilogy C.-E. A. Winslow, *Health on the Farm and in the Village: A Review and Evaluation of the Cattaraugus County Health Demonstration with Special Reference to Its Lessons for other Rural Areas* (New York: Macmillan, 1931); C.-E. A. Winslow, *A City Set on a Hill: The Significance of the Health Demonstration at Syracuse, New York* (Garden City, N.Y.: Doubleday, Doran, 1934); and C.-E. A. Winslow and Savel Zimand, *Health Under the "El": The Story of the Bellevue-Yorkville Health Demonstration in Mid-Town New York* (New York: Harper, 1937). See also Clyde V. Kiser, *The Milbank Memorial Fund: Its Leaders and Its Work, 1905–1974* (New York: Milbank Memorial Fund, 1975), 28–41; and H. R. O'Brien, "History of Public Health in Chautauqua, Cattaraugus and Allegany Counties," in William J. Dotty, Charles E. Congdon, and Lewis H. Thornton, *The Historic Annals of Southwestern New York* (New York: Lewis Historical Publishing, 1940), I: 164–6.

104 Newsholme, *Medicine and the State*, 275; and Newsholme, *Last 30 Years*, 363.

soon thereafter a report which the Fund published in its *Quarterly* and as a pamphlet.[105]

Within a few months of his visit came the first hint of trouble. Although the Cattaraugus County Medical Society had originally supported the county's application to join the demonstration project, it reversed itself in September 1926 and passed its first resolution criticizing the demonstration. Things were patched up temporarily, but in the fall of 1927 and during much of 1928 the Society denounced the demonstration both locally and at medical meetings elsewhere and sought to have it discontinued.[106] The criticism was often vague and polemical, but the medical society felt that the expansion of public health programs threatened the practices of its members. Objections were raised to the use of visiting public health nurses, to immunization by public health employees, and to the influence of lay officials. Local civic groups and the county board favored continuation of the demonstration, but the medical opposition alarmed the Milbank Fund's Technical Board. The Board feared that the statements of the Society and its officers would sour prospects for the expansion of public health work not only in Cattaraugus County but elsewhere. It perceived that the opposition came from a highly vocal minority of local practitioners led by the President of the county medical society, who had been employed by the demonstration as director of the county laboratory. The Board through its prestigious members first tried direct negotiations and then conciliation through the state medical society.

It was in the midst of this controversy that Newsholme returned to Cattaraugus County in May 1928. He reported to the Milbank Officers and Technical Board that he thought the demonstration was well administered and that the opposition from a few practitioners would fade away. He counseled the Board to continue its work and to avoid responding to the polemics.[107] It was Newsholme's comments on this occasion that led John Kingsbury, Secretary of the Fund, to invite him to undertake a major study with Milbank sponsorship. As Kingsbury reminded him, Newsholme had asserted that "it is the doctors who are the real obstacle to the progress of public health."[108] Kingsbury apparently hoped that armed with

---

105 Arthur Newsholme, "The New York Health Demonstrations in Syracuse and in Cattaraugus County," *Milbank Memorial Fund Quarterly Bulletin,* 4 (Oct. 1926), 49–66; and Arthur Newsholme, *The New York Health Demonstrations in the City of Syracuse and in Cattaraugus County* (New York: Milbank Memorial Fund, [1927]). The notes for some of Newsholme's speeches on this trip may be seen in Newsholme Papers, FA: D2(8).

106 This episode may be followed in Sterling Memorial Library, Yale University, Milbank Memorial Fund Records, Series I, Technical Board Minutes, Box XI, Folder 77, 461–7 (15 Sept. 1927), 476–8 (20 Oct. 1927), 489–98 (9 Nov. 1927), 501–2 (21 Nov. 1927), 522–3 (15 Dec. 1927), 540–4 (16 Feb. 1928), 558–60 (19 April 1928), and 577–81 (13 May 1928).

107 Newsholme, *Last 30 Years,* 303–4; and Milbank Papers, Technical Board Minutes, Box XI, folder 77, 577–81 (13 May 1928).

108 Kingsbury to Newsholme, 9 Nov. 1935, Kingsbury Papers, B–16, folder 2. Newsholme's record of how the invitation came about was not so colorful, Newsholme, *Last 30 Years,* 303, 304. Kingsbury also linked these studies to the medical opposition to the New York Health Demonstrations in his foreword to each of the volumes of Newsholme, *International Studies.* See Newsholme, *International Studies,* I: 7.

information from Europe, Newsholme, the eminent British authority and advocate of state medicine, could demonstrate this fact and build a case for fundamental change that would carry weight in the American health care debate. Newsholme would spend most of the next four years on the project.

With Milbank support Newsholme visited thirteen continental countries as well as several sites in the British Isles during 1929 and early 1930. Most of those continental visits were made on a four-month tour by car in the spring of 1929.[109] On this trip the Newsholmes and their chauffeur were joined by a secretary who knew several European languages. Along the way he interviewed health officials, collected reports, and observed services and facilities. The visits were necessarily brief and confined for the most part to major cities. Newsholme recognized that it was risky to form judgments on the basis of such limited experience. He argued that their travel by car gave them a more intimate look at the lives of the people than they would have had by train, and here and on other occasions during his retirement he insisted that his experience in public health allowed him to quickly grasp the significance of what he observed.[110] The fact remains that the study was hurriedly prepared, and that the farther east he traveled the more dependent Newsholme was upon the accounts he was given by the officials he interviewed.

This investigation resulted in his three-volume *International Studies on the Relation between the Private and Official Practice of Medicine* which appeared in 1931 and his *Medicine and the State* which was published the following year. From the first these volumes were planned as a set. *International Studies* would present the facts, while *Medicine and the State* would interpret them in the light of current medical problems.[111] Each continental nation occupied a chapter in one of the first two volumes of *International Studies,* and in these chapters Newsholme presented his findings for each nation under similar headings: sickness insurance, hospitals, midwifery, infant and child welfare, school medical work, the prevention of tuberculosis, and the prevention of venereal disease. In short he used the British administrative categories for public medical work to judge continental health services. The third volume of *International Studies,* by far the largest, was devoted entirely to the British Isles, with twenty of the book's twenty-eight chapters dealing with England and Wales. As he struggled to finish these descriptive volumes, his *International Studies,* Newsholme confided in frustration to Welch that while the subject was of the utmost importance, he recognized that the books would be "open to the accusation of being dull reading."[112] The first two volumes are certainly open to that charge. The recital of programs, benefits, and administrative arrangements in one nation after another has a soporific effect on

---

109 For their itinerary, see Newsholme, *Last 30 Years,* 347–8. The date of Newsholme's visit is given at the beginning of each chapter in Newsholme, *International Studies.* See also Newsholme to Kingsbury, 11 Feb. 1929, Kingsbury Papers, B–16, Newsholme folder 1.

110 Newsholme, *Last 30 Years,* 347; Newsholme, "New York Health Demonstrations," 49; and Newsholme, *International Studies,* I: 11.

111 Newsholme, *International Studies,* I: 11.

112 Newsholme to Welch, 20 Feb. 1931, Welch Papers.

the reader. But volume 3 is of another character entirely. Newsholme was now on familiar ground, and he provided what is probably the best single account of British health services written in the thirties. The concluding volume, *Medicine and the State,* is the volume Kingsbury wanted, a book concise enough and sweeping enough in its generalizations to be read by policymakers and members of foundation boards. This volume, like the first three, was written with the editorial assistance of the Milbank staff, and during its writing Kingsbury urged Newsholme to make stronger statements.[113] Kingsbury and Newsholme solicited Welch, who had encouraged the Fund to support the project, to write the foreword even before he had seen the completed manuscript.[114] Some years later Newsholme would tell Kingsbury that he was "prouder" of this book "than any other literary work undertaken by me."[115]

Newsholme held that the greatest problem facing medicine in the immediate future was the problem of correlating private and public medical services.[116] The primary goal of these books was to demonstrate that Europe was solving this problem. While Newsholme was convinced that Europe could teach America some things on this score, he was not uncritical of what he found on the Continent. He found that in Germany there was strong opposition to the national sickness insurance scheme from some private practitioners, and he quoted at length from a work by one of the scheme's medical critics.[117] He also recognized that in some places, Hungary most notably, the private family doctor had almost ceased to exist, although he believed that this was the result of the nation's postwar economic and social crisis rather than competition from public services.[118] After the Great War Hungary had rapidly expanded its social insurance as a "bulwark against Bolshevism" at the expense of neglecting essential public health services; in the process it had created a top-heavy system with a huge bureaucracy and costly central institutions.[119] Europe's experience also showed that generous insurance benefits provided in an ill-considered way could be damaging to medical care. In Poland the free choice of doctor and the easy access to specialists at ambulatories (outpatient clinics) meant that there was little continuity of care, no follow-up of patients, and the work of family medicine was seriously undermined.[120]

While health care provisions varied widely from one Continental nation to another, and while there were serious faults in some systems, Newsholme believed that Europe's experience had an important lesson for America. If the health needs

---

113 Kingsbury to Newsholme, 30 Nov. 1931, Kingsbury Papers, B–16, Newsholme folder 1. In this letter Kingsbury also tells Newsholme about the discussion at the Fund of the forthcoming book's title.
114 Newsholme to Welch, 13 Feb. 1932, Welch Papers; Welch to Newsholme, 24 Feb. 1932, ibid.; and Newsholme to Welch, 26 Feb. 1932, ibid.
115 Newsholme to Kingsbury, 9 Nov. 1939, Kingsbury Papers, B–16, Newsholme folder 3.
116 Here Newsholme quoted C. V. Chapin. Newsholme, *Medicine and the State,* 225.
117 Newsholme, *International Studies,* I: 171–80.
118 Ibid., II: 174–5, 184–6, 188.   119 Ibid., 186, 188, 194–5.   120 Ibid., 218–19, 220.

of the wage-earning population in modern society were to be adequately met, state support of medical services was needed, either as subsidies to institutions and to voluntary insurance, as was the practice in the Netherlands, Denmark, and Sweden, or as contributions to a compulsory national insurance scheme, as was the rule in Eastern Europe.[121] He reverted again to an historic or evolutionary explanation. The advancement of civilization and the development of moral sensibility meant that two postulates were now almost universally accepted: First, "The health of every individual is a social concern and responsibility," and second, "Medical care in its widest sense for every individual is an essential condition of maximum efficiency and happiness in a civilized community."[122] The cost of care was simply beyond the means of ordinary families. Both basic humanitarian concerns and the social cost of preventable and neglected illness compelled the public to step into the gap. "Health is worth whatever expenditure is efficiently incurred in its maintenance or to secure its return."[123]

He defended the principle of insurance for medical care and the necessity of making its provision compulsory, adding that insurance schemes could be structured so as to curb waste or abuse and to encourage prevention.[124] But he worried now about the moral effects of health insurance, of inadvertently encouraging a "doctor-seeking habit," or of creating a false sense of security that would stifle "that spirit of adventure in man which is a main condition of mental and moral progress," of eroding "the element of venture and daring" that is "needed for fullness of manhood."[125] Structural checks would go some way to preventing such dependency or abuse, but alone they would never suffice. Success with social insurance depended on a high sense of responsibility in both providers and recipients. The final chapter of *Medicine and the State* was entitled "Medicine and Character." Here Newsholme relied on the evolution of public morality and social conscience not only to combat social disease but to serve as the final protector of social insurance.[126]

Europe's experience also demonstrated that under the influence of new knowledge and social needs the distinctions between curative and preventive and between private and public medicine were breaking down. For the majority of people curative medicine was no longer exclusively the preserve of private practitioners. Nor was preventive medicine exclusively the duty of public authorities. The family physician must remain, Newsholme claimed, the basis of the health care system, but already he was unable to meet all the medical needs of his patients.[127] In the future his work must be coordinated with that of public – that is, voluntary and official – agencies and be financed collectively.

121 Newsholme, *Medicine and the State,* 24. For specific arrangements, see Newsholme, *International Studies,* I: 19–111.
122 Newsholme, *Medicine and the State,* 29, 43–4. And for the following, see ibid., 58–9, 244–5, 253–4.
123 Ibid., 53.   124 Ibid., 108–15, 137–40, 141, 144–7.
125 Ibid., 68, 111.   126 Ibid., 283.   127 Ibid., 41–3, 222–4.

Newsholme was perfectly aware that private physicians objected to supervision or to health care initiatives by public authorities. While he was at the Local Government Board the establishment of local authority infant-welfare centers and tuberculosis dispensaries in some places was met by opposition from medical practitioners, especially when full-time salaried medical officers were hired.[128] In *Medicine and the State* he answered the alarmist predictions of local medical societies. Judging from European experience, the major threats to the private general practice of medicine came from hospitals and specialists and not from public health departments.[129] The work undertaken recently by maternal and infant-welfare centers, by tuberculosis dispensaries, by school medical services, and by venereal disease clinics had previously gone undone and would still be undone were it not for the initiative of health departments. In England, Newsholme claimed, private medical practice experienced a net gain from the work of these centers as undetected cases were discovered and referred to practitioners and as public education in connection with these public services increased demand for private medical services.[130] But Newsholme was clearly glossing over difficulties. It could be argued that affiliating general practitioners with local authority clinics would both stimulate medical interest in prevention and provide a means of coordinating some of the work of these practitioners. But Newsholme as a civil servant had been skeptical of the competence and cooperation of private practitioners and had pressed for the appointment of full-time, salaried medical officers. While at the L.G.B. he had resisted the appointment of private general practitioners on a part-time basis to fill positions in local authority clinics, and in retirement he continued to maintain that experience had proved that such part-time appointments had not worked successfully.[131]

Newsholme and the Milbank Fund tried to forestall a hostile reception from medical readers. Welch told Newsholme that while they both realized that Kingsbury was "particularly disturbed" by events in Cattaraugus County, he was pleased to see that Newsholme had not dwelt on this "ephemeral side of a big subject."[132] Privately to Welch, Newsholme explained that he had made only

---

128 For early hints of this opposition while the administration of the Sanatorium Benefit was still being discussed, see the transcript of an interview between Metropolitan M.O.H. and L.G.B. officials, 30 Sept. 1912, P.R.O., MH 55/528. For samples of the B.M.A.'s position on full-time medical officers at infant-welfare centers, see "Maternity and Child Welfare," *Br. Med. J.* (1916), no. 1: 280–1; and "Maternity, Child Welfare, and a Ministry of Health," ibid., 1917, no. 1: 430–1. For the conflict over the appointment of full-time school medical officers in Brighton after Newsholme's departure, see Newsholme, *International Studies,* III: 367–73.

129 Newsholme, *Medicine and the State,* 20–1, 79–80, 233.

130 Newsholme, *International Studies,* III: 190–2, 207–10; and Newsholme, *Medicine and the State,* 191, 192–3, 197–8, 233–7.

131 See, for example, Arthur Newsholme, "Memorandum on Health Visiting and on Maternity and Child Welfare Centres," Newsholme, *Ann. Rep. Med. Off. L.G.B.,* 44 (1914–15): 8. For his views in retirement, see Newsholme, *International Studies,* III: 190; and Newsholme, *Medicine and the State,* 192.

132 Welch to Newsholme, 24 Feb. 1932, Welch Papers.

"veiled" reference to the opposition from local medical societies.[133] In print he tried to represent the problem as one of false appearances. In America physicians' antipathy toward "politics," he suggested, had produced a quiescence on the part of the majority that had permitted a small minority of medical activists to gain control of local medical societies and to misrepresent the profession.[134] He was confident that American experience would mirror Britain's. In Britain, initial hostility from medical professionals had given way to cooperation and improved health. "The history is one of steady emergence from a relatively narrow 'trades-union' point of view to a statesmanlike position, in which endeavour is made to place first the welfare of patients and the public, and to utilise every medical practitioner as a unit in maintaining and advancing the common health."[135] The Milbank Fund press release for *Medicine and the State* assured American readers that while Newsholme used the term "state medicine," he was not "a revolutionary in thought" and expected changes to come gradually.[136] Newsholme prepared short summaries of his argument and conclusions for both British and American medical journals.[137] His article for the *Journal of the American Medical Association* used nine postulates to argue for the inevitability of socialized medicine. By socialization, he explained, he meant provision of medicine services by both voluntary contributions and state activity.[138]

In the end it was the more modest but better publicized recommendations of the Committee on the Cost of Medicine Care and not Newsholme's reports which touched off the storm of controversy. Newsholme kept abreast of the work of the C.C.M.C. and corresponded regularly with C.-E. A. Winslow, its Vice-Chairman and Chairman of its Executive Committee. He even offered the committee the mass of reports he had collected.[139] Newsholme found the C.C.M.C.'s majority report too timid. He complained to Winslow about the use of the term "group purchase" instead of "insurance," the heavy reliance on group practice rather than on technical assistance for the general practitioner through public means, and the minor role recommended for the state by the majority.[140] Winslow conceded the last point but added, "If you could measure the violence of the storm which is breaking as a result of our very moderate recommendations, I think you would realize that we have gone quite far enough ahead of current

133 Newsholme to Welch, 8 March 1932, Welch Papers.
134 Newsholme, *Medicine and the State*, 276.
135 Ibid., 276.
136 Milbank Memorial Fund press release, 9 May 1932, Milbank Papers, Series I, Box XXII, folder 176.
137 Arthur Newsholme, "Medicine and the State," *Medical Officer*, 44 (1930): 249–52; and Arthur Newsholme, "The Relationship of the Private Medical Practitioner to Preventive Medicine," *J. Am. Med. Assn.*, 98 (1932): 1739–43.
138 Newsholme, "Relation of the Private Medical Practitioner," 1741.
139 Newsholme to Winslow, 24 Dec. 1930, Winslow Papers; and Newsholme to Winslow, 18 Oct. 1931, ibid.
140 Newsholme to Winslow, 17 Nov. 1931, ibid.; Newsholme to Winslow, 9 Jan. [1933, incorrectly dated 1932], ibid.; Newsholme to Winslow, 25 Feb. [1933, incorrectly dated 1932], ibid. See also Winslow to Newsholme, 10 March 1933, ibid.

medical opinion."[141] Newsholme was often the one to urge moderation, but in this case he continued to hold that the committee's majority report was too cautious. No system of insurance for the majority of the population would work without substantial tax assistance, and he continued to be skeptical that privately organized group practices either would work efficiently or would avoid costly duplication with other private or public providers.[142] The majority report's fundamental flaw was that it did not grow naturally out of what had previously existed.

In this last point Newsholme was probably right. Yet we may wonder how well his own proposals met that criterion. He took Britain as his model, but he recognized full well how slowly most features of current British health care had evolved and how differently things were organized on the other side of the Atlantic. With the benefit of hindsight we may suggest that he failed to understand the American situation. He underestimated the strength of voluntarism in America – this in spite of the fact that he was closely affiliated with an important private philanthropy – and he overestimated the attractiveness of state initiatives in health care. While he had some appreciation of the fact that Americans did not hold local public officials in high esteem, he seems to have felt, curiously, that inviting American general practitioners to serve as Medical Officers of Health in their own practices would be a tempting proposition. And, of course, Newsholme did not yet fully appreciate the political power of organized medicine in America. He would gain a greater appreciation of that power over the next few years.

The appearance of *International Studies* and *Medicine and the State* led to a final and more exciting assignment from the Milbank Fund, a chance to observe health work in the great social experiment of the age, the Soviet Union. The invitation came in June 1932 from John Kingsbury, who was planning to attend an international tuberculosis conference in the Hague in September and wanted Newsholme to join him in observing the health care system of the U.S.S.R. the previous month.[143] Newsholme was at first reluctant to go. His wife Sara was suffering from heart disease and was in poor condition. On the trip he would fret about her condition and several times nearly return prematurely.[144] He initially also doubted the usefulness of such a visit. "Seriously I don't think that advanced civilizations like those of U.S., Germany and Gt Britn. can learn much from a country recently emerged from serfdom. . . ."[145] He would change his mind once he had been there. Finally he simply could not resist going.

Their journey in the Soviet Union took them some 9,000 miles in about four weeks during August and September 1932.[146] They traveled from Moscow to

141 Winslow to Kingsbury, 28 Jan. 1933, ibid.   142 Newsholme, *Last 30 Years*, 354–9.
143 Kingsbury to Newsholme, 23 June 1932, Kingsbury Papers, B–79, folder 3.
144 Newsholme reminded Kingsbury of this and of her insistence that he go in spite of family objections. Newsholme to Kingsbury, 25 Sept. 1933, ibid., folder 10; and Newsholme to Kingsbury, 14 Oct. 1933, ibid., folder 11.
145 Newsholme to Kingsbury, 5 July 1932, ibid., folder 3.
146 For a map of their itinerary, see Newsholme and Kingsbury, *Red Medicine*, 19. For a short description of their route, see Newsholme, *Last 30 Years*, 377–9.

Leningrad and back to Moscow and then on a great loop to the east as far as Kazan, where they took a river boat on the Volga for four days to Stalingrad. From Stalingrad they traveled overland in the Caucasus as far south as Tiflis, the Georgian capital, and then on to the Black Sea where they sailed along the coast to Yalta and Sevastopol in the Crimea. The final leg of their trip took them north through the Ukraine and central Russia back to Moscow. Along the way they received preferential treatment, and they recognized that they were being shown the best the system had to offer. They were met by local health and party officials. A car and interpreter were put at their disposal, and they were taken to points of interest: a polyclinic and Pavlov's laboratory in Leningrad, a factory hospital and polyclinic in Gorky; a state collective farm in Georgia; sanatoriums and rest homes in the former palaces and mansions of Yalta; and recreational facilities, hospitals, and central health institutions in Moscow. Fitting in so much travel in such a short period meant that they could seldom stay in one place for more than two or three days. Much of their information came from interviews with officials.[147] Since neither Westerner knew Russian, they were dependent on the interpreters their hosts provided. The two visitors soon recognized that some of their interpreters' command of English was not very good. They also began to suspect that the replies to their questions were being emended by the interpreters, all of whom were state officials and some of whom were members of the Communist Party.[148] Still the two trusted their ability to sift the evidence they were shown and to arrive at a good understanding of the nation's health and health care provisions. They also studied recent accounts of the Soviet experiment by other Western observers.[149]

The volume resulting from the Newsholme–Kingsbury visit was the joint effort of minds that brought different talents and political sympathies to the work. Kingsbury made the book accessible. He hired a medical editor to revise the manuscript and to help enliven its prose.[150] He also enlisted the services of Margaret Bourke-White, who took Kingsbury's list of suggestions to the Soviet Union and produced some stunning photographs for the book.[151] The finished product is the most popular of Newsholme's publications. It is entirely narrative with almost no use of statistics. The prose is lively, and the book sports an arresting title, *Red Medicine: Socialized Health in Soviet Russia.* Newsholme at first opposed the title and only became reconciled to it when he saw that it attracted atten-

147 See, for example, Newsholme and Kingsbury, *Red Medicine,* 20–4, 56, 222–25.
148 Ibid., 4, 5–6, 13, 44–6.
149 For some impression of the extent to which they considered the views of others, see Kingsbury to Newsholme, 11 July 1932, Kingsbury Papers, B–79, folder 3; Kingsbury to Newsholme, 6 Dec. 1932, ibid., folder 4; Newsholme to Kingsbury, 15 Dec. 1932, ibid., folder 4; Kingsbury to Newsholme, 27 Jan. 1933, ibid., folder 5; Kingsbury to Newsholme, 1 March 1933, ibid., folder 6;
150 Kingsbury to Newsholme, 30 Dec. 1932, ibid., folder 4.
151 Margaret Bourke-White to Kingsbury, 22 Nov. 1932, ibid., folder 1.

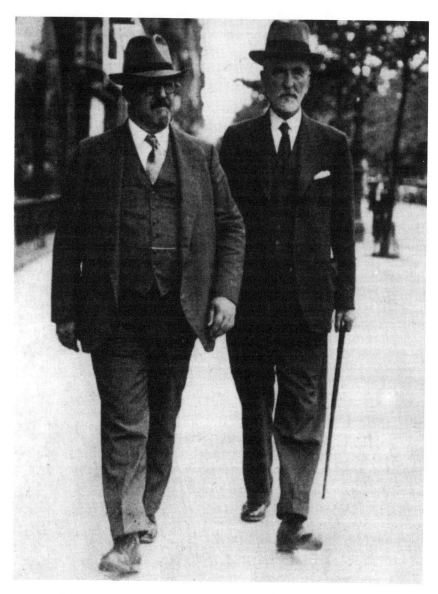

Illustration 12.1. Newsholme, on the right, and John Kingsbury in Berlin on their way to the Soviet Union, 1932. From Newsholme, *Last Thirty Years of Public Health,* facing p. 376.

tion.[152] He favored at first "Soviet Russia with Special Reference to Social Medicine,"[153] a title that shows perhaps the effects of a lifetime of reading blue books and M.O.H. annual reports.

There was much that the two Western observers could agree on. The Soviet Union had made remarkable progress in bringing a medically backward nation into the twentieth century. The scale and distribution of facilities, the expansion of the corps of health care workers, and the changes in the nation's vital statistics were all testimony to rapid modernization. They admired the Soviet goal of making comprehensive health care available to all as a basic government service in which the payment of fees and private profit had been banished.[154] They also could agree that many of the shortcomings they saw, shortages of doctors and supplies (especially in rural areas), poor dentistry, overwork and poor pay for doctors, were problems of development that would probably disappear with time. However, when it came to the Soviet system itself and the place of health services in it, the two parted company. Their differences are a microcosm of the liberal debate in the West over the Soviet experiment.

Kingsbury returned to America an admirer and in addresses began to use the Soviet example as a model of what could be accomplished if society collectively dedicated itself to improving its medical system. In November, after Kingsbury's return, Welch, whom Kingsbury had also invited to join the expedition to the U.S.S.R., arranged for Kingsbury to address the University Club at Johns Hopkins. Kingsbury talked for an hour and then talked even more enthusiastically for another hour about his slides. After the second hour he got some stiff questioning from faculty and from Senator Walcott. Kingsbury described the scene for Newsholme.

It was evident that there were doubting Thomases in this little after-meeting, doubtful indeed if I had really seen what I thought I had seen. Dr. Welch like a husky young football player took the ball on a forward pass and made touchdown after touchdown. He said to some of his colleagues on the Johns Hopkins faculty, "The trouble with you fellows is that you don't want to believe anything good about the Soviet system!" He repeatedly challenged them in this fashion and indeed, rebuked some of them for their closed minds. Wasn't this typical and yet extraordinary from a man of eighty-three?[155]

Winslow observed "John Kingsbury is so completely converted that it is difficult to get him to take much interest in anything less than a complete Soviet health program."[156]

152 Newsholme to Kingsbury, 8 Feb. 1933, ibid., folder 6; and Newsholme to Kingsbury, 16 April 1934, ibid., B–16, Newsholme folder 2.

153 Newsholme to Kingsbury, 18 April 1933, ibid., B–79, folder 7.

154 For these points of agreement, see Newsholme & Kingsbury, *Red Medicine*, 31, 212–13, 219, 265–71, 289–94.

155 Kingsbury to Newsholme, 6 Dec. 1932, Kingsbury Papers, B–79, folder 4. On Kingsbury's invitation to Welch to join the tour of the U.S.S.R., see Kingsbury to Newsholme, 11 July 1932, ibid., folder 3.

156 Winslow to Newsholme, Winslow Papers, 21 Dec. 1932, Winslow Papers.

Some of the criticism of the Soviet Union in the American press made Kingsbury bristle. Will Durant's articles in the *Saturday Evening Post,* for example, he considered "intellectually dishonest," and he denounced them in letters to Newsholme.[157] Kingsbury also discounted many of the stories of persecution in the Soviet Union, claiming to have learned from experience to distrust the accounts of Russian émigrés and the cabals of counterrevolutionaries in the United States, and here and on several other occasions he justified the use of harsh measures by quoting Sidney Webb, "Revolutions are like that." Need one look further, he asked, than the treatment of the Scottsboro boys or the Amritsar incident to show that "deplorable situations" can exist under American or British rule even without conditions of war and revolution?[158] In the later thirties, during the state trials and purges, Kingsbury would be convinced that the Soviet authorities had been compelled reluctantly to act by the existence of a huge "Trotsky-Fascist" conspiracy which threatened the existence of the new order.[159]

While Newsholme could share Kingsbury's admiration for the stated ends in the Soviet system, he had better instincts about Soviet means. He recognized that in Stalin's Russia not only were civil rights abused, but that the administrative system was so subservient to political ends that it was almost impossible to form an objective view of even basic economic or demographic conditions.

It is a very difficult thing to deal with a country which is determined to smash minorities, and which openly regards justice as a matter to be administered in the main with an eye to political ends. If to this is added justice administered secretly and without open trial, then even – as you know – Sidney Webb is obliged to protest.... Thanks for the Folio of Charts.... My difficulty is how far can we trust Russian statistics (Hello: *suspicious* again!!). If justice is regarded as a thing to be manipulated politically, why not also social statistics?[160]

Newsholme was horrified at the "class-hatred or at least class government, the constant preference to the worker, and the cruelty to the kulaks."[161]

Such differences were not easily reconciled, when it came time to write. By December 1932 Newsholme had prepared a first draft which Kingsbury considered unfair and unduly critical, and he insisted that Newsholme change it. He cited other Western authorities, most notably the Webbs, who had recently become ardent apologists for the Soviet Union, to convince Newsholme that he had misunderstood the Soviet system.[162] In the ensuing discussions the two compared their task to the painting of Oliver Cromwell's portrait. Newsholme

157 Kingsbury to Newsholme, 16 Dec. 1932 [appended to Kingsbury to Newsholme, 6 Dec. 1932], Kingsbury Papers, B–79, folder 4.
158 Kingsbury to Newsholme, 10 May 1933, ibid., folder 8.
159 Kingsbury to Newsholme, 11 Feb. 1937, ibid., B–16, Newsholme folder 3; and Kingsbury to Newsholme, 27 Jan. 1938, ibid.
160 Newsholme to Kingsbury, 18 April 1933, ibid., B–79, folder 7.
161 Newsholme to Kingsbury, 11 Jan. 1933, ibid., folder 5.
162 Kingsbury to Newsholme, 30 Dec. 1932, ibid., folder 4; Newsholme to Kingsbury, 31 Jan. 1933, ibid., folder 5; and Kingsbury to Newsholme, 27 Jan. 1933, ibid., folder 5.

insisted that the warts must be there.[163] Kingsbury claimed to have no objection to including the warts provided they belonged to their subject's face, but he saw no point in covering them with hair.[164] Under continual pressure from Kingsbury Newsholme rethought his account. In early February he went to see Harold Laski and the Webbs, and he submitted the manuscript with Kingsbury's objections to the Webbs for criticism.[165] Sidney Webb objected with particular vigor to Newsholme's comments on religious persecution and on the suppression of civil liberties, stoutly asserting that the Soviet Union was fundamentally no less democratic than the Western democracies. Newsholme's annotations show that he remained unconvinced.[166] "You escape scot free and are greatly praised," he told Kingsbury when he received the Webbs' critique, "I am wounded in many points, but not in any vital spot."[167] Newsholme was willing to defer to the Webbs' authority on Soviet government and administration, but he remained suspicious that their understanding was biased.

We must leave in warts here and there. That is my main dispute with Webb as I told him. On one point he has freely criticized the Russian system, i.e. for not allowing free discussion of the bigger issues; but apart from this – if I am to be frank – his articles in *Current History* give me the impression of suppression of unfavorable points, perhaps unconscious. I think we shall gain by avoiding this. Of course Webb's grasp of the governmental problem is exceptional and far-reaching, though here again I am not enamored like him of the machinery, unless administered by *ideal man*. It may very easily develop all the evils of the American Ward Boss system.[168]

Newsholme agreed to rewrite the work, narrowing his focus and toning down his criticism. Some weeks earlier Kingsbury had suggested a strategy for working out their differences. They should omit topics on which they strongly disagreed, unless the topic was really germane. During the rewrite he urged Newsholme to avoid comments on moral questions, a reference to Newsholme's objections to Soviet policy on divorce and abortion, or to "matters of administrative policy which have no direct bearing on our subject" including the confiscation of land and the treatment of the kulaks, but ironically he urged at the same time some discussion of Soviet advances in areas other than medicine: heavy industry, publishing, management of science.[169]

---

163 Newsholme to Kingsbury, 11 Jan. 1933, ibid., folder 5.
164 Kingsbury to Newsholme, 27 Jan. 1933, ibid., folder 5. For further rhetorical use of this analogy, see Newsholme to Kingsbury, 8 Feb. 1933, ibid., folder 6; Kingsbury to Newsholme, 20 Feb. 1933, ibid., folder 6; and Newsholme to Kingsbury, 3 March 1933, ibid., folder 5.
165 Newsholme to Kingsbury, 8 Feb. 1933, ibid., folder 6.
166 See Webb's annotations on the typescript draft, ibid., B–78, folder: *Red Medicine,* Notes by Sidney Webb: 49–50, 97–8.
167 Newsholme to Kingsbury, 16 Feb. 1933, ibid., B–79, folder 6.
168 Newsholme to Kingsbury, 3 March 1933, ibid.
169 Kingsbury to Newsholme, 1 March 1933, ibid. See also Kingsbury to Newsholme, 27 Jan. 1933, ibid., folder 5.

By April Newsholme had finished a new manuscript. Kingsbury would be pleased, he hoped, by his "total abstinence from moralizing." "It has been a struggle; but – unless you find an occasional 'slip' – I think I have been entirely 'objective.' "[170] Kingsbury sent the manuscript to two additional experts; he urged that a few more changes be made, and by June he realized that he had pushed Newsholme, who was having second thoughts about some of his concessions, as far as he could.[171] *Red Medicine* was ready for publication, some warts remaining.

The published work celebrates Soviet achievements in developing a comprehensive health system that united preventive and curative functions and was rapidly narrowing the gap between need and provision. It concluded, in fact, by judging Soviet medicine by two standards, the major deficiencies the final report of the Committee on the Cost of Medical Care had found in American medicine, and the postulates for a good health care system Newsholme had outlined in *Medicine and the State*. Kingsbury and Newsholme concluded that while Soviet medicine had not yet lived up to its promise, that promise placed it closer to realizing the ideals of state medicine than any other nation in the world.[172]

At the same time the book acknowledged some grave problems. Most serious, from a strictly medical standpoint, was the fact that a segment of the Soviet population was disenfranchised and not entitled to the services and benefits guaranteed to workers. These former bourgeois, landlords, nobles, kulaks, and tsarist officials were unlikely to have a ration card, to be entered on employment lists, or to receive advanced schooling. Kingsbury and Newsholme believed that these people eventually, although belatedly, received medical attention, although they conceded that they were unable to confirm this fact.[173] This is an instance of what Newsholme called class government, and it was symptomatic of other problems. Although the official Soviet line blaming the kulaks for the milk and meat shortages is repeated in the published volume, and the furiosity of some state actions is explained as the inevitable consequence of revolution, the text maintains that the Soviet secret police were as guilty of "secret and hateful operations" as the tsarist police, that "utter mercilessness" was used with the kulaks in the collectivism of land, and that a "war mentality" was maintained to keep people's enthusiasms at "fever heat."[174] Some of Newsholme's "moral" objections also remained. In a brief section the book mentions the State's suppression of religion and its attempts to elevate Bolshevism, "materialistic communism of an intolerant type," to the status of a quasireligion.[175]

To appreciate the salutary effect of Newsholme's caution one need only com-

---

170 Newsholme to Kingsbury, 1 April 1933, ibid., folder 7.
171 Victor O. Freebury to Newsholme, 13 June 1933, ibid., folder 9; Newsholme to Kingsbury, 27 May 1933, ibid., folder 8; and Kingsbury to Newsholme, 30 June 1933, ibid., folder 9.
172 Newsholme and Kingsbury, *Red Medicine*, 271–94.
173 Ibid., 189, 192–3, 225, 269–70, 276.
174 Ibid., 15, 77, 81, 83–4, 85, 94–6, 96–7.   175 Ibid., 131.

pare *Red Medicine* to other Western accounts that appeared before the Second World War. Perhaps the best comparison is to Henry Sigerist's *Socialized Medicine in the Soviet Union,* a work which, for all its author's interest and enthusiasm for the Soviet Union, was remarkably uncritical.[176] Newsholme wrote to Sigerist after the latter's book appeared, complimenting him on his production but chastising the author quite fairly for writing with a "missionary spirit" and for attempting to glorify the Soviet Union by belittling what was being done in the English-speaking world.[177] Seen in comparison, Newsholme and Kingsbury's book appears more remarkable for its caution and perceptiveness. Viewed from the perspective of nearly sixty years *Red Medicine* reflects not only the compromises worked out between its authors but more generally the ambivalence with which many liberals viewed the new Soviet State during the great depression. "Can a *modus vivendi* be found between the extremes of communism and the suicidal competitions of capitalist countries? The future of the world hangs largely on finding a satisfactory answer to this question."[178]

It is a tribute to Newsholme's and Kingsbury's mutual respect and affection that their friendship survived the ordeal of preparing *Red Medicine.* They in fact remained the closest of friends until Newsholme's death a decade later. Kingsbury expected a hostile reception to the book from organized medicine. The reviews, he told Newsholme, will be the occasion for another "brickbat to be hurled in my direction" from "my friend Fishbein," Morris Fishbein, the editor of the *Journal of the American Medical Association.*[179] In this prediction Kingsbury was correct.[180] But Kingsbury's outspoken defense of Soviet medicine continued, and he sometimes let his enthusiasm get the better of him, as at a talk in December 1933 before the League for Unity of the Medical Professions at the New School for Social Research. "Under the spell of that audience I cut loose a bit, and I must say they gave me a wonderful reception."[181] He made himself a target and something of a liability at the Milbank Fund. In April 1935 he was asked to resign.[182] As soon as Newsholme heard trouble was brewing, he wrote a sympathetic letter of advice. "Now as to your difficulties with the doctors – I want you to be willing to 'lie low' for a while. You may be reminded that this is a triangular affair." He drew a triangle with "Milbank Fund, espl. you" on one side, "The

176 Henry E. Sigerist, *Socialized Medicine in the Soviet Union* (New York: W. W. Norton, 1937). For a fine discussion of Sigerist's interpretation of Soviet medicine, see John Hutchinson, "Dances with Commissars: Sigerist and Soviet Medicine," in *Making Medical History: The Life and Times of Henry E. Sigerist,* ed. Elizabeth Fee and Theodore Brown, forthcoming.
177 Newsholme to Henry Sigerist, 9 Dec. 1937, Kingsbury Papers, B-19. See also Newsholme to Sigerist, 23 Nov. 1937, and Sigerist to Newsholme, 3 Dec. 1937, ibid.
178 Newsholme and Kingsbury, *Red Medicine,* 115.
179 Kingsbury to Newsholme, 13 Nov. 1933, Kingsbury Papers, B–79, folder 11.
180 Morris Fishbein, "The State and the Doctor," in *The Medical Profession and the Public: Currents and Counter-Currents containing Papers Read at a Joint Meeting of the College of Physicians of Philadelphia and the American Academy of Political and Social Science* (Philadelphia: 1934), 92.
181 Kingsbury to Newsholme, 16 Dec. 1933, Kingsbury Papers, B–79, folder 11.
182 Press Release 93, Milbank Papers, Series I, Box 22, folder 179.

organized trades Union of the Medl. Practitioners" on the second, and "The President's Policy." on the third. The doctors attack you, he advised Kingsbury, in trying to anticipate F.D.R.'s next move with his social security plan.[183] The following May Newsholme intervened to stop *The Lancet* from publishing an article critical of Kingsbury, explaining to Kingsbury that he wanted to avoid having him classed as an extremist so that F.D.R. might offer him an important post or so that after the storm blew over he might be reappointed at the Milbank Fund.[184]

Newsholme continued to share Kingsbury's bitterness over this dismissal and believed that his friend had been very badly treated.[185] However, the two continued to differ fundamentally about what the Soviet Union represented. "I know we disagree *toto caelo* in our views as to U.S.S.R.," Newsholme wrote to Kingsbury on one of many occasions that he gave advice on a manuscript.[186] His advice on these occasions shows us that their differences were matters of temperament as well as substance. Newsholme criticized Kingsbury's propensity for making statements which he should know would "arouse antagonism" and prevent readers from taking his case seriously. "A first class case such as you have in your paper, always gains *by understatement*. The classical instance of this is Baldwin's speech on [the abdication of King] Edward, which carried the whole British nation with him."[187]

Despite all his reservations about the Soviet health care system, Newsholme continued to hold that it had a lesson for the West. Together with his study of the continental health care systems, his trip to the Soviet Union had shown him that during his lifetime scientific and political change had created a new public health agenda, a State obligation to promote the health of all of its people, not merely to prevent specific diseases. The Soviet Union was the first country to recognize and to officially accept this change and to commit the state to its furtherance. "It is futile to minimise this by saying that in many parts of the U.S.S.R. the ideal has not been fulfilled. In *many other parts it has;* and the great fact is that the *means of its universal accomplishment exist in U.S.S.R. and nowhere else.* Take for instance V.D. where England approaches most nearly to U.S.S.R., and U.S.A. lags twenty (possibly it will be fifty) years behind."[188]

For the remainder of Newsholme's life, the two friends corresponded about international affairs and medical policy. They continued to have high hopes for the New Deal. When F.D.R. regularized trade relations with the Soviet Union, Newsholme showered the President with rare, from him, praise.

183 Newsholme to Kingsbury, 15 April 1935, Kingsbury Papers, B–16, Newsholme folder 2.
184 Newsholme to Kingsbury, 20 May 1936, ibid.
185 Newsholme to Kingsbury, 4 Sept. 1935, ibid; Kingsbury to Newsholme, 9 Nov. 1935, ibid.; and Newsholme to Kingsbury, 27 Nov. 1935, ibid.
186 Newsholme to Kingsbury, 8 Feb. 1938, ibid., Newsholme folder 3. Note that there are two letters with this date.
187 Newsholme to Kingsbury, 8 Feb. 1938, ibid. See both letters of this date.
188 Newsholme to Kingsbury, 1 March 1937, ibid.

What a wonderful man he is! So far he has successfully initiated a social revolution *by consent.* I hope this may continue. It is (next to U.S.S.R.) the biggest social experiment in history; and, unlike Russia, no force is involved. How different from Poland, Italy, and Germany! If it can be continued without infringing the principle of representative government (not necessarily in its present form, in which too often it is pseudo-representation) it will be an unequalled contribution to civilization. In Britain a somewhat similar evolution is taking place; but we crawl, while you jump![189]

They continued to hope in vain that Roosevelt would champion national health insurance. In June 1937 Kingsbury reported that the A.M.A., which Newsholme had christened a "self-centered ring of obstruction" was running scared and feared that F.D.R. would be their Lloyd George.[190] The next year when he heard that F.D.R. had appointed a committee, Newsholme thought this might be the signal that the Administration was going to act on health insurance. He added

It is a strange anomaly that over here the B.M.A. are once more pleading for extension of medical attendance under an insurance system for all with an income of less than £250 . . . while with you there is still the problem of the initial step. . . . But that will come soon.[191]

In the last year of his life Newsholme saw the Beveridge Report, and he wrote to Kingsbury in January 1943 endorsing its recommendations and praising its author.[192]

The decade between *Red Medicine* and the Beveridge Report was a time of increasing loneliness for Newsholme. It began with a terrible blow when Sara, his wife of fifty-two years, died of heart disease.[193] It continued with the loss of friends and members of his household and toward the end was exacerbated by his failing health and wartime restrictions on travel.[194] In the middle thirties he took William Henry Welch's advice and turned for therapy to writing his reminiscences. *Fifty Years in Public Health,* a volume that traced his career until he entered the Local Government Board, appeared in 1935. The sequel, *The Last Thirty Years in Public Health,* was published a year later.

This autobiographical pair was not his first venture into history. In the late twenties, perhaps encouraged by the example of Welch, the great partisan of

189 Newsholme to Kingsbury, 26 March 1934, ibid., Newsholme folder 2.
190 Newsholme to Homer Folks, 22 May 1937, ibid., Newsholme folder 3; and Kingsbury to Newsholme, 18 June 1937, ibid.
191 Newsholme to Kingsbury, 21 July 1838, ibid.
192 Newsholme to Kingsbury, 28 Jan. 1943, ibid. See also Janet Beveridge to Newsholme, 2 March 1943, ibid.
193 For Newsholme's terrible sense of loss, see Newsholme to Winslow, 24 Sept. 1933, Winslow Papers; Newsholme to Kingsbury, 24 Sept. 1933, Kingsbury Papers, B79, Folder 10; and Newsholme to Welch, 26 Sept. 1933, Welch Papers.
194 See, for example, his response to the discovery that his housekeeper had advanced breast cancer, in Newsholme to Kingsbury, 13 Dec. 1936, Kingsbury Paper, B–16, Newsholme folder 2. See also Newsholme to Kingsbury, 30 June 1937, ibid., Newsholme folder 3.

medical history whom he had seen interjecting historical examples into faculty discussions, Newsholme produced a two-volume general history of public health.[195] The results were not very satisfactory. *The Evolution of Preventive Medicine* and *The Story of Modern Preventive Medicine* are uninspired compilations, elementary and derivative, and need not be further noticed. *Fifty Years in Public Health* and *The Last Thirty Years in Public Health,* however, are much more useful. They contain information about Newsholme's early life and career which is available in no other place, but they leave the contemporary reader disappointed. The volumes were obviously written in haste without aids to memory other than a collection of reprints and a couple of travel diaries. Even more disappointing is Newsholme's reserve about past controversy and his deference to the sensibilities and reputations of former associates and their families. Soon after finishing *The Last Thirty Years,* Newsholme told Homer Folks that he had felt obliged to leave out much of what he would like to have written.[196] These two books do lack the detail, vividness, and candor of the good eyewitness account, and they add very little to the picture of the political and personal dynamics within either Whitehall or Town Hall than can be pieced together from public records. Following their publication he gave a few addresses, and one of these was published.[197] But the autobiography was for all intents and purposes his final public word.

By the late thirties he was suffering from high blood pressure, and his activities were more restricted. He made his final visit to America in the winter of 1937–8, living in Southern California. Thereafter he spent most of his time at home in Worthing on the Sussex Coast reading, writing letters, and entertaining occasional houseguests. Travel to London was now only for special events such as Beatrice Webb's eightieth birthday celebration at the London School of Economics.[198]

He retained a sense of civic responsibility and a desire to be useful. As war approached, at the age of eighty-two, he volunteered for service in civilian hospitals.[199] He was never called. He was assigned the task of housing a mother and four children from London during the conflict. He would have undertaken the assignment, but his doctor intervened to prevent it.[200] He stayed at home and recorded watching the dogfights over the coast and hearing bombs explode.[201] Throughout his nation's horrible struggle Newsholme remained cheerful and optimistic. He was confident not only of the eventual victory of the Allies but

---

195 Arthur Newsholme, *Evolution of Preventive Medicine* (Baltimore: Williams and Wilkins, 1927); and Arthur Newsholme, *The Story of Modern Preventive Medicine, Being a Continuation of the Evolution of Preventive Medicine* (Baltimore: Williams and Wilkins, 1929).
196 Newsholme to Homer Folks, 22 May 1937, Kingsbury Papers, B–16, Newsholme folder 3.
197 Newsholme, "Health Department in the Field of Medicine."
198 Webb, Diary, 19 May 1938, 52: 6479.
199 Newsholme to [Mabel] Kingsbury, 27 Jan. 1939, Kingsbury Papers, B–16, Newsholme folder 3.
200 Newsholme to John [Kingsbury], 9 Nov. 1939, ibid. See also Newsholme to Kingsbury, 31 Dec. 1938, ibid.
201 Newsholme to Kingsbury, 13 Sept. 1940 and 13 Nov. 1940, ibid.

confident that it would soon be possible to banish both war and poverty.[202] His letters to the Kingsburys became particularly affectionate during the war. He told them several times that he did not expect to see the war's end, and so he had no hope of ever seeing them again. In February 1941 his letters had begun to arrive typed or in another's hand writing, and as the months passed his signature gradually grew more illegible. By early 1943 it had become indecipherable, the obvious product of tortured effort. He died on May 17, 1943, at the age of eighty-six. His passing was marked in a modest way. He had outlived most of his generation and many of his younger colleagues, and his nation was preoccupied with war.

202 Newsholme to Kingsbury, 8 June 1919 and 30 March 1943, ibid.

13

Assessments of a career

During the last forty years several preoccupations have driven historians to examine the work of public health authorities in Britain. Most recently it has been the effort to explain the fall in mortality during the nineteenth century. The issue has been raised in its contemporary form by the well-known works of Thomas McKeown and associates, who grant to conscious human intervention – clinical medicine, public health, or social welfare – only a small part in the mortality decline before the twentieth century.[1] While conceding that the construction of sewage systems, the provision of protected water supplies, and vaccination for smallpox had some effect on human mortality and suggesting that spontaneous changes in the virulence of its agent accounted for the diminished mortality from scarlet fever, these authors have argued that only improvements in the standard of living, especially in nutrition, could account for the magnitude of the mortality decline. For some years historians accepted this analysis with little question, showing particular appreciation for McKeown's demonstration that clinical intervention could not possibly account for mortality decline on such a scale.[2] But recently they have turned their attention to the most debatable part of McKeown's thesis, the role played by mass intervention by public authorities.[3] So important has this issue become, that it dominates the

1 Thomas McKeown and R. G. Record, "Reasons for the Decline of Mortality in England and Wales during the Nineteenth Century," *Population Studies,* 16 (1962): 94–122; Thomas McKeown, "Medicine and World Population," *J. Chronic Diseases,* 18 (1965): 1076–7; Thomas McKeown, *The Role of Medicine: Dream, Mirage, or Nemesis?* (Princeton, N.J.: Princeton Univ. Press, 1979).
2 For an application of McKeown's analysis to America, see Judith Walzer Leavitt and Ronald L. Numbers, "Sickness and Health in America," in *Sickness and Health in America: Readings in the History of Medicine and Public Health,* ed. Leavitt and Numbers (Madison: Univ. of Wisconsin Press, 1978), 3–10; and Ronald L. Numbers, "History of Medicine: A Field in Ferment," *Reviews in American History;* 10 (1982), 259. For a more critical early use of McKeown's argument, see Robert Woods and John Woodward, "Mortality, Poverty and the Environment," in *Urban Disease and Mortality in Nineteenth-Century England,* ed. Woods and Woodward (London: Batsford Academic and Educational Press, 1984), 29–33.
3 Bill Luckin, "Evaluating the Sanitary Revolution: Typhus and Typhoid in London, 1851–1900," in *Urban Disease and Mortality in Nineteenth-Century England,* ed. Robert Woods and John Woodward (London: Batsford Academic and Educational Press, 1984), 102–19; Anne Hardy, "Urban Famine or Urban Crisis? Typhus in the Victorian City," *Medical Hist.,* 32 (1988): 401–25; Simon Szreter, "The Importance of Social Intervention in Britain's Mortality Decline c. 1850–1914: A Re-interpretation

discussion of public health in the new *Cambridge Social History of Britain*.[4] For England and Wales some of the most interesting recent work is by Simon Szreter and Anne Hardy.[5] They question McKeown's assumptions, criticize his exclusive reliance on national mortality figures, and contest his reading of those trends, particularly for tuberculosis, his key example, and argue that the work of local authorities in disease prevention was not only an important but a decisive component in the improvement of health that occurred after 1870.

One value of the work of Szreter and Hardy is that it changes the focus of historical discussions of public health to the period after 1870, when, they argue, the effects of public intervention are manifest, and to the local level, where such intervention was undertaken with great variation from local authority to local authority. Neither this period nor local public health initiatives have been emphasized in the historical literature until very recently. It is true, however, that the best general account of the history of public health in nineteenth-century Britain, Anthony Wohl's *Endangered Lives*,[6] anticipated both emphases, and that valuable monographs with both a local focus and an emphasis on the period after 1870 appeared thirty years or more ago.[7] But the terms in which the history of public health is considered are changing. Hardy's monograph on the experience of the Metropolitan local authorities is a particularly ambitious analysis of public initiatives and mortality trends that will undoubtedly be emulated in studies of other places. While this investigation of Newsholme's career was not undertaken to test the McKeown thesis, it has led me to agree that McKeown probably undervalued local authorities' public health initiatives in the late nineteenth century. No one, of course, would argue that Brighton in this period was a typical county borough. It was uncommonly prosperous, and it had especially strong social and professional ties to the Metropolis. It had an unusually high stake in a reputation for salubrity and, by the eighties, a Town Council committed to protecting that reputation. It also had in Arthur Newsholme an unusually active and able Medical Officer of Health. Brighton's Sanitary Department was certainly one of the administrative success stories of late-nineteenth-century public health. If not typical, Brighton's experience at least stands as an important example of what was possible for provincial local authorities.

of the Role of Public Health," *Social Hist. Med.*, 1 (1988), 1–37; Leonard G. Wilson, "The Historical Decline of Tuberculosis in Europe and America: Its Causes and Significance," *J. Hist. Med.*, 45 (1990): 366–96; Anne Hardy, *The Epidemic Streets: Infectious Disease and the Rise of Preventive Medicine, 1856–1900* (Oxford: Clarendon Press, 1993).

4 Virginia Berridge, "Health and Medicine," in *The Cambridge Social History of Britain, 1750–1950*, ed. F.M.L. Thompson (Cambridge: Cambridge Univ. Press, 1990) III, 191–203.

5 See esp. Hardy, *Epidemic Streets*; and Szreter, "Importance of Social Intervention."

6 Anthony S Wohl, *Endangered Lives: Public Health in Victorian Britain* (Cambridge, Mass.: Harvard Univ. Press, 1983).

7 William M. Frazer, *Duncan of Liverpool. Being an Account of the Work of Dr. W. H. Duncan Medical Officer of Health of Liverpool 1847–1863* (London: Hamish Hamilton, 1947); and Jeanne L. Brand, *Doctors and the State: The British Medical Profession and Government Action in Public Health, 1870–1912* (Baltimore: Johns Hopkins Univ. Press, 1965).

After a difficult political struggle Brighton began to improve its sewerage and water supply in the 1870s, and its typhoid mortality began the gradual, irregular decline that we would expect to follow the piecemeal improvement of these services. (See Illustration 5.1.) During Newsholme's tenure the town acted to improve the urban environment in other ways as well – through improved garbage collection (scavenging) and refuse removal, through closer supervision of the quality of foods sold in town, and through its early slum clearance projects. What is particularly interesting in the light of Szreter's and Hardy's reassessment is the evidence of how regularly Brighton's households, particularly working-class households, came in contact with the Sanitary Department. This contact was not confined to regular inspection of physical facilities – plumbing, water supply, complaints of nuisances, elimination of cesspools – although that work occupied a great deal of the Department's energy. It also included visits to every household following a death from a disease recognized as communicable and following every report of a notifiable disease. Such visits might result in orders for cleansings and disinfection, in the vaccination of contacts or in their temporary barring from school or from certain trades, or in the identification of new cases who might be removed to the isolation hospital or referred to a private physician or to the Sussex County Hospital. These visits also did much to expand Newsholme's appreciation of how infection spread in the community, and they eventually provided the basis for a system of surveillance which served as an early warning of dangers that might call for immediate action, such as the banning of the sale of milk from a certain farm. The Sanitary Department also made some attempt to change human behavior through its contacts with households. Its annual distribution of pamphlets on infant care and summer diarrhea, the instruction, supplies, and supervision that it gave to tuberculosis patients and their families, and its enforcement of the bylaws on subletting and overcrowding are obvious examples. I have made no attempt to estimate quantitatively the effect of such efforts on Brighton's morbidity and mortality, but the similarity of these activities to those Anne Hardy has found to have had a beneficial impact on mortality in the Metropolis is striking and highly suggestive.

Although Newsholme's career in Brighton is testimony to the breadth, vigor, and consistency of effort by some local authorities, it also demonstrates some of the barriers that existed to effective intervention. Some of these barriers were legal. Newsholme could not obtain authority, for example, to ban the sale of shellfish obtained from sewage-contaminated water, although he had reason to believe that their sale was responsible for serious illness in his town. Nor was he able to acquire authority to improve poor housing on a house-by-house basis as he wished. Other barriers were imposed by limitations of knowledge. Brighton failed in its attempt to control scarlet fever by isolating cases, because its officials did not understand the cause of the disease and could not accurately identify who was infected. Similarly, it is clear that Newsholme initially overestimated the benefit a tuberculosis patient would experience from a short period in a sanatorium, although his continued claim of public benefit from the instruction patients received in the institution is harder to assess. Finally, like all local authorities, Brighton lacked the resources and the will to confront adequately the housing problems its poorest citizens faced. In the short run its slum improvement projects seem to have forced those living in the worst conditions into even more crowded housing.

I fully endorse the suggestion that public health be studied through the work of local authorities, and I find Arthur Newsholme's career in Brighton every bit as illuminating as his tenure in Whitehall. His experience in Brighton illustrates how a successful public health program could be constructed. While the administrative history of the central health authority in the nineteenth century has been fairly well documented, we know much less about how local health authorities conducted their business. Newsholme's example makes it clear that in spite of familiar handicaps under which local health authorities worked – the absence of much compulsory health legislation, the lack of tenure for provincial M.O.H., local opposition to increases in the rates, and substantial protection for private property in law and administrative tradition, and so on – it is obvious that an M.O.H. of the late nineteenth century could innovate and act on a broad front, provided he could retain the support of his Sanitary Committee and Council. However, as Newsholme's conflict with the butchers shows, even comparatively secure M.O.H. could be vulnerable to pressure from vested interests.

Newsholme was certainly fortunate in his choice of local authority, but he was also a highly effective administrator. He cultivated the trust of his Committee and Council, and in Committee meetings and privately, always without public rancor, he applied continuous pressure for an incremental expansion of services. He was convincing because he could explain his preventive strategy in terms that were generally comprehensible and because he could regularly exhibit to Councillors and Aldermen improving mortality and morbidity rates. His frugality as an administrator certainly pleased his political superiors. Over the course of his career he significantly expanded the services his department offered with almost no increase in the size of his staff except at the borough sanatorium. He recognized the importance of marshaling professional authority in support of his programs. His own rise in the public health world was a help, and he was careful to bring to the attention of his Committee the signs of his professional recognition. He also learned the power of local example, and when he encountered opposition to his proposals, he gathered evidence from fellow M.O.H. of local authorities which had enacted the measure he was advocating. Closer to home, he cultivated good relations with local medical practitioners. He was assisted immensely in his relations with both the Council and with the local medical profession by the warm support he received from Joseph Ewart, among the most prominent medical men in the county and in turn Councillor, Alderman, and Mayor of Brighton. On more than one occasion Ewart proved a critical ally. Newsholme was careful to avoid antagonizing local practitioners. He participated in local medical society meetings, and he tried to ease practitioners' anxieties over innovations that his department sought. When a practitioner did not comply with the law (the issue was most often the failure to notify an infectious disease), Newsholme dealt with the matter privately and in a nonadversarial manner. He left Brighton before the opening of local authority clinics placed much greater strain on relations between health departments and local practitioners. He, of course, would do much to encourage the establishment of these clinics, and he grew very resentful of organized medicine's opposition. But that alienation was in the future.

While in Brighton, Newsholme expanded the scope of public health work in three principal directions. First, he worked to complete the original sanitary campaign against filth and organic waste by banishing cesspools from Brighton, by campaigning for a municipal destructor, or incinerator, and for better refuse collection; by enforcing higher environmental standards on places where animals were slaughtered and butchered; and by lobbying for a municipal abattoir under the continuous supervision of the Sanitary Department. Second, he enlarged the Sanitary Department's concern for infected food by initiating campaigns against tuberculous meat, sewage-contaminated shellfish, and milk contaminated by the unknown agent of scarlet fever. This work was more difficult than the first type of sanitary work both because the risk of consuming such food was neither certain nor uncontested and because, in acting against such risks, Newsholme needed to extend his authority beyond his town's boundaries and in so doing challenged the jurisdiction of neighboring local authorities and threatened strong commercial interests. It is testimony to his tenacity that he succeeded with milk and meat. Control of the sale of oysters eluded him. Third, and most important, under his tenure the Sanitary Department focused its attention to an increasing degree on infected individuals. Such new work was made possible by the adoption of compulsory notification of infectious diseases and by the system of voluntary notification of tuberculosis that Newsholme initiated in Brighton. Notification not only made possible surveillance of infection and tracing of cases, but it added weight to the strategy of preventing disease by treating it. The most tangible example of the Sanitary Department's expanded agenda is the reconstruction and increased use of the borough sanatorium. The changing mix of cases in the Sanatorium mirrors both local morbidity trends and the changes in the Sanitary Department's focus as the old scourges, smallpox, typhus, and typhoid, declined.

Local authorities not only acted on opportunities provided by permissive legislation and according to instructions sent to them by the central health authority, but they also cultivated new ideas and initiated programs that were later adopted by the nation. In Newsholme's career we can see how his publicizing within the M.O.H. world the hazards of sewage-contaminated shellfish led local authorities to pressure the Local Government Board to investigate this problem and to seek a remedy. Newsholme's career illustrates the way that local experience could help shape national health policy. He was unique in coming to the post of Medical Officer of the L.G.B. after serving as an M.O.H. for more than two decades, and several policy innovations he supported in Whitehall bear the mark of his local experience. The best example is probably his plan for a national tuberculosis service that owed much to what had been accomplished in Brighton. But in a more fundamental way, the tuberculosis program in Brighton seems to have served as the inspiration for his general goal of establishing unified, local medical systems under the supervision of M.O.H.

The recent historical interest in the work of local health authorities is a departure from the dominant scholarly tradition of the last forty years. Most studies of public health in that period have had a national or central focus. This was true of the influential biographies of pioneer administrators Edwin Chadwick or John Simon[8] and the studies of the central health authorities that they served.[9] Some of the most influential of this work has been inspired by an interpretation of administrative history most often associated with the work of Oliver MacDonagh.[10] MacDonagh found in the growth of nineteenth-century government a self-generating process led not by politicians, intellectuals, or moralists but by bureaucrats. Once in place, the inspectorate identified problems and proposed new legislative remedies which often resulted in more regulation and inspection and in an expansion of the civil service. It has been a very influential historical explanation. Royston Lambert's biography of John Simon and Roy McLeod's studies of the Local Government Board and of the Alkali Act Administration are examples of studies of public health and state medicine that were conceived within this framework.[11]

More recently historians have begun to question the adequacy of the model. Some have emphasized that even in the early and middle Victorian years, cultural and political forces were important in the growth of government's role in the public health.[12] MacDonagh's explanation is even less adequate for developments

8 S. E. Finer, *The Life and Times of Sir Edwin Chadwick* (London: Methuen, 1952); R. A. Lewis, *Edwin Chadwick and the Public Health Movement 1832–1854* (London: Longmans, Green, 1952); Anthony Brundage, *England's 'Prussian Minister': Edwin Chadwick and the Politics of Government Growth 1832–1854* (University Park: Pennsylvania State Univ. Press, 1988); Royston Lambert, *Sir John Simon 1816–1904 and English Social Administration* (London: MacGibbon and Fee, 1963).

9 C. Fraser Brockington, *Public Health in the Nineteenth Century* (Edinburgh and London: E. and S. Livingstone, 1965); Roy M. MacLeod, "The Anatomy of State Medicine: Concept and Application," in *Medicine and Science in the 1860s: Proceedings of the Sixth British Congress on the History of Medicine,* ed. F.N.L. Poynter (London: Wellcome Institute of the History of Medicine, 1968), 199–227; Roy M. MacLeod, "The Frustration of State Medicine, 1880–1899," *Medical Hist.,* 11 (1967): 15–40.

10 Oliver MacDonagh, "The Nineteenth-Century Revolution in Government: A Reappraisal," *Historical J.,* 1 (1958): 52–67; Oliver MacDonagh, *A Pattern of Government Growth, 1800–1860: The Passenger Acts and Their Enforcement* (London: MacGibbon and Kee, 1961); and Oliver MacDonagh, *Early Victorian Government 1830–1870* (New York: Holmes and Meier, 1977).

11 Lambert, *Sir John Simon;* Roy M. MacLeod, *Treasury Control and Social Administration: A Study of Establishment Growth at the Local Government Board 1871–1905,* Occasional Papers on Social Administration, no. 23 (London: G. Bell, 1968); and Roy M. MacLeod, "The Alkali Acts Administration, 1863–84: The Emergence of the Civil Scientist," *Victorian Studies,* 9 (1965): 85–112.

12 Pat Thane, "Government and Society in England and Wales, 1750–1914," in *The Cambridge Social History of Britain 1750–1950,* ed. F.M.L. Thompson (Cambridge: Cambridge Univ. Press, 1990), III, 18–21; and Brundage, *England's 'Prussian Minister.'*

in the late nineteenth and early twentieth centuries. There is much evidence that after 1870 civil servants played a less creative role in social policy; in fact it seems that in the Departments most involved with that policy, the Board of Education, the Home Office, and the L.G.B., specialist officials were denied access to policy makers and that senior officials in those Departments were quite resistant to change.[13]

Newsholme's public career demonstrates that there is much room for historical disagreement over the role of administrators in policy innovation in the late nineteenth and early twentieth centuries. Administrators could still exert considerable influence on policy. In Brighton Newsholme expanded municipal health services beyond recognition, seizing opportunities as they presented themselves and proposing pragmatic solutions to problems he could convince his Committee really existed. In Whitehall the career of Robert Morant, especially his role in framing the Education Act of 1902 and in establishing the School Medical Service, is likewise testimony to the force of strong civil servants in national policy formation. Once at the Local Government Board Newsholme worked to develop incrementally a national tuberculosis program using not fresh legislation but administrative means, the extension of existing legislation by administrative order. The innovative process for the tuberculosis program was characterized by a feedback mechanism in which local reaction to each stage was used to gauge whether the nation was ready for the next stage. But this deliberate, piecemeal administrative process was derailed by Lloyd George's National Health Insurance scheme. Furthermore, the Chancellor was not acting on a blueprint drawn up for him by the Department most interested in the issue to be addressed with legislation. In fact he kept that Department in the dark until the bill was nearly ready for presentation to the Cabinet. He found his own experts to design his scheme, and they worked under his direct supervision. Driven by political considerations, what is more, he did not rely on the established Department to administer the new insurance benefits but created a new, ad hoc, administration.

Far from being in control of changes in social policy during Newsholme's tenure in Whitehall, the civil servants of the L.G.B. were often playing catch-up – trying to secure first modification of the national insurance bill, then trying to implement the Sanatorium Benefit in ways that would not be merely a sham, then struggling to maintain local services during conditions of war, battling to protect their territory from an administrative rival, and jockeying themselves in preparation for the creation of the Ministry of Health. During the years of the Liberal government's social legislation, 1906–14, political forces dominated social policy formation, and then during the First World War, Lloyd George's preference to consult and to deal directly with interested parties was further strengthened by the

---

13 R. Davidson and R. Lowe, "Bureaucracy and Innovation in British Welfare Policy 1870–1945," in *The Emergence of the Welfare State in Britain and Germany,* ed. W. J. Mommsen (London: Croom Helm, 1981), 264–5, 269–72.

national emergency conditions.[14] One result was the weakening of the power of established bureaucracies to make policy innovations.

But to argue that under the Liberal Governments after 1906 and the wartime Coalition Government, civil servants were not the dominant force in policy innovation or in the growth of government is not to deny their force in social policy. Legislation must be implemented after all, and in that sphere civil servants continued to exercise great influence. Furthermore, the Medical Department of the Local Government Board continued to innovate using administrative means. Three new national medical services, for tuberculosis, for venereal disease, and for infant welfare, appeared during Newsholme's tenure at the L.G.B. Civil servants planned as well as administered all three programs, although political developments, the passage of National Insurance in particular, and wartime conditions had a strong influence on the shape these programs finally assumed. Of the three new services only the venereal disease service was planned de novo and initiated by special legislation. The other two depended on local experience and were begun by applying existing legislation, although their expansion was made possible with the assistance of special Exchequer grants.

The venereal disease service is the one least studied by historians and only now is attracting attention.[15] It is also the one which experts, such as Newsholme, had the greatest hand in shaping. Emergency wartime conditions and anxiety over the return of thousands of infected soldiers meant that the recommendations of the Royal Commission were enacted without the compromise and accommodation that usually accompanied policy formation, and that the service was speedily begun. In creating a service in which treatment was recognized as an essential part of prevention and in providing specialist diagnosis and treatment that was confidential, free of cost, and available regardless of place of residence through local authority clinics under the control of the M.O.H., the venereal disease service came the closest to realizing Newsholme's idea of what health services should look like under a unified local authority medical system. It is little wonder then that in retirement Newsholme was proudest of the venereal disease service.[16]

The state's tuberculosis program has fared rather badly at the hands of historians in recent studies.[17] It is blamed for devoting too many of its resources to building

---

14 John Turner, " 'Experts' and Interests: David Lloyd George and the Dilemmas of the Expanding State, 1906–19," in *Government and Expertise: Specialists, Administrators and Professionals, 1860–1919,* ed. Roy MacLeod (Cambridge: Cambridge Univ. Press, 1988), 205–23.

15 Recently the service has received some historical attention. See David Evans, "Tackling the 'Hideous Scourge': The Creation of the Venereal Disease Treatment Centres in Early Twentieth-Century Britain," *Social Hist. Med.,* 5 (1992): 413–33.

16 It was, for example, his favorite example of the superiority of British services to those available in America. See Newsholme, *Last 30 Years,* 367–70. See also Newsholme to Kingsbury, 1 March 1937, Kingsbury Papers, B–16, Newsholme folder 3; and Newsholme to Homer Folks, 22 May 1937, ibid.

17 F. B. Smith, *The Retreat of Tuberculosis 1850–1950* (London: Croom Helm, 1988), 103–8, 130, 238–9, 245–6; Linda Bryder, *Below the Magic Mountain: A Social History of Tuberculosis in Twentieth-Century Britain* (Oxford: Clarendon Press, 1988), 36–69; and Neil McFarlane, "Hospitals, Housing, and Tuberculosis in Glasgow," *Social Hist. Med.,* 2 (1989): 59–85.

and maintaining sanatoriums and for offering patients and their families little besides a dreary stay in such ineffectual institutions. Whether sanatoriums contributed to the decline of tuberculosis is a question which has been recently debated.[18] While that issue may not be settled, it is certain that Newsholme believed that institutional isolation was an important preventive measure. We have seen how he tried to demonstrate statistically its value by considering confinement in Poor Law institutions in the nineteenth century as a sort of unintended quarantine whose benefit he thought he could detect in the fall of tuberculosis mortality. I have discussed in Chapter 6 some important methodological weaknesses in these studies. However, the issue here is not whether Newsholme was correct in his inferences. In the present context it is the shape tuberculosis service assumed that is of greater interest. I have tried to demonstrate that Newsholme had a dominant role in initiating the state's tuberculosis policy, yet his plans for the gradual evolution of a comprehensive set of municipal services were foiled first by the Sanatorium Benefit of the National Insurance Act and then by the disruption of the Great War. What emerged after the war was a service both smaller and more narrowly focused on the sanatorium than Newsholme had intended.

The state's initiatives in child, infant, and maternal welfare from 1906 to 1919 have received much more historical attention than either the tuberculosis or the venereal disease services. Historians have viewed these initiatives in a variety of ways: as elements in the evolution of social insurance and early steps toward the welfare state,[19] as examples of the wartime governments' domestic and population policies,[20] or as part of a broader national policy toward women and children.[21] All of these studies place the developments they trace in the context of national population and strategic anxieties about military preparedness, national efficiency, imperial prowess, physical degeneration, changing fertility patterns, and eugenics. Newsholme does not figure largely in these accounts except as the author of major studies of infant mortality, which some of these authors use to describe the social and mortality problems Britain faced at the time.

Newsholme's role in the creation of the infant-welfare program is more difficult to characterize than the part he played in the other two new national programs. He produced the most comprehensive epidemiological studies of infant, child,

18 For example, see Wilson, "Historic Decline of Tuberculosis;" and the exchange of letters between Wilson and Bryder in *J. Hist. Med.*, 46 (1991): 358–68.
19 Bentley B. Gilbert, "Health and Politics: The British Physical Deterioration Report of 1904," *Bull. Hist. Med.*, 39 (1965): 143–53; and Bentley B. Gilbert. *The Evolution of National Insurance in Great Britain: The Origins of the Welfare State* (London: Michael Joseph, 1966), 102–58.
20 J. M. Winter, *The Great War and the British People* (Cambridge, Mass.: Harvard Univ. Press, 1986), 143–53, 189–204. See also J. M. Winter, "The Impact of the First World War on Civilian Health in Britain," *Economic Hist. Rev.*, 30 (1977): 487–507.
21 Deborah Dwork, *War Is Good for Babies and Other Young Children: A History of the Infant and Child Welfare Movement in England 1898–1918* (London and New York: Tavistock, 1987); Jane Lewis, *The Politics of Motherhood: Child and Maternal Welfare in England, 1900–1939* (London: Croom Helm, 1980); Carol Dyhouse, "Working-Class Mothers and Infant Mortality in England, 1896–1914," in *Biology, Medicine and Society 1840–1940*, ed. Charles Webster (Cambridge: Cambridge Univ. Press, 1981), 73–98; and Anna Davin, "Imperialism and Motherhood," *Hist. Workshop*, 5 (1978): 9–65.

and maternal mortality, writing five major reports in six years, years when there were very heavy demands on his time – negotiations on the Insurance Act and the Sanatorium Benefit, the launching of the tuberculosis program, and the burden of war work. These studies are remarkable for their scope, for their resistance to simple or narrow explanations for high infant or maternal mortality rates, and for their forceful insistence on the need for public action. It is clear that Newsholme was keenly concerned with the problem of infant mortality, and he had taken some action to try to reduce it while still in Brighton. But in Whitehall his department was slow to take initiative until challenged by a rival department. How much of this delay was due to administrative myopia or inertia among his superiors at the L.G.B. and how much to Newsholme's own decision to undertake epidemiology investigation before policy formation cannot now be determined with certainty.

I have argued in Chapter 11 that Newsholme had four fundamental purposes in undertaking his studies of infant and child mortality: (1) to demonstrate its magnitude and variation by place and social class; (2) as a result of (1), to suggest that infant and child mortality could be significantly reduced; (3) to prove that this mortality was not eugenic and hence that it ought to be reduced; (4) to place on local authorities the primary responsibility for the diminution of infant and child mortality in the immediate future. I also showed that a careful reading of Newsholme's works does not support the representation of his views in several recent historical accounts of the infant-welfare movement which claim that he placed primary responsibility for excessive infant deaths on the ignorance or carelessness of mothers or on their employment outside of the home. Here as elsewhere he resisted single-causal explanations of social problems just as he resisted reductionist models of infectious disease. Parental behavior unquestionably had a bearing on infant mortality, but many factors came into play including family income, overcrowded housing, and poor community sanitation. He certainly avoided blaming mothers for the nation's avoidable toll of young lives. The most potent causes of excessive infant mortality were to be found in the circumstances in which the urban working class was forced to live. Only local authorities could effectively remedy these circumstances. Effective public initiatives in industrial cities with high infant mortality not only would directly reduce infant mortality but it would encourage and enable working-class parents to nurture their children effectively.

Newsholme's tenure at the Local Government Board witnessed not only the founding of new national health services. It also saw major structural change with the establishment of the Ministry of Health.[22] Historians have often celebrated the new ministry. John Turner concluded that the creation of the Ministry was "one of the wartime coalition's best claims to achievement in social policy" and "one of

22 For standard histories of the establishment of the new ministry, see Bentley B. Gilbert, *British Social Policy 1914–1939* (Ithaca, N.Y.: Cornell Univ. Press, 1970), 98–161; and Frank Honigsbaum, *The Struggle for the Ministry of Health 1914–1919*, Occasional Papers on Social Administration No. 37 (London: G. Bell & Sons, 1970).

the least stuffy and most readily interventionist Ministries between the wars."[23] Frank Honigsbaum sees the creation of the new ministry as a long-overdue reform and the victory for a small group of dedicated and capable reformers. In agreement with the reformers themselves, Honigsbaum labels the L.G.B.'s history in public health as "disastrous."[24] Recently historians have begun to reassess both the L.G.B. in its last years and the performance of the Ministry of Health in late years. It is important first of all to notice that the Ministry of Health Act did not accomplish what the reformers wanted. The Act did not unite all health services in one ministry. It left lunacy and mental deficiency, industrial hygiene, and even the school medical service in the hands of other departments.[25] Although local authority health services expanded in the interwar period, the overlapping of services and their uncoordination within the public sector and between it and the voluntary sector continued.[26] Second, the Ministry did not prove to be a dynamic, innovative department after all. Robert Morant died in the spring of 1920. "Deprived of Morant," Charles Webster has observed, "the Ministry of Health became a career backwater staffed by second-rate minds suitable only to act as instruments of regulation."[27] Christopher Addison was dismissed at the end of March 1921. His clumsy and largely ineffective efforts at a postwar housing policy and his discourtesy toward colleagues had made him a political liability.[28] With Addison and Morant gone, but with Newman still in place, the new Ministry drifted back to the administrative style it had exhibited as the L.G.B.[29] No period in the interwar years witnessed the rapid innovation in health services that occurred in the years between 1906, when the school medical service was launched, and 1914, when Exchequer grants for infant-welfare work were announced by both the L.G.B. and the Board of Education.

More telling in any assessment of the Ministry of Health under Newman's tenure or of its performance in comparison to that of the L.G.B. in its later years are recent studies of infant, child, and maternal health in the interwar period by Jane Lewis and Charles Webster, which have revealed much neglect of basic physiological needs and low standards of health, especially in economically depressed areas.[30] The fiscal constraints of the Depression do not seem sufficient

23 John Turner, " 'Experts' and Interests," 216.   24 Honigsbaum, *Struggle*, 26, 9.
25 These defects were protested by M.O.H. "Ministries of Health Bill, 1918: Memorandum by Society of Medical Officers of Health," *Public Health,* 32 (1918–19): 51–2. See also Christine Bellamy, *Administering Central–Local Relations: The Local Government Board in Its Fiscal and Cultural Context* (Manchester: Manchester Univ. Press, 1988), 258.
26 Berridge, "Health and Medicine," 226–8, 230.
27 Charles Webster, "Conflict and Consensus: Explaining the British Health Service," *Twentieth Cent. Br. Hist.,* 1 (1990): 146.
28 Gilbert, *British Social Policy,* 134–58.   29 Bellamy, *Administering Central–Local Relations,* 258–9.
30 See, for example, Lewis, *Politics of Motherhood,* 43–50, 172–86; Charles Webster, "The Health of the School Child during the Depression," *The Fitness of the Nation – Physical and Health Education in the Nineteenth and Twentieth Centuries: Proceedings of the 1982 Annual of the History of Education,* ed. Nicolas Parry and David McNair (Leicester: History of Education Society, 1983), 76–81; Charles Webster, "Health, Welfare and Unemployment during the Depression," *Past and Present,* 109 (1985): 213–29; and Charles Webster, "Healthy or Hungry Thirties?" *Hist. Workshop,* 13 (1982): 117–19, 122–5.

explanations. These failures were also matters of priorities and of leadership. Not only does the Ministry seem not to have insisted on adequate standards of service or to have investigated in a timely manner complaints of ill-health caused by malnutrition, but it seems to have suppressed unfavorable information and to have attempted to silence critics within the public health service.[31]

It is tempting to offer the following summary characterization of interwar health policy: strict Treasury discipline, an inclination to evade problems until public outcry made further evasion impossible, the use of investigative committees and commissions to delay action, a minimum legislative response with maximum reliance on permissive powers, strict control of new services to give the impression of adequate response to need while actually providing services only on a token basis, a failure to distribute services according to need, and finally a preference for services maximizing the growth of medical bureaucracies, even when this involved inefficient use of resources.[32]

Given what we know about Newsholme's insistence on careful investigation of mortality and morbidity trends, it is highly unlikely that if his standards had been maintained in the new ministry, that ministry would have ignored regional and class differences in child health or that it would have refused to undertake an investigation of maternal mortality, as George Newman did, because it would have created a demand for medical services that the Ministry was not prepared to entertain.[33]

Such performance should make us suspicious of any trumpeting account of the founding of the Ministry of Health. It also makes the assessment of Newsholme that Newman recorded in his diary in December 1913: a " 'failure' – 'weak & vain' – an able man good at Brighton, weak at L.G.B."[34] sound particularly hollow and self-serving. Newman attributes that judgment to the Webbs, but since they make no mention of it, we have it only on his authority. There is little reason to believe that he kept it to himself during his negotiations with senior civil servants and ministers that led to his appointment to the new Ministry. This assessment of Newsholme is also reproduced by Frank Honigsbaum, who in charting the formation of the new Ministry passes on the views of its architects concerning their rivals. Honigsbaum, for example, accepting Newman's and Addison's low opinion of Newsholme, argues that Newsholme's twenty years of experience as an M.O.H. made him "unfit for service at the national level," and that his handling of the influenza epidemic in the autumn of 1918 was a primary reason why Newsholme was passed over for the chief medical post at the Ministry of Health.[35] I find little evidence for either claim. In this book I have tried to demonstrate that Newsholme's experience in Brighton contributed much to his success at the

31 Webster, "Healthy or Hungry Thirties?" 112–15; and Webster, "Health of the School Child," 76–81.
32 Webster, "Conflict and Consensus," 143.
33 Webster, "Health of the School Child," 80; Webster, "Healthy or Hungry Thirties," 122–3.
34 George Newman, Diary, 2 (18 Dec. 1913), P.R.O., MH 139/2. Hereafter cited as Newman, Diary.
35 Honigsbaum, *Struggle,* 70, 55, 51.

L.G.B. The second claim rests primarily on the "rigorous post-mortem examination" Newsholme allegedly underwent at the Royal Society of Medicine on November 13, 1918, and on several contemporary newspaper articles.[36] The discussion at the Society was lengthy, extending over two meetings and occupying over one hundred printed pages in the Society's proceedings.[37] Almost all of the discussion dealt with the epidemiology, clinical course, postmortem and bacteriological findings, or treatment of influenza, and many of the contributors were medical officers in the British, colonial, or American armed forces. Only two speakers addressed the actions taken by public health authorities in England, Newsholme and Major Greenwood, and their comments are the only two which Honigsbaum cites.[38] In the next to the last sentence in his comment Greenwood, then affiliated with the Ministry of Munitions,[39] pointed out that unlike the Local Government Board, the Ministry of Munitions had considered the possibility of an outbreak of influenza in the fall of 1918 and had sent a circular to its hostels advising that plans be made for removal and nursing of the sick. This is hardly a rigorous postmortem or a professional repudiation of Newsholme's leadership. Three items in the *Times* decry the fact that medical science did not know the cause of influenza and the lack of warning the nation received; they report a hostile question Hayes Fisher, the current L.G.B. President, answered in Parliament, and they supported the formation of a Ministry of Health to promote research and team work; one explicitly endorsed Rhondda's proposal to base the new Ministry on the L.G.B.[40] Obviously the great pandemic of 1918–19 was a disaster for all combatant nations. It may be true, as some historians have recently argued, that Britain might have made better provision for its sick during the outbreak,[41] but there really was little that civil authorities could have done in wartime conditions to halt the spread of the disease, and most contemporaries did not blame the nation's public health authorities. As we saw in Chapter 10, even George Newman, not one to miss a chance to criticize Newsholme, maintained that civil and military authorities had done all that they could have done during the pandemic.[42] Much more probable reasons why Newman got the job at the new ministry include Newsholme's age and Newman's close alliance with Morant.

Honigsbaum may be right that Newsholme's advocating a unified local authority health service alarmed the medical profession. He also may be right that Newsholme lacked political astuteness, if by that we are to understand that he had the temerity to criticize Lloyd George's nearly finished plan for national health insurance and to insist on defects in the plan that experience would soon confirm

36 Ibid., 51, 78.
37 "Discussion on Influenza," *Proc. Roy. Soc. Med.,* 12 (1918–19): 1–102.
38 "Discussion on Influenza," 1–18, 21–4.
39 "Major Greenwood, D.Sc., F.R.C.P., F.R.S.," *Br. Med. J.* (1949), no. 2: 877.
40 *Times,* 28 Oct. 1918, 7; ibid., 29 Oct. 1918, 7; ibid., 30 Oct. 1918, 7.
41 Sandra M. Tomkins, "The Failure of Expertise: Public Health Policy in Britain during the 1918–19 Influenza Epidemic," *Social Hist. Med.,* 3 (1992), 437, 444, 452–3.
42 George Newman, *Ann. Rep. Med. Off. L.G.B.,* 48 (1918–19), 11–13.

or that Newsholme lacked Newman's skill in or taste for intrigue. But I question Honigsbaum's reading of the competition between the Board of Education and the L.G.B. and between Newman and Newsholme. Surviving papers of the two boards call into question his suggestion that the Board of Education was ready to cede infant-welfare work to the L.G.B. in 1913 or 1914 but only contested the territory to protect the interests of voluntary societies that had requested its help.[43] That is what Newman sometimes claimed, but the manuscript record belies it. Departmental papers also enable us to better understand Newsholme's administrative schemes for comprehensive infant programs that were drawn up during the interdepartmental conflict,[44] and they provide reason to be cautious in accepting too readily Newman's and Addison's judgments of Newsholme and the L.G.B.

In considering the competition between the Board of Education and the L.G.B. or the creation of the Ministry of Health, we should resist the temptation to see these episodes in strictly personal terms, as reflections of rivalries between individuals or as demonstrations of personal competence and failure. There can be no doubt that both Newsholme and Newman were able, energetic, and influential medical officers. The struggle in which they found themselves was created in part by administrative and political circumstances. I find quite helpful the recent suggestion of Christine Bellamy that some of the blame for these struggles and for the difficulties of creating the Ministry of Health must fall on the leadership of the Liberal Party.[45] By bypassing the L.G.B. in social policy initiatives, Lloyd George increased already fragmented administrative arrangements and necessitated a new ministry to achieve consolidation, and by insisting, as he did, that all significant opposition be removed by negotiation before the Ministry of Health Bill be presented, he made Addison's task in bringing forward the bill nearly impossible. Further, the party allowed a rising faction (including Addison), which "possessed both a deep partisan suspicion of the officials of the Local Government Board and low confidence in the capacity and enthusiasm of the local authorities as the instruments of social change" to undermine the Board's authority, to drive its already low status lower and to provoke the sort of disruptive competition that developed.[46]

In comparison to the amount of historical attention paid to health policy and administration or to the effects of public health initiatives on mortality or morbidity, the professionalization of public health or its scientific content has been rather neglected. Dorothy Porter has studied the struggles of Medical Officers of Health to construct a profession of preventive medicine.[47] This study of Newsholme's

---

43 Honigsbaum, *Struggle*, 20–3. Honigsbaum relied instead on papers of the Ministry of Reconstruction and of the War Cabinet.
44 Ibid., 29, 33.
45 For the following comments, see Bellamy, *Administering Central–Local Relations*, 250–4.
46 Ibid., 252.
47 Dorothy E. [Watkins] Porter, "The English Revolution in Social Medicine 1889–1911," (University of London: unpublished Ph.D. dissertation, 1984), esp. 189–214. See also Steven J. Novak, "Professionalism and Bureaucracy: English Doctors and the Victorian Public Health Administration," *J. Social Hist.*, 6 (1973): 440–62.

career adds little to what she has concluded. Newsholme was an active member of the Society of Medical Officers of Health – President, Member of the Council, and twice Editor of *Public Health* – and an examiner for the Diploma in Public Health at London, Oxford, and Cambridge universities. He was not conspicuous, however, in some activities usually associated with professionalization, such as the effort to win tenure for provincial Medical Officers of Health. Newsholme never had tenure in Brighton. He did not actively campaign for it while an M.O.H., and there is no evidence that once in Whitehall he worked to change the L.G.B.'s traditional indifference to the issue.

Margaret Pelling's study of the medical understanding of cholera and fever throws a good deal of light on the activities of the central health authority and its officials in the 1840s and 1850s, and Christopher Hamlin's research on water analysis and the water supply of British cities offers an illuminating case study of problems encountered in applying science to a particularly troublesome set of urban problems.[48] But there has been no general historical analysis of the reception and application of the germ theory in British preventive medicine or public health. Bruno Latour has recently asserted that in France hygienists were among the first to embrace Pasteur's ideas of disease causation and became some of his most vociferous partisans.[49] Newsholme's career suggests that a different process was at work in Britain. Newsholme was never hostile or indifferent to the new theory. We have seen that even in the eighties his popular works on hygiene accept the notion that microorganisms may cause specific diseases. He also acted on this conviction, in 1897 opening a municipal hygienic laboratory for bacteriological analysis and then introducing specific preventive measures against tuberculosis predicated on the conviction that the bacillus that Koch had identified was the disease's cause. But the picture that emerges from Newsholme's work as an M.O.H. is a gradual addition of new ideas and techniques to older ones. We have seen how, over a twenty-year period, nonspecific environmental factors slowly gave way to specific microbial agents in Newsholme's discussion of typhoid fever and in the priorities he set for disease prevention. We have also observed how his most ambitious epidemiological studies of the middle and late 1890s were premised on the conviction that the experimental medicine of his day, for all its success in the discovery of specific microbial agents of disease, could not explain the epidemic phenomena of infectious diseases. In order to explain why a particular disease was epidemic at a particular time and place, one needed to consider environmental factors like groundwater and rainfall.

48 Margaret Pelling, *Cholera, Fever and English Medicine 1825–1865* (Oxford: Oxford Univ. Press, 1978); Christopher Hamlin, *A Science of Impurity: Water Analysis in Nineteenth Century Britain* (Berkeley and Los Angeles: Univ. of California Press, 1990); and Christopher Hamlin, "Politics and Germ Theories in Victorian Britain: The Metropolitan Water Commissions of 1867–9 and 1892–3," in *Government and Expertise: Specialists, Administrators and Professionals, 1860–1919,* ed. Roy MacLeod (Cambridge: Cambridge Univ. Press, 1988), 110–27.

49 Bruno Latour, *The Pasteurization of France,* trans. Alan Sheridan and John Law (Cambridge, Mass.: Harvard Univ. Press, 1988), 13–58.

Recent scholarship has demonstrated that the nineteenth-century British public health enterprise owed much to the data and to the statistical methods emanating from the General Register Office in London.[50] In Newsholme's opinion the M.O.H.'s most basic task was monitoring the health of the people and discovering conditions that threatened health. The gathering of vital data and their statistical analysis must be the starting point for informed, responsible administration. His own contributions are in the mainstream of British vital statistics and epidemiology. His admiration for the work of William Farr, the first statistical superintendent of the G.R.O., was no coincidence, and the several editions of Newsholme's *Elements of Vital Statistics* helped to make those entering public health conversant with the statistical methods Farr had pioneered. Like Farr and his successors, Newsholme used registration and census data to determine mortality patterns and to study the relationship of those patterns to conditions of life – age, martial status, occupation, population density, housing, income, and so forth. Like Farr, Newsholme considered the life table the best criterion of a population's physical well-being, and he recognized the dangers in the use of crude mortality rates for comparative purposes. He followed Farr in his techniques of correcting for differences in the age structure of the populations he compared through the use of standardized mortality rates, using the entire nation, its healthy districts – another Farr device – or its rural areas as standard populations. The methods the practitioners of this modest statistical art used were not mathematically sophisticated, but they did much to elucidate the conditions favorable to disease and the means by which it spread. They also helped to mobilize public opinion and to encourage action. We have seen how Newsholme repeatedly used the vital statistics of his town and then of his nation to urge specific public initiatives.

Circumstances – the advent of disease notification, most notably – permitted Newsholme and his contemporaries to go beyond Farr and to bring morbidity within the realm of official statistics. Prompt notification of cases forged a direct link between the statistical functions of the local health authority and its administrative activity. The same notification slip not only added to the columns of figures in Health Department ledgers, but it might prompt an immediate visit by an official. This new information enabled Newsholme to undertake some of his most novel epidemiological work – his studies of milk-borne scarlet fever, of contaminated shellfish and typhoid fever, and of familial infection in tuberculosis. Despite this important enlargement in the statistical base from which Newsholme and his generation worked, the epidemiological studies that his contemporaries in public health undertook were almost entirely based on mass population data. Newsholme made almost no use of clinical data in his epidemiology. The excep-

50 Simon Szreter, "The GRO and the Public Health Movement in Britain, 1837–1914," *Social Hist. Med.*, 4 (1991): 435–63; Fred Lewes, "The GRO and the Provinces in the Nineteenth Century," ibid., 479–96; Edward Higgs, "Disease, Febrile Poisons, and Statistics: The Census as a Medical Survey, 1841–1911," ibid., 465–78; John M. Eyler, "Mortality Statistics and Victorian Health Policy: Program and Criticism," *Bull. Hist. Med.*, 50 (1976): 335–55; and John M. Eyler, *Victorian Social Medicine: The Ideas and Methods of William Farr* (Baltimore and London: Johns Hopkins Univ. Press, 1979).

tions are his few studies of "return cases" of scarlet fever and diphtheria at the Brighton Sanatorium.

This statistical enterprise, so basic to the public health movement and so well established by 1900, did not go uncontested. The most serious intellectual challenge came from Karl Pearson and his associates who wielded more powerful mathematical tools than the vital statisticians and the Medical Officers of Health and who had different views of human nature and society. Newsholme and Pearson and other biometricians quarreled over statistical methods and interpretations, but the fundamental differences between them were as much political as professional. Statistics for Newsholme were always tools for public health work, the most basic of social reforms. Health – the stamina to work and to compete – in a free society was a fundamental right. Newsholme was convinced that physical well-being and the social and economic success which accompanied it were neither accidental blessings nor determined primarily by heredity. Instead they were largely the results of conditions of life over which society had a considerable influence and in which it had a great interest. His own liberal faith in social reform was focused and found a more articulate voice during the discussions of physical degeneration and national prowess that followed the Boer War. Newsholme's own experience in investigating the physical conditions in Brighton's slums had made him receptive to the revelations of social investigators such as Rowntree, who demonstrated the precarious conditions in which unskilled labor lived. From his own experience as an M.O.H. he had also learned the biological and social costs of postponed or inadequate medical attention. His association with the Webbs encouraged him to translate his social concerns and administrative experience into policy recommendations. The result was his plan for a unified local authority health service in which the health department would provide a wide array of preventive and therapeutic services for the working class and would supervise the work of most practitioners who served that class. His object was not only to make timely medical care available to all so that communicable disease could be discovered and its spread halted and so that the progressive loss of physical capacity which accompanied neglected illness could be ended; he also hoped to end the isolation of general practitioners by providing for them expert pathological and consultant services. This solution gained strength from his belief that to an increasing degree in the future it would be impossible to draw a line between preventive work and therapeutic work. No experience did more to cement that notion than his work in Brighton with tuberculosis. The national venereal disease service he helped design was its most complete embodiment.

The logic of his own arguments eventually carried him far from his original conception of the state's obligations in matters of health. He initially opposed the British scheme of national insurance on principle. Not only did it operate independently of the local authority's public health initiatives, but it seemed to ignore prevention and stress palliation, and it did nothing to change the conditions in which general practitioners worked. As we have seen, through the twenties Newsholme continued to criticize the British scheme and to suggest changes. But his experiences abroad caused him to reassess the place health insurance could occupy. His research on national medical systems, which resulted in *International Studies* and *Medicine and the State,* encouraged him to think of state medicine rather than public health. Properly administered, publicly subsidized and supervised health insurance could not only cure and palliate, but it could also be a major contributor to preventive work by bringing to medical attention conditions whose future damage could be limited. His plan called for rethinking of the state's role in health. By the middle thirties, after his visit to the Soviet Union, he criticized most American public health officials, such as Winslow, and some British officials for taking too narrow a view of their work. The job of state medicine was not only the prevention of disease but it included the promotion of health in all citizens.[51]

I have tried to suggest that at their core Newsholme's motives were moral. Sometimes, it is true especially late in his life, he could sound prudish when discussing sexuality, marriage, and alcohol. But to dismiss his pronouncements on such occasions as the cranky ideas of an old man, as some of his younger contemporaries apparently did, would be a great mistake. Society's obligation to prevent disease and premature death and to relieve suffering did not, in his opinion, spring only from its economic, strategic, or political interests. It was rooted, he believed, in a basic moral obligation human beings had to one another and that society owed to even its most helpless members. As such, it was the foundation for his liberal convictions and his reform agenda. It lies behind small episodes such as his editorials on conditions in the concentration camps during the Boer War or his campaign to see that Brighton made provision to rehouse its poorest and least influential residents by including common lodging houses in its housing schemes. On a larger scale it is seen in his objections to the civil rights abuses in the Soviet Union, and in his opposition to statistical studies that he was convinced were designed to shift the blame for disease or disability from society to the individual through the guise of heredity. But there were limits to what the state could do, and moral obligations fell on individuals as well as on society. Through environmental reform, through adequate health care provision, through universal education, society could do much to improve human welfare, but in the type of society that he was willing to conceive, Newsholme believed, for example, that children would get the care and nurturing they needed only when parents met their responsibilities. In a free society, only responsible choices, only behavioral changes, could solve some health problems whose roots lay beyond the realm of state interference.

---

51 Newsholme to Kingsbury, 1 March 1937, Kingsbury Papers, B–16, Newsholme folder 3. It has been argued that even in Britain a narrow view of state medicine as the prevention or treatment of specific diseases was also common in the interwar years. Jane Lewis, *What Price Community Medicine? The Philosophy, Practice and Politics of Public Health since 1919* (Brighton: Wheatsheaf Books, 1986), 1–4, 15–34.

SELECT BIBLIOGRAPHY

I. MANUSCRIPTS AND PUBLIC RECORDS

Alan M. Chesney Medical Archives, Johns Hopkins University
    School of Hygiene and Public Health, Dean's Office Correspondence
    William Henry Welch Papers
American Philosophical Society Library
    Raymond Pearl Papers
Bodleian Library, Oxford University
    Christopher Addison Papers
British Library
    John Burns Papers
British Library of Political and Economic Science, London School of Economics
    William J. Braithwaite Papers
    Sidney and Beatrice Webb, Local Government Collection
    Beatrice Webb, Diary
    Passfield Papers
British Medical Association Library
    Medico-Political Committee minutes and documents
    Central War Committee Papers
East Sussex County Record Office, Lewes
    Brighton Corporation. Proceedings of the Committees Report Books
        Proceedings of the Sanitary Committee
        Register of Slaughter Houses
    Brighton, Hove and Sussex Hospitals Board, scrapbook and minute book.
House of Lords Record Office
    David Lloyd George Papers
John Hay Library, Brown University
    Charles V. Chapin Papers
Library of Congress
    John A. Kingsbury Papers
London School of Hygiene and Tropical Medicine Library
    Arthur Newsholme Papers
National Library of Medicine
    James Angus Doull Papers
Public Record Office, Kew
    Board of Education Papers (ED)

Cabinet papers (CAB)
Ministry of Health Papers (MH)
Ministry of Pensions Papers (PIN)
Ministry of Reconstruction Papers (RECO)
Treasury papers (T)
Sterling Memorial Library, Yale University
    Charles-Edward Amory Winslow Papers
    Milbank Memorial Fund Papers
University College Library, London
    Karl Pearson Papers
Wellcome Institute for the History of Medicine, London
    George Newman Papers

II. BRITISH STATUTES

29 & 60 Vict., C. 90: The Sanitary Act, 1866.
31 & 32 Vict., C. 130: The Artizans and Labourers Dwelling Act, 1868 [Torrens Act].
35 & 36 Vict., C. 79: Public Health Act, 1872.
38 & 39 Vict., C. 36: The Artizans and Labourers Dwellings Improvement Act, 1875 [Cross Act].
38 & 39 Vict., C. 55: The Public Health Act, 1875.
38 & 39 Vict., C. 83: Local Loans Act, 1875.
38 & 39 Vict., C. 89: Public Works Loans Act, 1875.
47 & 48 Vict., C. 262: Brighton Improvement Act, 1884.
52 & 53 Vict., C. 72: Infectious Disease (Notification) Act, 1889.
53 & 54 Vict., C. 34: Infectious Disease (Prevention) Act, 1890.
53 & 54 Vict., C. 70: Housing of the Working Classes Act, 1890.
56 & 57 Vict., C. 68: Isolation Hospitals Act, 1893.
59 & 60 Vict., C. 137: Brighton Corporation Water Act, 1896.
59 & 60 Vict., C. 221: Brighton Corporation Act, 1896.
62 & 63 Vict., C. 8: Infectious Disease (Notification) Extension Act, 1899.
1 Edw. 7, C. 8: Isolation Hospitals Act, 1901.
1 Edw. 7, C. 224: Brighton Corporation Act, 1901.
2 Edw. 7, C. 17: Midwives Act, 1902.
7 Edw. 7, C. 17: Notification of Births Act, 1907.
8 Edw. 7, C. 107: London County Council (General Powers) Act, 1908.
1 & 2 Geo. 5, C. 48: Finance Act, 1911.
1 & 2 Geo. 5, C. 55: National Insurance Act, 1911.
3 & 4 Geo. 5, C. 23: Public Health (Prevention and Treatment of Disease) Act, 1913.
3 & 4 Geo. 5, C. 37: National Insurance Act, 1913.
5 & 6 Geo. 5, C. 64: Notification of Births (Extension) Act, 1915.
7 & 8 Geo. 5, C. 21: Venereal Disease Act, 1917.
8 & 9 Geo. 5, C. 29: Maternity and Child Welfare Act, 1918.
10 & 11 Geo. 5, C. 10: National Health Insurance Act, 1920.

III. PARLIAMENTARY COMMISSIONS AND DEPARTMENTAL
COMMITTEES (HOUSE OF COMMONS SESSIONAL PAPERS UNLESS
OTHERWISE NOTED)

1895, XXXV. C. 7703 & 1896, XLVI, C. 7992: *Report and Papers of the Royal Commission Appointed to Inquire into the Effect of Food Derived from Tuberculous Animals on Human Health.*

1898, XLIX, C. 8824, 8831: *Report and Papers of the Royal Commission Appointed to Inquire into the Administrative Procedures for Controlling Danger to Man through the Use as Food of the Meat and Milk of Tuberculous Animals.*

1899, X, [172]: (Lords Papers) *Report from the Select Committee on the Oysters Bill.*

1903, XXX, Cd. 1507, 1508: *Report and Papers of the Royal Commission on Physical Training in Scotland.*

1904, XXXIII, Cd. 2175, 2210, 2186: *Reports and Papers of the Interdepartmental Committee on Physical Deterioration.*

1904, XXXVII, Cd. 1884: *Fourth Report and Papers of the Royal Commission on Sewage Disposal.*

1904, XXXIX, Cd. 2092: *Interim Report of the Royal Commission on Tuberculosis.*

1907, XXXVIII, Cd. 3322: *Second Interim Report of the Royal Commission on Tuberculosis.*

1909, XLIX, Cd. 4483: *Third Interim Report of the Royal Commission on Tuberculosis.*

1909, XXXVII, Cd. 4499: *Report of the Royal Commission on the Poor Laws and Relief of Distress.*

1909, LXXI, Cd. 4508: *Report of the British Delegates to the International Congress on Tuberculosis Held at Washington from 21 September to 3rd October, 1908.*

1910, XLIX, Cd. 5068: *Report of the Royal Commission on the Poor Laws and Relief of Distress,* Appendix Vol. 9, Evidence Relating to Unemployment.

1911, XLII, Cd. 5761: *Final Report of the Royal Commission on Tuberculosis.*

1912–13, XLVIII, Cd. 6164, 6641, 6654: *Reports and Papers of the Departmental Committee on Tuberculosis.*

1916, XV, Cd. 8200: *Final Report of the Committee on Retrenchment in the Public Expenditure.*

1916, XVI, Cd. 8189, 8190: *Final Report and Papers of the Royal Commission on Venereal Diseases.*

1919, XXX, Cmd. 317: *Report of the Inter-departmental Committee Appointed to Consider and Report upon the Immediate Practical Steps Which Should Be Taken for the Provision of Residential Treatment for Discharged Soldiers and Sailors suffering from Pulmonary Tuberculosis and for Their Re-introduction into Employment, Especially on the Land.*

IV. OFFICIAL REPORTS

Brighton Corporation. *Proceedings of the Town Council.*

Brighton Corporation. Medical Officer of Health, *Annual Reports on the Health, Sanitary Condition, &c. of the Borough of Brighton.*

Quarterly Report of the Medical Officer of Health.

Brighton Corporation, Sanitary Committee. Duties of the Medical Officer of the Sanatorium (Brighton [1890]).

Instructions to Nurses [at the Brighton Sanatorium] (Brighton, n.d.).

Rules & Regulations [for consumptive patients treated under the Hedgcock Bequest] (Brighton, n.d.).

Brighton Corporation, Francis J. Tillstone, Town Clerk. *Duties of Head Porter* [of the Brighton Sanatorium] (Brighton, 1890).

Duties of the Matron [of the Brighton Sanatorium] (Brighton, 1890).

Canada, Department of National Health and Welfare. *Health Insurance in Great Britain, 1911–1948,* Social Security Series, Memorandum No. 11 (Ottawa, 1952).

England and Wales, Board of Education. *Annual Reports of the Chief Medical Officer of the Board of Education.*

England and Wales, General Register Office. *Annual Reports of the Registrar-General of England and Wales.*

England and Wales, Local Government Board. *Annual Reports of the Local Government Board.*

Minutes of Discussion at a Conference on the Treatment and Cure of Venereal Diseases (London: HMSO, 1918).

Report of the Special Work of the Local Government Board Arising out of the War, B.P.P. 1914–16, XXV, Cd. 7763.

England and Wales, Medical Officer of the Local Government Board. *Annual Reports of the Medical Officer of the Local Government Board.*

Supplements to the Annual Report of the Medical Officer of the Local Government Board

to 24th *Ann. Rep.* (1894–95): *Report and Papers on the Cultivation and Storage of Oysters and Certain Other Mollusks in Relation to the Occurrence of Disease in Man* (H. Timbrell Bulstrode, et al.) B.P.P. 1896, XXXVII, C. 8214.

to 39th *Ann. Rep.* (1909–10): *Infant and Child Mortality* (Arthur Newsholme), B.P.P. 1910, XXXIX, Cd. 5263.

to 40th *Ann. Rep.* (1910–11): *Report on Isolation Hospitals* (H. Franklin Parsons), B.P.P. 1912–13, XXXVI, Cd. 6342.

to 42nd *Ann. Rep.* (1912–13): *Second Report on Infant and Child Mortality* (Arthur Newsholme), B.P.P. 1913, XXXII, Cd. 6909.

to 43rd *Ann. Rep.* (1913–14): *Third Report on Infant Mortality Dealing with Infant Mortality in Lancashire* (Arthur Newsholme et al.), B.P.P. 1914, XXXIX, Cd. 7511.

to 44th *Ann. Rep.* (1914–15): *Maternal Mortality in Connection with Childbearing and Its Relation to Infant Mortality* (Arthur Newsholme), B.P.P. 1914–16, XXV, Cd. 8085.

to 45th *Ann. Rep.* (1915–16): *Report on Child Mortality at Ages 0–5 in England and Wales* (Arthur Newsholme), B.P.P. 1917–18, XVI, Cd. 8496.

England and Wales, Ministry of Health. *Annual Reports of the Ministry of Health.*

Annual Reports of the Chief Medical Officer of the Ministry of Health.

Great Britain, Privy Council, *Report as to the Practice of Medicine and Surgery by Unqualified Persons in the United Kingdom,* B.P.P. 1910, XLIII, Cd. 5422.

Greenhow, Edward Headlam, "The Results of an Inquiry in the Different Proportions of Death Produced by certain Diseases in Different Districts in England," in *Papers Relating to the Sanitary State of the People of England,* B.P.P. 1857–8, XXIII, 1–164.

Johnstone, R. W. *Report on Venereal Diseases,* B.P.P. 1913, XXXII, Cd. 7029.

Wandsworth, Metropolitan Borough of, Board of Works, *Report on the Sanitary Condition of the Several Parishes Comprised in the Wandsworth District by the Medical Officers of Health.*

V. NEWSPAPERS

Brighton Gazette
Brighton Herald
Daily News [London]
Daily Telegraph [London]
Manchester Guardian
Morning Post [London]
Olean Evening Times
Sussex Daily News
The Times

VI. PUBLISHED WORKS BY NEWSHOLME OTHER THAN
OFFICIAL REPORTS

"About Civilization and the Survival of the Fittest," *Brighton Herald*, 14 Oct. 1893.
"Abstract of a Lecture on the Prevention of Tuberculosis," *Polyclinic*, 4 (1901), 77–8.
"An Account of the System of Voluntary Notification of Phthisis in Brighton, and of the Treatment and Training of Patients in Its Isolation Hospital," *Tuberculosis*, 4 (1906–7): 226–42. With H. C. Lecky.
"Address on Neo-natal Mortality," *Lancet* (1920) no. 1: 1097–1101.
"Address on Neo-natal Mortality," *Mother and Child*, 1 (1920): 3–15.
"Address on Possible Medical Extensions of Public Health Work," *Journal of State Medicine*, 9 (1901): 538–55.
"An Address on Social Evolution and Public Health," *Lancet* (1904), no. 2: 1330–6.
"An Address on Some Aspects of Maternity and Child-welfare Work," *Lancet* (1918), no. 2: 1–3.
"An Address on the Present Position of the Tuberculosis Problem," *Lancet* (1926), no. 1: 1021–6.
"An Address on the Relative Rôles of Compulsion and Education in Public Health Work," *Lancet* (1922), no. 2: 219–23.
"An Address on the Spread of Enteric Fever by Means of Sewage-Contaminated Shellfish," *British Medical Journal* (1896), no. 2: 639–44.
"Alcohol and Public Health," in *The Drink Problem in Its Medico-Sociological Aspects*, ed. T. N. Kelynack (London: Methuen, 1907), 122–51.
"Alleged Physical Degeneration in Towns," *Public Health*, 17 (1904–5): 293–300.
"The Bearing of School-attendance upon the Spread of Infectious Diseases," *Transactions of the Sanitary Institute*, 11 (1890): 100–8.
"The Better Use of Vital Statistics in Public Health Administration," *Quarterly Publication of the American Statistical Association*, 17 (1921): 815–25.
"Bills of Mortality in South Africa," *British Medical Journal* (1901), no. 1: 160–2, 221–2.
"Brighton as a Health Resort," *Illustrated Medical News*, 5 (5 Oct. 1889): 2–4.
The Brighton Life Table (Brighton, 1893).
Can Human Life Be Prolonged and Disease Be Prevented? (Onondaga, N.Y.: Onondaga Health Association, 1926).
"The Causes of the Past Decline in Tuberculosis and the Light Thrown by History on Preventive Measures for the Immediate Future," *Charities*, 21 (1908–9): 206–29.

"The Causes of the Past Decline in Tuberculosis and the Light Thrown by History on Preventive Measures for the Immediate Future," *Trans., Sixth International Congress on Tuberculosis* (Washington, D.C., 1908), Suppl. *A Series of Public Lectures*, 80–109.

"The Children's Charter of Health," *Public Health*, 20 (1907–8): 161–3.

The Climatic and Other Advantages of Brighton (Brighton: Brighton Publicity Association, [c. 1906]).

"The Community and Social Hygiene," in *Foundations of Social Hygiene* (London: British Social Hygiene Council, 1926), 107–28.

"The Concentration Camps in South Africa," *British Medical Journal* (1901), no. 2: 1423–4.

"The Condemnation of the Meat of Tuberculous Animals," *Public Health*, 5 (1892–3): 4–6.

"A Contribution to the Study of Epidemic Diarrhoea," *Public Health*, 12 (1899–1900): 139–211.

"The Control of Conception," in *Sexual Problems of To-day*, ed. Many Scharlieb (London: Williams and Norgate, 1924), 147–72.

"The Control of Measles," *Public Health*, 10 (1897–8): 308–11.

"The Decline of Human Fertility in the United Kingdom and Other Countries as Shown by Corrected Birth-rates," *Journal of the Royal Statistical Society*, 69 (1906): 34–87. With T.H.C. Stevenson.

"The Decline in the Registered Mortality from Syphilis in England. To What Is It Due?" *Journal of Social Hygiene*, 12 (1926): 513–23.

The Declining Birth-Rate: Its National and International Significance (London: Cassell, 1911).

"Discussion on Influenza," *Proceedings of the Royal Society of Medicine*, 12 (1918–19): 1–18.

"A Discussion on the Administrative Prevention of Tuberculosis," *British Medical Journal* (1902), no. 2: 438–40.

"A Discussion on the Co-Ordination of the Public Medical Services," *British Medical Journal* (1907), no. 2: 656–60.

"A Discussion on the Means of Preventing the Spread of Infection in Elementary Schools," *British Medical Journal* (1899), no. 2: 589–90.

"A Discussion on the Preventive and Remedial Treatment of Tuberculosis," *British Medical Journal* (1899), no. 2: 1158.

"Disease Records as an Indispensable Means of Disease Prevention," *Proceedings of the International Conference on Health Problems in Tropical America* (Boston: United Fruit Company, 1924), 940–5.

Domestic Economy: Comprising the Laws of Health in Their Application to Home Life and Work (London: Swan Sonnenschein, 1902). With Margaret Eleanor Scott.

"Domestic Infection in Relation to Epidemic Diarrhoea," *Journal of Hygiene*, 6 (1906): 139–48.

"The Duties and Difficulties of Sanitary Inspectors," *Sanitary Record*, n.s. 10 (1888–9): 411–14.

Elementary Hygiene, 2nd ed. (London, 1893).

The Elements of Vital Statistics (London, 1889).

The Elements of Vital Statistics, 3rd ed. (London, 1899).

The Elements of Vital Statistics in Their Bearing on Social and Public Health Problems, new ed. (London: George Allen and Unwin, 1923).

"The Enemies of Child Life," *Nineteenth Century*, 83 (1918): 76–98.

"Enteric Fever and Shell-fish," *Public Health*, 10 (1897–8): 390–1.

"Epidemic Diarrhoea, Municipal Scavenging, Rainfall, and Temperature," *Public Health,* 15 (1902–3): 654–5.

Epidemic Diphtheria: A Research on the Origin and Spread of the Disease from an International Standpoint (London, 1898).

"Epidemic Influenza and Medical Officers of Health," *Medical Press,* n.s. 106 (1918): 368–9.

"The Epidemiology of Diphtheria," in *The Bacteriology of Diphtheria,* ed. G.H.F. Nuttall and G. S. Graham-Smith (Cambridge: Cambridge Univ. Press, 1908), 53–81.

"The Epidemiology of Rheumatic Fever," *Practitioner,* 66 (1901): 11–21.

"The Epidemiology of Scarlet Fever in Relation to the Utility of Isolation Hospitals," *Transactions of the Epidemiological Society of London,* n.s. 20 (1900–1): 48–69.

"The Epidemiology of Smallpox in the Nineteenth Century," *British Medical Journal* (1902), no. 2: 17–26.

Evolution of Preventive Medicine (Baltimore: Williams & Wilkins, 1927).

"An Explanation of the Supposed Increase of Cancer Mortality in This Country," *British Medical Journal* (1898), no. 1: 74–5.

Fifty Years in Public Health: A Personal Narrative with Comments (London: George Allen & Unwin, 1935).

"Four and a Half Years' Experience of the Voluntary Notification of Pulmonary Tuberculosis," *Journal of the Sanitary Institute,* 24 (1903): 253–60.

A General Description of the History of Isolation Accommodation Provided by the Borough, with a More Detailed Account of Improved Accommodation now Provided by the Corporation (Brighton, 1898). With Francis J. C. May.

"The Graphic Method of Constructing a Life Table Illustrated by the Brighton Life Table, 1891–1900," *Journal of Hygiene,* 3 (1903): 297–324.

"The Growth of Social Insurance in Great Britain," *Proceedings of the Institute of Medicine* [Chicago], 6 (1927): 133–48.

"The Health Department in the Field of Medicine from the Standpoint of Experience in England," *American Journal of Public Health,* 27 (1937): 1089–93.

"The Health of Scholars: With Special Reference to the Education Code and the Board of Education Act, 1899," *Journal of the Sanitary Institute,* 21 (1900): 269–79.

Health Problems in Organized Society: Studies in the Social Aspects of Public Health (London: P. S. King, 1927).

"The Historical Development of Public Health Work in England," *American Journal of Public Health,* 9 (1919): 907–18.

Hughes Science Readers, no. 1–4, ed. Arthur Newsholme [no. 1 & 2 by Richard Balchin, no. 3 & 4 by Arthur Newsholme] (London, 1883–4).

Humane Slaughtering and the Public Health (London: Model Abattoir Society, 1923).

Hygiene: A Manual of Personal and Public Health (London, 1884).

"An Improved Method of Calculating Birth-Rates," *Journal of Hygiene,* 5 (1905): 175–84, 304–10. With T.H.C. Stevenson.

"Inaugural Address on Private Medical Practice and Preventive Medicine," *Lancet* (1926), no. 2: 893–7.

"Infantile Mortality: A Statistical Study from the Public Health Standpoint," *Practitioner,* 75 (1905): 489–500.

"The Influence of Civilization upon the Survival of the Fittest," *Annual Report of the Brighton & Sussex Natural History and Philosophical Society* (1894), 5–12.

"The Influence of Soil on the Prevalence of Pulmonary Phthisis," *Practitioner,* 66 (1901): 206–13.

"The Influence of the Drinking of Alcoholic Beverages on the National Health," in *Alcohol and the Human Body,* ed. Victor A. H. Horsley and Mary D. Sturge, 5th ed. (London: Macmillan, 1915), 317–26.

"Influenza from a Public Health Standpoint," *Practitioner,* 78 (1907): 118–23.

"Influenza from a Public Health Standpoint," *Practitioner,* 102 (1919): 6–11.

"An Inquiry into the Principal Causes of the Reduction in the Death-rate from Phthisis during the Last Forty Years, with Special Reference to the Segregation of Phthisical Patients in General Institutions," *Journal of Hygiene,* 6 (1906): 304–84.

"International Aspects of Alcoholism with Special Reference to Prohibition in America" [abstract] *British Medical Journal,* 1921, no. 2: 660.

International Studies on the Relation between the Private and Official Practice of Medicine with Special Reference to the Prevention of Disease, 3 vols. (London: George Allen and Unwin, 1931; Baltimore: Williams & Wilkins, 1931).

"An Introductory Address on the Relation of the Medical Practitioner to Preventive Measures against Tuberculosis," *Lancet* (1904), no. 1: 282–6.

"Introductory Remarks on Epidemic Catarrhs and Influenza," *Lancet* (1918), no. 2: 689–93.

The Last Thirty Years in Public Health: Recollections and Reflections on my Official and Post-Official Life (London: George Allen and Unwin, 1936).

Lessons on Health: Containing the Elements of Physiology and Their Application to Hygiene (London, 1890).

"The Life Work of Sir John Simon," *Journal of Hygiene,* 5 (1905): 1–6.

"Local Authorities and Sanatoria for Consumption," *Practitioner,* 68 (1902): 79–88.

"The Lower Limit of Age for School Attendance," *Practitioner,* 79 (1907): 593–607.

"The Lower Limit of Age for School Attendance," *Proceedings of the Second International Congress on School Hygiene* (London, 1908), II: 612–22.

"The Lower Limit of Age for School Attendance: A Plea for the Exclusion of Children under Five Years of Age from Public Elementary Schools," *Public Health,* 14 (1901–2): 576–83.

"Man's Advance throughout the Ages," *Medical Press,* n.s. 120 (1925): 442–4.

"The Measurement of Progress in Public Health: with Special Reference to the Life and Work of William Farr," *Economica,* 3 (1923): 186–202.

"Medicine and the State," *Medical Officer,* 44 (1930): 249–52.

Medicine and the State: The Relation between the Private and Official Practice of Medicine with Special Reference to Public Health (London: George Allen and Unwin, 1932; Baltimore: Williams and Wilkins, 1932).

"Memorandum as to the Connection between the Consumption of Shell-fish Contaminated by Sewage and Infectious Disease," *Public Health,* 10 (1897–8): 421–4.

"Midwifery Work and Social Welfare," *Maternity and Child Welfare,* 7 (1923): 181–5.

"The Milroy Lectures on the Natural History and Affinities of Rheumatic Fever: A Study in Epidemiology," *Lancet* (1895), no. 1: 589–96, 657–65.

"The Milroy Lectures on the Natural History and Affinities of Rheumatic Fever" [abstract] *British Medical Journal* (1895), no. 1: 527–8, 581–3.

The Ministry of Health (London and New York: G. P. Putnams, 1925).

"The Moral Aspects of Social Hygiene," *Hibbert Journal,* 22 (1923–4): 279–93.

"The Moral Aspects of Social Hygiene," *Journal of Social Hygiene*, 10 (1924): 513–32.

"National Changes in Health and Longevity," *Quarterly Publication of the American Statistical Association*, 17 (1920–1): 689–719.

"The National Importance of Child Mortality," *Journal of the Sanitary Institute*, 31 (1910): 326–48.

"A National System of Notification of Sickness," *British Medical Journal* (1895), no. 2: 529–31.

"A National System of Notification of Sickness," *Public Health*, 8 (1895–6): 106–8.

"A National System of Notification and Registration of Sickness" [abstract] *Lancet* (1895), no. 2: 1560–4.

"A National System of Notification and Registration of Sickness," *Journal of the Royal Statistical Society*, 59 (1896): 1–28.

"A National System of Notification and Registration of Sickness," *Medical Press*, n.s. 60 (1895): 658–61.

"New Light on the Drink Problem," *Contemporary Review*, 125 (1924): 438–44.

The New York Health Demonstrations in Syracuse and in Cattaraugus County (New York: Milbank Memorial Fund, 1927).

"The New York Health Demonstrations in Syracuse and in Cattaraugus County," *Milbank Memorial Fund Quarterly Bulletin*, 4 (1926): 49–66.

"The Non-participation of the Higher Ages in the Improved Expectation of Life in England," *Public Health*, 5 (1892–3): 340–2.

"A Note on the Causes of the Historical Reduction of Leprosy," *Proceedings of the International Conference on Health Problems in Tropical America* (Boston: United Fruit Company, 1924), 791–5.

"Notes on Sanitary Administration," *Public Health*, 12 (1899–1900): 833–40.

"Notification of Consumption: Its Pros and Cons. Remarks Introductory to a Discussion on the Prevention of Phthisis," *Journal of the Sanitary Institute*, 21 (1900): 49–54.

"Notification of Infectious Diseases," *Public Health*, 10 (1897–8): 227–30.

"The Notification of Phthisis Pulmonalis," *Practitioner*, 67 (1901): 26–36.

"Notification of Tuberculosis in Great Britain: A Historical Note," *British Medical Journal* (1943), no. 2: 75–6.

"Nursing as an Instrument of Public Health," *Medical Officer*, 19 (1918): 77–8.

"Occupation and Mortality," *Transactions of the Sanitary Institute*, 14 (1893): 81–101.

"On a Doubtful Case of Recurrent Small-pox," *British Medical Journal* (1896), no. 2: 1031.

"On an Outbreak of Scarlet Fever and Scarlatinal Sore Throat Due to Infected Milk," *Public Health*, 19 (1906–7): 756–72.

"On an Outbreak of Sore Throats and of Scarlet Fever Caused by Infected Milk," *Journal of Hygiene*, 2 (1902): 150–69.

"On Child Mortality at the Ages 0–5 Years, in England and Wales," *Journal of Hygiene*, 16 (1917): 69–99.

"On the Alleged Increase of Cancer," *Proceedings of the Royal Society of London*, 54 (1893–4): 209–42. With George King.

"On the Death Rates and Causes of Death in Enumeration Districts, with Special Reference to the Conditions of Housing," *Public Health*, 4 (1991–2): 226–31.

"On the Study of Hygiene in Elementary Schools," *Public Health*, 3 (1890–1): 134–6.

"Our Premises Challenged," in *National Physical Training: An Open Debate*, ed. J. B. Atkins (London: Isbister, 1904), 101–16.

"Physical Inspection," *Journal of the Sanitary Institute*, 26 (1905): 64–8.

"The Place of the Alcohol Question in Social Hygiene," *British Journal of Inebriety*, 26 (1928): 58–73.

"Pneumonia from a Public Health Standpoint," *Practitioner*, 64 (1900): 46–55.

"The Possible Association of the Consumption of Alcohol with Excessive Mortality from Cancer," *British Medical Journal* (1903), no. 2: 1529–31.

"Poverty and Disease, as Illustrated by the Course of Typhus Fever and Phthisis in Ireland," *Proceedings of the Royal Society of Medicine*, 1 (1908), pt. 1, Epidemiology Section, 1–44.

"Poverty in Town Life," *Practitioner*, 69 (1902): 682–94.

"The Pre-school Child and Tuberculosis," *Mother and Child*, 2 (1921): 222–3.

"Presidential Address on the Relative Roles of Compulsion and Education in Public Health Work," *Journal of the Royal Sanitary Institute*, 43 (1922–3): 82–96.

"The Prevention of Phthisis with Special Reference to its Notification to the Medical Officer of Health," *Public Health*, 11 (1898–9): 309–22.

The Prevention of Tuberculosis (New York: E. P. Dutton, 1908).

"The Problems of Ventilation, with Special Reference to Schools," *Practitioner*, 66 (1901): 562–6.

Prohibition in America and Its Relation to the Problem of Public Control of Personal Conduct (London: P. S. King, 1921).

"Protracted and Recrudescent Infection in Diphtheria and Scarlet Fever," *Medico-Chirugical Transactions*, 87 (1904): 549–93.

"Protracted and Recrudescent Infection in Diphtheria and Scarlet Fever, *Public Health*, 16 (1903–4): 690–723.

Public Health and Insurance: American Addresses (Baltimore: Johns Hopkins Univ. Press, 1920).

"The Public Health Aspects of Summer Diarrhoea," *Practitioner*, 69 (1902): 161–80.

"Public Health Authorities in Relation to the Struggle against Tuberculosis in England," *Journal of Hygiene*, 3 (1903): 446–67.

"Public Health Education," *Hospital and Health Review*, n.s. 1 (1921): 5–10.

"Public Health Progress in England during the Last Fifty Years," *Commonhealth*, 6 (1919): 295–316.

"The Rates of Mortality in the Concentration Camps in South Africa," *British Medical Journal* (1901), no. 2: 1418–20.

Red Medicine: Socialized Health in Soviet Russia (Garden City, N.Y.: Doubleday, Doran, 1933). With John A. Kingsbury.

"The Relation of the Dental Profession to Public Health," *British Dental Journal*, 24 (1903): 533–45.

"The Relation of Vital Statistics to Sanitary Reform," *Lancet* (1902), no. 1: 1755–8.

"The Relation of Vital Statistics to Sanitary Reform," *Medical Magazine*, n.s. 11 (1902): 360–72.

"The Relations of Tuberculosis to War Conditions. With Remarks on Some Aspects of the Administrative Control of Tuberculosis," *Lancet* (1917), no. 2: 591–5.

"The Relationship of the Private Medical Practitioner to Preventive Medicine," *Journal of the American Medical Association*, 98 (1932): 1739–43.

"The Relative Importance of the Constituent Factors Involved in the Control of Pulmonary Tuberculosis," *Transactions of the Epidemiological Society of London*, n.s. 25 (1905–6): 31–112.

"Remarks on the Causation of Epidemic Diarrhoea, Introducing the Discussion on Professor Delépine's Paper," *Transactions of the Epidemiological Society of London,* n.s. 22 (1902–3): 34–42.

"Remarks on the Conduct of Central and Local Government Authorities in England," *American Journal of Public Health,* 9 (1919): 581–3.

"Retrospect and Outlook on the Tuberculosis Problem," *Medical Officer,* 25 (1921): 209–11.

School Hygiene: The Laws of Health in Relation to School Life (London, 1887).

"The School in Relation to Tuberculosis," *Proceedings of the Second International Congress on School Hygiene* [London, 1907] (London, 1908), vol. 2, 426–30.

The Second Brighton Life Table (Brighton: Brighton Corporation, 1903). With T.H.C. Stevenson.

"Shell-fish and Infection," *Journal of Sanitary Institute,* 25 (1904): 454–62.

"The Social Aspects of the Alcohol Problem," *Practitioner,* 113 (1924): 216–25.

"Some Anomalies of Local Public Health Administration," *Lancet* (1925), no. 1: 1279–82.

"Some Aspects of Heredity," *Annual Report of the Brighton & Sussex Natural History and Philosophical Society* (1895), 5–8.

"Some Conditions of Social Efficiency in Relation to Local Public Health Administration," *Public Health,* 22 (1909–10): 403–14.

"Some Considerations on Tuberculosis," *Transactions of the Sixteenth Annual Meeting of the National Tuberculosis Association* (St. Louis, 1920), 483–6.

"Some International Aspects of Alcoholism with Special Reference to Prohibition in America," *British Journal of Inebriety,* 19 (1922): 93–113.

"Some Problems of Preventive Medicine of the Immediate Future," *Canadian Practitioner and Review,* 44 (1919): 201–14.

"Some Public Health Aspects of 'Birth Control'," in *Medical Views on Birth Control,* ed. James Marchant (London: Martin Hopkinson, 1926), 132–50.

Special Report on Overcrowding, on the Clearing of Insanitary Areas, and on the Provision of Housing Accommodation by the Town Council (Brighton: Brighton Corporation, 1904).

"The Spread of Enteric Fever and Other Forms of Illness by Sewage-Polluted Shellfish," *British Medical Journal* (1903), no. 2: 295–7.

"The Spread of Enteric Fever by Means of Sewage Contaminated Shell-fish," *Journal of the Sanitary Institute,* 17 (1896): 389–411.

"The Statistics of Cancer," *Practitioner,* 62 (1899): 371–84.

The Story of Modern Preventive Medicine, Being a Continuation of the Evolution of Preventive Medicine (Baltimore: Williams & Wilkins, 1929).

"A Study of the Relation between the Treatment of Tubercular Patients in General Institutions and the Reduction in the Death-Rate from Tuberculosis," *Rapports Congrès International de la Tuberculose* (Paris, 1905), 413–37.

The Role of 'Missed' Cases in the Spread of Infectious Diseases (London & Manchester: Sherratt & Hughes, 1904).

"Things That Matter in Public Health," *Journal of the Royal Sanitary Institute,* 44 (1923–4): 1–9.

Treatise on Public Health and Its Applications in Different European Countries, by Albert Palmberg, translated and section on England by Arthur Newsholme (London: Swan Sonnenschein & Co., 1893).

"Tuberculosis in Relation to Milk Supply," *Proceedings of the Brighton and Sussex Medico-Chirugical Society* (4 March 1897), 83–9.

"Tuberculosis in Relation to Milk Supply," *Practitioner,* 66 (1901): 675–83.

"Tuberculosis: Its Causes and the Means of Stamping it Out," *Sanitary Record*, n.s. 19 (1897): 172–4, 198–200.

"Typhoid Fever from Defective Workmanship," *Sanitary Record*, n.s. 6 (1884–5): 351–2.

"United States Points the Way toward Increased Life Period," *Nation's Health*, 8 (1926): 679–80.

"The Utility of Isolation Hospitals in Diminishing the Spread of Scarlet Fever. Considered from an Epidemiological Standpoint," *Journal of Hygiene*, 1 (1901): 145–52.

"Vital Statistics," *Encyclopaedia Medica*, 14 vols. (New York: Longmans Green, 1903), vol. 13: 398–413.

"Vital Statistics and Their Relation to Sanitary Reform," *Proceedings of a Conference on Sanitary Progress and Reform* (Manchester: Manchester and Salford Sanitary Association:, 1902), 64–74.

"The Vital Statistics of Peabody Buildings and Other Artisans' and Labourers' Block Dwellings," *Journal of the Statistical Society of London*, 54 (1891): 70–99.

"Vital Statistics: Their Better Use in Public Health Administration," *Lancet* (1921), no. 2: 833–6.

"The Voluntary Notification of Phthisis in Brighton: Including a Comparison of Results with Those Obtained in Other Towns," *Journal of the Sanitary Institute*, 28 (1907): 26–35.

"The Waste of Life and Efficiency in South Africa," *British Medical Journal* (1901), no. 1: 165–6.

"The Work of the Red Cross Organizations in Relation to the Preventive Medicine of the Future," *Boston Medical and Surgical Journal*, 181 (1919): 473–7.

VII. PUBLISHED WORKS BY OTHER AUTHORS

Abel-Smith, Brian. *The Hospitals 1800–1948: A Study in Social Administration in England and Wales* (Cambridge, Mass.: Harvard Univ. Press, 1964).

Acheson, Roy. "The British Diploma in Public Health: Birth and Adolescence," in *A History of Education in Public Health: Health That Mocks the Doctor's Rules*, ed. Fee, Elizabeth and Roy M. Acheson. (Oxford and New York: Oxford Univ. Press, 1991), 44–82.

Acton, William. "The Death Drains at Brighton," *Lancet* (1860), no. 2: 522.

Addison, Christopher. *Four and a Half Years: A Personal Diary from June 1914 to January 1919*, 2 vols. (London: Hutchinson, 1934).

"Arthur Newsholme, K.C.B., M.D. Lond., F.R.C.P.," *Lancet* (1943), no. 1: 696.

Ashby, Hugh T. *Infant Mortality* (Cambridge: Cambridge Univ. Press, 1915).

Ayers, Gwendoline M. *England's First State Hospitals and the Metropolitan Asylums Board 1867–1930* (Berkeley and Los Angeles: Univ. of California Press, 1971).

Bailey-Denton, J. "Report on the Brighton Sewage," *Lancet* (1882), no. 2: 196–8.

Beaver, M. W. "Population, Infant Mortality and Milk," *Population Studies*, 27 (1973): 243–59.

Bellamy, Christine. *Administering Central–Local Relations, 1871–1919: The Local Government Board in Its Fiscal and Cultural Context* (Manchester: Manchester Univ. Press, 1988).

Bernstein, George L. *Liberalism and Liberal Politics in Edwardian England* (Boston: Allen and Unwin, 1986).

Berridge, Virginia. "Health and Medicine," in *The Cambridge Social History of Britain 1750–1950*, ed. F.M.L. Thompson (Cambridge: Cambridge Univ. Press, 1990), vol. 3, 171–242.

"Blood-Poisoning at Brighton," *Lancet* (1882), no. 1: 536, 625, 669.

Bloomfield, Arthur L. *A Bibliography of Internal Medicine: Communicable Diseases* (Chicago: Univ. of Chicago Press, 1958).

Blyth, A. Wynter. *A Manual of Public Health* (London, 1890).

Braithwaite, William J. *Lloyd George's Ambulance Wagon*, ed. Henry N. Bunbury (London: Methuen, 1957).

Brand, Jeanne L. *Doctors and the State: The British Medical Profession and Government Action in Public Health, 1870–1912* (Baltimore: Johns Hopkins Univ. Press, 1965).

Brandt, Allan. *No Magic Bullet: A Social History of Venereal Disease in the United States since 1880* (New York: Oxford Univ. Press, 1985).

"Brighton and the Registrar-General's Mortality Statistics," *Lancet* (1881), no. 2: 1061.

"Brighton and the Registrar-General's Mortality Statistics," *Lancet* (1882), no. 1: 37–8,

"Brighton Mortality Statistics," *Lancet* (1882), no. 1: 699–700, 760–1.

"Brighton Sewage," *Lancet* (1882), no. 2: 33–5, 192.

Bristowe, John Syer. *A Treatise on the Theory and Practice of Medicine* (London, 1876).

Broadbent, William. "A Note on the Transmission of the Infection of Typhoid Fever by Oysters," *British Medical Journal* (1895), no. 1: 61.

Brockington, C. Fraser. *Public Health in the Nineteenth Century* (Edinburgh and London: E. & S. Livingstone, 1965).

Brown, Kenneth D. *John Burns* (London: Royal Historical Society, 1977).

Brundage, Anthony. *England's 'Prussian Minister': Edwin Chadwick and the Politics of Government Growth 1832–1854* (University Park: Pennsylvania State Univ. Press, 1988).

Bryder, Linda. *Below the Magic Mountain: A Social History of Tuberculosis in Twentieth-Century Britain* (Oxford: Clarendon Press, 1988).

Cabot, Hugh. *The Doctor's Bill* (New York: Columbia Univ. Press, 1935).

Caiger, F. Foord. "Scarlet Fever," in *A System of Medicine*, 8 vols. ed. Thomas Clifford Allbutt, (London and New York: Macmillan, 1900), vol. 2, 122–78.

Carr, A. S. Comyns, W. H. Stuart Garnett, and J. H. Taylor. *National Insurance* (London: Macmillan, 1912).

Cassedy, James H. *Charles V. Chapin and the Public Health Movement* (Cambridge, Mass.: Harvard Univ. Press, 1962).

Clarke, Peter. *Liberals and Social Democrats* (Cambridge: Cambridge Univ. Press, 1978);

Collini, Stefan. *Liberalism and Sociology: L. T. Hobhouse and Political Argument in England 1880–1914* (Cambridge: Cambridge Univ. Press, 1979).

Cormack, Una. *The Royal Commission on the Poor Laws, 1905–09 and the Welfare State* (London: Family Welfare Assn., 1953).

"The Corporation of Brighton v. 'The Lancet'," *Lancet* (1882), no. 1: 1093.

Crowther, M. A. "Paupers or Patients?: Obstacles to Professionalization in the Poor Law Medical Service before 1914," *Journal of the History of Medicine and Allied Sciences*, 39 (1984): 33–54.

Cullen, M. J. "The Making of the Civil Registration Act of 1836," *Journal of Ecclesiastical History*, 25 (1974): 39–59.

Dale, Anthony. *Fashionable Brighton 1820–1860*, 2nd ed. (Newcastle-upon-Tyne: Oriel, 1967).

Davidson, R., and R. Lowe. "Bureaucracy and Innovation in British Welfare Policy 1870–1945," in *The Emergence of the Welfare State in Britain and Germany*, ed. W. J. Mommsen (London: Croom Helm, 1981), 263–95

Davies, Celia. "The Health Visitor as Mother's Friend: A Woman's Place in Public Health, 1900–14," *Social History of Medicine* 1 (1988): 39–59.

Davin, Anna. "Imperialism and Motherhood," *History Workshop*, 5 (1978): 9–65.

Dean, George. "A Typhoid Carrier of Twenty-Nine Years' Standing," *British Medical Journal* (1908), no. 1: 562–3.

Delépine, S. "The Bearing of Outbreaks of Food Poisoning upon the Etiology of Epidemic Diarrhoea," *Transactions of the Epidemiological Society of London*, n.s. 22 (1902–3): 11–33.

"Discussion on Influenza," *Proc. Roy. Soc. Med.*, 12 (1918–19), 1–102.

Dowling, Harry F. *Fighting Infection: Conquests of the Twentieth Century* (Cambridge, Mass.: Harvard Univ. Press, 1977).

Dickens, P., and P. Gilbert. "Inter-war Housing Policy: A Study of Brighton," *Southern History*, 3 (1981): 210–31.

Dolman, Claude E. "Max Joseph von Pettenhofer," *Dictionary of Scientific Biography*, 10: 558–60.

Doty, William J., Charles E. Congdon, and Lewis H. Thornton. *The Historic Annals of Southwestern New York*, 3 vols. (New York: Lewis Historical Publishing, 1940).

"The Drainage and Sewage of Brighton," *Lancet* (1882), no. 1: 1000–1.

"The Drainage of Brighton," *Lancet* (1882), no. 2: 74.

Dwork, Deborah. *War Is Good for Babies and Other Young Children: A History of the Infant and Child Welfare Movement in England 1898–1918* (London and New York: Tavistock, 1987).

Dyhouse, Carol. "Working-Class Mothers and Infant Mortality in England, 1896–1914," in *Biology, Medicine and Society 1840–1940,* ed. Charles Webster (Cambridge: Cambridge Univ. Press, 1981), 73–98.

Eade, Peter. "Typhoid Fever and Oysters and Other Mollusks," *British Medical Journal* (1895), no. 1: 121–2.

Eckstein, Harry. *The English Health Service: Its Origins, Structure, and Achievements* (Cambridge, Mass: Harvard Univ. Press, 1958).

Ensor, R.C.F. *England 1870–1914* (Oxford: Clarendon Press, 1936).

Evans, David. "Tackling the 'Hideous Scourage': The Creation of the Venereal Disease Treatment Centres in Early Twentieth-Century Britain," *Social History of Medicine*, 3 (1992): 413–33.

Ewart, Joseph. "A Brief Review of Recent Sanitary Legislation," *Transactions of the Epidemiological Society of London*, n.s. 10 (1890–1): 1–21.

A Digest of the Vital Statistics of the European and Native Armies in India; Interspersed with Suggestions for the Eradication and Mitigation of the Preventable and Avoidable Causes of Sickness and Mortality amongst Imported and Indigenous Troops (London, 1859).

"Fever Cases in General Hospitals," *Lancet* (1887), no. 1: 195.

"Inaugural Address of Session 1891–92," *Trans. Epidem. Soc. London*, n.s. 11 (1891–2): 1–26.

The Sanitary Condition and Discipline of Indian Jails (London, 1860).

Eyler, John M. "The Conceptual Origins of William Farr's Epidemiology: Numerical Methods and Social Thought in the 1830s," in *Times, Places, and Persons: Aspects of the History of Epidemiology,* ed. Abraham M. Lilienfeld (Baltimore: Johns Hopkins Univ. Press, 1980), 1–21.

"The Epidemiology of Milk-borne Scarlet Fever," The Case of Edwardian Brighton," *American Journal of Public Health*, 76 (1986): 573–84.

"Mortality Statistics and Victorian Health Policy: Program and Criticism," *Bulletin of the History of Medicine*, 50 (1976): 335–55.

"Policing the Food Trades: Epidemiology, Hygiene, and Public Administration in Edwardian Brighton," in *History of Hygiene: Proceeding of the 12th International Symposium on the Comparative History of Medicine – East and West*, ed. Yosio Kawakita, Shizu Sakai, and Yasuo Otsuka (Tokyo: Ishiyaku EuroAmerican, 1991), 193–225.

"Poverty, Disease, Responsibility: Arthur Newsholme and the Public Health Dilemmas of British Liberalism," *Milbank Quarterly*, 67, Suppl. 1 (1989): 109–26.

"Scarlet Fever and Confinement: The Edwardian Debate over Isolation Hospitals," *Bulletin of the History of Medicine*, 61 (1987), 1–24.

"The Sick Poor and the State: Arthur Newsholme on Poverty, Disease, and Responsibility," in *Framing Disease: Studies in Cultural History*, ed. Charles E. Rosenberg and Janet Golden (New Brunswick, N.J.: Rutgers Univ. Press, 1992), 276–96; reprinted in *Doctors, Politics and Society: Historical Essays*, ed. Dorothy Porter and Roy Porter (Amsterdam: Rodopi, 1993), 188–211.

Victorian Social Medicine: The Ideas and Methods of William Farr (Baltimore and London: Johns Hopkins Univ. Press, 1979).

Falkus, Malcolm. "The Development of Municipal Trading in the Nineteenth Century," *Business History*, 19 (1977): 134–61.

Farr, William. *Vital Statistics: A Memorial Volume of Selections from the Reports and Writings of William Farr, M.D., D.C.L., C.B., F.R.S.*, ed. Noel A. Humphreys (London, 1885).

Farrant, Sue, K. Fossey, and A. Peasgood. *The Growth of Brighton and Hove 1840–1939* (Falmer, Sussex: Centre for Continuing Education, University of Sussex, 1981).

Fee, Elizabeth. *Disease and Discovery: A History of the Johns Hopkins School of Hygiene and Public Health, 1916–1939* (Baltimore and London: Johns Hopkins Univ. Press, 1987).

Fee, Elizabeth, and Roy M. Acheson. ed., *A History of Education in Public Health: Health that Mocks the Doctors' Rules* (Oxford and New York: Oxford Univ. Press, 1991), 44–82.

" 'Fever' in Brighton," *Lancet* (1881), no. 2: 881.

Finer, S. E. *The Life and Times of Sir Edwin Chadwick* (London: Methuen, 1952).

Fox, Daniel M. *Health Policies, Health Politics: The British and American Experience 1911–1965* (Princeton, N.J.: Princeton Univ. Press, 1985).

Fraser, A. Means. "Is the Hospital Isolation of Scarlet Fever Worth While?" *Public Health*, 16 (1903–4): 208–19.

Freeden, Michael. *The New Liberalism: An Ideology of Social Reform* (Oxford: Clarendon Press, 1978).

Friend, D. B. & Co. *Brighton Almanack*, 1894.

Gilbert, Bentley B. *British Social Policy 1914–1939* (Ithaca, N.Y.: Cornell Univ. Press, 1970).

The Evolution of National Insurance in Great Britain: The Origins of the Welfare State (London: Michael Joseph, 1966).

"Health and Politics: The British Physical Deterioration Report of 1904," *Bulletin of the History of Medicine*, 39 (1965): 143–53.

Gilbert, Edmund W. *Brighton: Old Ocean's Bauble* (London: Methuen, 1954).

"The Growth of Brighton," *Geographical Journal*, 114 (1949): 30–52.

Glass, D. V. *Numbering the People: The Eighteenth-Century Population Controversy and the Development of Census and Vital Statistics in Britain* (Farnborough, Hants.: D. C. Heath, 1973).

Gordon, Mervyn H. "The Cause of Return Cases of Scarlet Fever," *British Medical Journal* (1902), no. 2: 445–6.

Greenwood, F. J. "Women as Sanitary Inspectors and Health Visitors," in *Women Workers in Seven Professions: A Survey of their Economic Conditions and Prospects*, ed. Edith J. Morley (London: George Routledge, 1914), 221–34.

Hamlin, Christopher. "Politics and Germ Theories in Victorian Britain: The Metropolitan Water Commissions of 1867–9 and 1892–3," in *Government and Expertise: Specialists, Administrators and Professionals, 1860–1919*, ed. Roy MacLeod (Cambridge: Cambridge Univ. Press, 1988), 110–27.

A Science of Impurity: Water Analysis in Nineteenth Century Britain (Berkeley and Los Angeles: Univ. of California Press, 1990).

Hardy, Anne. *The Epidemic Streets: Infectious Disease and the Rise of Preventive Medicine, 1856–1900* (Oxford: Clarendon Press, 1993).

"Public Health and the Expert: The London Medical Officers of Health 1856–1900," in *Government and Expertise: Specialists, Administrators and Professionals, 1860–1919*, ed. Roy MacLeod (Cambridge: Cambridge Univ. Press, 1988), 128–42.

"Urban Famine or Urban Crisis? Typhus in the Victorian City," *Medical History*, 32 (1988): 401–25.

Hart, Ernest. "The Influence of Milk in Spreading Zymotic Disease," *Transactions of the International Medical Congress*, 7th session, 5 vols. (London, 1881), vol. 4, 528–39.

Hayward, T. E. "A Series of Life-Tables for England and Wales for Each Successive Decennium from 1841–50 to 1881–90, Calculated by an Abbreviated Method," *Journal of the Royal Statistical Society*, 64 (1901): 636–41.

Hennock, E. P. *British Social Reform and German Precedents: The Case of Social Insurance 1880–1914* (Oxford: Clarendon Press, 1987).

Fit and Proper Persons: Ideal and Reality in Nineteenth-Century Urban Government (Montreal: McGill-Queen's Univ. Press, 1973).

"The Origins of British National Insurance and the German Precedent 1880–1914," in *The Emergence of the Welfare State in Britain and Germany 1850–1950*, ed. W. J. Mommsen (London: Croom Helm, 1981), 84–106.

Higgs, Edward. "Disease, Febrile Poisons, and Statistics: The Census as a Medical Survey, 1841–1911," *Social History of Medicine*, 4 (1991): 465–78.

Hillier, Alfred. "The Prospect of Extinguishing Tuberculosis. Based on the Researches of Koch, Flügge, Frankel, Niven, and Others," *Public Health*, 15 (1902–3): 301–19.

Himmelfarb, Gertrude. *The Idea of Poverty: England in the Early Industrial Age* (New York: Alfred A. Knopf, 1984).

Hirst, J. D. "A Failure 'Without Parallel': The School Medical Service and the London County Council 1907–12," *Medical History*, 25 (1981): 281–300.

Hobson, J. A. *The Crisis in Liberalism: New Issues of Democracy* (London: P. S. King, 1909).

Problems of Poverty: An Inquiry into the Industrial Condition of the Poor, 8th ed. (London: Methuen, 1913).

Hogben, Lancelot. "Major Greenwood 1880–1949," *Obituary Notices of the Fellows of the Royal Society*, 7 (1950–1): 139–54.

Honigsbaum, Frank. "Christopher Addison: A Realist in Pursuit of Dreams," in *Doctors, Politics and Society: Historical Essays*, ed. Dorothy Porter and Roy Porter (Amsterdam and Atlanta: Rodopi, 1993), 229–46.

The Struggle for the Ministry of Health 1914–1919, Occasional Papers on Social Administration, no. 37 (London: G. Bell, 1970).

Hume, Edgar Erskine. *Max von Pettenhofer: His Theory of the Etiology of Cholera, Typhoid Fever, & and Other Intestinal Diseases, A Review of His Arguments and Evidence* (New York: Paul B. Hoeber, 1927).

Hutchinson, John. "Dances with Commissars: Sigerist and Soviet Medicine," in *Making Medical History: The Life and Times of Henry E. Sigerist,* ed. Elizabeth Fee and Theodore Brown, forthcoming.

Huxley, Thomas Henry. *Evolution and Ethics and Other Essays* (New York, 1899).

Kebbell, William. "The Drainage of Brighton," *Lancet* (1862), no. 2: 404.

Popular Lectures on the Prevailing Diseases of Towns: Their Effects, Causes, and the Means of Prevention (Brighton, 1848).

Kent, William. *John Burns: Labour's Lost Leader* (London: Williams and Norgate, 1950).

Kevles, Daniel J. *In the Name of Eugenics: Genetics and the Uses of Human Heredity* (New York: Alfred A. Knopf, 1985).

King, Lester S. *Medical Thinking: A Historical Preface* (Princeton, N.J.: Princeton Univ. Press, 1982).

Kiser, Clyde V. *The Milbank Memorial Fund: Its Leaders and Its Work 1905–1974* (New York: Milbank Memorial Fund, 1975).

Lambert, Royston. *Sir John Simon 1816–1904 and English Social Administration* (London: MacGibbon and Fee, 1963).

Langley, John. *Always a Layman* (Brighton: Sussex Society for Labour History, 1976).

Latham, Baldwin. "The Relation of Ground Water to Disease," *Quarterly Journal of the Royal Meteorological Society,* 17 (1891): 1–18.

Ledingham, Alexander, and J.C.G. Ledingham. "Typhoid Carriers," *British Medical Journal* (1908), no. 1: 15–17.

Ledingham, J.C.G. "The Typhoid Carrier Problem, with Some Experiments on Immunity in Carriers," *British Medical Journal* (1908), no. 2: 1173–5.

Ledingham, J.C.G., and J. A. Arkwright. *The Carrier Problem in Infectious Diseases* (London: Edward Arnold, 1912).

Lewes, Fred. "The GRO and the Provinces in the Nineteenth Century," *Social History of Medicine,* 4 (1991): 479–96.

Lewis, Jane. *The Politics of Motherhood: Child and Maternal Welfare in England, 1900–1939* (London: Croom Helm, 1980).

What Price Community Medicine? The Philosophy, Practice and Politics of Public Health since 1919 (Brighton: Wheatsheaf Books, 1986).

"London-by-the-Sea," *London,* 6 June 1895, 429–33.

Loudon, Irvine. *Death in Childbirth: An International Study of Maternal Care and Maternal Mortality 1800–1950* (Oxford: Clarendon Press, 1992).

"Maternal Mortality: 1880–1950. Some Regional and International Comparisons," *Social History of Medicine,* 1 (1988), 183–228

"Obstetric Care, Social Class, and Maternal Mortality," *British Medical Journal,* (1886), no. 2: 606–8.

"On Maternal and Infant Mortality 1900–1960," *Social History of Medicine,* 4 (1991), 29–73.

Luckin, Bill. "Evaluating the Sanitary Revolution: Typhus and Typhoid in London, 1851–

1900," in *Urban Disease and Mortality in Nineteenth-Century England,* ed. Robert Woods and John Woodward (London: Batsford Academic and Educational Press, 1984), 102–19.

Lyster, Robert A. "Sickness Insurance and Public Health," *British Medical Journal* (1911), no. 1: 507–8.

McBriar, A. M. *An Edwardian Mixed Doubles: The Bosanquets versus the Webbs. A Study in British Social Policy 1890–1929* (Oxford: Clarendon Press, 1987).

McCleary, G. F. *The Early History of the Infant Welfare Movement* (London: H. K. Lewis, 1933).

MacDonagh, Oliver. *Early Victorian Government 1830–1870* (New York: Holmes and Meier, 1977).

"The Nineteenth-Century Revolution in Government: A Reappraisal," *Historical Journal,* 1 (1958): 52–67.

A Pattern of Government Growth, 1800–1860: The Passenger Acts and Their Enforcement (London: MacGibbon and Kee, 1961).

McFarlane, Neil. "Hospitals, Housing, and Tuberculosis in Glasgow," *Social History of Medicine,* 2 (1989): 59–85.

MacKenzie, Donald A. *Statistics in Britain 1965–1930: The Social Construction of Scientific Knowledge* (Edinburgh: Edinburgh Univ. Press, 1981).

McKeown, Thomas. "Medicine and World Population," *J. Chronic Diseases,* 18 (1965): 1076–7.

The Role of Medicine: Dream, Mirage, or Nemesis? (Princeton, N.J.: Princeton Univ. Press, 1979).

McKeown, Thomas, and R. G. Record. "Reasons for the Decline of Mortality in England and Wales during the Nineteenth Century," *Population Studies,* 16 (1962): 94–122.

MacLeod, Roy M. "The Alkali Acts Administration, 1863–84: The Emergence of the Civil Scientist," *Victorian Studies,* 9 (1965): 85–112

"The Anatomy of State Medicine: Concept and Application," in *Medicine and Science in the 1860s: Proceedings of the Sixth British Congress on the History of Medicine,* ed. F.N.L. Poynter (London: Wellcome Institute of the History of Medicine, 1968), 199–227.

"The Frustration of State Medicine, 1880–1899," *Medical History,* 11 (1967): 15–40.

Treasury Control and Social Administration: A Study of Establishment Growth at the Local Government Board 1871–1905, Occasional Papers on Social Administration, no. 23 (London: G. Bell, 1968).

"Major Greenwood, D.Sc., F.R.C.P., F.R.S.," *British Medical Journal* (1949), no. 2: 877–9.

Marland, Hilary. "A Pioneer in Infant Welfare: The Huddersfield Scheme 1903–1920," *Social History of Medicine,* 6 (1993), 25–50.

Marriott, Edward Dean. "The Passing of the Isolation Hospital," *Sanitary Record,* n.s. 26 (1900): 71, 85, 124, 157–8, 175–6, 199–200.

"Scarlet Fever – The Case against Hospital Isolation," *Sanitary Record,* n.s. 25 (1900): 118–19.

Mason, J. Wright. "Secondary and Return Cases of Scarlatina," *Public Health,* 10 (1897–8): 218–21.

Millard, C. Killick. "The Etiology of 'Return Cases' of Scarlet Fever," *British Medical Journal* (1898), no. 2: 614–18.

"The Etiology of 'Return Cases' of Scarlet Fever," *British Medical Journal* (1902), no. 2: 441–5.

"The Hospital Isolation of Scarlet Fever: Some Points of Uncertainty," *Public Health,* 14 (1901–2): 285–94.

"The Influence of Hospital Isolation in Scarlet Fever: An Appeal to Statistics," *Public Health,* 13 (1900–1): 462–93.

Morgan, Kenneth, and Jane Morgan. *Portrait of a Progressive: The Political Career of Christopher, Viscount Addison* (Oxford: Clarendon Press, 1980).

Musgrave, Clifford. *Life in Brighton from Earliest Times to the Present* (London: Faber and Faber, 1970).

Newman, George. *Infant Mortality* (London: Methuen, 1906).

Niven, James. "Poverty and Disease," *Proceedings of the Royal Society of Medicine,* 3 (1910), pt. 2, Epidemiology Section, 1–44.

Novak, Steven J. "Professionalism and Bureaucracy: English Doctors and the Victorian Public Health Administration," *Journal of Social History,* 6 (1973): 440–62.

Numbers, Ronald L. "History of Medicine: A Field in Ferment," *Reviews in American History,* 10 (1982): 245–63.

Owen, David. *English Philanthropy 1660–1960* (Cambridge, Mass.: Harvard Univ. Press, 1964).

Pearson, Karl. "The Check to the Fall in the Phthisis Death-rate since the Discovery of the Tubercle Bacillus and the Adoption of Modern Treatment," *Biometrika,* 12 (1918–19): 374–6.

Darwinism, Medical Progress, and Eugenics: The Cavendish Lecture, 1912, Eugenics Laboratory Lecture Series, IX (London: Dulau, 1912).

Eugenics and Public Health (London: Dulau, 1912).

The Fight against Tuberculosis and the Death-rate from Phthisis (London: Dulau, 1911).

A First Study of the Statistics of Pulmonary Tuberculosis (London: Dulau, 1907).

"The Intensity of Natural Selection in Man," *Proceedings of the Royal Society of London,* ser. B, 85 (1912): 469–76.

Tuberculosis, Heredity and Environment (London: Dulau, 1912).

Pelling, Margaret. *Cholera, Fever and English Medicine 1825–1865* (Oxford: Oxford Univ. Press, 1978).

Peterson, M. Jeanne. *The Medical Profession in Mid-Victorian England* (Berkeley: Univ. of California Press, 1978).

Pike's Brighton and Hove Blue Book, 1891.

Pooley, Colin G. "Housing for the Poorest Poor: Slum-clearance and Rehousing in Liverpool, 1890–1918," *Journal of Historical Geography,* 11 (1985): 70–88.

Porter, Dorothy. " 'Enemies of the Race': Biologism, Environmentalism, and Public Health in Edwardian England," *Victorian Studies,* 34 (1991): 159–78.

[Watkins], Dorothy. "The English Revolution in Social Medicine, 1889–1911" (University of London: unpublished Ph.D. dissertation, 1984).

"Stratification and Its Discontents: Professionalization and Conflict in the British Public Health Service," in *A History of Education in Public Health: Health that Mocks the Doctors' Rules,* ed. Elizabeth Fee and Roy M. Acheson (Oxford and New York: Oxford Univ. Press, 1991), 83–113.

Porter, Dorothy, and Roy Porter. "The Enforcement of Health: The British Debate," in *AIDS: The Burdens of History,* ed. Elizabeth Fee and Daniel M. Fox (Berkeley: Univ. of California Press, 1988), 97–120.

"Recent Brighton Mortality Statistics," *Lancet* (1882), no. 2: 66.

"Report on the Drainage of Brighton, with a Chemical and Microscopical Analysis Illustrative of the Pollution of the Sea and Well Waters," *Lancet* (1862), no. 2: 397.

"Report of *The Lancet* Sanitary Commission on the Drainage of Brighton," *Lancet* (1868), no. 2: 383.

Richardson, Benjamin Ward. "A Biographical Dissertation," in *The Health of Nations: A Review of the Works of Edwin Chadwick*, 2 vols. (London, 1887).

"The Medical History of England: The Medical History of Brighton," *Medical Times and Gazette* (1864), no. 1: 649–52, 673–9, 697–703.

"Report on the Sanitary Condition of the Borough of Brighton," *Lancet* (1882), no. 2: 747–63.

Rowntree, B. Seebohm. *Poverty: A Study of Town Life* (London: Macmillan, 1902).

Rumsey, Henry W. *Essays and Papers on Some Fallacies of Statistics Concerning Life and Death and Disease with Suggestions Towards an Improved System of Registration* (London, 1875).

Scatterty, William. "Hospital Isolation," *Public Health,* 17 (1904–5): 356–64.

Searle, G. R. *Eugenics and Politics in Britain 1900–1914* (Leyden: Noordhoff, 1976).

The Quest for National Efficiency: A Study in British Politics and Political Thought, 1899–1914 (Oxford: Basil Blackwell, 1971).

Semmel, Bernard. *Imperialism and Social Reform: English Social-Imperial Thought 1895–1914* (Cambridge, Mass.: Harvard Univ. Press, 1960).

Sigerist, Henry E. *Socialized Medicine in the Soviet Union* (New York: W. W. Norton, 1937).

"The Sewage of Brighton," *Lancet* (1882), no. 1: 617.

Simon, John. *English Sanitary Institutions, Reviewed in Their Course of Development, and in Some of Their Political and Social Relations* (London, 1890).

"Sir Arthur Newsholme, K.C.B.," *Nature,* 151 (1943): 635–6.

"Sir Arthur Newsholme, K.C.B., M.D., F.R.C.P.," *British Medical Journal* (1943), no. 1: 680–1.

"Sir Arthur Newsholme, K.C.B., M. D., F.R.C.P.," *St. Thomas's Hospital Gazette,* 41 (1943): 92.

Smith, F. B. *The Retreat of Tuberculosis 1850–1950* (London: Croom Helm, 1988).

Sutcliffe, Anthony. "The Growth of Public Intervention in the British Urban Environment during the Nineteenth Century: A Structural Approach," in *The Structure of Nineteenth Century Cities,* ed. James H. Johnson and Colin G. Pooley (London and Canberra: Croom Helm, 1982), 107–24.

Swithinbank, Harold, and George Newman. *Bacteriology of Milk* (London: John Murray, 1903).

Szreter, Simon R. S. "The Genesis of the Registrar-General's Social Classification of Occupations," *British Journal of Sociology,* 35 (1934), 522–46.

"The GRO and the Public Health Movement in Britain, 1837–1914," *Social History of Medicine,* 4 (1991): 435–63

"The Importance of Social Intervention in Britain's Mortality Decline c. 1850–1914: A Re-interpretation of the Role of Public Health," *Social History of Medicine,* 1 (1988), 1–37.

Tarn, J. N. "Housing in Liverpool and Glasgow: The Growth of Civic Responsibility," *Town Planning Journal,* 39 (1968–9): 319–34.

Taylor, A. J. "The Taking of the Census, 1801–1951," *British Medical Journal* (1951), no. 1: 715–20.

Taylor, Iain C. "The Insanitary Housing Question and Tenement Dwellings in Nineteenth-century Liverpool," in *Multi-storey Living: The British Working-class Experience,* ed. Anthony Sutcliffe (London: Croom Helm, 1974), 41–87.

Thane, Pat. "Government and Society in England and Wales, 1750–1914," in *The Cambridge Social History of Britain 1750–1950,* ed. F.M.L. Thompson (Cambridge: Cambridge Univ. Press, 1990), vol. 3, pp. 1–61.

Thorn, R. Thorn. "The Administrative Control of Tuberculosis: The Harben Lectures for 1898," *Public Health,* 11 (1898–9): 201–5.

Thresh, John C. "The Utility of Isolation Hospitals," *Lancet* (1906), no. 1: 1058–60.

Tomkins, Sandra M. "The Failure of Expertise: Public Health Policy in Britain during the 1918–19 Influenza Epidemic," *Social History of Medicine,* 3 (1992): 435–54.

Turner, John. " 'Experts' and Interests: David Lloyd George and the Dilemmas of the Expanding State, 1906–19," in *Government and Expertise: Specialists, Administrators and Professionals, 1860–1919,* ed. Roy MacLeod (Cambridge: Cambridge Univ. Press, 1988), 203–23.

Walford, Edward. "The Influence of Hospital Isolation upon Scarlet Fever in Cardiff," *Public Health,* 16 (1903–4): 676–86.

Walton, John K. *The English Seaside Resort: A Social History 1750–1914* (Leicester: Leicester Univ. Press, 1983).

Webb, Beatrice. *The Diary of Beatrice Webb,* III, 1905–1924, "The Power to Alter Things," ed. Norman and Jeanne MacKenzie (Cambridge, Mass.: Belknap, 1984).

  Our Partnership, ed. Barbara Drake and Margaret I. Cole (London: Longmans, Green, 1948).

  "The Relation of Poor-Law Medical Relief to the Public Health Authorities," *Public Health,* 19 (1906–7): 129–38.

Webb, Sidney, and Beatrice Webb. *The Letters of Sidney and Beatrice Webb,* II, 1892–1912. ed. Norman MacKenzie (Cambridge: Cambridge Univ. Press., 1978).

  The State and the Doctor (New York: Longmans, Green, 1910).

Webster, Charles. "Conflict and Consensus: Explaining the British Health Service," *Twentieth Century British History,* 1 (1990): 146.

  "The Health of the School Child during the Depression," *The Fitness of the Nation – Physical and Health Education in the Nineteenth and Twentieth Centuries: Proceedings of the 1982 Annual of the History of Education,* ed. Nicolas Parry and David McNair (Leicester: History of Education Society, 1983), 70–85

  The Health Services since the War, I: Problems of Health Care, The National Health Service before 1957 (London: HMSO, 1988).

  "Health, Welfare and Unemployment during the Depression," *Past and Present,* 109 (1985): 204–29.

  "Healthy or Hungry Thirties?," *History Workshop,* 13 (1982): 110–29.

Wheatley, James. "The Desirability of an Inquiry into the Effect of Hospital Isolation of Scarlet Fever, and the Form an Inquiry Should Take," *Public Health,* 16 (1903–4): 355–9.

Wilson, George A. *Handbook of Hygiene and Sanitary Science,* 3rd ed. (Philadelphia, 1880).

Wilson, Leonard G. "The Historical Decline of Tuberculosis in Europe and America: Its

Causes and Significance," *Journal of the History of Medicine and Allied Sciences,* 45 (1990): 366–96.

"The Historical Riddle of Milk-Borne Scarlet Fever," *Bulletin of the History of Medicine,* 60 (1986): 321–42.

Winslow, C.-E.A. "Arthur Newsholme: 1857–1943," *Medical Care,* 3 (1943): 290.

The Conquest of Epidemic Disease: A Chapter in the History of Ideas (Princeton, N.J.: Princeton Univ. Press, 1944).

Health on the Farm and in the Village: A Review and Evaluation of the Cattaraugus County Health Demonstration with Special Reference to Its Lessons for Other Rural Areas (New York: Macmillan, 1931).

Winter, J. M. *The Great War and the British People* (Cambridge, Mass.: Harvard Univ. Press, 1986).

"The Impact of the First World War on Civilian Health in Britain," *Economic History Review,* 30 (1977): 487–507.

Wohl, Anthony S. *Endangered Lives: Public Health in Victorian Britain* (Cambridge, Mass.: Harvard Univ. Press, 1983).

The Eternal Slum: Housing and Social Policy in Victorian London (London: Edward Arnold, 1977).

"The Housing of the Working Classes in London 1815–1914," in *The History of Working-Class Housing: A Symposium,* ed. Stanley D. Chapman (Newton Abbott: David and Charles, 1971), 13–53.

Woods, Robert, and John Woodward. "Mortality, Poverty and the Environment," in *Urban Disease and Mortality in Nineteenth-Century England,* ed. Robert Woods and John Woodward (London: Batsford Academic and Educational Press, 1984), 19–36.

Yelling, J. A. *Slums and Slum Clearance in Victorian London* (London: Allen and Unwin, 1986).

INDEX